OPERATIVE GYNECOLOGIC LAPAROSCOPY

PRINCIPLES AND TECHNIQUES,

Second Edition

CAMRAN R. NEZHAT, M.D., FACOG, FACS
Director, Stanford Endoscopy Center for Training and Technology
Clinical Professor of Surgery and Obstetrics and Gynecology
Stanford University School of Medicine
Stanford, California

ALVIN M. SIEGLER, M.D., D.SC., FACOG
Professor Emeritus
Department of Obstetrics and Gynecology
State University of New York, Health Sciences Center
Brooklyn, New York

FARR R. NEZHAT, M.D., FACOG, FACS
Clinical Professor of Obstetrics and Gynecology
Stanford University School of Medicine, Stanford, California
Department of Gynecologic-Oncology
The Mount Sinai Hospital
New York, New York

CEANA H. NEZHAT, M.D., FACOG, FACS
Associate Clinical Professor of Obstetrics and Gynecology
Stanford University School of Medicine, Stanford, California
Director, Center for Special Pelvic Surgery
Atlanta, Georgia

DANIEL S. SEIDMAN, M.D.
Associate [illegible]
Department of C[illegible]
Sheba Medica[illegible]
Sackler School of M[illegible]
Tel [illegible]

ANTHONY A. LUCIANO, M.D., FACOG
Professor of Obstetrics and Gynecology
University of Connecticut School of Medicine
Director, Center for Fertility and Reproductive Endocrinology
New Britain General Hospital
New Britain, Connecticut

OPERATIVE GYNECOLOGIC LAPAROSCOPY

PRINCIPLES AND TECHNIQUES

Second Edition

Ca
Alv... ...iegler, M.D., D.Sc.
Farr R. Nezhat, M.D.
Ceana Nezhat, M.D.
Daniel S. Seidman, M.D.
Anthony A. Luciano, M.D.

McGRAW-HILL
Medical Publishing Division

New York St. Louis San Francisco Auckland Bogota Caracas
Lisbon London Madrid Mexico City Milan Montreal
New Delhi San Juan Singapore Sydney Tokyo Toronto

McGraw-Hill

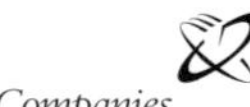

A Division of The McGraw-Hill Companies

Operative Gynecologic Laparoscopy:
Principles and Techniques, 2/e

1234567890 QWR QWK 09876543210

ISBN 0-07-105431-6

This book was set in Caslon type by Progressive Information Technologies. The editors were Martin J. Wonsiewicz, Susan R. Noujaim, and Karen G. Edmonson. The production supervisor was Richard Ruzyoka. Quebecor World/Kingsport was printer and binder.

This book is printed on acid-free paper.

Library of Congress Cataloging-in-Publication Data

Operative gynecologic laparoscopy: principles and techniques / Camran R. Nezhat . . . [et al.].—2nd ed.
p. ; cm.
Includes bibliographical references and index.
ISBN 0-07-105431-6
1. Generative organs, Female—Endoscopic surgery. 2. Laparoscopic surgery. I. Nezhat, Camran.
[DNLM: 1. Genital Diseases, Female—surgery. 2. Surgical Procedures, Laparoscopic.
WP 660 O613 2000]
RG104.7.O64 2000
618.1′059—dc21

99-088759

To our families, who have encouraged our medical and surgical careers since their inception.

CONTENTS

Forewords to the First Edition

Dr. Nezhat's textbook on endoscopic surgery is a timely contribution and has all the trappings of being extremely successful. The competition is keen at this point in time with regards to textbooks and atlases on endoscopic surgery but none will rival Dr. Nezhat's.

In the past decade, gyneclogic surgery, because of endoscopic surgery, has undergone a tremendous revolution. There are few cases now remaining in the gynecologist's surgical armamentarium that cannot be carried out through an endoscopic approach. Many of these changes are due to the courage, innovativeness, and technical skill of Dr. Camran Nezhat. Just as in Star Trek, he dared to go where no man went before and, by doing this, he opened up unimagined vistas to endoscopic surgeons all over the world. For his courage, Camran has over the years suffered, but he has persevered.

This book brings to a culmination many of Dr. Nezhat's techniques, innovations and most importantly, thought processes. All of the characteristics necessary for an excellent textbook of surgery are included. The text is well-written, provocative, clear, and demonstrates editorial consistency. The Illustrations are superb and would provide the novice in endoscopic surgery with enough information to carry out many of the procedures proposed.

I've chosen as an illustrative chapter, the chapter on endometriosis. It demonstrates many of the things that have been conjured up by Dr. Nezhat and have become part of what we do as endoscopic surgeons. These include hydrodissection, ureteric resection, reanastomosis with a stapler. If one could learn all of the techniques suggested in the chapter on endometriosis, one could become, as Dr. Nezhat has, a master endoscopic surgeon.

The book is encyclopedic in that it covers not only all surgical techniques, but also various kinds of equipment, laser and electrosurgical physics, adhesion formation, and most importantly, complications.

Dr. Nezhat has synthesized his years of experience in this text. It will become a classic in the field and is a testimony to his skill, intelligence, and perseverance.

Alan DeCherney, M.D.
Louis E. Phaneuf Professor and Chairman
Department of Obstetrics and Gynecology
Tufts University
Boston, Massachusetts

Excellence in any human activity always commands admiration and respect. In the case of surgical techniques, excellence commands not only the admiration and respect of professional colleagues, but the gratitude of patients as well. Those who have had the opportunity to see the "Nezhat Orchestra" operate and simultaneously conduct the endoscopic operating team, recognize that they have seen a performance of excellence. It is a unique combinaion of manual dexterity, innovation, creativity, and team work.

The rapid proliferation of laparoscopic procedures in the last two decades originated in gynecology, but crossed the borders of this discipline to several other applications below and above the diaphragm. Many new devices have been introduced into the armamentarium of the endoscopic operating room. However, if there was a single factor that contributed to the increased interest, quality of patient care, and education of new generations of surgeons, it was the incorporation of video equipment as an integral part of the standard endoscopic set. This was promulgated and pioneered by Dr. Camran Nezhat. In so doing, the secrets behind the curtain of the "single eye-single hand" procedures were revealed and broadened the horizons of operative laparoscopy.

In this book. "The Nezhats" review the instrumentation and general principles of laparoscopy and elucidate the management of various procedures in gynecology and gastrointestinal and genitourinary surgery. The uniformity of text and illustration format of this book contribute to the clear message that comes from the "Nezhat School of Laparoscopic Surgery," and is complementary to the high quality educational video-library that originated in the same school.

I regard it as an honor to have this opportunity to be associated with this special project that will find an important place in the literature of our specialty.

Yona Tadir. M.D.
Department of Surgery
Beckman Laser Institute & Medical Clinic
Irvine, California

Forewords to the Second Edition

Once again the Nezhats have provided, in their Second Edition, an excellent text in operative gynecologic laparoscopy. Not only has this group been clinically active and leaders in the field for many years, but the fact that they document their experiences and techniques is extremely laudatory. They have been not only innovators, demonstrating great creativity and imagination, but have studied their patients prospectively and retrospectively to draw conclusions based on experience and numbers of cases. Their knowledge of the technology that they employ i.e. lasers, electrosurgery, Harmonic scalpel instrumentation, is profound and they freely share it in this text.

The scope of the book covers all aspects of the leading surgical procedure in gynecology that can be carried out by endoscopy. Areas covered include adhesiolysis, ovarian cystectomy, ectopic pregnancy, operations on the uterus, but there are also portions on anesthesia and office microlaparoscopy, to site a few. The authors have made a tremendous number of revisions, demonstrating their care to detail, their awareness of this rapidly changing and developing field.

It is great that this group has produced a second edition since there are many changes that have occurred because the first edition including work on stress incontinence and the revisiting of presacral neurectomy. Each chapter is well referenced. Any surgical text must have excellent illustrations as does this one. This text is an excellent atlas as well.

I found this a comprehensive text for its knowledge, informative because of its insight and imagination, and practical because of its illustrations and explanations. This is a proud testimony to a work well done.

Alan H. DeCherney, M.D.
Professor and Chairman
Department of Obstetrics and Gynecology
UCLA School of Medicine

Drs. Nezhat embody the entire spectrum of current knowledge regarding laparoscopy. This book is a reference book in laparoscopy for advanced surgeons and beginners alike. The Nezhat's genius in the operating room is reflected in the writing of this book, especially in descriptions of new techniques and the lucid explanations of the advantages of laparoscopy over laparotomy in a growing list of gynecologic procedures.

As a gynecologist from Germany, I began promoting laparoscopy in 1963. At that time the current thinking was that laparoscopy was only performed by gastroenterologists and hepatologists under local anesthesia, and was a procedure to be avoided by all gynecologists. It was believed that turning the laparoscope towards the lower pelvis instead of the upper abdomen would be too dangerous. Structures such as the aorta, common iliac veins, intestines, and ureters were of great concern. There were fatal complications in early gynecologic laparoscopy cases, rendering the procedure obsolete in gynecology at the beginning of the 1960's. Because of these negative connotations and in order to market this innovative technology, I changed the name to “”Pelviscopy”. My scientific publications and my books were printed under this name.

Dr. Camran Nezhat never criticized any of my elaborate endoscopic procedures. Instead, with his genius, he widened the operative field, creating new techniques, employing new instruments, and apparatuses. In my opinion, with the cooperation of his two brothers, Camran Nezhat has enlivened and enriched the entire field of surgical laparoscopy.

Since its inception, endoscopy has changed and the authors have written about a new endoscopic world. The general surgeons have now accepted surgical laparoscopy completely. Years ago, if a gynecologist was unlucky in a pelviscopic procedure, the surgeons condemned this person as an unethical surgeon, who used techniques which were as yet unproven and against the current surgical rules.

This book is indeed a bible in surgical laparoscopy. At the end of each chapter an extended bibliography is included. A lengthy chapter is dedicated to complications and how they can be avoided. This is invaluable to all: Everbody can use it: the clinician, student, scientist, and lawyer. This manual should not be missed in any library.

On June 30, 1980 I performed a laparoscopic appendectomy, which ultimately opened the door for general surgeons to perform endoscopic surgery, especially since the appendix was a holy grail of surgery. Today Drs. Nezhat's book opens a new door to a whole new era of endoscopic surgery.

Prof. Dr. h.c. mult. Kurt Semm

PREFACE

The rationalization for writing a second edition to Operative Gynecologic Laparoscopy was conceived because the authors became cognizant of the meaningful changes that have occurred in laparoscopic techniques and equipment and gynecologic procedures carried out laparoscopically. Fundamental facts about electrosurgery, lasers, and laparoscopy were included again because we believe that the surgeon must be acquainted with these techniques to be able to employ them successfully during laparoscopic procedures. A chapter on the current state of the art of equipment has been written, although we appreciate the fact that changes in instruments will continue to evolve. The anesthesia chapter was rewritten by Dr. Lindsy Vokach-Brodsky who has cited some of the physiologic changes that occur during laparoscopy as a result of the position of the patient and the use of abdominal insufflation. It is important for the gynecologist also to be alerted to the signs of potential danger and their management.

The inclusion of a new chapter on office microlaparoscopy is justified because the advent of smaller-diameter laparoscopes with better optical qualities has facilitated successful diagnostic and operative procedures that can be carried out safely in a well-equipped office. Every chapter describing specific operations has been revised to include technologic advances to make the operative procedure easier and safer. The principles for preventing and treating pelvic adhesions are described, as well as the advantages of laparoscopic pelvic operations over laparotomy for many gynecologic abnormalities.

The laparoscopic treatment of most ovarian cysts is reasonable as long as the gynecologist is aware of the specific restrictions delineated in the book. The techniques for ovarian cystectomy and the laparoscopic removal of an ovarian remnant are described and illustrated. Endometriosis is one of the most common diseases affecting women in the childbearing age, and the authors have devoted themselves to the treatment of this disorder. The chapter on endometriosis is illustrated profusely and referenced carefully.

Reconstructive tubal operations by laparoscopy to cure infertility caused by tubal obstruction have evolved from the state of the art to the standard of care. The results of such operations seem to support this observation. Almost all tubal pregnancies can be managed laparoscopically.

The many laparoscopic classifications of hysterectomy confirm the acceptance of this new method for the removal of the uterus. An essential element for success is training in and experience with complex endoscopic procedures. This operation requires gynecologists to take advantage of all their skills to prevent ureteral and vascular injuries. The authors have described the technique of laparoscopic hysterectomy in a stepwise plan to enable gynecologists to minimize the risk to their patients and facilitate the procedure and share their final opinion as regard to the role of the laporoscope in hysterectory in the year 2000. Myomectomy and myolysis under laparoscopic guidance are techniques that have been reported in the literature. Their indications, limitations, and technique are described in this text. Laparoscopic-assisted myomectomy (LAM), its indication and advantages are described also.

The role of laparoscopy in the surgical treatment of gynecologic malignancy has become an acknowledged procedure in most departments of obstetrics and gynecology. A meaningful change from initial doubt has been caused by the recognized advantages of laparoscopic lymphadenectomy over laparotomy.

Genuine stress urinary incontinence is a common complaint of many women, and it is correctable by the endoscopic approach. Results appear to be comparable with those from a laparotomy. The choice of the proper patient with a careful preoperative evaluation is important.

The cause of pelvic pain often can be located by laparoscopic examination of the pelvis, and the abnormalities can be corrected. In some patients who appear to have minimal disease, a laparoscopic presacral neurectomy can relieve the discomfort. Although the long-term efficacy of uterosacral ablation is inconclusive, the technique is being used by many gynecologists and is relatively easy.

Complications can and do occur even with minor laparoscopic operations. It is important to minimize their occurrence, recognize their existence when they occur, and be able to manage them successfully. The authors have written about each of these untoward events in the sequence described above to lessen the sequelae.

Every chapter has had its references revised. The colored illustrations were done by Dr. Mauritzo Rosati from his observations of many of the operative procedures. His skillful renditions of more than 100 operations have enriched our book, and the authors are grateful to him for his patience and proficiency. We continue to be grateful to Charles Boyter and Christopher Wikoff for their line drawings and attention to detail.

ACKNOWLEDGMENTS

We thank Maryam Vega, Judy Leet, Bahana Nezami, Kymberly Gruyter for their administrative support. Ethicon Endo Surgery, Ethicon Inc., and Ethicon Gynecare (divisions of Johnson & Johnson) have helped defray some of the costs of this book. Mr. Nat Russo originally was responsible for this book and deserves special thanks. We thank Mr. Nat Russo of the Patherton Publishing Group, and Mr. Martin Wonsiewicz of McGraw-Hill for assistance in the development of this book. We deeply appreciate the exceptional effort patience, and outstanding ability of Ms. Susan Noujaim and Karen G. Edmonson in collating effectively the material for this book.

We are indebted to Drs. Vokach-Brodsky & Tazuke for their research in developing the chapters on Anesthesia, Oncology & Pregnancy. Finally we owe a special thanks and gratitude to Drs. Kevin Smith & Mary Jacobson for their tireless assistance in preparation, of this 2nd Edition.

CONTRIBUTORS

Lindsey Vokach-Brodsky, MB, chB [Chapter 6]
Department of Anesthesia
Stanford University Medical Center
Stanford, California

Salli Tazuke, M.D. [Chapter 21]
Department of Reproductive Endocrinology and Infertility
Stanford University Medical Center
Stanford, California

Daniel Tobias, M.D. [Chapter 16]
Clinical Assistant Professor
University of Medicine and Dentistry of New Jersey
Newark, New Jersey;
Attending Physician
Women's Cancer Center
Morristown Memorial Hospital
Morristown, New Jersey

SECTION I

1

Introduction

In the early decades of the twentieth century, physicians developed an interest in exploring body cavities with various forms of specula and optical instruments. Almost a century before, in 1807, Bozzini[1] described a light conductor in which a candle served as the illumination for a special "vase-like" instrument whose purpose was to enable physicians to explore the cavities of various organs. At that time, the medical profession was opposed to this type of "curiosity." Such investigations began again in 1880 when Nitze[2] developed the cystoscope. The new instrument was passed into the bladder so that the physician could locate bladder stones and remove them without the need for an abdominal incision. In 1901, Kelling[3] reported his findings from a celioscopic examination of a living dog after a pneumoperitoneum had been created with filtered air. Jacobaeus[4] coined the term *laparoscopy* after having explored the peritoneal cavity in human beings by "direct" insertion of a Nitze cystoscope without a pneumoperitoneum. He described the use of the laparoscope in 17 patients who had ascites. Kelling and Jacobaeus should be regarded as the pioneers of early laparoscopy.

The technique of abdominal entry was varied and controversial. The early laparoscopes were primitive, the lens systems were of an inferior quality, and adequate light and image transmission could be achieved only with wide lenses that required large-bore telescopes. Distally placed incandescent lightbulbs generated heat within the abdominal cavity and had the disconcerting habit of failing at the critical point of a procedure. In 1938, Veress[5] described a new needle for inducing pneumothorax for the treatment of tuberculosis, and this instrument currently is used most frequently for the creation of a pneumoperitoneum. Ruddock[6] described a good optical system that included a built-in biopsy forceps with a capability for electrocoagulation. He reported on its use in over 2000 patients. Apparently, the first gynecologic report was published by Hope[7] on the use of the laparoscope for the diagnosis of tubal pregnancy. In the same year, Anderson[8] suggested tubal fulguration as a method for tubal sterilization but did not describe any cases. Decker[9] achieved good observation of the pelvic organs with patients in the knee-chest position by using a culdoscope. Indeed, this endoscopic method was practiced almost exclusively in the United States for the next 25 years. In 1941, Power and Barnes[10] reported doing tubal sterilization by coagulating the isthmic portions of the fallopian tubes under laparoscopic control. In France, Palmer[11] adopted the deep Trendelenburg position and designed a forceps for ovarian biopsy. In 1947, he published the results of his first 250 laparoscopic operations. Laparoscopy and other endoscopic procedures attained wider acceptance after the introduction in 1952 of the "cold light" idea by Fourestier and colleagues.[12] In the same year, Hopkins and Kapany[13] in Britain introduced fiberoptics to the field of endoscopy. Frangenheim[14] and Albano and Cittidini[15] incorporated the new techniques of laparoscopy and published their findings in textbooks on that subject. The first book published in English was written by Steptoe,[16] who described the instruments available at that time. Details of many endoscopic procedures, including tubal sterilization, ovarian biopsy, uterine suspension, appendectomy, and lysis of adhesions, were included. Books by Bruhat,[17] Semm,[18] and Gomel[19] also included discussions on laparoscopy, culdoscopy, hysteroscopy, and gynecography.

In response to the worldwide interest in sterilization and population control with the use of the laparoscope and concern about potential complications, the American Association of Gynecologic Laparoscopists was formed in 1972. The initial enthusiasm for laparoscopy was based largely on the fact that for the first time female sterilization was available at a reasonable cost and that the procedure could be accomplished in most women on an outpatient basis.

Advanced operative endoscopy represents a continuation of those early developments and was adopted by other specialists besides gynecologists, including general surgeons, urologists, and vascular surgeons. The evolution of diagnostic and operative laparoscopy has been reviewed by Semm,[20] Azziz,[21] San Filippo,[22] Donnez,[23] and Nezhat and associates.[24] Those authors discussed essential instruments, the utility of multiple puncture sites, insufflation equipment, light sources, endoscopic photography, and the use of videomonitors for endoscopic procedures.

Articulated arms had been used for monitoring, documenting, and videotaping of the procedures.[25] Operating directly from the visual field provided by a videomonitor was presented, promulgated, and reported by Nezhat and colleagues.[26] Tadir and coworkers[27] noted that increased interest in laparoscopic surgery was undoubtedly the incorporation of video equipment as an integral part of the standard endoscopic set enthusiastically promoted by Nezhat. This was also the main contributing factor to laparoscopic cholecystectomy.

To facilitate the procedure, Bruhat, Tadir, and Daniell described the use of the laser laparoscope and Semm developed pelviscopy. Nezhat added the laser to the videolaparoscope for doing videolaseroscopy.[28–36] Technologic improvements and surgical advances accelerated the development of videolaparoscopy as a safe, effective, and reasonable alternative to laparotomy. Those advances enabled surgeons and assistants to stand comfortably while observing a monitor that provided a magnified view of the operative field. Small diameter laparoscopes that offer good resolution and light intensity have made laparoscopy suitable for patients who cannot withstand general anesthesia.[37] Small diameter scopes allow laparoscopy to be done as an office procedure.[38]

Some new laparoscopic operative techniques have been criticized because of their rapid and uncontrolled introduction.[39] However, surgical research often impedes the ability to introduce new operations using the long-established multiphase, randomized, and "blinded" standards employed for new medications.[40] Randomization from the first patients has been advocated in surgical trials.[41] This is an unrealistic recommendation because even experienced surgeons must do a new operation several times before they feel competent in it and it can be compared realistically to a conventional procedure.[42]

Randomized controlled trials are considered the "gold standard" of evidence based studies.[43] Data from early large uncontrolled series attesting to the efficacy and safety of many common laparoscopic operations gradually are being supplemented by results from randomized trials.[44] However, the use of randomized trials does not always prove the merits of laparoscopic procedures. For example, a critical review assessing the results of 12 randomized controlled trials on laparoscopic appendectomy in adults found that only half of them showed an advantage over the endoscopic approach.[45] While the postoperative complication rates were similar, more wound infections followed the laparotomy and more intraabdominal abscesses occurred after laparoscopic appendectomy. Differences in positive (the endoscopic approach) trials concerned subjective and controversial outcomes, and the flaw in negative trials was their lack of power. The authors found that no conclusions could be reached about the advantages of either laparotomy or laparoscopy.

The use of placebo or "sham operations" is another issue that is raised whenever the operative outcome is the alleviation of pelvic pain.[46] Although it is possible to randomize patients to either an operative or a diagnostic laparoscopic procedure,[47] patients are reluctant to participate. Since manufacturers are not required by regulatory agencies to sponsor controlled studies, another major obstacle is funding. Insurers may not reimburse patients or pay physicians for "research" operations.

The role of operative laparoscopy continues to be redefined.[48] Many conditions, such as pregnancy,[48,49] obesity,[50] severe adhesions,[51] previous laparotomies,[52] abdominal cancer,[53] abdominal hernia,[54] hypovolemic shock,[55] and bowel perforation with generalized peritonitis,[56] are no longer contraindications. Complications such as injury to the ureter[57] or major blood vessels[58,59] can be managed safely laparoscopically by an experienced endoscopist. Technologic innovations are expanding the potential of laparoscopy.

Training

The surgeon must learn hand, eye, and foot coordination to optimize the options available with trocars that contain the videolaparoscope, graspers, suction-irrigator, and bipolar forceps. The surgeon uses one hand to control the videolaparoscope and the other to manipulate selected instruments. With the foot control, either the laser placed through the operative channel of the laparoscope or the bipolar forceps inserted through an ancillary trocar can be started. Alternatively, with an assistant holding the videolaparoscope, the surgeon may use instruments in both hands for procedures such as suturing and cutting. Surgeons must learn monocular depth perception, as does an individual with sight in only one eye who wants to operate a motor vehicle safely. The loss of depth perception initially may hamper inexperienced trainees as well as experienced laparoscopists when they evaluate experimental video equipment purporting to provide binocular depth perception.[21] Proficient videolaparoscopists work successfully in three dimensions, using cues displayed on a two-dimensional screen.

A structured laparoscopic skills course for junior surgical residents that stresses knot tying and suturing is an effective way to develop dexterity and significantly improve the performance of laparoscopic tasks. Such training seminars could enhance the development of basic operative skills in a cost-effective manner.

It is often difficult to assess the learning curve for laparoscopic operations. Laparoscopic colectomy, which usually is done in a laparoscopically assisted fashion, is technically one of the most challenging endoscopic procedures. It is not mastered easily by the average surgeon and requires a skilled team for its successful completion. Conversion to laparotomy has been necessary in about 25 percent of patients in collected series.[60] With experience, decreases were found in hospital stay, need for conversion, and complications.[61] A retrospective study assessed the impact of the learning curve of one surgeon on term pregnancies after laparoscopic salpingostomy for tubal infertility. The successes were associated significantly and positively with the surgeon's experience.[62] Patient selection criteria should be emphasized during didactic teaching and the preceptorship process.

Surgical training can be divided into three sequential phases (Table 1-1). The first phase is based on reading material such as this textbook and courses that offer didactic lectures and laboratory sessions.[63] These laboratory classes must include the use of a pelvic trainer on dry models and animal parts. While animal parts such as pig bladders and bovine uteri offer some advantages for the training of an inexperienced surgeon, they are not ideal, as the tissues do not bleed and thus the need to achieve continuous hemostasis is not addressed. The best laboratory training is offered by doing closely guided procedures in live animals. Beyond the ethical objections expressed by some trainees, the use of live animal models is limited mostly by its substantial cost.

The second phase of training is the observation stage, where the surgeon views or assists at laparoscopic operations on patients. Viewing pretaped procedures is an important part of didactic learning but is no substitute for direct observation.

The third stage and most critical phase is for the trainee to work under the supervision and guidance of a skillful preceptor. The trainee is responsible for the selection of the patient, the preoperative preparation, and the postoperative management. The preceptor should allow the trainee to do most or all of the operation. Locating highly experienced preceptors who are ready to provide time-consuming direct supervision is

TABLE 1-1. Phases of Surgical Training in Accordance with the Guidelines for Attaining Privileges in Gynecologic Operative Endoscopy Set by the Society of Reproductive Surgeons

Phase I. A formal didactic course which includes supervised laboratory experience with a pelvic trainer and live animals

Phase II. An observation period in which the trainee views or assists in several endoscopic operations at the appropriate clinical skill level

Phase III. A preceptorship under the direct supervision of an experienced surgeon with recognized competence

Source: Azizz.[63]

difficult. Scheduling many patients during the preceptorship is not easy. In 1990, 50 percent of gynecologists in practice 8 years or longer did only one major operation or less a week.[64] Telesurgery may offer surgeons much-desired global access to surgical specialists.[65] An endoscopic specialist at a central site can guide a relatively inexperienced surgeon during a laparoscopic procedure in an effective and safe manner.

In the new millennium, the growing dominance of managed care may redefine the role of the gynecologists.[66,67] Residents are required to do more primary care and as a result are less exposed to advanced gynecologic operations. Improvements in medical imaging and the development of more effective medical treatments, such as methotrexate for ectopic pregnancy, have further decreased the need for some operations. More procedures are being done on an outpatient basis and under reimbursement restrictions imposed by managed care companies. The increasing complexity of advanced operative laparoscopy and the difficulty of obtaining sufficient surgical training and maintaining the patient volume needed to do them well have raised concerns regarding the ability to train gynecologic surgeons adequately. The need to set up a unique subspecialty in advanced gynecologic laparoscopic surgery should be considered.

The creation of a new subspecialty training program in advanced laparoscopic surgery could benefit urogynecology, pelvic reconstructive surgery, reproductive surgery, and oncologic surgery.[68] The recognition of gynecologic oncology as a subspecialty of obstetrics and gynecology in 1972 resulted in the incorporation of many surgical procedures previously not considered to be within the realm of operating gynecologists. Among these procedures are major intestinal and urologic operations that often are done during primary therapy for a specific gynecologic malignancy, to manage recurrent disease, or to treat complications related to the cancer or its treatment.[69] Similarly, advanced laparoscopic operations currently have evolved to include the most complex intestinal and urologic procedures for the treatment of benign conditions such as severe endometriosis and adhesions.[70,71] The establishment of structured and exhaustive training programs in gynecologic laparoscopy will enable incorporation into routine practice of the full potential of this minimal-access approach, with its inherent benefits to the patient.

The process of surgical training, certification, and credentialing was described by Azizz[63] as a continuous process that culminates in the acquisition of the necessary knowledge and skills, the documentation of those skills, and the assignment of operative privileges by a hospital or another operating facility. Documenting the surgeon's skill in laparoscopic operations should minimize liability in the event of a malpractice suit. Most institutions maintain that such certification is essential for their own protection in case litigation arises. This contention is supported by experience showing that courts generally have found hospitals and staff members negligent if a negative outcome occurs where no appropriate and reasonable control measures have been instituted.

Guidelines for attaining privileges in gynecologic operative endoscopy were proposed by the Society for Reproductive Surgeons and approved by the Board of Directors of the American Society of Reproductive Medicine. The guidelines presuppose that the applicant is eligible or certified by the American Board of Obstetrics and Gynecology, has been granted privileges to do diagnostic laparoscopy and laparoscopic tubal sterilization, and has demonstrated competence in those techniques. Additionally, to be granted privileges for gynecologic operative laparoscopy, the applicant must submit evidence of the satisfactory completion of a recognized formal didactic course that includes supervised experience in a laboratory with a pelvic trainer or live animal models. Also, the applicant must observe or assist on several appropriate operations and perform a number of procedures under the supervision of an experienced preceptor.

The Society for Reproductive Surgeons has proposed stratifying all laparoscopic procedures into three levels[72]: procedures not requiring additional training, procedures requiring additional training, and procedures requiring significant additional training (Table 1-2). This classification is similar to groupings proposed by others and is of importance to surgeons from a medicolegal perspective. The logic behind such categorization of the expert level is to substitute the commonly held practice in which many hospitals demand documentation of training for a single specific procedure, such as laparoscopic hysterectomy or laparoscopic bladder neck suspension. This type of narrow certification places a significant burden on the individual surgeon and, in light of the rapid developments in operative laparoscopy, is not practical. As an example of these swift changes, Azizz suggested in 1995 that hysterectomy and myomectomy should be classified under "innovative experimental operative laparoscopic procedures."[63]

TABLE 1-2. Stratification of Laparoscopic Procedures According to the Level of Additional Training Required as Suggested by the Society of Reproductive Surgeons

Procedures not requiring additional training (level 1)
Laparoscopic sterilization
Needle aspiration of simple cysts
Ovarian biopsy
Minor adhesiolysis
Partial salpingectomy for tubal pregnancy
Linear salpingostomy for tubal pregnancy
Endoscopic surgery for the American Fertility Society (AFS), stage I and stage II endometriosis
Procedures requiring additional training (level 2)
Laparoscopic division of uterosacral ligaments
Adhesiolysis for moderate or severe adhesions or adhesions involving the bowel
Laser or diathermy drilling to ovaries for polycystic ovarian syndrome
Neosalpingostomy for hydrosalpinx
Salpingectomy or salpingo-oophorectomy
Endoscopic management of endometrioma and ovarian cystectomy
Laparoscopically assisted vaginal hysterectomy
Endoscopic surgery for AFS stage III and IV endometriosis
Appendectomy
Procedures requiring significant additional training (level 3)
Pelvic lymphadenectomy
Extensive pelvic side wall dissection
Presacral neurectomy
Dissection of an obliterated pouch of Douglas
Bowel surgery
Retropubic bladder neck suspension
Hernia repair
Ureteral dissection

Source: Society for Reproductive Surgeons, American Fertility Society.[72]

However, 2 years later, those procedures were no longer placed in the "experimental" category.[73]

Despite explicit guidelines in respect to eligibility to perform laparoscopic operations, concern remains regarding the appropriateness of the training currently offered to new trainees.[74] This concern has led to the establishment of a reproductive surgery fellowship program by the Society for Reproductive Surgeons.

When endoscopic training is acquired during residency, certification of surgical skill becomes the responsibility of the program director. It is more common for the advanced training to be acquired after residency by practicing gynecologists, thus complicating the issue of certification and credentialing. The responsibility of certifying competency is an ethical and legal burden. Consequently, it has been common practice for postresidency credentialing to be related closely to the granting of privileges by a hospital.[28] The American College of Obstetricians and Gynecologists has issued a policy statement outlining general credentialing guidelines for endoscopic surgery.[75]

References

1. Bozzini P. *Der Lichtleiter oder Beschreibung einer einfachen Vorrichtung un ihrer Anwendung zur Erleuchtung inner Hohlen und Zwischenrauma des lebenden animalischen Korpers*. Weimar: Landes Industrie, Comptoir, 1807.
2. Nitze M. Uber eine neue Beleuchtungsmethode der Hohlen des menlischen Korpers. *Wein Med Presse* 1879; 20:251.
3. Kelling G. Uber Osophagoskopie, Gastroskopie und Zolioscopie. *Munch Med Wochenschr* 1902; 49:21.
4. Jacobeaus H. Uber die Moglichkeit, die Zystoskopie bei Untersuchung seroser Hohlun-

gen anzuwneden. *Munch Med Wochenschr* 1910; 57:2090.

5. Veress J. Neues instrument zur Ausfuhrung von Brust-oder Bauchpumktionen und Pneumothorax behandlung. *Dtsch Med Woschenschr* 1938; 64:1480.
6. Ruddock JC. Peritoneoscopy. *West J Surg* 1934; 42:392.
7. Hope R. The differential diagnosis of ectopic gestation by peritoneoscopy. *Surg Gynecol Obstet* 1937; 64:229.
8. Anderson ET. Peritoneoscopy. *Am J Surg* 1937; 35:36.
9. Decker A, Cherry T. A new method in the diagnosis of pelvic disease. *Am J Surg* 1944; 64:40.
10. Power FH, Barnes AC. Sterilization by means of peritoneoscopic tubal furguration: A preliminary report. *Am J Obstet Gynecol* 1941; 41:1038.
11. Palmer R. La coeloscopie gynecologique, ses possibilities et ses indications actualles. *Semin Hop Paris* 1954; 30:441.
12. Fourestier M, Gladau A, Voulmiere J. Perfectionments de l'endoscope medicale. *Presse Med* 1952; 60:1292.
13. Hopkins HH, Kapany NS. Flexible fiberoscope using static scanning. *Nature* 1954; 173:39.
14. Frangenheim H. *Die Laparoskopie und die Culdoscopie in der Gynakologie*. Stuttgart: Thieme, 1959.
15. Albano V, Cittidini E. *La celioscopia in Ginologia*. Palermo: Denaro, 1962.
16. Steptoe PC. *Laparoscopy in Gynaecology*. Edinburgh: Livingstone, 1967.
17. Bruhat MA, Mage, G, Pouly, JL. *Operative Laparoscopy.* McGraw-Hill, 1992.
18. Semm K. *Atlas of Gynecologic Laparoscopy and Hysteroscopy*. Philadelphia: Saunders, 1975.
19. Gomel V. *Laparoscopy and Hysteroscopy in Gynecologic Practice*. Chicago: Yearbook, 1995.
20. Semm K. *Operative Manual: Endoscopic Abdominal Surgery*. Chicago: Yearbook, 1987.
21. Azziz R. *Practical Manual of Operative Laparoscopy and Hysteroscopy,* 2nd ed. New York: Springer-Verlag, 1997.
22. San Filippo JS, Levine RL. *Operative Gynecologic Endoscopy,* 2nd ed. Semm K. *History of Operative Gynecologic Endoscopy.* New York: Springer-Verlag, 1996, pp 3–17.
23. Donnez, J, Nisolle M. *An Atlas of Laser Operative Laparoscopy and Hysteroscopy.* Parthenon Pub Group, 1996.
24. Nezhat C, Nezhat F, Nezhat CH, et al. Laparoscopic surgery, in Niederhuber, JE ed., *Fundamentals of Surgery*. Stamford, CT.: Appleton & Lange, 1997.
25. Phillips JM, Kott DF. Increased mobility with an articulated lens, in *Gynecologic Endoscopy Photography,* 1977.
26. Nezhat C, Crowgey SR, Garrison CP. Surgical treatment of endometriosis via laser laparoscopy. *Fertil Steril* 1986; 45:778.
27. Tadir Y, Fisch B. Operative laparoscopy: A challenge for general gynecology? *Am J Obstet Gynecol* 1993; 169:10.
28. Martin DC. Clinical use of lasers, in Hunt R, ed., *Atlas of Female Infertility Surgery.* 2d ed. St. Louis: Mosby Year Book, 1992.
29. Bruhat MA, Mage, G, Manhes M. Use of the CO_2 laser via laparoscopy, in Kaplan I, ed., *Proceedings of the Third International Congress for Laser Surgery.* Tel Aviv: 1979. Qui-Paz.
30. Tadir Y et al. Laparoscopic CO_2 laser sterilization, in Semm K, Mettler L, eds., *Human Reproduction.* Amsterdam: Excerpts Medicus, 1981.
31. Tadir Y et al. Laparoscopic application of CO_2 laser, in Atsumi K and Numsakui N, eds., *Proceedings of the Fourth Congress of the International Society for Laser Surgery.* Tokyo: Japanese Society for Laser Medicine, 1981.
32. Daniell JF, Pittaway DE. Use of the CO_2 laser in laparoscopic surgery: initial experience with the second puncture technique. *Infertility* 1982; 5:13.
33. Daniell JF: The CO_2 laser in infertility surgery. *J Reprod Med* 1983; 28:265.
34. Daniell JF: Laparoscopic salpingostomy: Early clinical results (abstract). *Laser Surg Med* 1983; 3:161.
35. Semm K. Course of endoscopic abdominal surgery, in Semm K, Frederich ER, eds., *Operative Manual for Endoscopic Abdominal Surgery*. Chicago: Yearbook, 1987.
36. Nezhat C, Crowgey SR, Nezhat F, Videolaseroscopy for the treatment of endometriosis associated with infertility. *Fertil Steril* 1989; 51:237.
37. Almieda OD, Val-Galls JM. Conscious sedation in microlaparoscopy. *J Am Assoc Gynecol Laparosc* 1997; 4:591.

38. Palter SF, Olive DL. Office microlaparoscopy under local anesthesia for chronic pelvic pain. *J Am Assoc Gynecol Laparosc* 1996; 3:359.
39. Seidman DS, Nezhat C. Is the laparoscopic bubble bursting? *Lancet* 1996; 347:542.
40. Hoerton R. Surgical research or comic opera: Questions, but few answers. *Lancet* 1996; 347:984.
41. Chalmers TC. Randomization of the first patient. *Med Clin North Am* 1975; 59:1035.
42. Nezhat FR, Nezhat CH, Seidman DS, Nezhat CR. Operative laparoscopy: Redefining the limits. *J Soc Laparoendosc Surg* 1997; 1(3):213.
43. Saskett DL, Rosenberg WMC, Gray JAM, et al. Evidence based medicine: What is and what isn't: It's about integrating individual clinical expertise and the best external evidence. *Br Med J* 1996; 312:71.
44. Nagele F, Molnar BG, O'Conor H, Magos AL. Randomized studies in endoscopic surgery—Where is the proof? *Curr Opin Obstet Gynecol* 1996; 8:281.
45. Slim K, Pezet D, Chipponi J. Laparoscopic or open appendectomy? Critical review of randomized, controlled trials. *Dis Colon Rectum* 1998; 41:398.
46. McLeod RS, Wright JG, Solomon MJ, et al. Randomized controlled trial in surgery: Issues and problems. *Surgery* 1996; 119: 483.
47. Sutton CJG, Ewen SP, Whielaw N, Haines P. Prospective, randomized, double-blind, controlled trial of laser laparoscopy in the treatment of pelvic pain associated with minimal, mild, and moderate endometriosis. *Fertil Steril* 1994; 62:696.
48. Tazuke S, Nezhat FH, Nezhat CH, et al. Laparoscopic management of pelvic pathology during pregnancy. *J Am Assoc Gynecol Laparosc* 1997; 4:605.
49. Nezhat FR, Tazuke S, Nezhat CH, et al. Laparoscopy during pregnancy: A literature review. *J Soc Laparosc Surg* 1997; 1:17.
50. Singh KB, Haddleston HT, Nandy I. Laparoscopic tubal sterilization in obese women: Experience from a teaching institute. *South Med J* 1996; 89:56.
51. Kaali SG, Bartfai G. Direct insertion of the laparoscopic trocar after a earlier laparotomy. *J Reprod Med* 1988; 33:739.
52. Shrimer BD, Dix J, Schemeig RE Jr, et al. The impact of previous abdominal surgery on outcome following laparoscopic cholecystectomy. *Surg Endosc* 1995; 9:1085.
53. Nezhat C, Seidman DS, Nezhat F, Nezhat CH. Laparoscopic surgery for gynecologic cancer, in Szabo Z, Lewis JE, Fantini GA, eds., *Surgical Technology International IV*. San Francisco: Universal Medical Press, 1995.
54. Stoker DL, Spiegelhalter DJ, Singh R, et al. Laparoscopic versus open inguinal hernia repair: Randomized prospective trial. *Lancet* 1994; 343:1243.
55. Soriano D, Yefet Y, Oelsner G, et al. Operative laparoscopy for management of ectopic pregnancy in patients with hypovolemic shock. *J Am Assoc Gynecol Laparosc* 1997; 4:363.
56. O'Sullivan GC, Murphy D, O'Brien MG, Irelans A. Laparoscopic management of generalized peritonitis due to perforated diverticula. *Am J Surg* 1996; 171:432.
57. Nezhat C, Nezhat F. Laparoscopic repair of resected ureter during operative laparoscopy to treat endometriosis: A case report. *Obstet Gynecol* 1992; 80:543.
58. Nezhat F, Brill A, Nezhat C, Nezhat C. Traumatic hypogastric artery bleeding controlled with bipolar desiccation during operative laparoscopy. *J Am Assoc Gynecol Laparosc* 1994; 1:2.
59. Nezhat C, Childers J, Nezhat F, et al. Major retroperitoneal vascular injury during laparoscopic surgery. *Hum Reprod* 1997; 12:480.
60. Schirmer BD. Laparoscopic colon resection. *Surg Clin North Am* 1996; 76:571.
61. Senagore AJ, Luchtefeld MA, Mackeigan JM. What is the learning curve for laparoscopic colectomy? *Am Surg* 1995; 61:681.
62. Dunphy BC, Shepard S, Cooke ID: Impact of the learning curve on term delivery rates following laparoscopic salpingostomy for infertility associated with distal tubal occlusive disease. *Hum Reprod* 1997; 12:1181.
63. Azizz R. Training, certification and credentialing in gynecologic operative endoscopy. *Clin Obstet Gynecol* 1995; 38:314.
64. Park RC, Bryon JW. Confronting troublesome gynecological surgery trends. *Contemp OB/GYN* 1994; 39:83.
65. Schulman PG, Docime SG, Selch W, et al. Telesurgical monitoring: Initial clinical experience. *Surg Endosc* 1997; 11:1001.
66. Russell KP. The obstetrician-gynecologist as a primary care physician: What's in a name? *Obstet Gynecol Surv* 1995; 50:329.

67. Dunn LJ. The obstetrician and gynecologist—generalist, specialist, subspecialist? *Am J Obstet Gynecol* 1995; 172:1188.
68. Seidman DS, Nezhat F, Hezhat CH, Nezhat C. Gynecologic operative laparoscopy: New training programs are needed, in Szabo Z, Lewis JE, Fantini GA, eds., *Surgical Technology International VI.* San Francisco: Universial Medical Press, 1997.
69. Barnhill D, Doering D, Remmenga S, et al. Intestinal surgery performed on gynecologic cancer patients. *Gynecol Oncol* 1991; 40:38.
70. Seidman DS, Nezhat C, Nezhat F, Nezhat CH. Laparoscopic interstinal procedures, in Azizz R, Murphy AA, eds., *Practical Manual of Operative Laparoscopy and Hysteroscopy,* 2d ed. New York: Springer-Verlag, 1997.
71. Nezhat CH, Seidman DS, Nezhat F, et al. Laparoscopic management of intentional and unintentional cystotomy. *J Urol* 1996; 156:1400.
72. Society for Reproductive Surgeons, American Fertility Society. Guidelines for attaining privileges in gynecologic operative endoscopy. *Fertil Steril* 1994; 62:118.
73. Azizz R. Training, certification, and credentialing in gynecologic operative endoscopy, in Azizz T, Murphy AA, eds., *Practical Manual of Operative Laparoscopy and Hysteroscopy,* 2d ed. New York: Springer-Verlag, 1997.
74. Keye WRE Jr. Hitting a moving target: Credentialing the endoscopic surgeon. *Fertil Steril* 1994; 62:1115.
75. American College of Obstetricians and Gynecologists. *Credentialing Guidelines for New Operative Procedures.* ACOG Committee Opinion 146. Washington, D.C.: ACOG, 1994.
76. Tadir Y, Fisch B,. Operative laparoscopy: A challenge for general gynecology? *Am J Obstet Gynecol* 1993 Volume 169. No. 1 p. 7–12.

2

The Informed Consent and Malpractice

A surgeon is required by law and bound by moral and ethical standards to explain a planned operation, its risks, and the expected outcome to the patient preoperatively. The purpose of this chapter is to (1) provide a guide for discussing a proposed laparoscopic operation with the patient and (2) describe the informed consent as it relates to laparoscopy.

Diagnostic laparoscopy has gained widespread acceptance among gynecologic and general surgeons, but patients' expectations and the actual results from advanced operative laparoscopic procedures frequently do not coincide. For example, some patients believe that lasers are essential for a thorough operation, although most surgeons acknowledge that scissors and electrosurgical instruments are equally effective. Patients tend to consider laparoscopic procedures minor operations. This idea is reinforced by terms such as *same-day surgery, Band-Aid surgery, minimal invasive surgery*, and *laser surgery*. Patients and physicians underestimate the risks of complex operative endoscopy, which are potentially as serious as those associated with laparotomy.

The Informed Consent

Since 1914, surgeons have been required to obtain a patient's written consent before an operative procedure. This process allows the patient to participate in decisions with an understanding of the factors relevant to the proposed operation. The proper consent requires that the patient be informed of the diagnosis, the proposed treatment, the probability of success, alternative forms of therapy, and the risks of the planned operation. The information should be precise and presented understandably. Audiovisual material can be used to supplement the physician's explanation. This exchange forms an intrinsic part of the doctor-patient relationship. Through these discussions, the physician can make intraoperative decisions that are consistent with the patient's desires and goals. The circumstances under which the consent is obtained are also important. The patient should not be under the influence of a medication that might interfere with his or her rational judgment.

Although the principle of obtaining an informed consent is the same in any operation, the following discussion concerns issues in laparoscopic procedures. Operative laparoscopy often is done immediately after a diagnostic laparoscopy. Sometimes a precise diagnosis cannot be made preoperatively, particularly in infertile women and those complaining of pelvic pain. The preoperative discussion should include possible diagnoses because some infertile patients have no clinical evidence of adhesions, endometriosis, or pelvic abnormalities, and significant disease that is found laparoscopically requires an extensive operation. Anticipated procedures should be explained so that the patient has realistic expectations about the type and duration of the anesthesia, the planned operation, and the length of hospitalization. The surgeon provides information about the procedure's chance of success and the possible need for follow-up therapy. If a patient declines the proposed operation, alternatives are described. Patients undergoing operations for the relief of pelvic pain require extensive preoperative evaluation and counseling because these women may be disappointed if they experience postoperative pain.

Postoperative complaints after laparoscopic operations vary with the type of procedure[1] and are influenced by the geographic setting.[2] For example, expectations regarding pain and discomfort postoperatively may differ between women in Europe and America and can be influenced culturally. Most women are informed that they can return to normal activity within a week after advanced operative procedures and a few days after a diagnostic laparoscopy.

If the findings provide a range of options, the patient can elect to have only diagnostic laparoscopy. A woman suspected of having an ectopic pregnancy needs to understand the relative risks and benefits of expectant or medical management and salpingectomy or salpingostomy. Her obstetric history, clinical findings, and desire for fertility and acceptance as well as the financial availability of assisted reproductive technology influence the type of operation. Myomectomies done by laparoscopy can be associated with bleeding or injury to adjacent organs, and a laparotomy may be required. The patient should be made aware of the possible risk of uterine rupture in future pregnancies.[3] When initial laparoscopy reveals severe pelvic adhesions or when there is a known history of severe endometriosis, particularly in women with cul-de-sac obliteration, the risk of complications, especially bowel injury, is increased. The importance of the laparoscopic surgeon's experience in such cases is stressed.

Ideally, most questions are answered in the physician's office during the preoperative consultation, but the patient should be given ample time preoperatively to discuss additional concerns, such as fertility, in case intraoperative decisions affect future childbearing. If the abnormalities cannot be corrected laparoscopically, some patients will request a laparotomy under the same anesthesia, while others will want to schedule a laparotomy later.

Adequacy of the Informed Consent

Legal standards define the adequacy of an informed consent.[4] With the majority rule, disclosure is decided by a professional medical standard on the basis of the customary disclosure practices of physicians in the same specialty. The minority rule requires physicians to divulge the risks that a prudent patient needs to understand to make a decision. The minority rule has been modified to either a subjective test or the informational requirements of a specific patient: the plaintiff.

The consumers' movement in health care and the proliferation of consumer-directed information, including the Internet information "superhighway," have contributed to the growing participation of patients in medical decision making.[5] This new attitude is consistent with both the ethical principle of patient autonomy and the legal requirement of informed consent. Patients are not expected to be passive and compliant and are encouraged to participate in surgical decision making. The traditional unilateral process of informed consent is evolving into one of informed collaborative choice.[5,6] More patient participation and opportunity for choice of treatment options will improve patient satisfaction and may decrease the risk of malpractice claims.[7,8]

Patient communication must be free from inappropriate outside influences to obtain adequate informed consent.[9] Studies have shown that physicians often fail during the informed consent process to communicate pertinent information, including the rationale of the procedure, its benefits and risks, and alternative procedures.[10] Failure to share information with the patient is a major barrier to informed consent. The process of decision making and the importance of patient participation are recognized in many fields of medicine.[9,11] Appropriately, the American College of Obstetricians and Gynecologists' computer-based interactions series has developed a program that provides insight on clinical decision making.[12] When asked to provide informed consent, many patients lack the self-confidence needed to make complex decisions about the operation. The rushed setting, the fear of limited access to costly care in the managed care era, and the difficulty of putting into perspective the risks of nontreatment often prevent the patient from reaching a thoughtful decision in considering an operation. It is essential to provide the patient with simple and accurate information in a comfortable and safe environment.

Sensitivity to the patient and a commonsense approach to the informed consent are practical. Good communication is essential and is encouraged. The patient expects her physician to assess the problem, propose treatment, and address her concerns with compassion. Patients are anxious preoperatively; the physician can ease that apprehension by carefully explaining the procedure's anticipated consequences. When describing the frequency of complications, one should use terms such as *rare, uncommon*, and *unusual*. One should not attempt to provide precise complication rates. It is important to explain the precautions that will be taken to lessen the risks. Additional consent is required for photographic documentation.

Exceptions to the Informed Consent

Clinical conditions such as life-threatening situations can create exceptions to a full disclosure. Other possible exceptions are an unconscious patient and a situation in which the risks of failure to treat are greater than the risks of treatment. Whenever possible, the patient's family should be informed. Obtaining an informed consent implies that the patient is competent to give it. No clear standard exists for competency, but patients with severe mental retardation or psychiatric disorders, and those intoxicated by drugs or alcohol are unable to give an informed consent. Criteria for discovering incompetency include inability to make decisions, making decisions for irrational reasons, irrational decision, and inability to know, appreciate, or understand the information provided. If the physician believes a patient is partially or totally incompetent, it is important to involve the family, a guardian, or even the courts to get a proper informed consent. A patient can waive her right for full disclosure of the risks, but the reasons must be documented and discussed with the family. However, the physician should not decide that disclosing some or all of the risks would upset the patient and prevent her from making a rational decision. Such a claim can be difficult to prove. The courts may view the physician's self-interest as an overriding factor.[13]

Malpractice (Civil Liability)

Regardless of the type or route of the surgical procedure, the basis for malpractice is the same. Most cases begin after the patient experiences an unanticipated unfavorable result.[14] Operations more likely to result in a lawsuit are those in which the doctor did not discuss with the patient the possibility of an adverse outcome.[14] Knowing when to stop a complicated procedure represents common sense and good judgment. Despite proper training and skill, sequelae can occur. To prevent untoward results, gynecologists must improve their competence in operative laparoscopy with postgraduate courses and by gradually undertaking increasingly complex procedures. The cause of the complication should be explained to the patient. When the surgeon does not communicate adequately, the patient may seek another physician to explain the untoward result. Physicians should be restrained in criticizing colleagues unless all the facts are known. In a review of adverse outcomes, less than 2 percent resulted in a malpractice claim.[15]

Proof of Malpractice

The elements needed to legally prove malpractice are as follows:

1. *Duty*. The physician's duty in a legal sense is decided by the community standard of practice for a particular procedure.
2. *Dereliction of duty (negligence)*. Negligence is a deviation from the accepted standard of care, custom, or common practice. It can result from several acts or failures to act, including failure to conduct adequate examinations and tests, careless execution of medical and surgical procedures, inappropriate prescription or administration of drugs, inadequate monitoring of the patient, failure to refer patients to other specialists as needed, and unethical conduct that harms a patient.
3. *Damage and direct causality*. If injury results, the patient needs to prove that the negligence was the proximate cause of the damage.

As operative laparoscopy becomes more complex, the levels of experience and expertise vary widely. Often, the standard of care is not defined clearly. Surgeons must be aware of their level of skill, as some laparoscopic operations may be done safely by laparotomy. In other instances, a colleague with more endoscopic experience can help or the patient can be referred to a more accomplished endoscopist.

The relation between the number of malpractice claims and personal, educational, and practice characteristics was studied in a sample of 427 surgeons, including 115 gynecologists.[16] Surgeons who were terminated because of a high number of claims were found to be less likely to have completed a fellowship, belong to a clinical faculty, be members of professional societies, have specialty board certification, or be in a group practice. These findings were interpreted to suggest that manifest exemplary modes of professional peer relationships and responsible clinical behavior are likely to be related to a lower rate of malpractice claims.

Audiotape analysis has identified significant differences in the communication actions of no-claims and claims physicians in primary care. Compared with claims primary care physicians, no-claims primary care physicians used more statements of orientation, laughed and used humor more, tended to use more facilitation, and spent more time in routine visits. Interestingly, a similar association between communication behaviors and malpractice claims was not found for surgeons.[17]

CONSENT TO LAPAROSCOPIC SURGERY

Patient's Name____ Date______________________________

I authorize and direct ________________________________M.D., and/or associates or assistants of his or her choice to treat the condition/s believed to exist in my case.

The laparoscope, a surgical instrument similar to a telescope is inserted through a small incision in the belly button. The abdomen is distended with a gas called carbon dioxide. The scope allows the doctor to visualize the pelvic organs and allows other instruments to be used under direct vision. Small second, third and fourth incisions are occasionally made at the pubic hairline for scissors, coagulator, or laser to perform major closed surgery at laparoscopy.

Hysteroscopy (the use of a small optical tube that is inserted through the vagina into the uterus without incision to visualize the uterine cavity) is usually performed with laparoscopy in order to determine: (1) the size and depth of the uterine cavity; (2) the presence of congenital abnormalities within the uterus, such as a septum that divides the inside of the uterus, or a double uterus; (3) the presence of polyps or fibroid tumors in the uterine cavity; (4) whether specific abnormalities of the endometrium (lining of the uterus) are present, e.g. hyperplasia (build up lining of the uterus), tuberculosis, or cell changes that indicate early cancer. D&C (dilatation and curettage) may also be performed if indicated.

Video and/or pictures may be taken during surgery and used to show you what was seen and done. They are also used for teaching other patients and other surgeons these techniques.

Your doctor performs advanced laparoscopic surgery that includes procedures considered investigational and may include modified instrumentation. These are relatively new techniques not commonly undertaken elsewhere and can include laparoscopic oophorectomy, hysterectomy, and tubal reversal. Laparoscopic treatment of ovarian neoplasms, benign or malignant is considered investigational.

Antibiotics, anticoagulants, and other medications may be used with surgery to aid in healing. These medications are not labeled (neither approved nor disapproved) by the FDA for adhesion prevention.

Although laparoscopy is generally an outpatient procedure, you may be asleep from 1-4 hours, occasionally longer.

1. Plan to avoid any activities that will require concentration for at least 2 days.
2. You can usually return to work and moderate activities by the third day.
3. You may need 1-3 weeks to return to heavy activities and for full recovery.

Shoulder pain from the carbon dioxide gas and abdominal distention are common. Your throat may be sore from the endotracheal tube. About 1 in 40 patients are admitted for overnight stay due to nausea, drowsiness, or pain.

Complications from laparoscopic surgery are very uncommon, but they do sometimes occur. It is also possible that because of complications, or because of the discovery of life-threatening abnormalities, immediate major abdominal surgery might be necessary. The chance of severe complications such as hysterectomy, colostomy, paralysis, or death is rare. With respect to your life, this operation is six times safer than driving a car and two to three times safer than being pregnant.
Some of the possible complications are the same as those of regular surgery. Complications include bleeding; infection, particularly of the navel; generalized disease; inflammation of the lining of the abdomen; injury to the stomach or intestines; gas embolism to the lining from the carbon dioxide; abnormal gas collections underneath the skin and in the chest; ruptures or hernias in the surgical wound and through the breathing muscles (diaphragm); burns on the skin of the abdomen and inside the abdomen; damage to the kidney and urinary system; blood clots in the pelvis and lungs; damage to the kidney and urinary systems; blood clots in the pelvis and lungs; and allergic and other bad reactions to one or more substances used in the procedure.

Some of the complications of this procedure may require major surgery; some of the complications can cause poor healing wounds, scarring and permanent disability, and very rarely, some of the complications can even cause death.

The alternative procedure to the laparoscopic surgery is major surgery. However, this alternative method also carries the same risks, and requires a much longer period to recover and more pain and discomfort. Therefore, in those patients in whom laparoscopic surgery is possible, the procedures provide the patient with diagnosis and treatment at low risk and less discomfort. Your doctor cannot and does not guarantee the success of this procedure, but believes that the procedure is in your best interest.

I further understand that during the course of the operations or treatment, unforeseen conditions may be revealed requiring an extension of the original procedure/s or different procedures than those specifically discussed. I hereby authorize the above named surgeon, his or her associates, and assistants to perform such other laparoscopic surgical procedures and if necessary laparotomy (abdominal surgery) and to remove any tissue or organs that may be necessary or medically desirable as determined by the surgeons professional judgement. This authority shall extend to treatment of conditions not previously known by my physicians.

My signature below constitutes my acknowledgment: 1. that I have read or had read to me the contents of this form, 2. that I understand and I agree to the foregoing, 3. that the proposed operation/s or procedure/s have been satisfactorily explained to me including possible risks and alternatives, 4. that I have all the information that I desire and have had ample opportunity to ask questions on specific points, 5. and that I hereby give my authorization and consent.

DO NOT SIGN THIS FORM UNLESS YOU HAVE READ IT, UNDERSTAND IT, AND AGREE WITH WHAT IT SAYS.

Date: Signature:

Time: Witness:

Figure 2-1. This consent form is used for laparoscopic operations.

PHOTOGRAPH CONSENT AND RELEASE FORM

I, _______________________, hereby irrevocably authorize ____________________, their successors, assigns, and those acting with their permission upon their authority to copyright, use and publish for art, advertising, medical, trade, commercial and other lawful purpose, any depiction or likeness for me or which I may be included in whole or part, including, but not limited to, motion pictures, video tapes and still photographs, and further including any composite photograph or photograph distorted in character or in form, and any motion picture or video tape edited by addition thereto or deletion of any part thereof, whether in conjunction with my name, a fictitious name or no name, or any reproduction or variation thereof by whatever medium made, taken at ____________________ Hospital during the period of ________________________.

I hereby waive any right which I may have to inspect or approve any such photograph, motion picture, video tape or other likeness or the use to which it is put, and acknowledge that except for the consideration recited I shall receive no payment or remuneration for the use of any such photograph, motion picture, or video tape or likeness.

I hereby release ____________________ their successors and assigns, and those acting with their permission and upon their authority, of and from every liability, responsibility and claim which may arise by reason of any exercise of the authority granted above or any blurring, distortion, alteration, optical illusion, or use in composite form, whether intentional or otherwise, which may occur or result in the taking or publication of such photograph, motion picture, video tape or other likeness unless it can be shown that publication ____________________ thereof was for the purpose of subjecting me to conspicuous ridicule, scandal or indignity.

I understand that my tape(s) may be used for medical studies and instructional purposes for the advancement and increased expertise of videolaseroscopy.

The condition of the pelvis will be videotaped before, in some parts during, and after the procedure. This tape could be misplaced or erased. If I personally receive a tape, it will be an edited version, approximately 5-10 minutes in length, and the ____________________ and staff cannot be held responsible for any mechanical failure that might occur during the original filming or reproduction of the video.

______________________________	______________________________
SIGNATURE	DATE
______________________________	______________________________
WITNESS	DATE

Figure 2-2. Photographic consent and release form.

CONSENT AND APPLICATION FOR OBSERVATION OF MEDICAL PROCEDURE RELEASE AND INDEMNITY

PATIENTS CONSENT TO OBSERVER

I hereby authorize____________________Hospital to permit the presence of such observers as they may deem fit while I am undergoing surgery, childbirth, examination, or other treatment or diagnostic procedure at the Hospital. I hereby consent to being observed by any such persons.

This consent and authorization is expressly limited to the following conditions:

____

____

____

______________________		______________________	
Patient's Signature	Date/Time	Witness	Date/Time
Patient's Representative	Date/Time	Patient unable to consent because______________________	

I. OBSERVER'S REQUEST AND RELEASE

I ________________________, hereby request ____________________ Hospital to permit me to observe certain medical and/or surgical procedures to be performed at the Hospital. I understand that I will be under the physician's direct supervision and agree to follow the physician's instructions to abide by all Hospital rules and regulations governing such observations. I recognize that I will be under the supervision of the physician, and not the hospital.

In consideration for the physician and hospital allowing me to observe, I hereby expressly release the physician, the hospital, their agents and employees of and from any and all claims, damages, responsibilities and liabilities which may arise, directly or indirectly, from or in connection with my activities at the Hospital. I further agree to indemnify and hold harmless the physician, the hospital, their agents and employees from and against any and all claims, liabilities and damages arising directly or indirectly out of or in connection with my observation of medical and/or surgical procedures at the Hospital.

If I am under eighteen years of age, my parent or legal guardian has consented to my observation of the medical and/or surgical procedures and agrees to release, indemnify and hold harmless the physicians, the hospital, their agents and employees from and against any and all claims, liabilities and damages arising directly or indirectly out of or in connection with my observation of medical and/or surgical procedures at the Hospital.

______________________		______________________	
Observer	Date	Witness	Date
Parent or Guardian	Date	Witness	Date

II. PHYSICIAN'S INDEMNITY FOR OBSERVER

I have agreed to let______________________ (the "observer") accompany me during certain medical and/or surgical procedures at the Hospital and to observe such procedures. I agree that I will be completely responsible for the Observer and that he or she will be within my control at all times and will abide by all Hospital rules and regulations relating to his or her observing such procedures at the hospital.

In consideration of the Hospital's permitting the observer to accompany me, I agree to indemnify and hold harmless the hospital, its agents and employees from and against any and all claims, liabilities and damages arising, directly or indirectly, out of or in connection with the observation by such observer of medical and/or surgical procedures at the Hospital.

______________________		______________________	
Physician	Date	Witness	Date

Figure 2-3. A sample consent and application form for observation of medical procedures release and indemnity.

Malpractice cases usually are caused by delayed diagnosis, failure to recognize a complication, or inadequate treatment. Many injuries can be identified intraoperatively and repaired. For instance, delayed recognition of bowel injury can result in a catastrophic outcome of a complication that could have been repaired during the primary operation. Once the injury is identified, the physician can either repair it or seek proper consultation.[18] Failure to call for consultation and inappropriate repair of a laparoscopic injury have been recognized as a major cause of litigation.[19] Patients who complain postoperatively of increasing abdominal pain should be examined promptly, and their clinical condition should be evaluated. Postoperative infection is rare, and a careful examination is needed to discover the cause of fever. Significant abdominal discomfort and vomiting postoperatively can be associated with an incisional hernia even in small 5-mm ports that are left unsutured.[20] Hypotension caused by intraoperative hemorrhage is managed by promptly diagnosing and locating the vascular injury, obtaining hemostasis, and replacing blood as needed.[21,22]

Doing an appendectomy incidental to other authorized abdominal and pelvic operations is acceptable, as the long-term benefits of appendectomy have been shown in women with chronic pelvic pain even when the appendix is histologically normal.[23] However, the physician can be liable for assault and battery if proper consent is not obtained. If a complication arises, the lack of consent can become the source of a malpractice claim.

Medical errors that harm patients should be brought to their attention. Such full disclosure is clearly in the best interest of patients because it allows them to understand what has occurred and gain appropriate compensation for the harm they have suffered.[24] However, not infrequently surgeons find it difficult to admit errors, especially to those who have been harmed by them. Yet physicians' ethical responsibilities sometimes differ from their legal and risk-management responsibilities. It is therefore argued that the physician must continue to respect the patient and communicate honestly with him or her throughout the relationship even if the patient has been injured. Moreover, offering an apology for harming a patient should be considered one of a surgeon's ethical responsibilities. Monetary compensation alone should not be offered as a charitable gesture; instead, it should be accompanied by an apology to demonstrate the responsibility of the physician to the trusting patient. Full and honest disclosure of errors is most consistent with the mutual respect and trust patients expect from their physicians.

Avoiding Malpractice

While it is impossible to guarantee that a surgeon can avoid malpractice claims, Roberts and colleagues[8] suggest several steps to reduce the risk:

1. Engage in good-quality careful medical practice.
2. Be sure that you are trained adequately before attempting a diagnostic procedure or treatment.
3. Refer a patient to other physicians for care or consultation if the care required is not within your area of expertise.
4. Make sure that your knowledge is current, especially in the rapidly advancing areas of diagnostic and operative laparoscopy.
5. Do the procedure only if the facility in which care is given is equipped to provide good emergency care if a complication occurs during treatment.
6. When using nonstandard treatments (those not generally condoned and employed by the medical community), exercise caution.
7. Obtain adequate informed consent. Sample consent forms are illustrated below (Figures 2-1, 2-2, and 2-3).

References

1. Azizz R, Steinkampf MP, Murphy A. Postoperative recuperation: Relation to the extent of endoscopic surgery. *Fertil Steril* 1989; 51:1061.
2. Semm K: *Operative Manual for Endoscopic Abdominal Surgery*. Chicago: Year Book, 1987.
3. Stenchever MA. Too much informed consent? *Obstet Gynecol* 1991; 77:631.
4. Meisel A. The "exceptions" to the informed consent doctrine: Striking a balance between competing values in medical decision making. *Conn Med* 1981; 45:107 (pt 1) and 45:27 (pt 2).
5. Barr JR. Following a few simple rules may help prevent malpractice claims. *Can Med Assoc J* 1991; 114:355.
6. Localio AR, Lawhters AG, Brennan TA, et al. Relation between malpractice claims and adverse events due to negligence: Results of the Harvard Medical Practice Study III. *N Engl J Med* 1991; 325:245.
7. Mills HM. Medical lessons from malpractice cases. *JAMA* 1963; 183:1073.
8. Roberts DK, Shane JA, Roberts ML. *Confronting the Malpractice Crisis: Guidelines*

for the Obstetrician-Gynecologist. Kansas, City: Eagle Press, 1985.

9. Pelosi MA III, Pelosi MA. Spontaneous uterine rupture at thirty-three weeks subsequent to previous superficial laparoscopic myomectomy. *Am J Obstet Gynecol* 1997; 177:1547.
10. Gambone JC, Reiter RC. Hysterectomy: Improving the patient's decision making process. *Clin Obstet Gynecol* 1997; 40:868.
11. DiMatteo MR. The physician-patient relationship: Effects on the quality of health care. *Clin Obstet Gynecol* 1994; 37:149.
12. Ballard-Reisch DS. A model of participative decision making for physician-patient interaction. *Health Comm* 1990; 2:91.
13. Greenfield S, Kaplan R, Ware JE. Expanding patient involvement in care: Effects on patient outcomes. *Ann Intern Med* 1985; 102:520.
14. Wagener J, Taylor SE. What else could I have done? Patients' responses to failed treatment decisions. *Health Psychol* 1986; 5:481.
15. Honde CJ, Reiter RC. Decision making in women's health care. *Obstet Gynecol* 1994; 37:162.
16. Wu WC, Pearlman RA. Consent in medical decision making: The role of communication. *J Gen Intern Med* 1988; 3:9.
17. Gambone JC, Reiter RC, Pitts J. *Interactions: Programs in Clinical Decision Making*. American College of Obstetricians and Gynecologists. Hamilton, Ontario: Decker Electronic Publishing, 1996.
18. Adamson TE, Baldwin DC Jr, Sheehan TJ, Oppenberg AA. Characteristics of surgeons with high and low malpractice claims rates. *West J Med* 1997; 166:37.
19. Levinson W, Roter DL, Mullooly JP, et al. Physician-patient communication: The relationship with malpractice claims among primary care physicians and surgeons. *JAMA* 1997; 277:553.
20. Sutton CJG. Medico-legal implications of keyhole surgery. *Medico-Legal J* 1996; 64:101.
21. Nezhat C, Nezhat F, Seidman DS, Nezhat C. Incisional hernias after operative laparoscopy. *J Laparoendosc Adv Surg Tech* 1997; 7:111.
22. Seidman DS, Nasserbakht F, Nezhat F, et al. Delayed recognition of iliac artery injury during laparoscopic surgery. *Surg Endosc* 1996; 10:1099.
23. Nezhat C, Childers J, Nezhat F, et al. Major retroperitoneal vascular injury during laparoscopic surgery. *Hum Reprod* 1997; 12:480.
24. Protopapas A, Shushan A, Hart R, et al. Is laparoscopic appendectomy a gynaecological procedure? *Lancet* 1998; 351:500.

SECTION II

3

Equipment

Successful operative laparoscopy requires the proper basic and specialized equipment to make difficult procedures technically possible and safe. Most operations can be done with two or three forceps, a suction-irrigator probe, a bipolar electrocoagulator, and a CO_2 laser. With the rapid growth of operative laparoscopy, disposable, semireusable, and reusable instruments have become available. In selecting the appropriate instruments, their cost and effectiveness should be considered because too many instruments clutter the field and increase operative time.

With videolaseroscopy, the operation is observed by the surgeon and operating room staff on video monitors. The CO_2 laser is used through the operative channel of the laparoscope for cutting and establishing hemostasis of small blood vessels.[1] Electrocoagulation with a bipolar forceps is used to control bleeding from larger vessels. These instruments enable surgeons to increase the diversity of laparoscopic procedures. Some of them have multiple functions, while others are specialized. Most are designed to fit through trocar sleeves between 2 and 33 mm in diameter. A description of sub-2-mm laparoscopes and surgical instruments is provided in Chap. 8.

Disposable and Reusable Instruments

Several factors must be considered in choosing instruments, such as initial cost, cost per use, ease of use, and reliability.[2] Reusable instruments require initial and maintenance expenses, handling, sterilizing, sorting, and storing. For some reusable instruments, such as scissors, reliability declines with use, and they are replaced periodically. Others, such as claw forceps, do not become less efficient, and their construction and materials allow a certain level of indelicate handling.

A Canadian study found that the cost of reprocessing instruments varied from $2.64 (Canadian) to $4.66 for each disposable laparoscopic instrument.[3] Purchases of 10 commonly reused disposable laparoscopic instruments cost $183,279, and the reprocessing cost was estimated at $35,665 for the study period. Not reusing disposable instruments would have cost $527,575 in the same period. Disposable laparoscopic instruments were reused 1.7 to 68 times each. Under carefully monitored conditions and strict guidelines, reuse of disposable laparoscopic equipment can be cost-effective.[3] The use of reusable hook electrosurgical instruments was less expensive than that of their limited-reuse counterparts. Surgeons were very satisfied with this type of instrument. The authors noted that attempts to compare the cost of laparoscopic instruments are limited by rapid evolution in design and the availability of many types of devices.[4]

A cost analysis of single-use compared with reusable laparoscopic instruments could be done through an examination of the charges or prices in the health care providers' bill, not the actual costs. For reasons related to the structure of medical care reimbursement for surgical procedures, the price of a disposable instrument often is not related to the cost of its manufacture and distribution. A patient may be charged as much as three times the hospital's cost for each disposable instrument used.[2] Growing competition among hospitals and the expanding application of global fees have resulted in a reconsideration of the use of some disposable instruments.

A review of all laparoscopic and thoracoscopic procedures done over 4 years in which disposable laparoscopic instruments were reused revealed no complications related to malfunction of disposable instruments.[5] These instruments can be reused safely under strict guidelines.[5] However, not following the "single use" recommendation of the manufacturer can create a litigation risk in case of malfunction. Disposable instruments cost as much as $100 to $200 each. The expenditure required for disposable trocars has been estimated to be seven times higher than that for reusable trocars.[6] The use of a stapler can add $1000 to $3000 to the operation, thus offsetting the cost savings achieved by laparoscopy. The higher charge for laparoscopic hysterectomy is attributed mostly to the added expense of disposable instruments.[7,8] The assertion that the use of disposable instruments, especially staples, saves money by reducing operating time is not true.[8]

The main advantages of disposable instruments are sharpness and a theoretically reduced risk of transmission of disease. Environmental concerns arise with respect to their disposal and biodegradability. There is no evidence that reusable instruments increase the low risk of infection associated with laparoscopy.[6] The safety of reusing disposable instruments suggests that a combination of selected disposable and reusable equipment makes the most sense. Some manufacturers offer "resposable" instruments that combine disposable components with reusable parts, such as scissors with reusable handles and single-use blades.

The Basic Instruments

The Laparoscope

The endoscope can view the abdominal and pelvic cavity and is the most important piece of equipment. It must be in optimal condition. Although the diameter of laparoscopes varies from 2 to 12 mm and the angle of view varies from 0 to 90 degrees, the most commonly used laparoscopes are straight diagnostic (Figure 3-1A) and angled operative laparoscopes (Figure 3-1B, and 3-1C). Microlaparoscopes are described in Chap. 8. A direct 10-mm, 0-degree diagnostic laparoscope and an 11-mm, 0-degree operative laparoscope with a channel for the CO_2 laser are preferable (Figure 3-2, A and B). The image transmitted by the diagnostic scope is better. The operative channel requires a reduction in the size of the lens system and the number of fiberoptic bundles. With a Hopkins rod lens system, the shaft of the laparoscope contains quartz rods with concave ends that provide excellent clarity. This type of lens rarely is dislodged during handling. A recent advance in the operative laparoscope design is the Spacemaker II surgical balloon dissector (General Surgical Innovations, San Jose, CA). This device creates a predictably shaped operating space while providing observation during insertion and dissection for specialized procedures such as bladder neck suspension (Figure 3-2C). Endoscopes are either rigid or flexible. Most rigid scopes are focused with the camera coupler. With a videoscope (camera and scope together), either there will be a focus control on the scope or the focus will occur automatically inside the camera. The image is magnified and appears larger on the monitor.

Flexible scopes rely on many fiberoptic bundles. As the image is magnified, so are the bundles, making the ends of the bundles visible along with the image. The scopes are relatively fragile, and small cracks allow water to seep through the lens and distort the image.

Primary Trocars

Reusable and disposable trocars are constructed of a combination of metal and plastic (Figure 3-3, A and B). A feature common to all of them is a flapper or trumpet valve that is designed to prevent gas leakage as the laparoscope or other instruments are removed from the abdomen. With reusable trocars, this mechanism creates friction on the laparoscope. After a prolonged procedure, the trocar moves with the laparoscope. This phenomenon causes inadvertent removal of the trocar from the abdominal cavity and a loss of pneumoperitoneum. When the spring is removed from the valve, there is less friction and that problem can be avoided. A feature of disposable cannulas is a retention screw (Ethicon) (Figure 3-4A), an expansion device like an umbrella (Dexide, Inc., Fort Worth, TX) or an inflatable balloon (Marlow Surgical Technologies, Willoughby, OH) (Figure 3-4B). The balloon can tamponade abdominal wall bleeding that can obscure the operating field. The SpaceSEAL Balloon Tip Cannula (General Surgical Innovations, San Jose, CA) incorporates an adjustable atraumatic foam locking pad for increased port stabilization (Figure 3-4C). A radially expanding outer sheath has been developed to allow safer

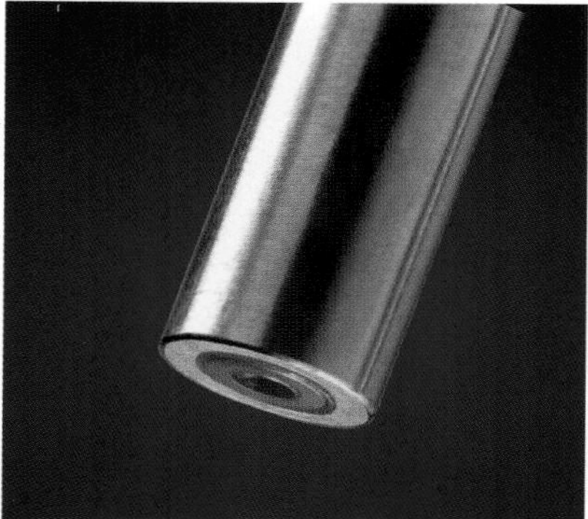

A

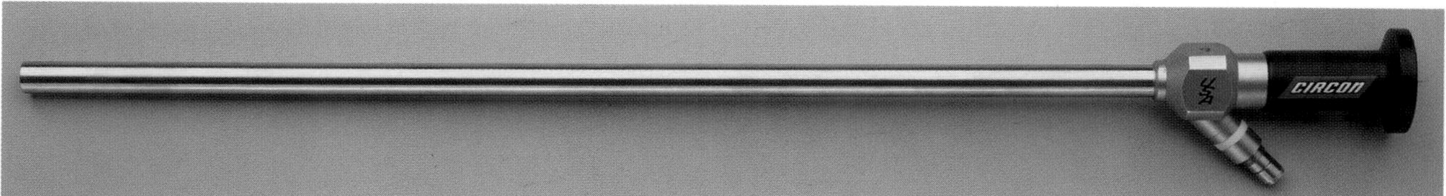

B

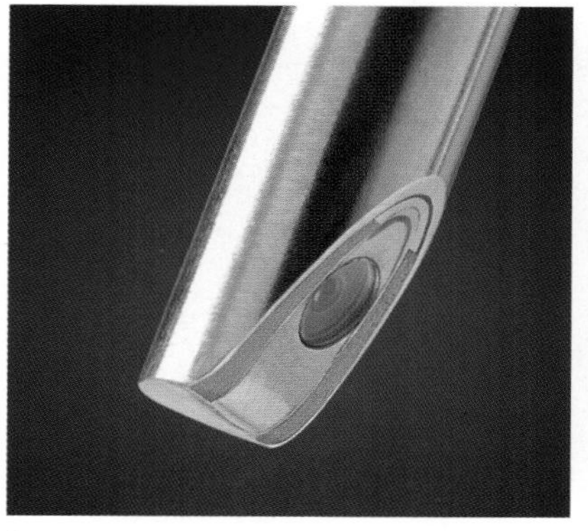

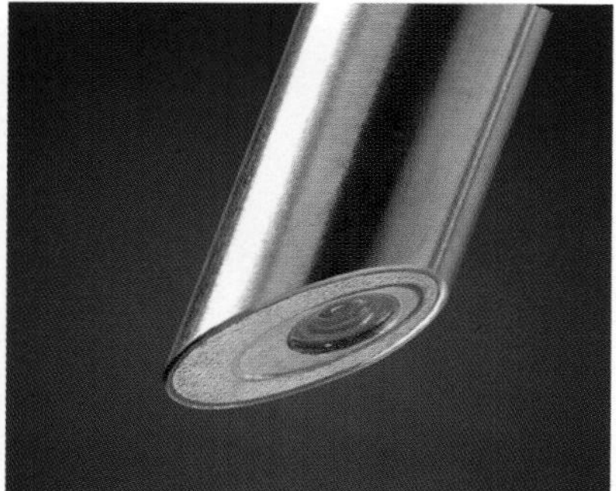

C

Figure 3-1. **A.** A 5-mm straight diagnostic laparoscope. **B.** A 10-mm diagnostic laparoscope. **C.** Angled laparoscopes.

trocar insertion (Step[tm], InnerDyne, Sunnyvale, CA). The radially expanding dilation is supposed to leave a 50 percent smaller scar while securely anchoring the cannula and virtually eliminating abdominal wall bleeding (Figure 3-5).

Another approach to improve the safety of primary trocar insertion is the observing or optical trocar (Optiview, Ethicon) (Figure 3-6). The inner trocar of this trocar is hollow except for a clear plastic conical tip with two external ridges. The trocar-cannula assembly is passed through tissue layers to enter the operative space under direct vision from a 10-mm 0-degree laparoscope placed into the trocar. Initial experience suggests that this technique represents a safe alternative to Veress needle placement when laparoscopic access could be hazardous or difficult.[9,10] The optical device requires some additional training so that the operator can identify the various anatomic layers upon entry into the abdomen through the contact view. This device is no substitute for proper training, and its cost-effectiveness for an experienced laparoscopist is doubtful.

A fiberglass optic-equipped safety needle has been developed for visually controlled access in laparoscopic procedures. This device can allow immediate diagnosis of small bowel perforation by endoscopy.[11]

Various disposable trocar tips are available. Spring-loaded safety shields (Ethicon) retract into the cannula as the trocar is inserted into the abdomen. This exposes the sharp trocar for entry

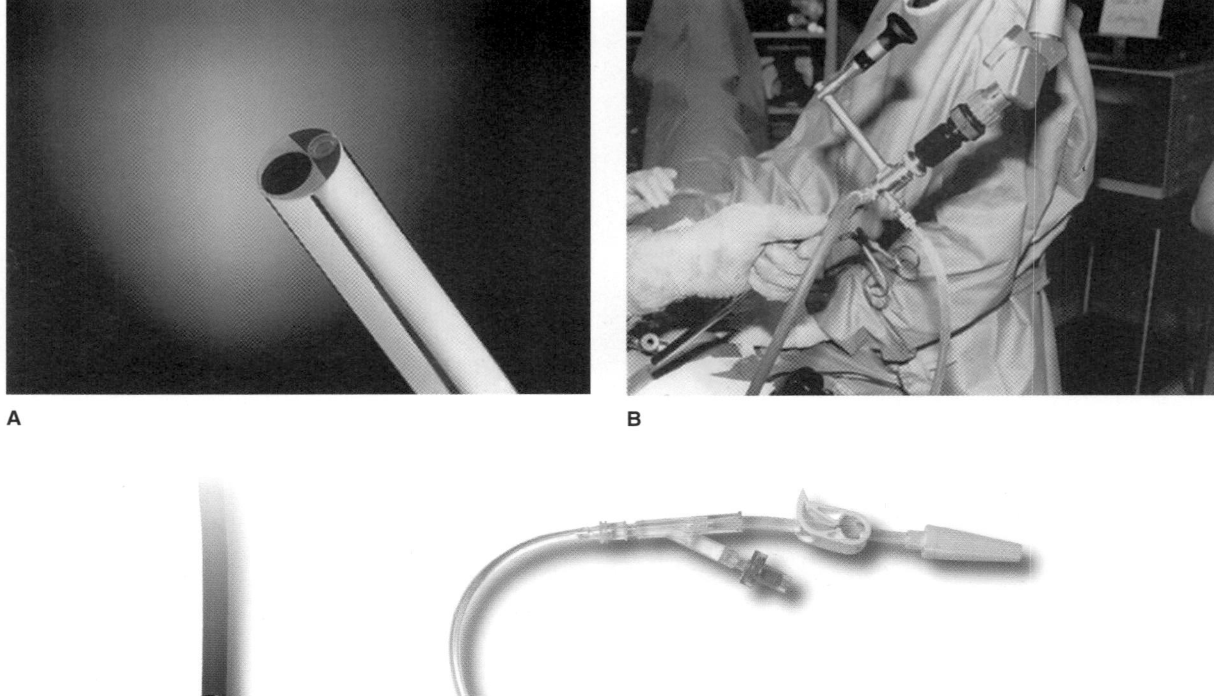

Figure 3-2. **A.** The laser laparoscope has two channels: one for the CO_2 laser and one for the light source. **B.** The CO_2 laser is connected to the operative channel of the laparoscope. **C.** The Spacemaker II balloon dissector provides observation during insertion and dissection.

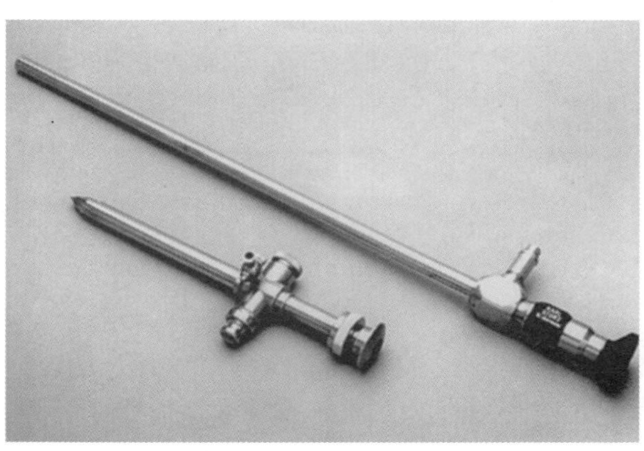

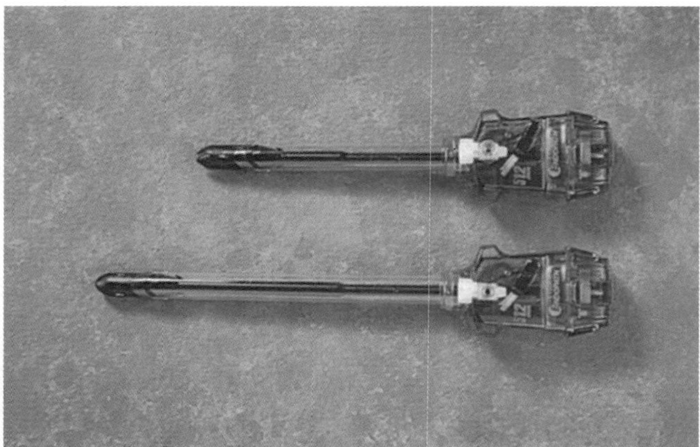

Figure 3-3. **A.** A reusable 11-mm trocar with a 10-mm laparoscope. **B.** Tristar 10-mm and 12-mm disposable trocars (Ethicon).

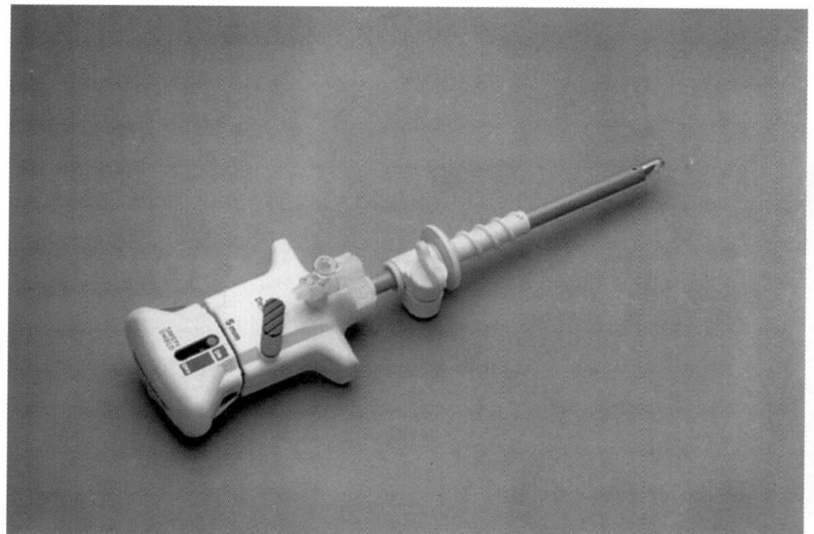

A

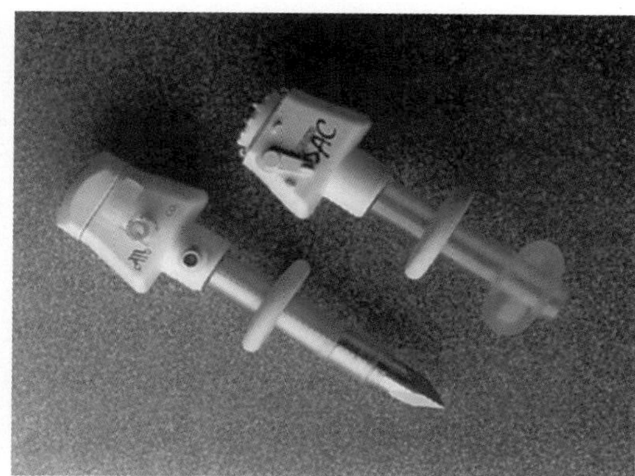

B

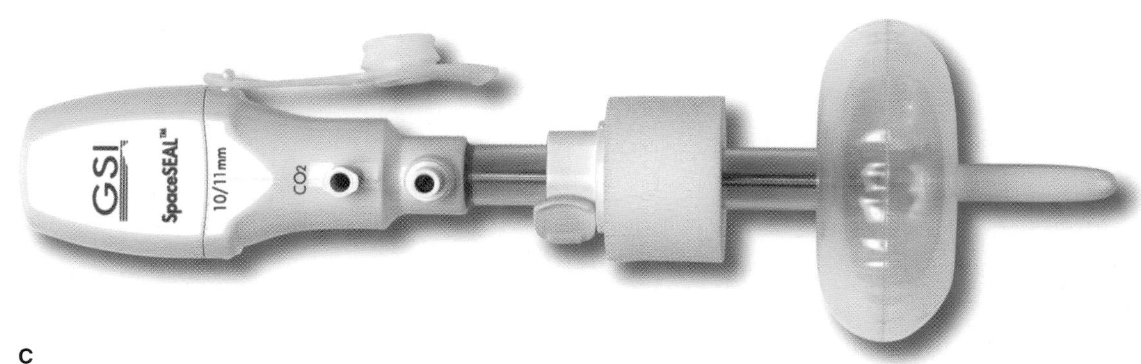

C

Figure 3-4. **A.** A 5-mm trocar with a retention screw (Ethicon). **B.** A trocar with an inflatable balloon (Marlow Surgical Technologies). **C.** A trocar with an inflatable balloon and an adjustable foam locking pad (General Surgical Innovations).

and automatically releases the plastic shield inside the peritoneal cavity to cover the sharp tip and protect intraabdominal organs. Another trocar uses the same principle as the Veress needle. The trocar tip has a hollow core with a spring-loaded blunt stylet (Dexide). After the peritoneal cavity is penetrated, the blunt stylet moves beyond the tip to prevent injury. Bullet tip disposable trocars (Ethicon) lessen the possibility of tissue being caught between the trocar and the sleeve. In the presence of adhesions to the anterior abdominal wall, under the umbilicus, the reusable devices have no proven advantage.

Secondary Trocars

Reusable and disposable accessory trocars and sleeves come in a variety of lengths and range in diameter from 2 to 30 mm; the most common size is 5 mm. Some are threaded and are screwed into the abdominal wall, making them relatively immobile during manipulation. The use of "fascial screws" is associated with an increased incidence of omental and bowel herniation after laparoscopy.[12]

Veress Needle

Disposable and reusable Veress needles consist of a blunt-tipped, spring-loaded inner stylet and a sharp outer needle (Figure 3-7). As the needle passes through the abdominal layers, the stylet retracts to allow penetration into the peritoneal cavity. The absence of tissue resistance allows the blunt stylet to protrude. A lateral hole on this stylet enables CO_2 gas to be delivered intraabdominally. The disposable

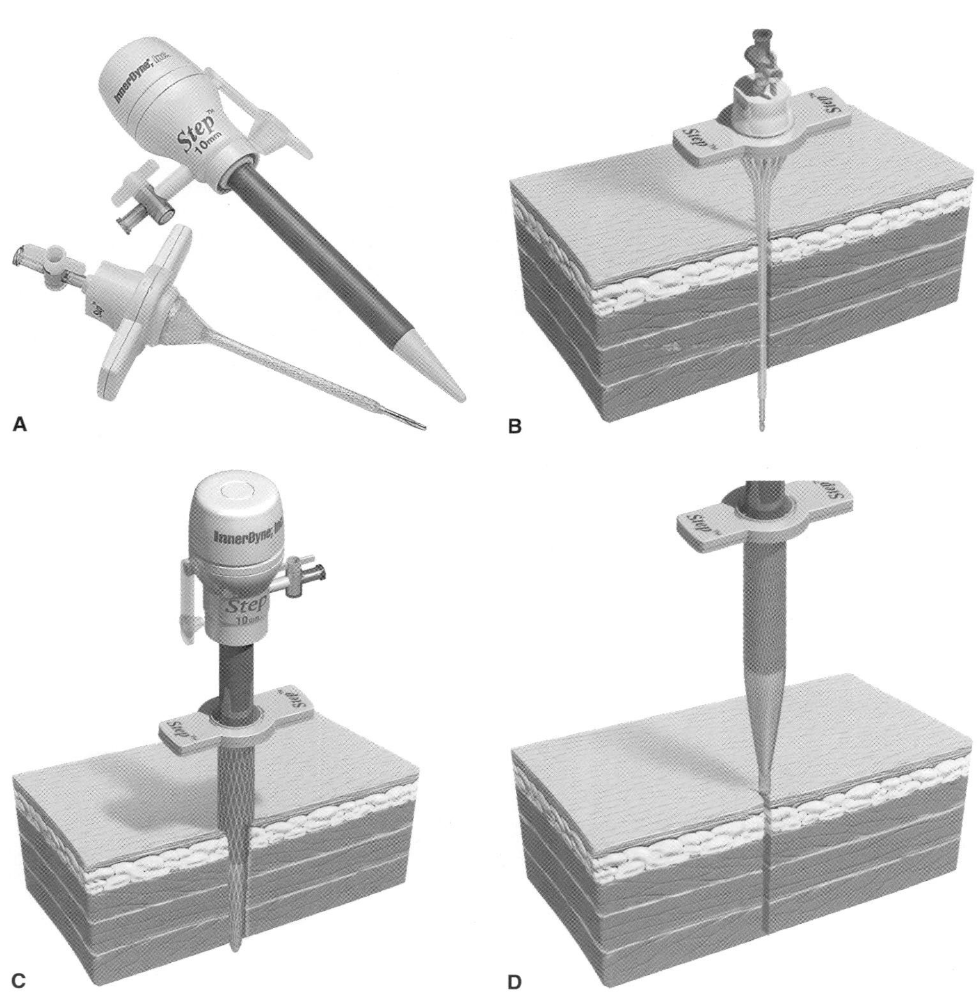

Figure 3-5. **A.** A radially expanding 10-mm cannula/dilator. **B.** After insufflation, intraabdominal entry is made by using an insufflation and access needle with a radially expandable sleeve. The needle is withdrawn, leaving the expandable sleeve in place. **C.** A tapered blunt dilator is inserted, expanding the sleeve and tissue tract. Radial dilation of the tract splits each layer of tissue along a path of least resistance. **D.** After the cannula is removed, a small slitlike defect remains when the layers of muscle in the abdominal wall collapse.

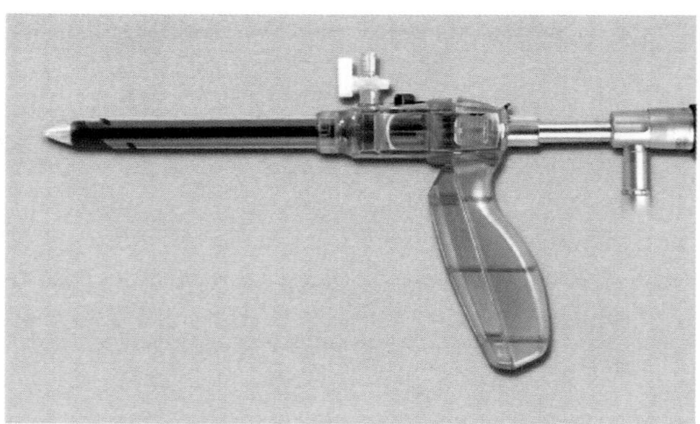

Figure 3-6. An optical trocar.

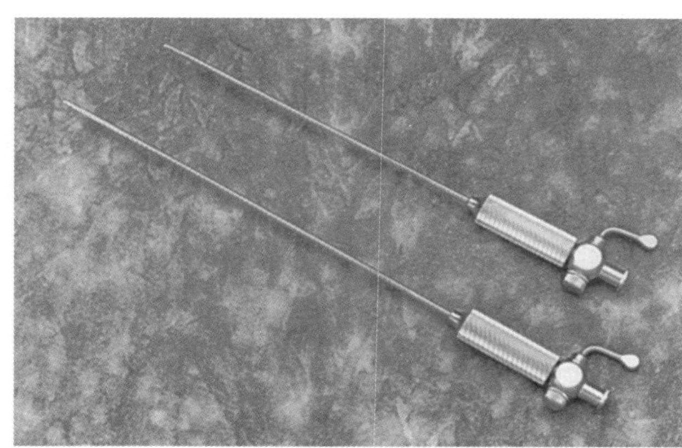

Figure 3-7. Reusable Veress needles.

Veress needle has several added safety points related mainly to the sharp tip of the outer needle and the smooth operation of the spring mechanism.

Insufflator

To adequately observe the contents of the abdominal and pelvic cavity, the abdomen is distended with insufflated CO_2. Some operations require an automatic electric insufflator (Figure 3-8, A and B) that can deliver up to 15 L of gas per minute or two insufflators that each deliver 9 to 10 L of gas per minute. The insufflator compensates for changes in intraabdominal pressure. To avoid complications such as subcutaneous emphysema, intraabdominal pressures should not exceed 16 mm Hg. Although a mechanical abdominal wall lifter can replace a pneumoperitoneum, complications, including femoral nerve injury, have been reported with this device. The Thermoflator (Karl Storz, Culver City, CA) uses the Optitherm heating system to warm CO_2 gas (37°C/99°F) immediately before it enters the patient's abdominal cavity, and this may help maintain body temperature, decrease the risk of hypothermia, and reduce endoscope fogging (Figure 3-8C).

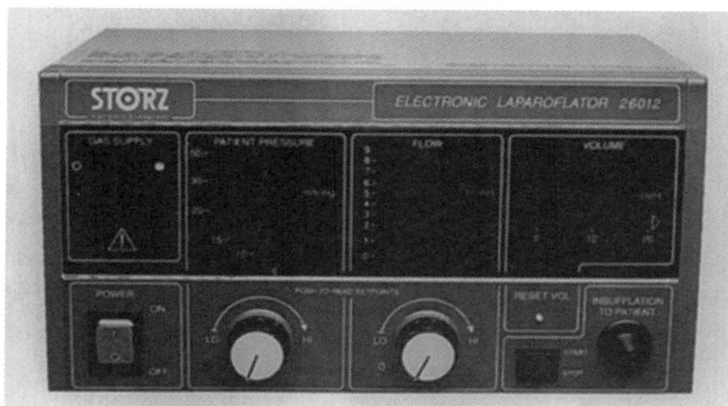

A

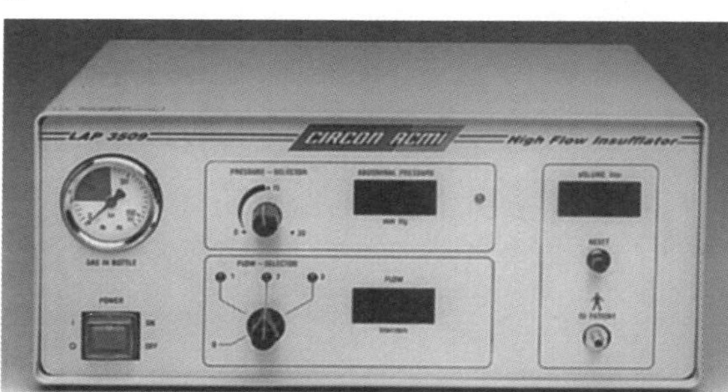

B

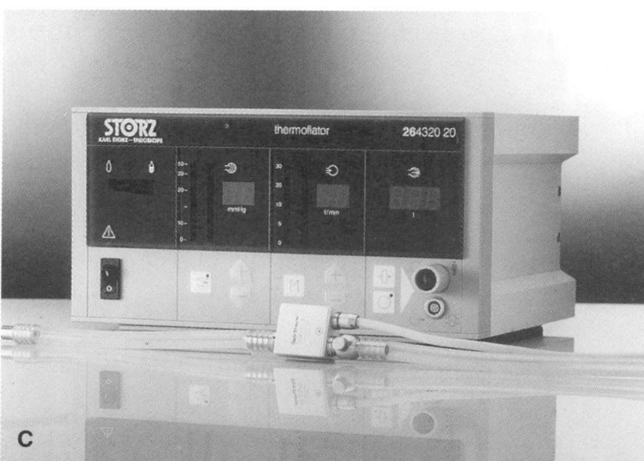

C

Figures 3-8. **A.** and **B.** Automatic insufflators deliver up to 10 L (Karl Storz) and 9 L per minute (Circon). **C.** The Thermoflator (Storz) warms CO_2 gas(37°C/99°F) immediately before it enters the patient's abdominal cavity.

The Light Cord

The light cord is as important as a high-resolution camera and a precision scope. If light does not move properly from the light source to the scope through the cord, the value of the camera is limited and images are poor. Light dispersed evenly across the cord's diameter is preferred. Light cords are either fiberoptic or liquid-filled. Fiberoptic cables are available in varying lengths (6, 8, and 10 feet) with little light loss. Light cords are fragile and should not be wound into small bundles. Liquid-filled light guide cables transmit more light and are more durable than fiberoptic cables. They are more expensive, produce more heat at their connection to the endoscope, and are limited to a standard 6-foot length.

Light Sources

All light sources use xenon, halogen, or mercury bulbs. Each type generates light of a different color and intensity. The most common bulbs are halogen and xenon, with xenon available in 150, 175, and 300 W (Figure 3-9). Xenon bulbs generate a

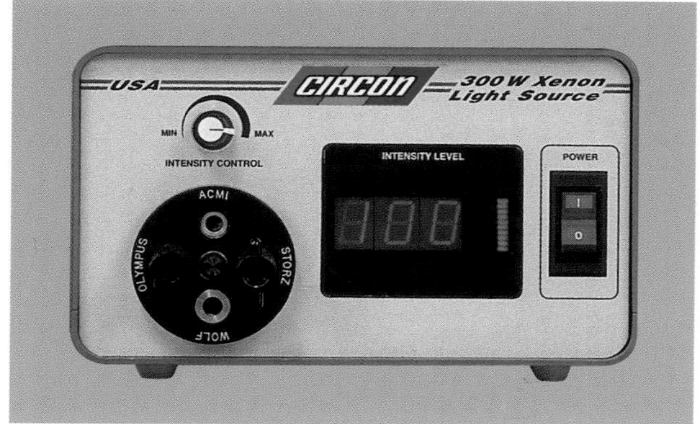

Figure 3-9. Xenon light source by Circon.

higher intensity of light, last longer, and are more expensive to replace. They provide consistent levels of light intensity and can generate even higher levels of light as needed.

Suction-Irrigator Probe and Hydrodissection Pump

A suction-irrigator probe is a versatile instrument (Figure 3-10). Controlled suction and irrigation enhance observation and improve operative technique. This device serves as an extension of the surgeon's fingers, serves as a backstop for the CO_2 laser, and helps with hydrodissection, division of tissue planes and spaces, lavage, blunt dissection, and smoke and fluid evacuation. A properly designed suction-irrigation system has the following characteristics (Figure 3-10):

1. The trumpet valve is designed ergonomically and versatile so that electrosurgical accessories, lasers, and hand instruments can be inserted through the probe (Figure 3-11, A and B).
2. The trumpet valve is easy to use and provides constant control of fluid or suction, including valve regulation, rather than an on/off mechanism.
3. The internal valve diameters are large enough to allow blood and tissue to pass easily through the canister and provide sufficient irrigation flow.
4. Probe tips are smooth, strong, and nonreflective so that they can be used for blunt dissection and serve as a backstop for the CO_2 laser (Figure 3-12).
5. The irrigation pump provides precise and variable irrigation pressures.

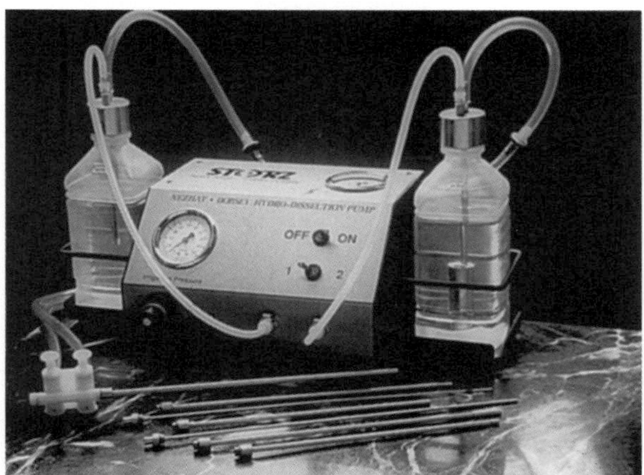

Figure 3-10. Nezhat-Dorsey suction-irrigator pump and probes.

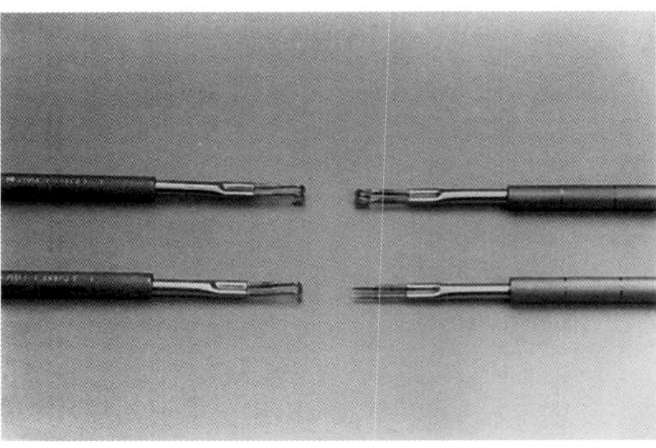

A

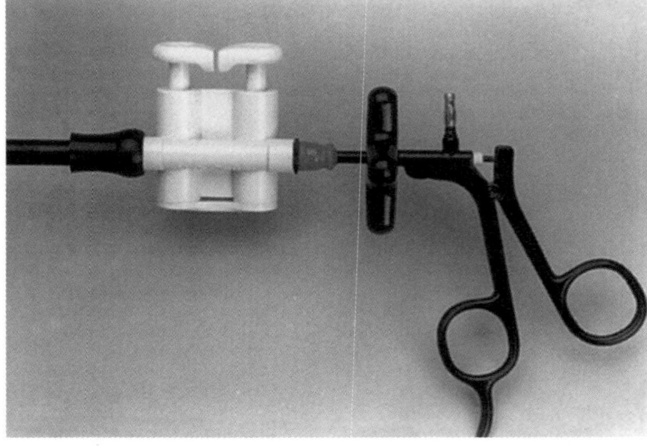

B

Figure 3-11. A. Nezhat-Dorsey hydodissection suction-irrigator probes with different electrosurgical accessories. **B.** A hydrodissection probe can accommodate hand instruments.

A trumpet valve can incorporate a metered adjustment feature, allowing smoke evacuation without manual intermittent depression of the suction piston. To begin smoke evacuation, a control

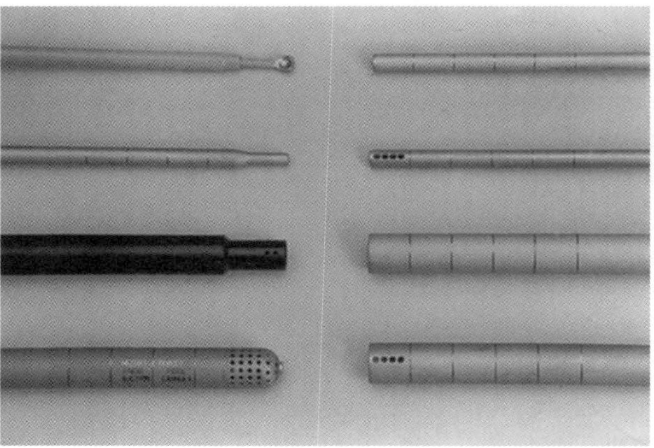

Figure 3-12. Different size probe tips are smooth and nonreflective and can be used for blunt dissection and as laser backstops.

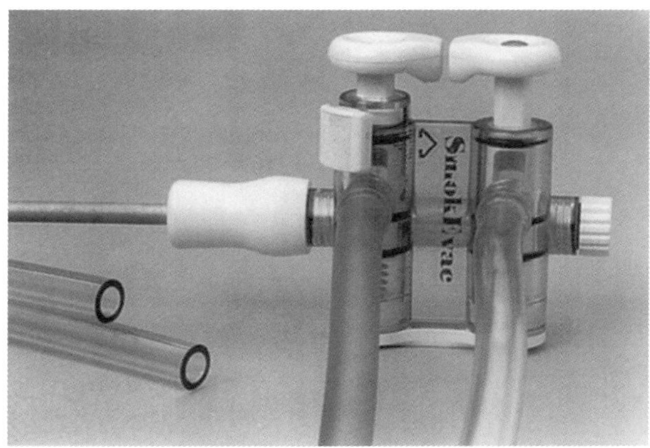

Figure 3-13. A trumpet valve has a control-metered adjustment pad that permits smoke evacuation.

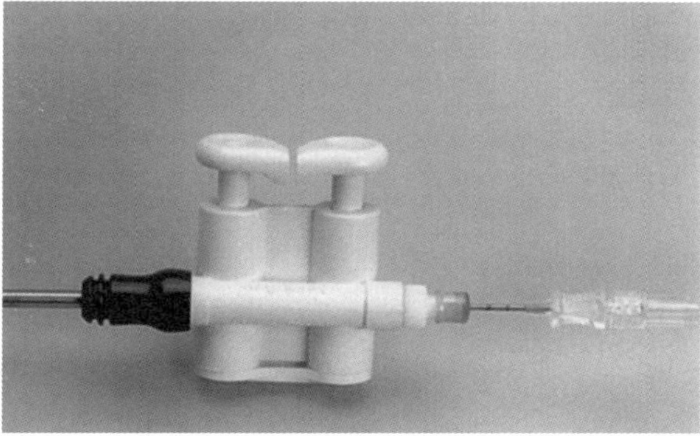

Figure 3-15. The aspiration-injection needle is inserted through the back of the trumpet valve. At the distal end of the needle, there is a Luer-Lock that allows connection to a syringe so that suction and irrigation are not interrupted.

pad is rotated counterclockwise by the surgeon, allowing variable evacuation up to 10 L per minute (Figure 3-13). Additional suction capability can be accessed by depressing the suction piston button. Laser or electrosurgical accessories inserted through the rear access port simultaneously can be combined with smoke evacuation, maintaining a clear field of vision. Several probe tips are available in various lengths and shapes (Figure 3-14). A quick mechanism disconnect probe tip speeds the changing of the tips. An aspiration-injection needle accessory with nonfenestrated 5-mm/28-cm probe tips allows precise closed-chambered aspiration of ovarian cysts or injection of fluid (Figure 3-15). This system has reusable probe tips. Although the pump can deliver fluid with a pressure up to 775 mm Hg, 300 mm Hg is used for routine irrigation (Figure 3-16). Higher pump pressures are used to dissect areas near the bowel, bladder, major blood vessels, and ureters. The irrigation fluid consists of warmed 1-L bottles of lactated Ringer's solution (Travenol Laboratories, Deefield, IL), and wall suction is used as the aspirated material initially enters a Vac-Rite canister. A laser plume filter removes particles that might clog the wall suction. A higher pneumatically powered pump pressure with adjustable pulsations has been developed (American Hydro-Surgical Instruments System II Pump). It incorporates the effectiveness

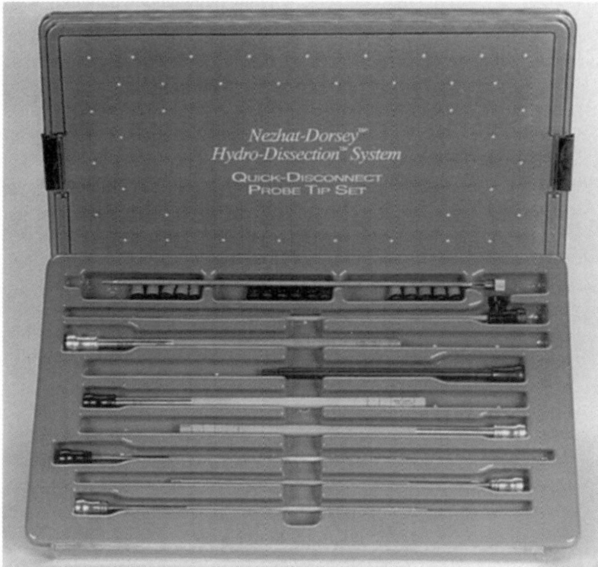

Figure 3-14. Designed specifically for use with the Nezhat-Dorsey hydrodissection system, the "Quick-Disconnect" probe tip set contains one 5-mm probe tip without irrigation holes, one Micro-Probe tip, one 10-mm probe tip with irrigation holes, one suction cannula, one instrument insert probe, 12 instrument insert adapters, and six "Quick-Disconnect" adapters. All probe tip sets are available in 23-cm, 28-cm, and 33-cm lengths.

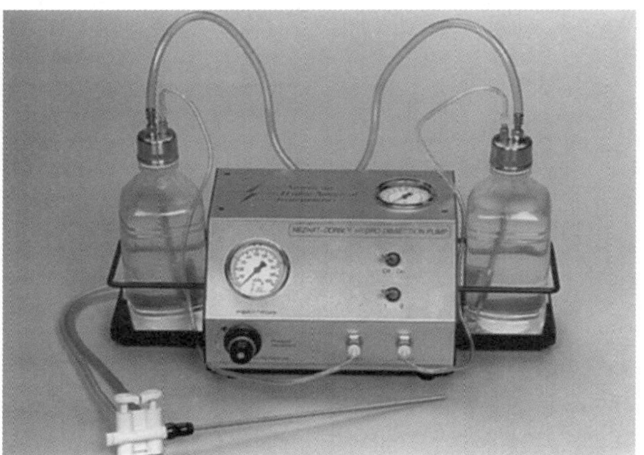

Figure 3-16. The hydrodissection pump holds two bottles of irrigation fluid and delivers up to 775 mm Hg or 300 mm Hg for routine irrigation that is provided by pressurized CO_2 connected to the bottles.

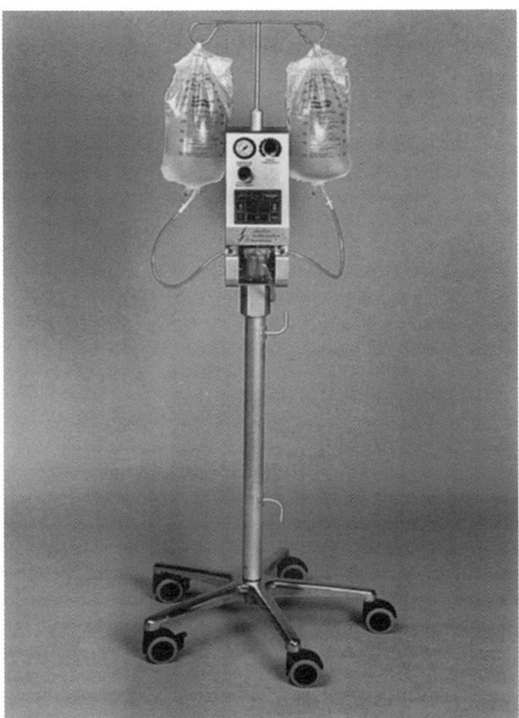

Figure 3-17. The System II Pump (American Hydro-Surgical Instruments) uses bag irrigation as effectively as pressurized pump irrigation.

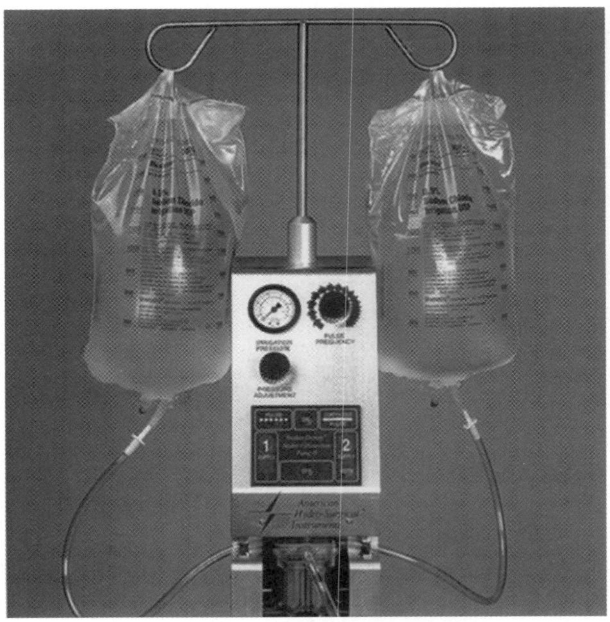

Figure 3-18. The System II Pump (American Hydro-Surgical Instruments) has a "pump cartridge chamber" into which a disposable cartridge is inserted.

and convenience of bag irrigation with the precision and effective delivery of pressurized pump irrigation (Figure 3-17). It does not use electric current, electronics, or any type of computer software but offers irrigation control. It has a "pump cartridge chamber" into which a disposable cartridge is inserted (Figure 3-18). As compressed gas does not contact the irrigation fluid at any time, this design eliminates the potential for procedural contamination during setup and the possibility of inadvertently entering the abdominal cavity.

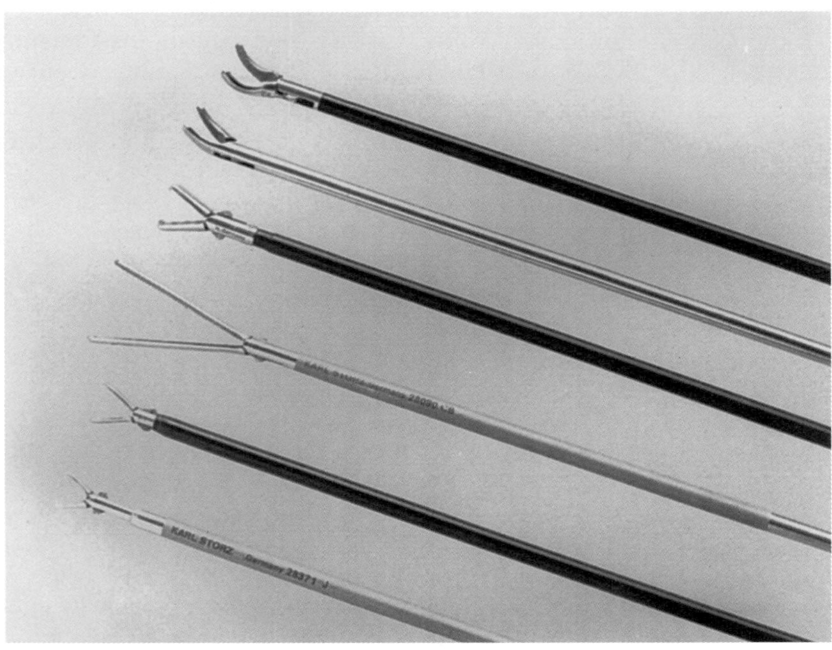

Figure 3-19. Straight and curved laparoscopic grasping forceps.

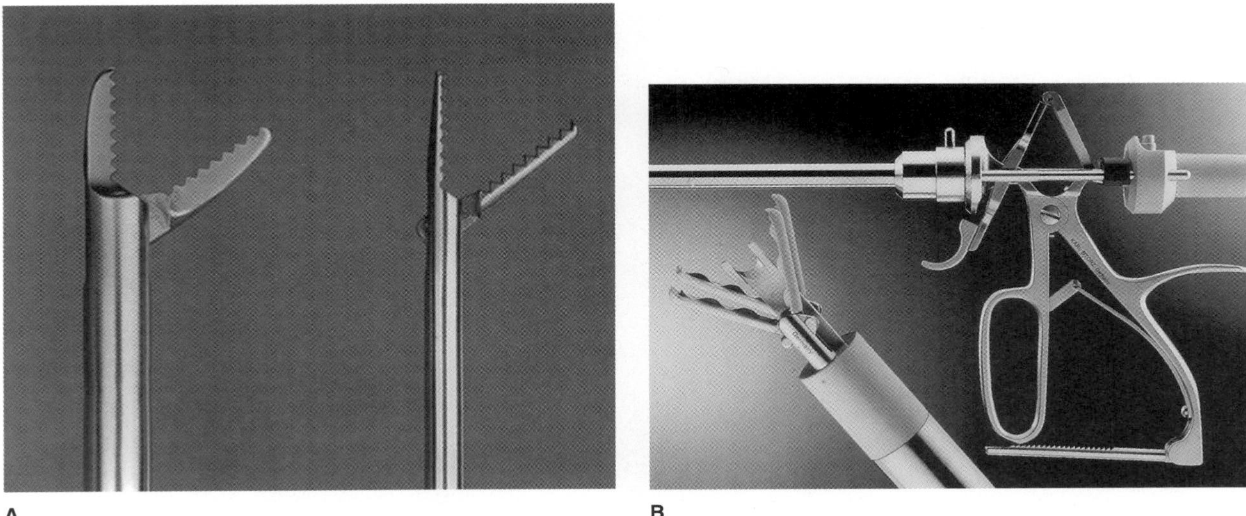

Figure 3-20. **A.** Serrated jaws of 5-mm (left) and 3-mm (right) needle holders. **B.** The Remorgida 3-in-1 bipolar forceps (Storz).

Irrigation bags replace bottled solutions. As the bag is depleted, it collapses on itself, stopping the pump and alerting the staff to switch to the second fluid supply. The fluid is delivered in a continuous flow or in a pulsed irrigation mode. The rates of pulsation and irrigation pressure are adjustable. The latter setting ranges from 0 to 2500 mm Hg. Pulsatile irrigation cleanses the surgical site more effectively than does normal continuous flow, enabling a more thorough removal of blood clots and char. The use of irrigation fluid warmed to 39°C has been advocated to decrease this drop in core temperature commonly observed in laparoscopy.[13]

Forceps

Atraumatic and grasping forceps with jaws are available in sizes from 3 to 10 mm (Figure 3-19). Atraumatic stabilization of structures is important in many procedures, and several types of forceps are available for this purpose. The preferred type is medium-sized with a rounded tip and serrated jaws. It can grasp tissue for exposure, act as a blunt probe with the jaws closed, affect traction with the jaws open for more tissue surface area, serve as a needle holder, and tie sutures (Figure 3-20A).

Forceps can grasp tissue and remove tissue from the peritoneal cavity. Those made of titanium with a polished finish can serve as a backstop for the CO_2 laser, while others have monopolar electrocoagulating ability. The Remorgida 3-in-1 bipolar forceps (Karl Storz, Culver City, CA) features two jaws of atraumatic grasping teeth and a scalpel-like blade between the forceps, enabling surgeons to grasp, cut, and coagulate tissue with one instrument (Figure 3-20B). Creating a neosalpingostomy in a hydrosalpinx requires two grasping forceps for traction and countertraction. Fine forceps are used for delicate work such as ovariolysis, fimbrioplasty, and tubal exploration during salpingostomy for ectopic pregnancy (Figure 3-21).

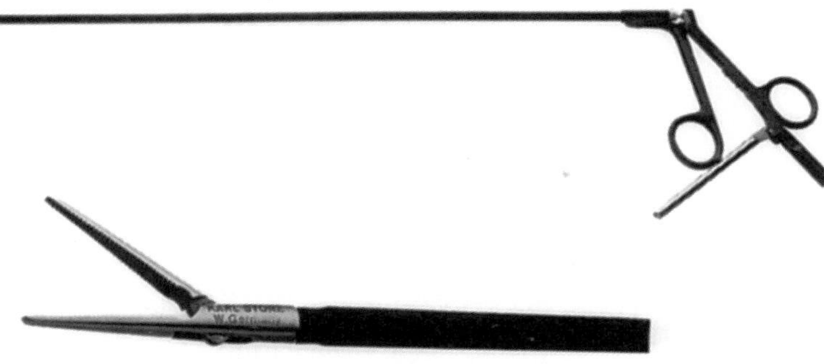

Figure 3-21. Fine forceps can be used for delicate procedures such as ovariolysis, fimbrioplasty, and tubal exploration for ectopic pregnancy.

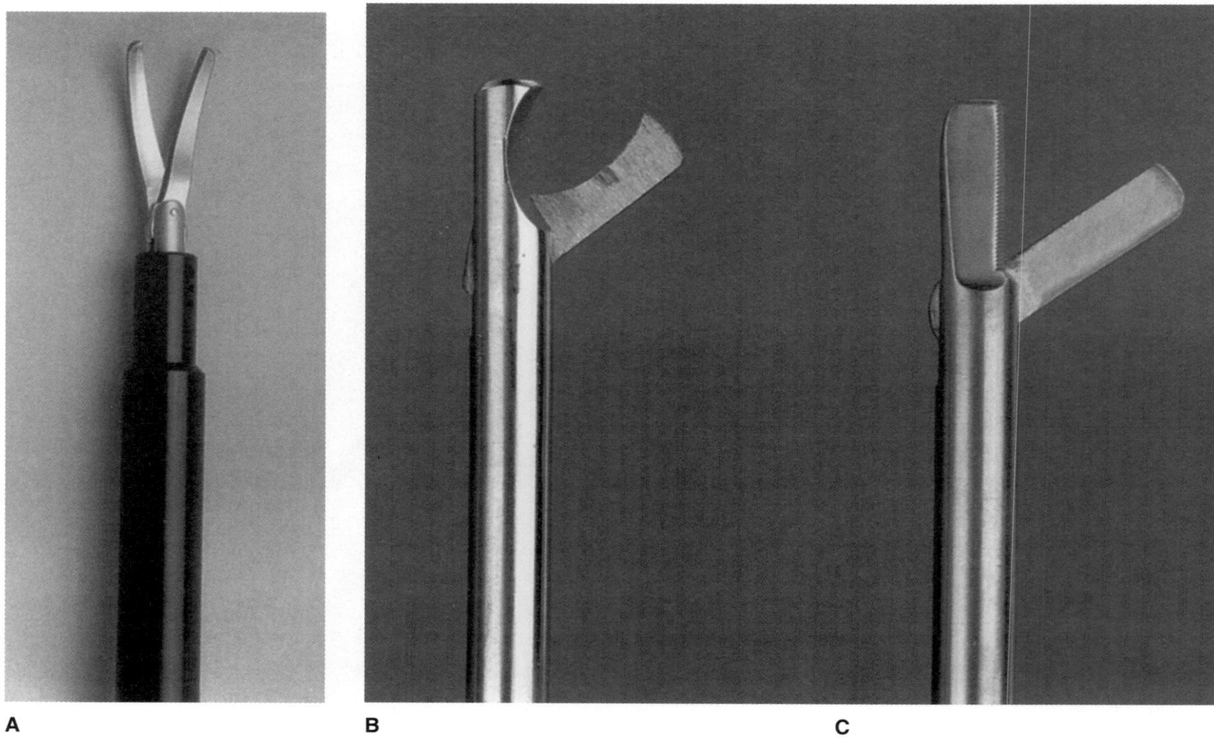

Figure 3-22. Laparoscopic scissors. **A.** Curved. **B.** Hooked. **C.** Straight.

Scissors

This instrument is curved, straight, or hooked (Figure 3-22, A, B, and C). Some have an electrical adapter so that they can be combined with unipolar or bipolar electrocoagulation (Figure 3-23). Scissors are inserted into the secondary trocar under direct observation to avoid injury to pelvic structures. Hooked scissors have overlapping tips and can cause damage even when closed. Scissors can lyse adhesions, divide coagulated tissue, cut sutures, and open a fallopian tube for salpingostomy. If they become dull, they are discarded because sharpening is ineffective. Disposable scissors are particularly useful for patients who have extensive adhesions.

Biopsy Forceps

These instruments can sample suspected endometrial implants, ovarian lesions, and peritoneum (Figure 3-24). The jaws should be sharp and overlap when closed to avoid tearing tissue and causing unnecessary bleeding. Some have a small tooth on the upper or lower jaw and are ideal for taking a tissue sample from hard or slippery surfaces (Figure 3-25). Bleeding from the biopsy site is controlled by a defocused laser or bipolar electrocoagulation.

Electrosurgical Generator and Bipolar Forceps

The primary instrument used for hemostasis during operative laparoscopy is the bipolar electrocoagulator (Figure 3-26). One should prepare and test this instrument before the operation begins because it is essential for hemostasis during oophorectomy, hysterectomy, or even bowel resection to desiccate the mesenteric artery. Several types of bipolar forceps are available (Figures 3-26 and 3-27, A and B). Fine

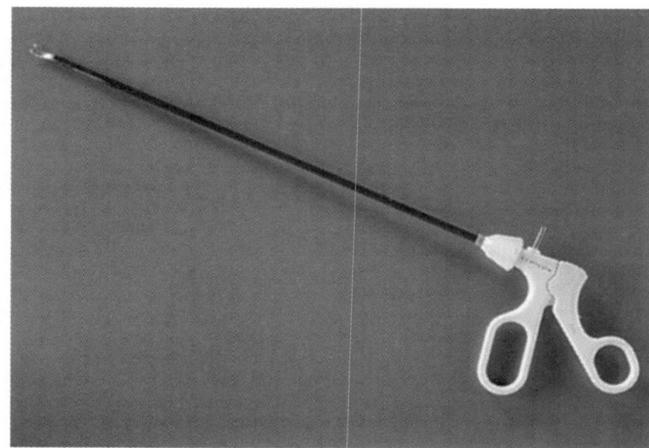

Figure 3-23. Laparoscopic scissors have unipolar electrocoagulation capability.

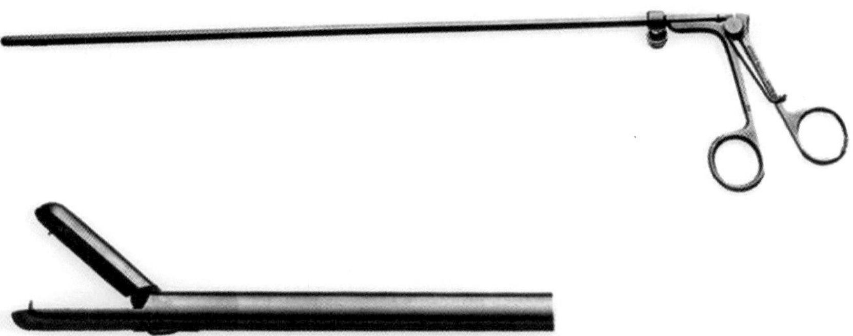

Figure 3-24. A 5-mm biopsy forceps is used to obtain tissue from endometrial ovarian implants.

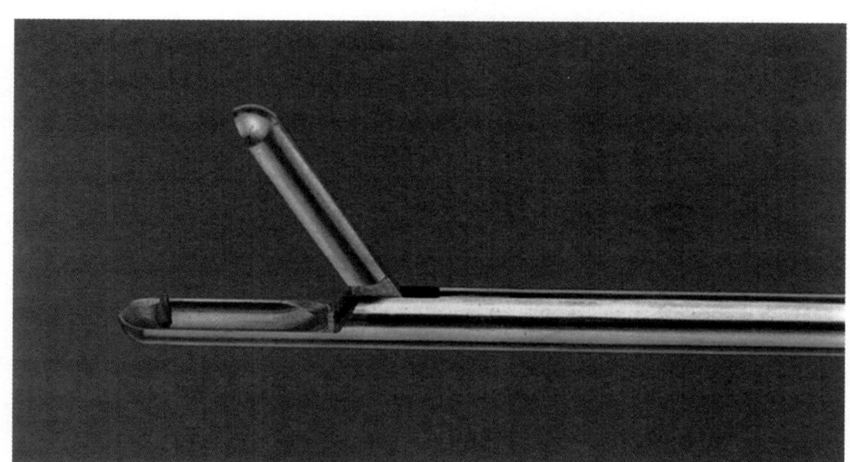

Figure 3-25. A biopsy forceps has small teeth on the upper and lower jaws to biopsy hard and slippery tissue surfaces.

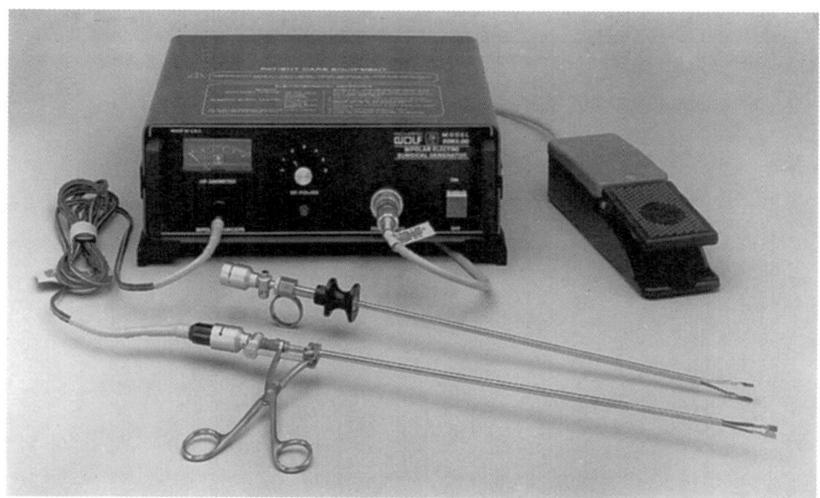

Figure 3-26. An electrogenerator with different types of bipolar forceps.

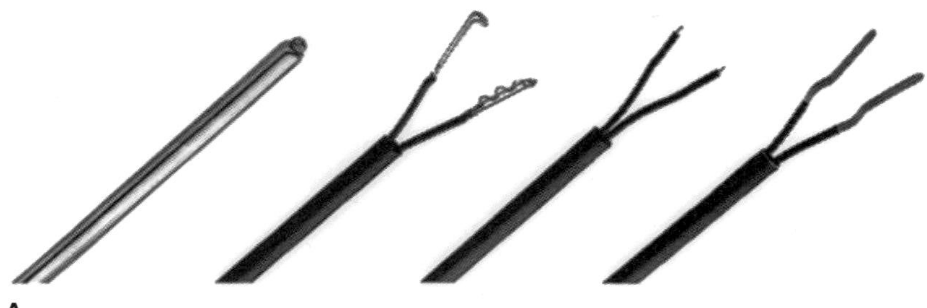
A

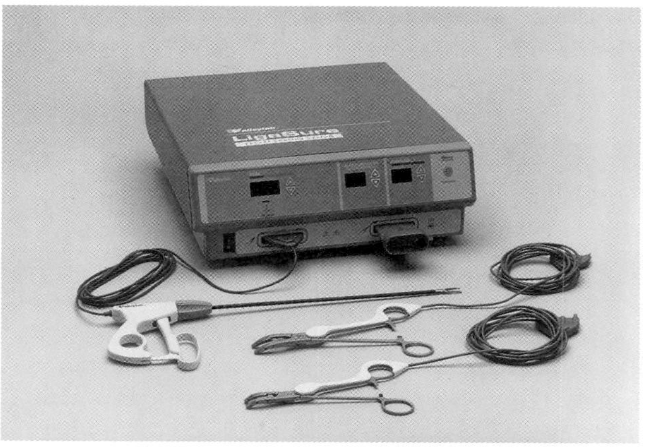

B

Figure 3-27. **A.** Bipolar forceps with different tips are seen with a coagulating probe (left). **B.** A LigaSure generator is shown with instruments for laparoscopic and open operations (Valley Lab).

tips are used for coagulating small blood vessels during delicate operations involving the tubes, bowel, or ureter. Flatter jaws are appropriate for use on large blood vessels or pedicles, including the uterine artery and the infundibulopelvic ligaments. A 3-mm bipolar forceps is available and is useful for tubal coagulation under local anesthesia. The LigaSure vessel-sealing technology (Valley Lab, Boulder, CO) available for laparoscopic and open procedures uses bipolar electrosurgery with a feedback-controlled output to achieve a seal on vessels up to 7 mm in diameter (Figure 3-27B).

Specialized Instruments

Claw-Tooth and Spoon Forceps

These 10-mm graspers require a 10- to 11-mm sleeve and are used during myomectomy to remove large pieces of tissue such as a section of tube and ovary or an ectopic pregnancy (Figure 3-28).

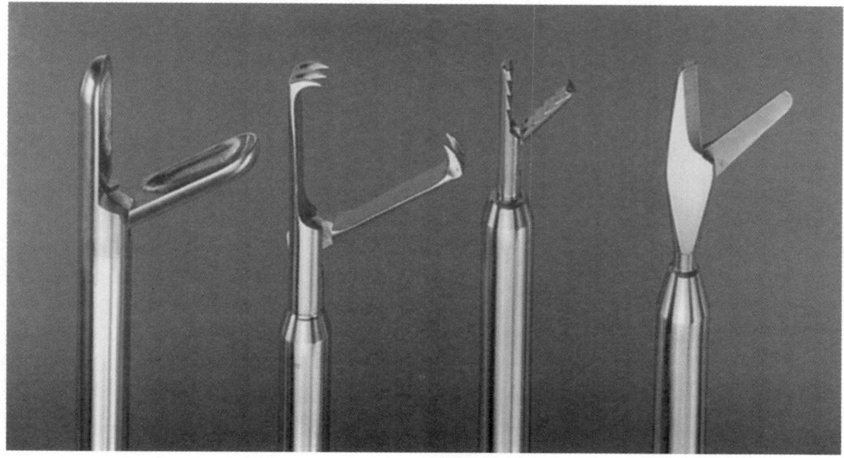

Figure 3-28. Different 10-mm instruments are used during operative laparoscopy. From left to right: spoon forceps, claw graspers, serrated grasper, and scissors.

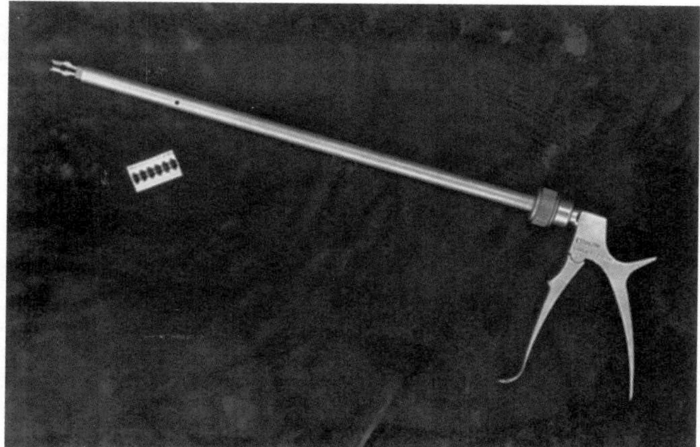

Figure 3-29. A reusable 10-mm laparoscopic clip applicator with clips.

Clips

Laparoscopic clip applicators are used through 5- to 11-mm sleeves for reapproximation of peritoneal surfaces or hemostasis of medium-sized vessels. A disposable loaded applicator and reusable single clip applicators are available (Figures 3-29 and 3-30).

Linear Stapler

The stapler designed for gynecologic use is similar to the one used for bowel operations and fits through a 12-mm trocar sleeve[14] (Figure 3-31). Ethicon and U.S. Surgical produce endoscopic surgical staplers with different designs, but their function is essentially the same. The available staplers are disposable and can be reloaded with cartridges for use in gynecologic, general, and thoracic surgery (Figure 3-32). Each cartridge contains 54 (Ethicon) or 48 (U.S. Surgical) titanium staples that are arranged in two sets of triple-staggered rows. The instrument also contains a push bar knife assembly, which cuts between the two sets of triple rows, ligating both ends of the incised tissue. The cut line usually is shorter than the staple line. For example, the laparoscopic linear cutter 35 (Ethicon) cut line is approximately 33 mm with a staple line of 37 mm.

Tissue to be clipped is placed on stretch with grasping forceps, and the Endoclip applicator's jaws are placed at the desired incisional site. When fired, it simultaneously places six rows of small titanium clips and cuts along the center, leaving three rows of clips on the edge of each pedicle (Figure 3-33). This instrument is used to seal blood vessels and cut pedicles but should be used with caution. Several complications have resulted from the use of this device.[15]

Myoma Screw

When one is doing a laparoscopic myomectomy, it is difficult to stabilize a smooth, hard fibroid. Five- and 10-mm myoma screws allow the surgeon to

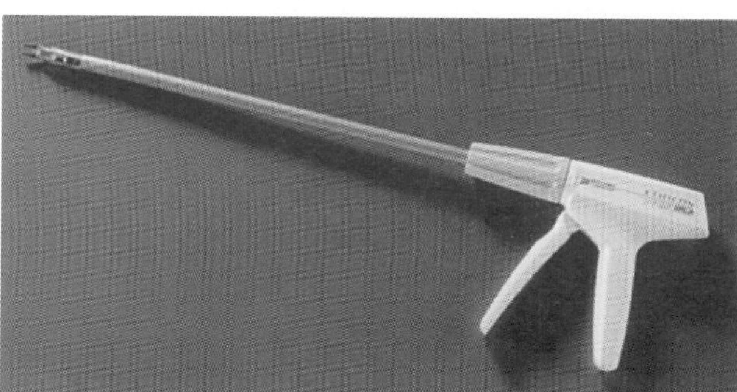

Figure 3-30. A disposable loaded 10-mm laparoscopic clip applicator.

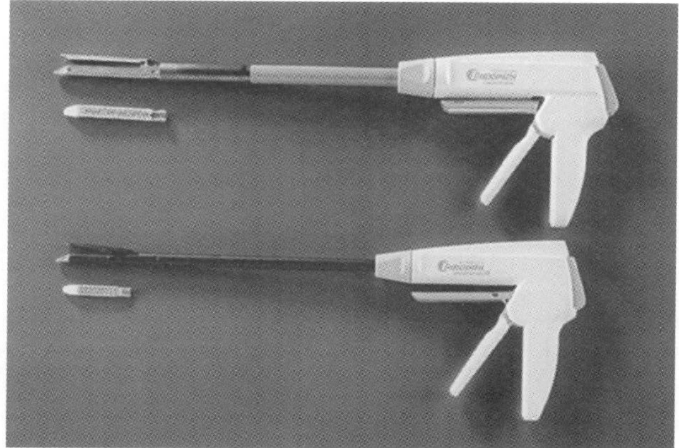

Figure 3-31. Endo-path linear cutters (Ethicon) are used in intestinal operations and gynecologic laparoscopy.

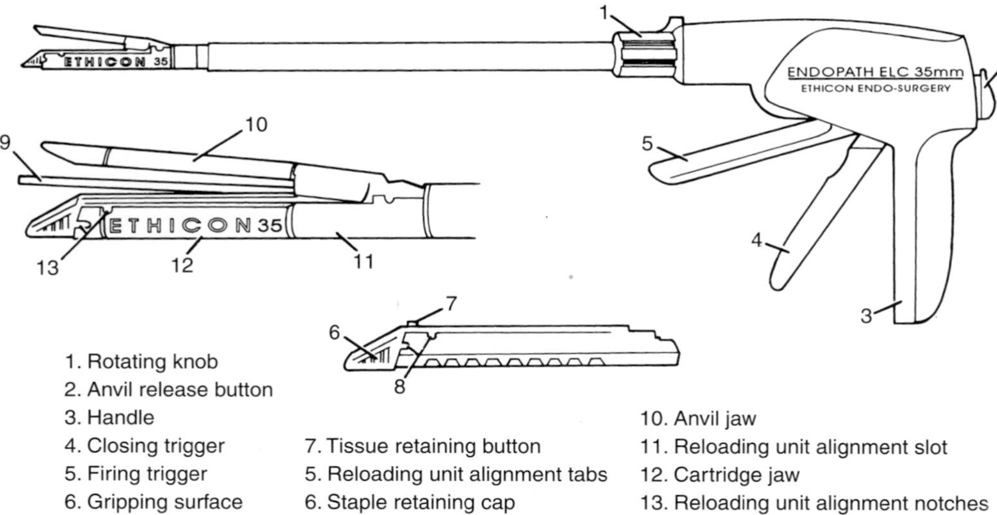

Figure 3-32. Schematic representation of the Endo-path linear cutter 35 (ELC 35, Ethicon).

maneuver the myoma and apply traction with improved visibility and access (Figure 3-34).

Morcellator

Morcellators grasp, core, and cut the tissue to be removed into small bits. These fragments are forced into the hollow part of the instrument. It is designed for the removal of fragments of myomas and ovaries through 5- or 10-mm trocar sleeves or through a colpotomy incision. If the removal of a large myoma is attempted, the effort to morcellate it mechanically may outweigh the amount of time saved, particularly if the myoma is calcified.

Electromechanical morcellators such as the Steiner Electromechanical Morcellator (Karl Storz, Tuttlingen, Germany) consist of a motor-driven cutting cannula that can be inserted directly into the peritoneal cavity or introduced through a standard trocar (Figure 3-35). Tissue is morcellated and removed by applying uniform traction and varying the speed and direction of the cannula's rotation. This technique facilitates the rapid removal of even large sections of tissue through the minimal access ports.

Carter and McCarus[16] compared electromechanical to manual morcellation in doing laparoscopic myomectomies. The use of the electromechanical morcellator reduced the average time for extraction of myomas less than 100 g by 15 minutes and 401 to 500 g by 150 minutes on average. The average time saved for all myomectomies was 53 minutes. It was estimated that with operating room charges of $10 per minute, the $14,000 cost of the morcellator was recovered by the twenty-first case. The authors concluded that electromechanical morcellation results in significant time savings compared with the manual technique, with financial savings accruing rapidly after the twenty-first case.

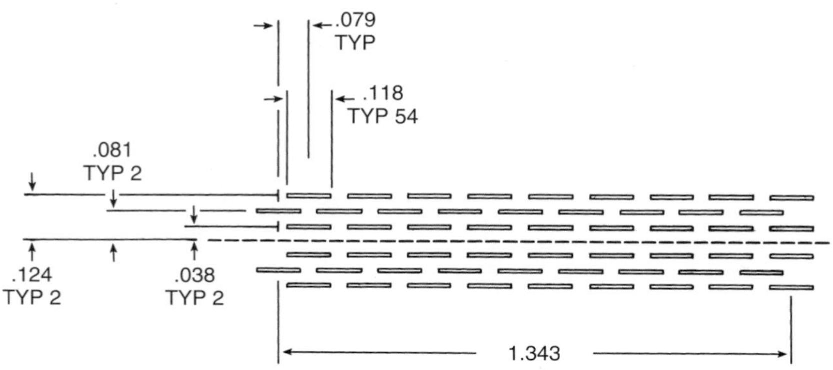

Figure 3-33. The stapler can place six rows of small titanium staples (54 staples).

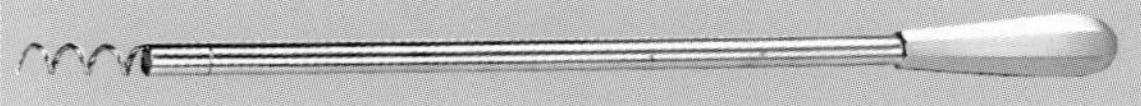

Figure 3-34. A myoma screw (Circon).

The Serrated Edged Macro Morcellator (S.E.M.M.) has been used during laparoscopic myomectomy.[17] It allows rapid morcellation of even large myomas, up to 418 g, and their removal by means of a 15-mm trocar. This morcellator has been used extensively in Germany to do endoscopic intrafascial supracervical hysterectomy.[18] It is available with a battery-operated motor (WISAP Moto-Drive) in diameters of 10, 15, 20, and 24 mm.

A powered disposable morcellator (Gynecare, Sunnyvale, CA) has been used successfully during laparoscopic supracervical hysterectomy to morcellate the entire uterus for easy removal through a 15-mm cannula (Figure 3-36).[19]

The use of the automatic tissue morcellator does not interfere with proper histologic evaluation of solid pediatric malignant tumors in which accurate histologic assessment is important for prognosis and staging.[20]

Specialized Graspers

Three-pronged forceps specifically designed to atraumatically immobilize adnexal structures[21] hold the ovary, while four-pronged forceps are designed to hold fallopian tubes. The force applied by the prongs is adjustable and is maintained by tightening a screw in the handle. Three-pronged graspers with teeth also are available. Large spoon forceps are used to extract tissue excised during the procedure.

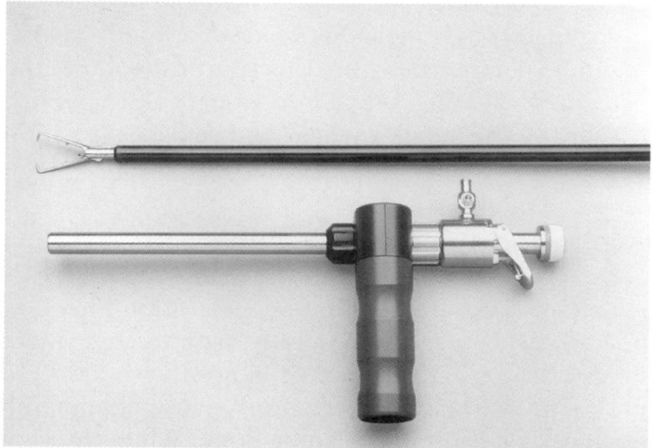

Figure 3-35. Steiner Electromechanical Morcellator (Storz).

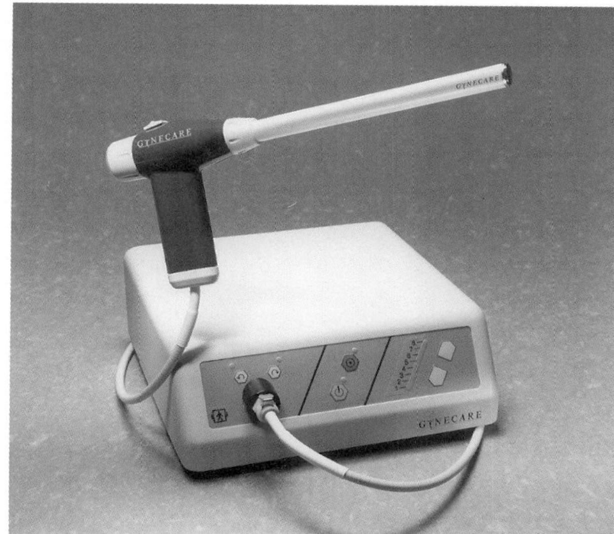

Figure 3-36. The Diva powered disposable morcellator (Gynecare).

Laparoscopic Specimen Retrieval Bag

To simplify the retrieval of specimens from the abdominal cavity and avoid contamination of the abdominal and pelvic cavity with cyst contents, a disposable retrieval bag (Endopouch, Ethicon) has been developed (Figure 3-37). It is composed of a flexible plastic bag with a cannula, introduction sleeve, and introduction cap (Figures 3-38 through 3-44). The bag is pushed by hand into the introducer before being loaded into a 10-/11-mm trocar (Figures 3-38 and 3-39A). During loading, the cannula should not be pulled to retract the Endopouch bag. The introducer cap and introducer sleeve are inserted into the abdomen through the trocar (Figure 3-39B). The introducer cap should remain flush against the top of the trocar. The cannula is pushed until the bag is exposed fully. A closed grasper is used to expand the bag opening

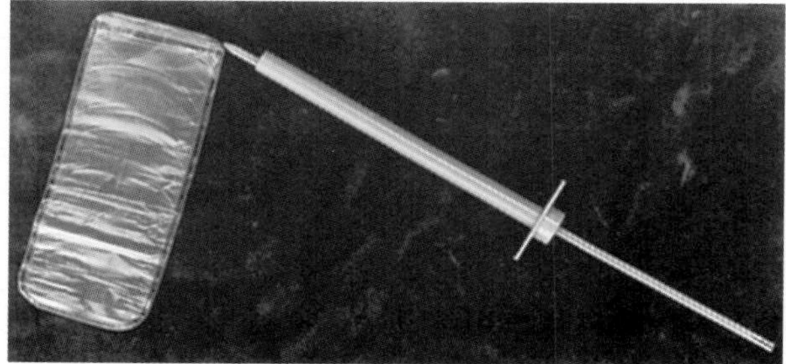

Figure 3-37. Specimen retrieval bag (Endopouch, Ethicon).

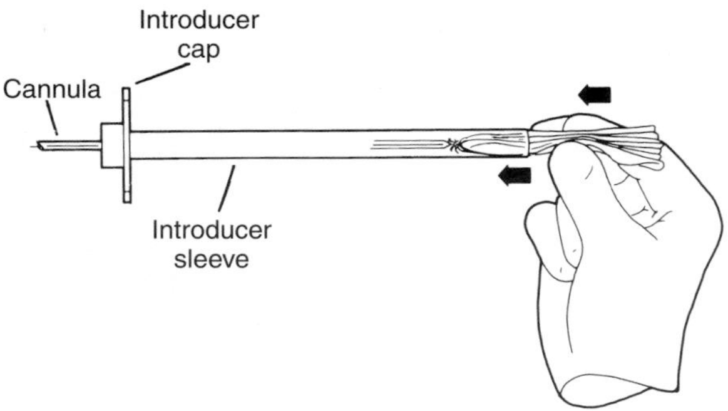

Figure 3-38. The bag is put into the introducer.

(Figure 3-40). A specimen is placed in the bag (Figure 3-41A), and the cannula is broken at the scored point (Figure 3-41B), allowing the suture to be pulled through the cannula and closing the top of the bag (Figure 3-42). The bag is retracted to the base of the trocar sleeve by carefully pulling the suture strand. Small masses are retracted into the introducer and extracted through the trocar sleeve. If the bag and contents cannot be extracted, the bag is pulled into the trocar until resistance is felt (Figure 3-43). The trocar is removed, and the bag

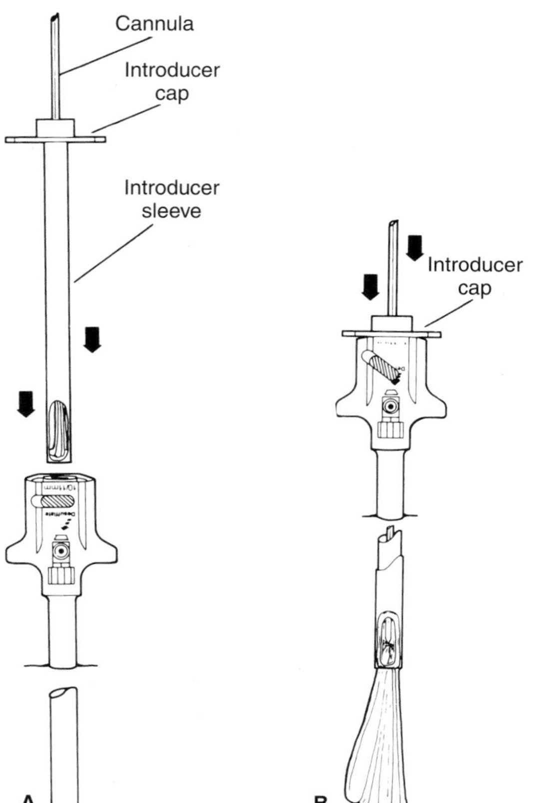

Figure 3-39. A. The introducer is placed into the trocar. **B.** The bag can be pushed into the abdominal cavity.

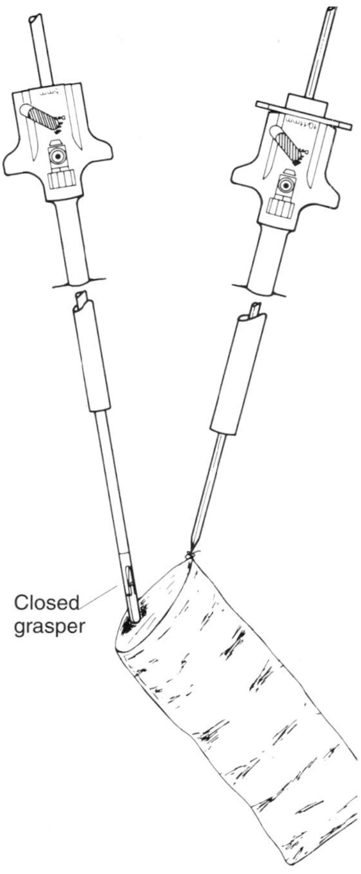

Figure 3-40. A closed grasper is used to open the bag.

is brought to the incision. The contents are aspirated or removed with forceps (Figure 3-44). A larger incision may be required to remove the bag with its contents from the body.

Instruments for Trocar Port Dilation

Occasionally a 10- or 12-mm instrument must be inserted through incisions made for 5-mm instruments. Dilator rods for this purpose allow the placement of a 10- or 12-mm trocar. The operator withdraws the smaller trocar and replaces it with a larger one.

Aspiration-Injection Needle

A 16- or 22-gauge calibrated aspiration-injection needle can be used to precisely aspirate and inject fluids (Figure 3-45). When it is used with a 28-cm probe tip without fenestrations, close-chambered ovarian cyst aspiration can be done. When the suction is started and the probe tip is placed on tissue, suction-retraction of that tissue results. The needle

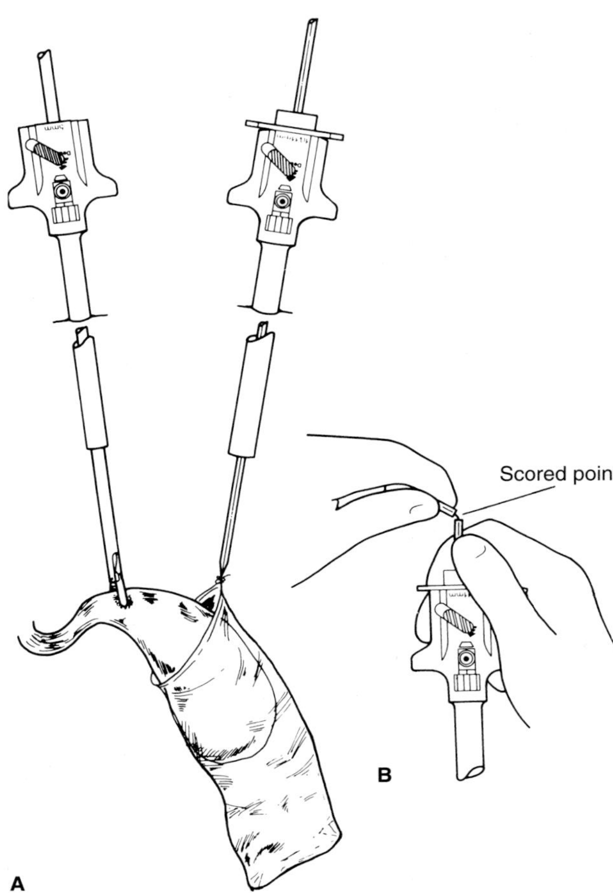

Figure 3-41. **A.** The specimen is placed in the bag. **B.** The cannula is broken at the scored point.

Figure 3-42. The bag is closed around the specimen.

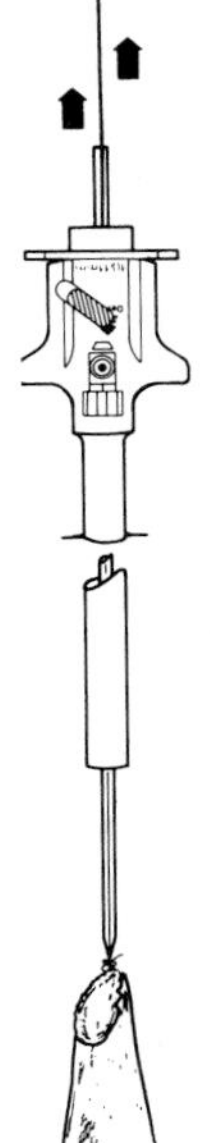

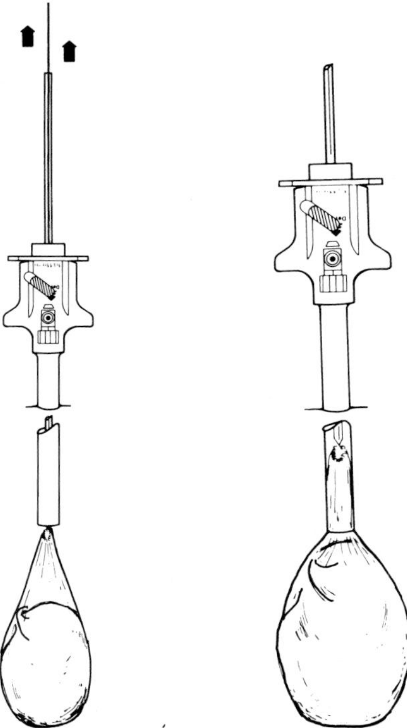

Figure 3-43. The bag is pulled to the base of the trocar sleeve until resistance is felt.

is inserted into the cyst, and leakage of contents is avoided. The 2-cm exposed portion of the needle is etched with 0.5-cm markings to accurately gauge tissue penetration. When a 60-mL syringe is attached to the needle, the fluid from the aspirated cyst is sent for cytologic examination.

This needle also is used to inject dilute vasopressin into the base of fibroids before myomectomy or into the mesosalpinx or tube before salpingostomy for tubal pregnancy. A syringe is attached to the needle by a connecting tube before injection to verify that intravascular injection does not occur.

Figure 3-44. The specimen is pulled to the abdominal wall and aspirated.

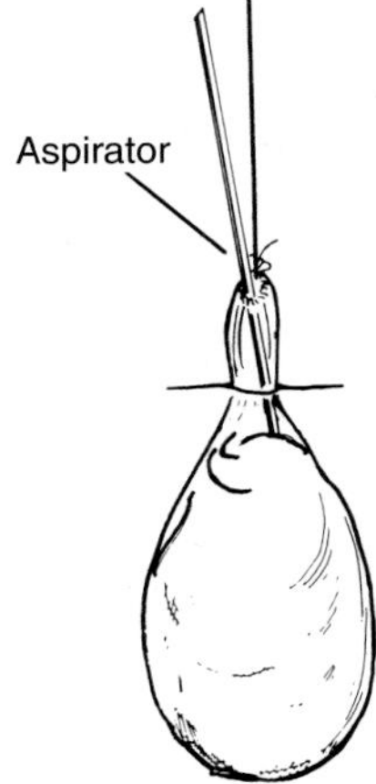

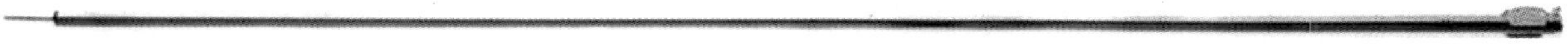

Figure 3-45. A laparoscopic aspiration-injection needle is used for aspiration of ovarian cysts (16- or 18-gauge), injection of diluted vasopressin in the base of a myoma, or hydrodissection (22 gauge).

Uterine Manipulators

Safe, effective endoscopy requires adequate mobilization and stabilization of the uterus and associated organs. Various combinations of uterine sounds, cannulas, and dilators are available. The most useful types of manipulators are the HUMI (Unimar, Wilton, CT) and the Cohen cannula in combination with a single-toothed tenaculum applied to the anterior cervical lip (Figure 3-46). The HUMI has a balloon at its tip to minimize the chance of uterine perforation, but when uterine manipulation is vigorous, the HUMI can twist within the uterine cavity, making it difficult to stabilize the uterus. The Cohen cannula is inserted as far as the internal os and is rigid, allowing excellent control of the uterine position. Although a large acorn tip limits its uterine entry, the cervix may dilate, resulting in uterine perforation by the acorn tip. It is crucial to monitor the position of uterine manipulators continually.

Valtchev and Papsin[22] (Conkin Surgical Instruments, Ltd., Toronto, Canada) devised an instrument consisting of an acorn-shaped head with a cannula connected to a rod by an articulation point. This arrangement allows the angle between the rod and the cannula to be changed, providing various degrees of uterine anteversion, which is adjusted with a screw. The Hulka tenaculum and sound combination is a good uterine manipulator but lacks a channel for chromopertubation.

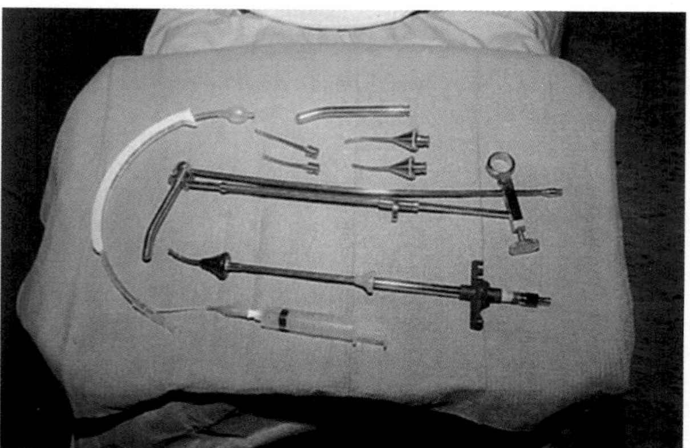

Figure 3-46. Three different uterine manipulators: HUMI, Cohen cannula, and Valtchev cannula.

More elaborate systems specifically designed to simplify total laparoscopic hysterectomy are available. For instance, the Koh Colpotopmizer system (Cooper Surgical) is devised to be used with the RUMI uterine manipulator and consists of a vaginal extender to delineate the vaginal fornices and a pneumo-occluder (Figure 3-47).[23]

Another uterine manipulator that includes a vaginal cup to define the dissecting plane of colpotomy, as well as to prevent the loss of pneumoperitoneum, is the Vcare uterine manipulator (Conmed, Utica, NY) (Figure 3-49).

Ceana Glove

Laparoscopic procedures that involve incision of the vaginal apex result in the loss of the pneumoperitoneum. A simple cost-effective technique has been developed by Ceana Nezhat that effectively preserves pneumoperitoneum. Two 4-inch by 4-inch sponges are folded (Figure 3-48) and submerged in sterile water or saline for several seconds. The sponges are placed in a latex surgical

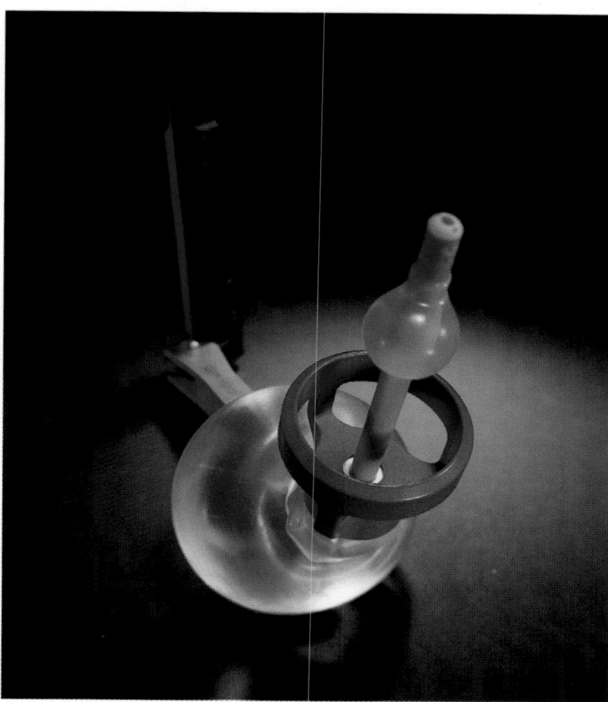

Figure 3-47. The Koh Colpotopmizer system.

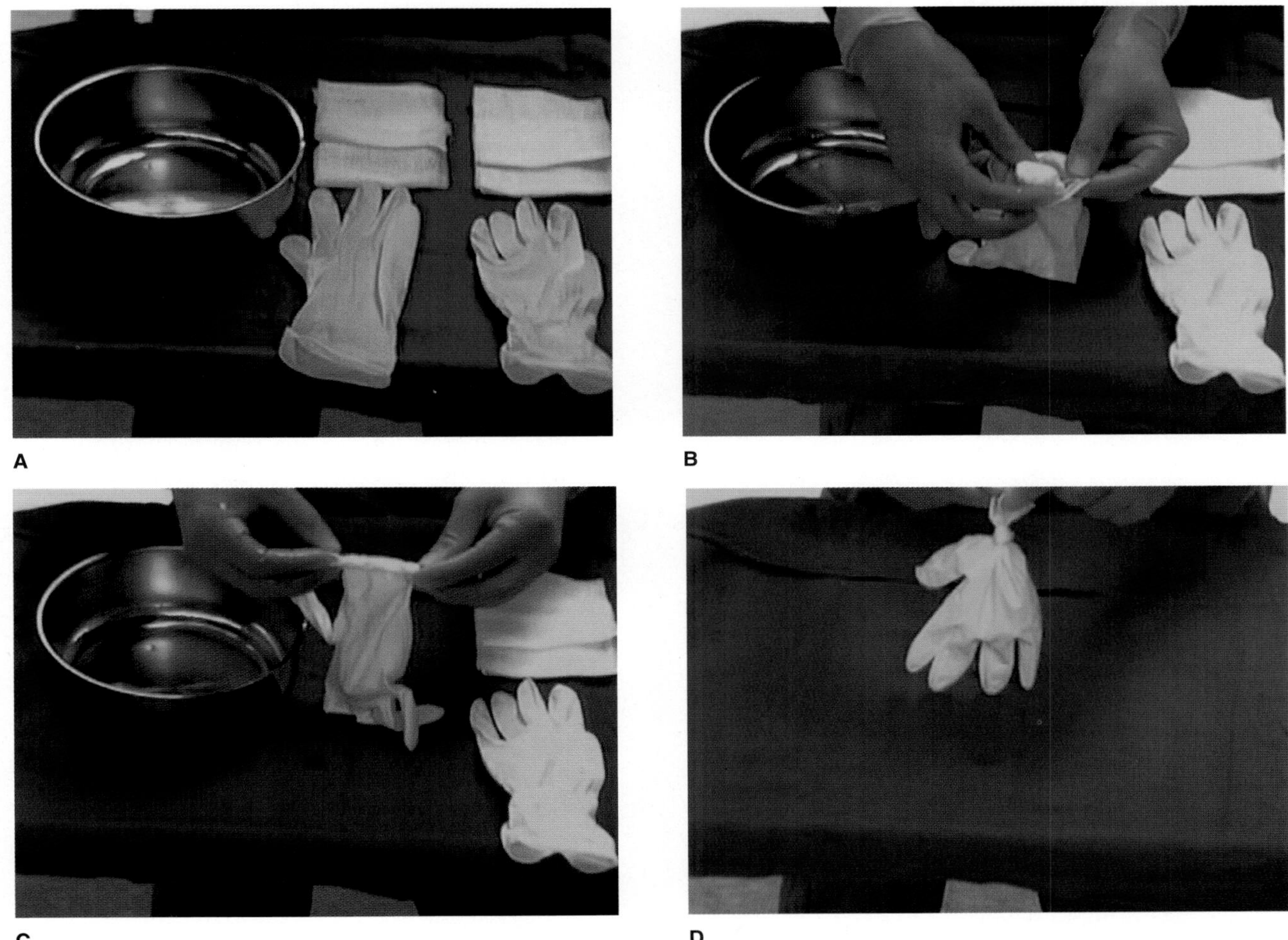

Figure 3-48. The Ceana glove. **A.** The materials for a Ceana glove are available in the operating room and can be prepared easily. **B.** Two 4 × 4 sponges are folded and emerged in sterile water. **C.** They are inserted inside a sterile glove. **D.** The glove is closed at the top, and is placed in the vagina to block the loss of pneumopertioneum.

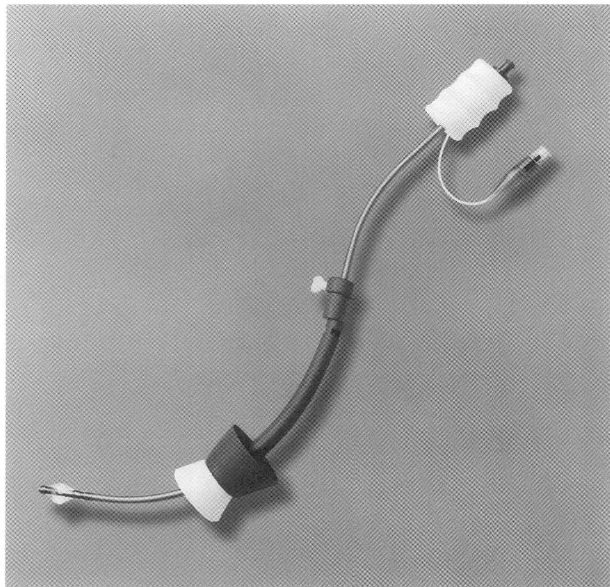

Figure 3-49. The Vcare uterine manipulator.

glove, usually trapping some air in the glove fingers[3-7] (Figure 48, B and C. The top of the glove is tied shut and placed in the vagina or minilaparotomy incision, acting as a flexible air block for preservation of pneumoperitoneum (Figure 3-48D). This device, which is called the Ceana glove, is available in any operating room and has been found to be both safe and effective in numerous laparoscopic procedures.

Instruments for Port Closure

The use of a new device for the closure of subcutaneous tissue in laparoscopic sites was reported by Airan and Sandor.[24] The use of such instruments is gaining in popularity with the widening recognition of the risk of incisional hernia at trocar sites. It is similar to the device described as the Carter Thomason device.[25] Both instruments operate as a needle and a grasper that serve as a suture passer. The conical suture passer guide frequently aids in introducing the suture at the proper angle for the closure of fascia, muscle, and peritoneum. The conical guide has the additional benefit of maintaining pneumoperitoneum once the laparoscopic trocar has been removed. The Carter Thomason suture passer (Figure 3-50) has been recommended for use without the guide if that is deemed more appropriate, for instance, in ligating epigastric arteries. Since the proper closing of the abdominal layers occasionally presents a challenge, the growing interest in instruments designed to assist the surgeon is encouraged. The J-needle allows for port closure that incorporates all layers of the abdominal wall under direct observation (Figure 3-51).

Endoscopic Ultrasound

Intraoperative ultrasound has gained an established role in many surgical procedures. Laparoscopic ultrasound and thoracoscopic ultrasound are the latest modes of intraoperative sonography. They have been introduced mainly to overcome the two major drawbacks of laparoscopy: the ability to show only the surface of the organs and the lack of manual palpation of the anatomic structures. The technology, new indications, and results of intraoperative and laparoscopic ultrasound were reviewed by Bezzi and associates[26] during more than 500 operative procedures. Intraoperative ultrasound and laparoscopic ultrasound are helpful in confirming preoperative studies and acquiring new data not available otherwise. An important role of these techniques is to ascertain the anatomy of the involved organs, thus providing guidance for surgery. Both techniques play an important role in surgical decision making, particularly with respect to hepatic, biliary, and pancreatic malignancies. In some series, the rate of major changes in the surgical strategy can be as high as 38 percent. A relatively new application of intraoperative ultrasound is the ability to do interstitial therapy for tumors at the time of the initial surgery. This can be useful, for example, in patients undergoing liver resection when other unresectable lesions are found in a different segment or in the contralateral lobe. Finally, laparoscopic sonography plays an important role in staging abdominal neoplasms, providing more information than do preoperative imaging and laparoscopic exploration. This feature can be used to effectively stage gastrointestinal malignancies, pancreatic carcinomas, and abdominal lymphomas. It may be expected that a variety of open procedures will be done with videolaparoscopic monitoring and will need guidance from laparoscopic sonography. In the future, the staging of abdominal neoplasms may be improved by laparoscopy combined with laparoscopic ultrasound. A cost-benefit analysis of these techniques and a comparison with preoperative tests should be carried out. High-resolution images can be obtained to delineate abnormalities such as suspected ovarian cysts and uterine myomas. Endoscopic ultrasound is a new instrument that allows the surgeon to evaluate and define pelvic abnormalities suspected at laparoscopy.

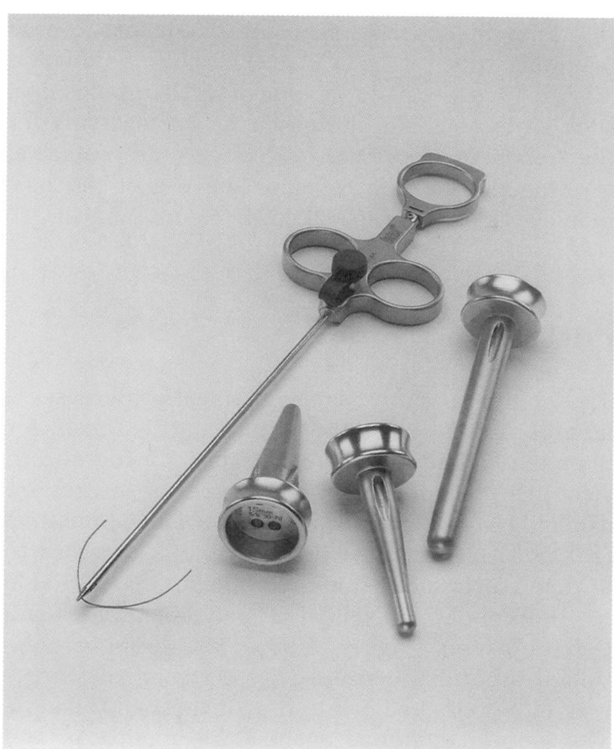

Figure 3-50. The Carter-Thomason device.

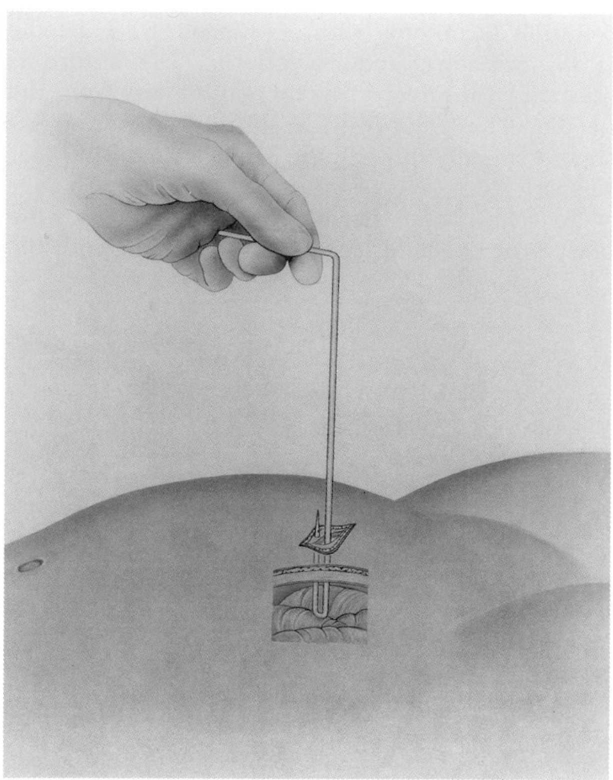

Figure 3-51. A J-needle.

Endoscopic ultrasound may augment the diagnosis of subtle pathologic findings during laparoscopy.[27,28]

Harmonic Scalpel

The ultrasonically activated vibrating blade of the harmonic scalpel (Ethicon) moves longitudinally at

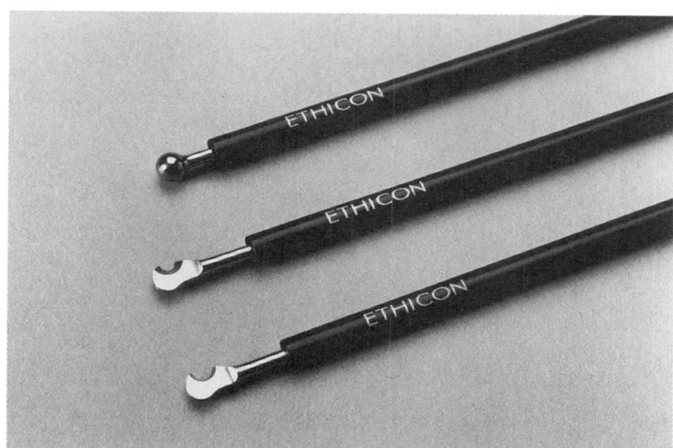

A

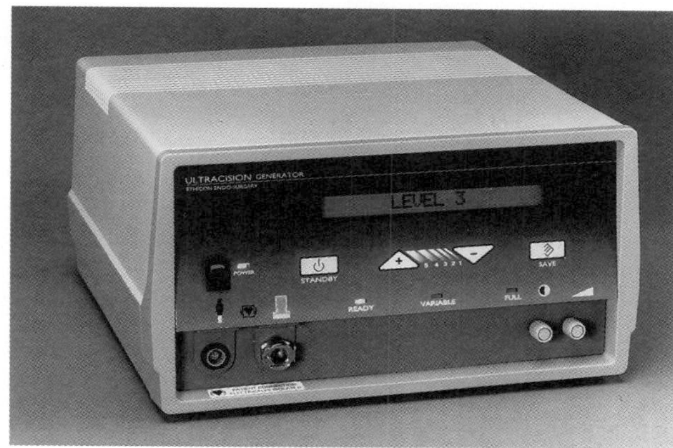

B

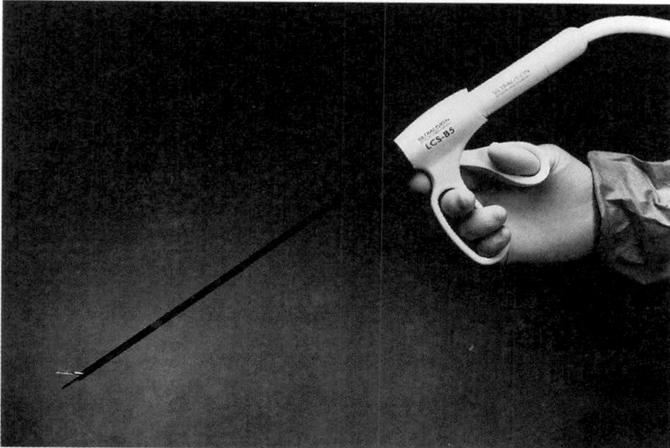

C

Figure 3-52. The harmonic scalpels (Ethicon) **(A)** and generator **(B)**. Interchangeable attachment for the harmonic scalpel **(C)**.

55,000 vibrations per second, cutting tissue while simultanoeusly providing hemostasis. The vibration of the ultrasonic scalpel is thought to generate low heat at the incision site. This combination of vibration and heat causes the proteins to denature (Figure 3-52, A and B). The harmonic scalpel may limit the number of steps required for desiccation and transection of vascular pedicles such as the infundibulopelvic ligaments, reducing overall operating time. It is available in both 5-mm and 10-mm sizes. Several additional interchangeable tips, such as those useful during linear salpingotomy for the treatment of ectopic pregnancies, are available, allowing the surgeon to tailor the use of the harmonic scalpel to the specific task (Figure 3-52C).

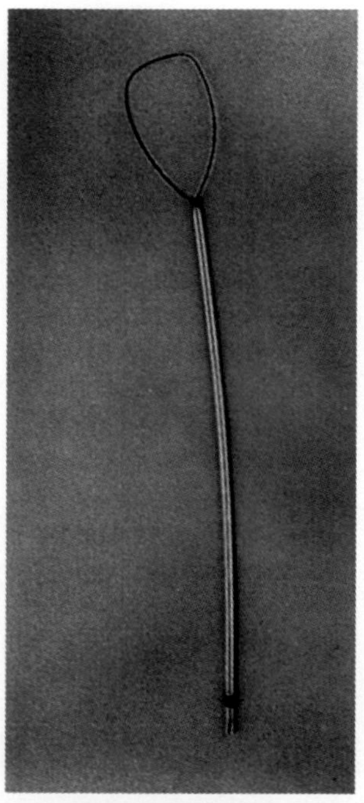

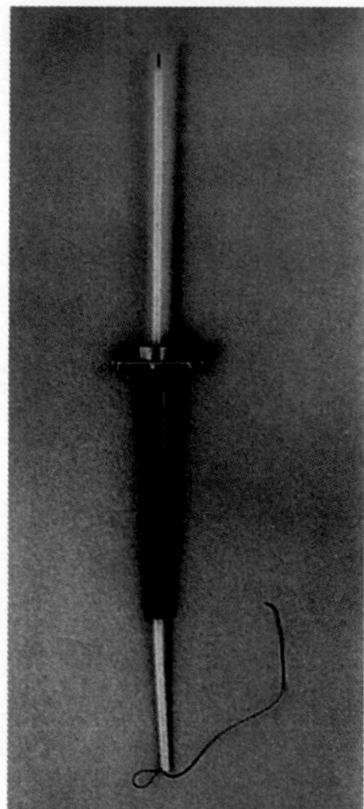

Figure 3-53. **A.** Endoloop suture, a pretied slipknot, is attached to a rigid disposable applicator. **B.** It is inserted into the trocar sleeve

Sutures

The ability to suture laparoscopically increases a laparoscopist's versatility. Suturing is used for hemostasis and to oppose tissues during reconstructive procedures. Different types of sutures are available for endoscopic use. The Endoloop (Ethicon) suture, a preformed slipknot attached to a rigid, disposable 5-mm applicator, is available in 0-chromic, polyglactin, polydioxanone, and polypropylene (Figure 3-53). The loop is positioned around the pedicle by grasping the structure to be removed and pulling it through the loop. The loop is tightened against the applicator, and the suture is cut with scissors or the laser beam against a backstop.

Suture material is available with a straight or curved swaged needle specifically designed for laparoscopic use. It is available in 0-chromic catgut, 4-0 polydioxanone with a swaged ST-4 needle (PDS, Ethicon), and polyglactin. The suture is grasped with forceps several centimeters from the needle. The grasper with suture is inserted intraabdominally through the 5-mm accessory trocar sleeve.

To place the needle intraabdominally, the grasper or needle driver is removed along with the

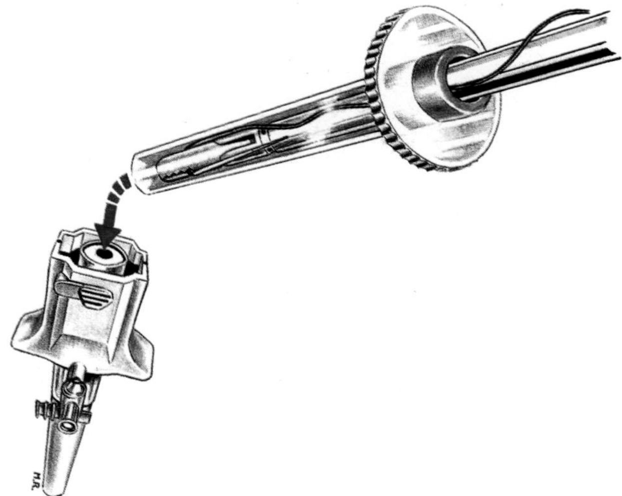

Figure 3-54. The needle holder is inserted into the introducer. The introducer is placed into a 5-mm sleeve.

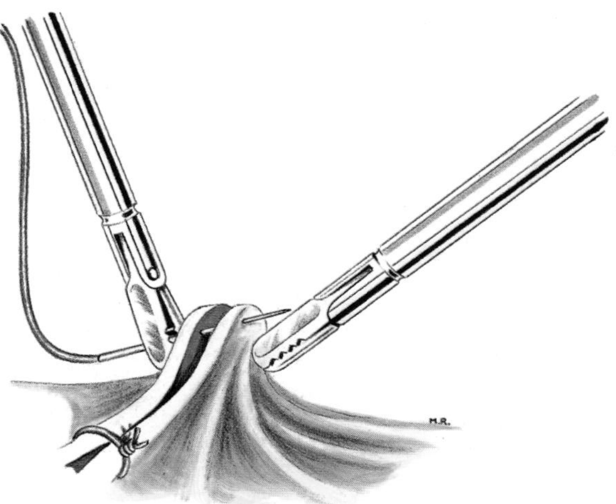

Figure 3-55. The needle driver was placed into a contralateral sleeve. The needle was advanced into the abdominal cavity and passed from the holder to the driver. While the needle was steadied with the driver, the holder was repositioned to the desired location. The needle was tapped with the driver to lock it into a right-angle position. The needle is rearmed with the driver. The driver is used to pass the needle through the tissue and then grasp the tip and pass the needle to the holder.

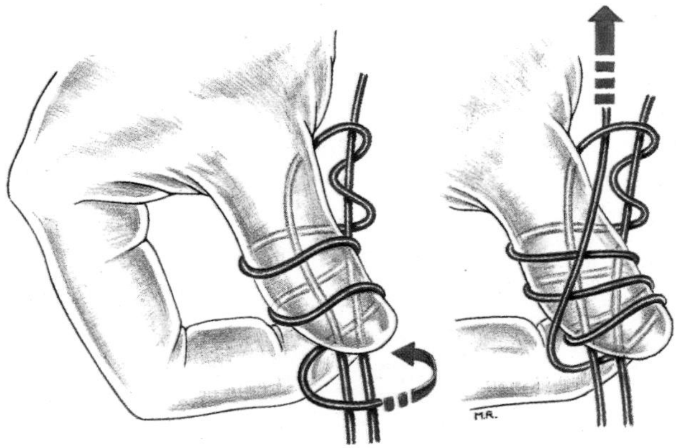

Figure 3-57. Three revolutions are made around both suture strands with the free end of the suture (left). The tail of the suture is inserted through the first loop (right). The tail of the suture is inserted through the first loop directly above the surgeon's thumb.

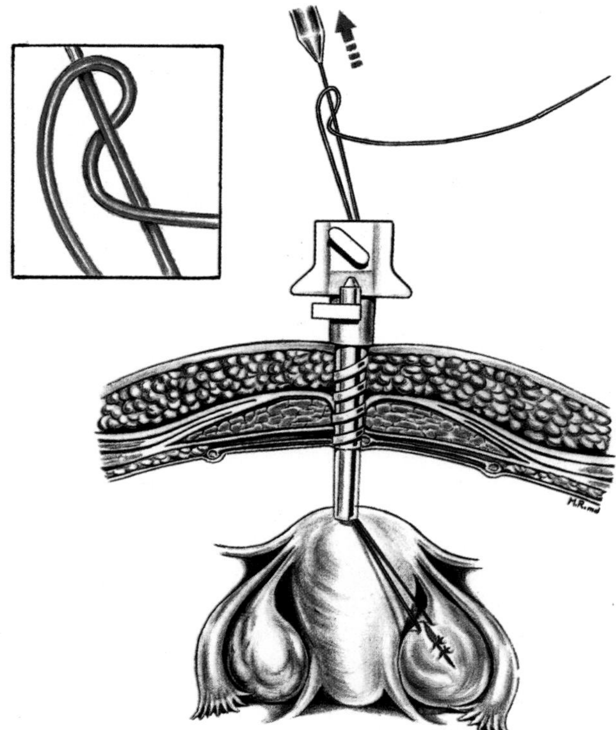

Figure 3-56. The needle holder and excess suture lines were withdrawn from the abdominal cavity through the introducer. (An assistant covers the introducer channel to prevent the loss of pneumoperitoneum). After the surgeon cuts the suture beneath the swage point, a single throw knot is made with the two suture ends (inset).

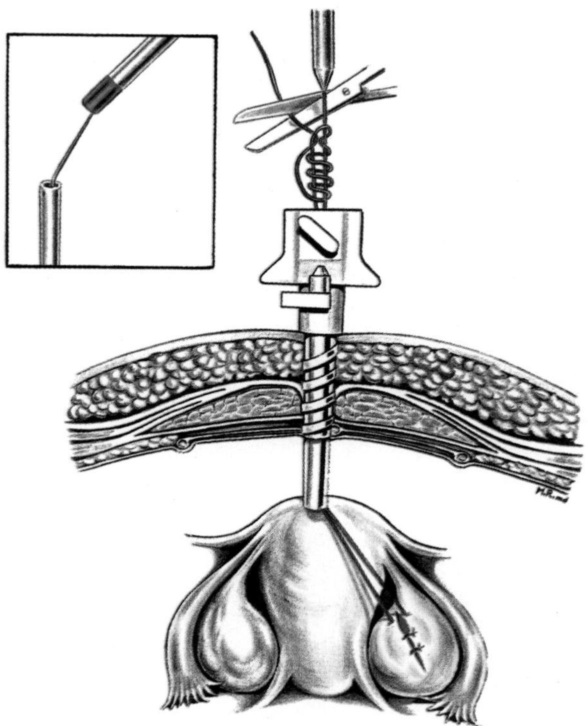

Figure 3-58. The suture tail is cut about 0.6 cm above the knot. The end of the Endoknot shaft is snapped out at the colored band (*inset*), allowing the shaft to slide the knot downward. Placing the shaft perpendicular to the knot lessens suture breakage and ensures knot security.

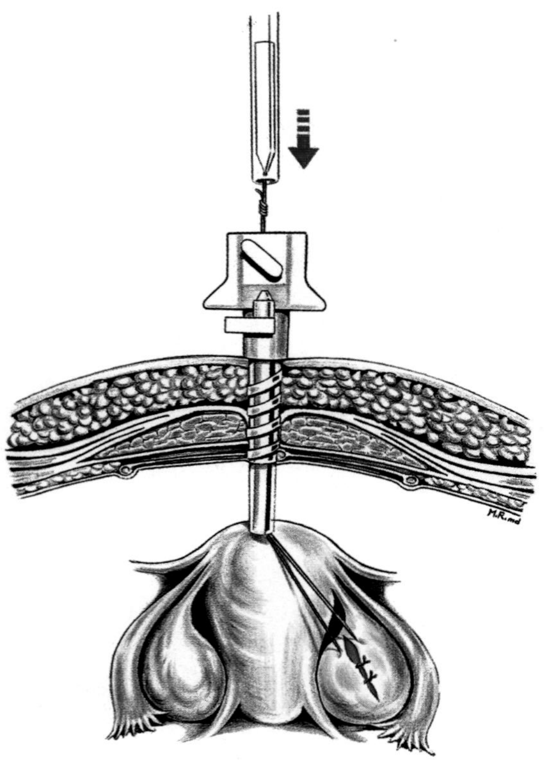

Figure 3-59. The Endoknot cannula acts as an integral knot pusher for placement of the formed knot.

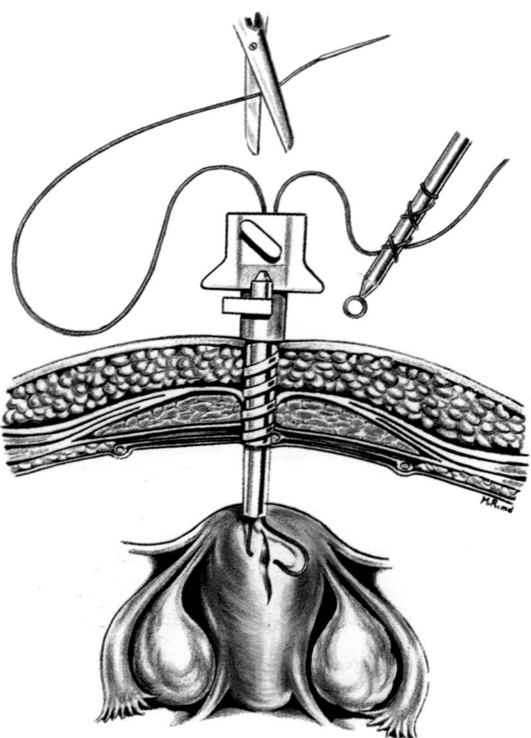

Figure 3-61. The needle and suture are placed in the 3-mm suture introducer. After the needle is passed through the tissue, the needle and suture are brought out of the cannula and the suture is cut.

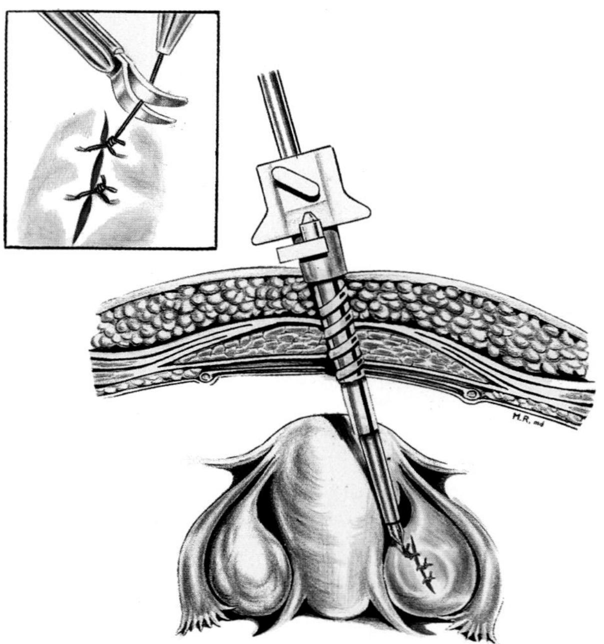

Figure 3-60. The scissors, inserted through the contralateral trocar, are used to cut the knot (*inset*). The pretied Endoknot consists of synthetic absorbable suture material with a hollow plastic tube that is narrowed at one end and scored at the other. The center of the plastic tube has a 4-0 stainless steel suture that is looped at the narrow end and swaged at the surgical needle. The scored end of the device serves as the handle. The primary advantage of this device is that the knot is preformed and does not have to be made manually by the surgeon.

trocar sleeve, which remains around the grasper's shaft. The suture is grasped about 5 cm from the needle, and the grasper is reintroduced with the trocar sleeve into the suprapubic incision site. The needle follows the grasper into the abdominal cavity. A needle larger than a CT-1 is awkward to use intraabdominally. Once the suture is placed, several techniques can be used to secure the knot. An Endoloop (Ethicon) with a premade knot is tightened around the pedicle with the plastic knot pusher. Other types of extracorporeal knots are the Duncan[29] and clinch knots, but their closure depends on a single knot that may slip. The knot may not slide because of suture friction. Tissue trauma can result from the suture being pulled in opposite directions through transfixed tissue as the needle is withdrawn from the abdomen when a sliding knot is applied.

Intracorporeal knotting is difficult and requires practice. An instrument-tying method employed within the abdomen uses two forceps and suture material. The suture can get caught in the articulation point of the forceps and break. However, variations of the fisherman's clinch knot prevent some

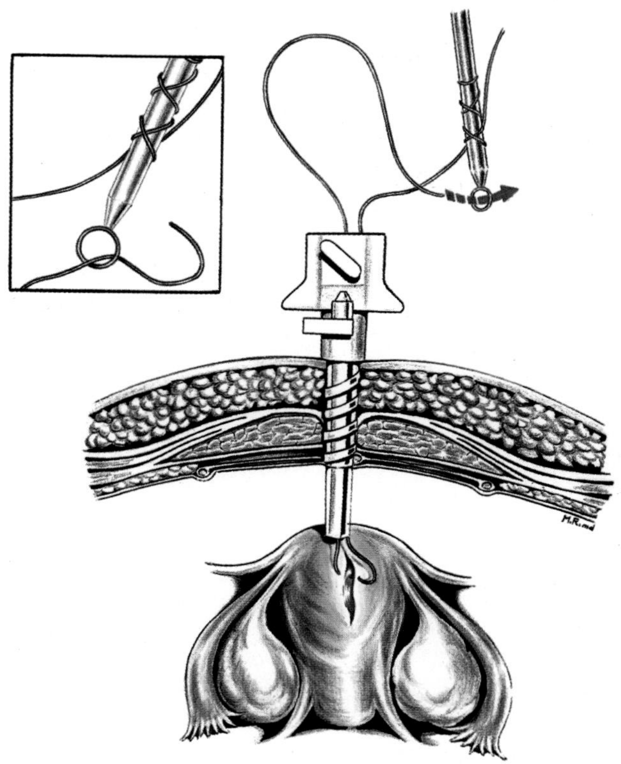

Figure 3-62. About 5 cm of the longest end of the suture is pushed through the wire loop near the tapered end of the cannula. The inset shows a close-up of this process.

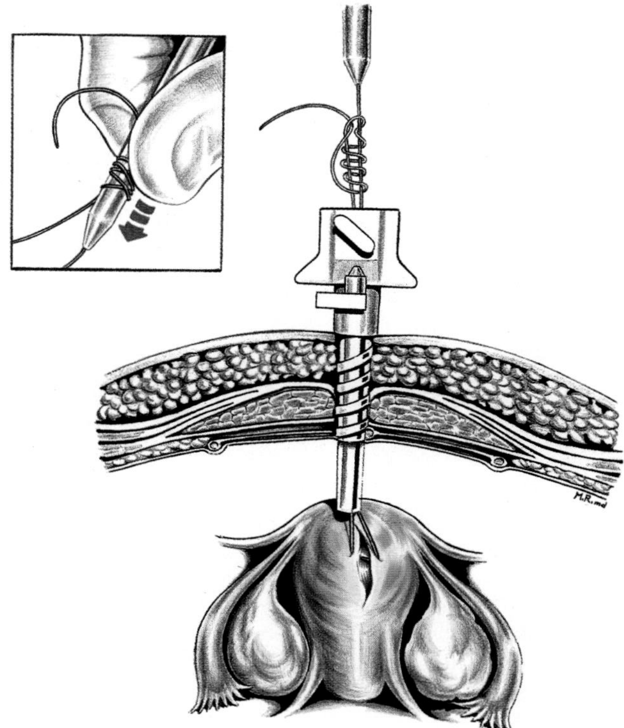

Figure 3-64. The pretied slipknot is pushed off the conical end of the cannula (*inset*). The excess suture is trimmed at the end of the slipknot. The slipknot is pushed into the trocar and onto the tissue to be sutured.

difficulties. The use of the knot pusher was described originally in 1972.[30] The principles of this instrument do not differ from those of tying sutures deep in the pelvis, where the surgeon uses a finger to push and secure the knot.

Extracorporeal knot tying simplifies laparoscopic suturing. Instruments that help this process include a needle holder, needle driver, suture introducer, and scissors. A suture is loaded into the needle holder, holding the suture below the swage point so

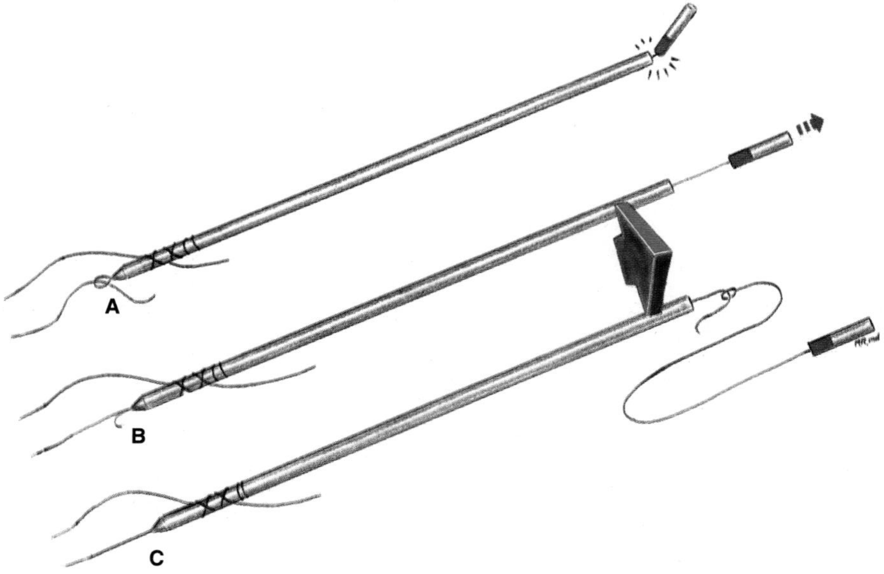

Figure 3-63. The scored end of the cannula A. is snapped off. The wire suture is pulled completely through B. The scored end is discarded C.

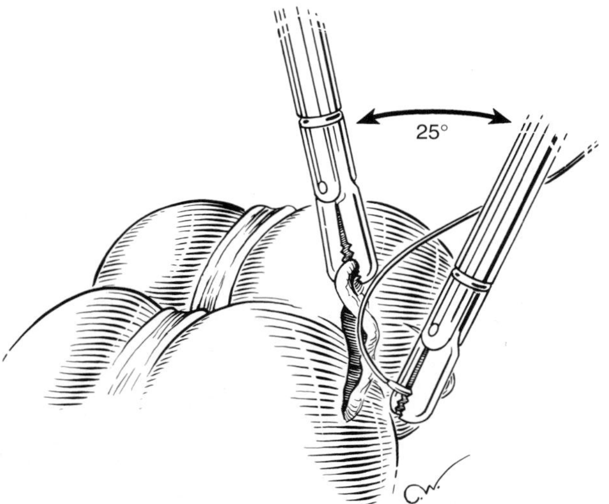

Figure 3-65. After the needle is positioned, it is grasped with the needle holder.

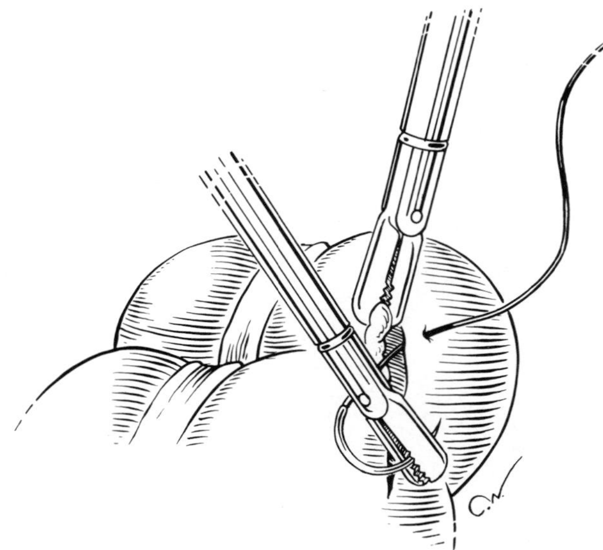

Figure 3-67. The graspers hold the needle, and the needle holder applies counterpressure on the tissue.

that the needle will collapse into the introducer. The needle holder is inserted into the introducer (Figure 3-54). The introducer is placed into a 5-mm trocar, and the needle driver is placed into a contralateral trocar. A needle is advanced into the abdominal cavity and passed from the holder to the driver. While the needle is steadied with the driver, the holder is repositioned to the desired location. The needle is tapped with the driver to lock it into a right-angle position. The needle is rearmed with the driver. A driver is used to pass the needle through the tissue, and then grasp the tip and pass the needle to the holder (Figure 3-55). To reduce the risk of pulling the suture out of the tissue,

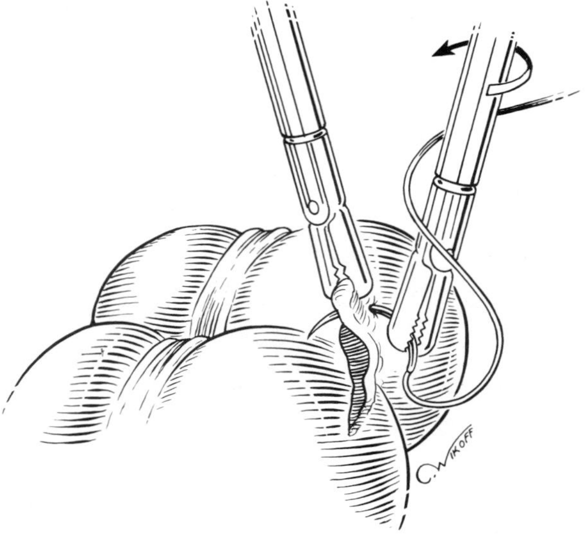

Figure 3-66. While grasping forceps hold the tissue being sutured, the suture is inserted through the tissue.

tension on the suture line is kept to a minimum. The holder, needle, and excess suture line are withdrawn from the abdominal cavity through the introducer. An assistant covers the introducer channel to maintain a pneumoperitoneum (Figure 3-56). The surgeon cuts the suture below the swage point and makes a single-throw knot with the two suture ends. The knot is held securely with the thumb and third finger while three revolutions are made around both suture strands with the free end of the suture (Figure 3-57). The tail of the suture is inserted through the first loop directly above the assistant's hand. After the tail is passed through the loop, the operator pulls up on the tail to form the knot and cuts the tail approximately 0.6 cm above the knot. The end of the Endoknot shaft is snapped off at the colored band, allowing the shaft to slide the knot downward (Figure 3-58). Placing the shaft perpendicular to the knot reduces suture breakage and ensures knot security. The Endoknot cannula is placed in the introducer (Figure 3-59). When the surgeon pulls back on the small end piece of the Endoknot shaft while sliding the plastic shaft forward, the knot is allowed to move forward as the loop decreases in size. The Endoknot cannula acts as an integral knot pusher for placement of the formed knot. Scissors inserted through the contralateral trocar are used to cut the excess suture. The procedure for pretied knot is similar to the technique described above except for forming the knot (Figures 3-60 through 3-64). Intracorporeal knot tying is used during microsurgery and fine

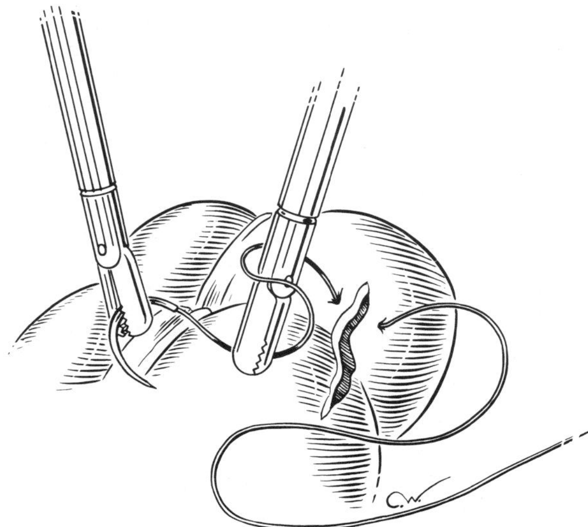

Figure 3-68. The needle is removed from the tissue. Enough suture is pulled through to form a knot, leaving a sufficient tail.

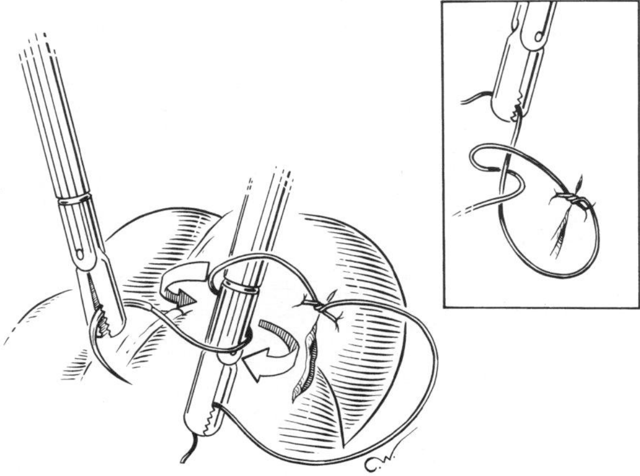

Figure 3-69. The needle is grasped with a grasping forceps, and two or three loops are made around the needle holder. The free end of the suture is grasped with the needle holder and brought inside the formed loops (*inset*).

suturing. It is more difficult and time-consuming than extracorporeal knot tying. The instructions for introducing the needle and suture into the abdomen are the same as those for extracorporeal knot tying. The needle and the entire suture are placed in the abdominal cavity. After the needle is positioned, it is grasped with the needle holder (Figure 3-65). While the grasping forceps apply pressure to the tissue being sutured, the suture is inserted through the tissue (Figure 3-66). Graspers hold the needle, and the needle holder applies counterpressure to the tissue (Figure 3-67). The needle is removed from the tissue. Enough suture to form a knot is pulled through, leaving a sufficient tail (Figure 3-68). The needle is grasped with a grasping forceps, and two or three loops are made around the needle holder. The free end of the suture is grasped with the needle holder and brought inside the formed loops (Figure 3-69), and using both grasping forceps and the needle holder, the suture is tied over the tissue. Additional knots are applied over the suture, reversing the direction of the sutures with each successive knot.

Laparotomy-Type Instruments

Babcocks, atraumatic bowel grasping forceps, Allis clamps, and Metzenbaum scissors have been adapted for laparoscopic use. The acquisition of these instruments depends on whether they will improve a procedure's efficiency.

Standard grasping forceps hold needles for most procedures, but stronger needle holders are necessary if precise placement is required and for suturing thick tissue (i.e., myometrium or periosteum). Some needle holders have handles similar to those used in laparotomy (Figure 3-70). Straight and curved narrow tip needle holders are available for fine intraabdominal suturing (Figure 3-71).

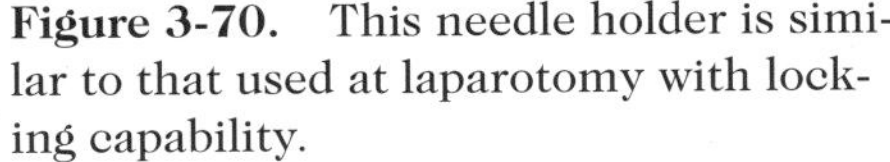

Figure 3-70. This needle holder is similar to that used at laparotomy with locking capability.

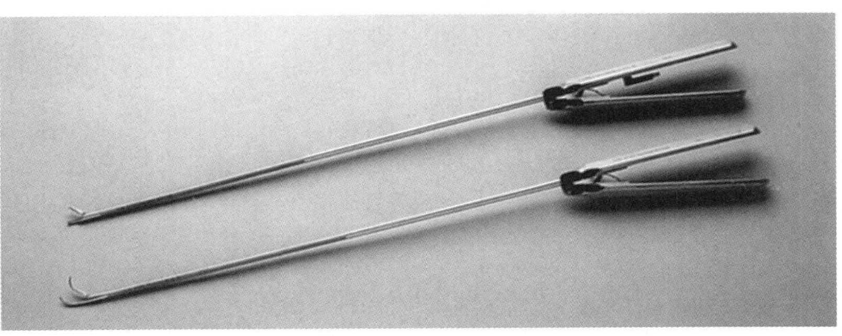

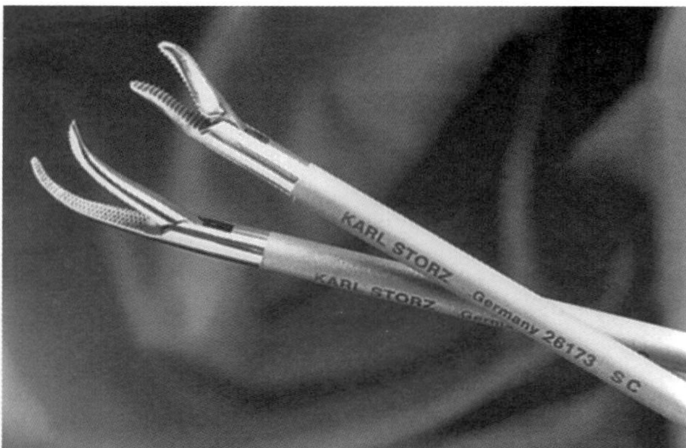

Figure 3-71. Curved and straight fine serrated tips provide a better grip of straight or curved needles.

The Camera

The camera includes the camera head with its cable and the camera control unit (CCU) or camera controller. The cable is plugged into the camera controller. The lens on the medical camera is called a coupler. The coupler screws onto the camera head and is available in several sizes that magnify the image. A 35-mm coupler will produce a larger image on the monitor than will a 28-mm coupler. With a direct coupler, the image travels directly to the camera. With a beam splitter, part of the image travels to the camera and part travels to a porthole or eye cup. The porthole allows the surgeon to view the image directly.

Couplers are mounted and fixed on the camera head. Removable couplers allow the purchase of a camera with interchangeable direct couplers and beam splitters. The removable coupler provides flexibility and economy. Being removable is a potential problem because the coupler is screwed to the camera head, and if it is not attached securely or if its O-ring is worn, liquids may seep between the coupler and the camera head, causing internal fog. A coupler with internal fog is not usable and must be repaired. A fixed coupler eliminates this problem.

Most cameras are either a single chip or a 3-chip and are equal in quality. The production of a unique video camera (Circon) has proprietary Red-Green-Blue (RGB) 24-bit digital enhancement circuits. The signals coming from the charged coupled device (CCD) sensor are sampled at equal time intervals, and the amplitude of each sample is classified into a discrete level system and converted to a binary code. All the video information is encoded into a stream of noise-free digital numbers. These numbers are used as variables in mathematical equations (algorithms) to manipulate and shift in time and value through digital signal processing. Digital electronics are the leading edge in video technology and will be the new standard of performance just as digital compact discs have replaced LP records and audiocassettes. Digital signals take up less bandwidth than do the analog signals currently in use. Moreover, digitally processed signals can be applied to 3-chip and high-definition television (HDTV).

Another breakthrough in medical cameras is "chip-on-a-stick," a technology that combines the camera and the scope on one piece of equipment. The camera chip is taken out of the camera head and placed at the distal end of the scope. This technology does away with the optical lenses an image passes through when the chip is in the camera head. Chip-on-a-stick cameras require less light than do standard cameras because light is not lost in the light cord and rod lens.

One feature of the camera head is its ability to manipulate peripheral equipment by using buttons to accomplish a variety of tasks, including activation of the video printer and videocassette recorder (VCR). Some cameras have a single button to start both the video printer and the VCR. With a main control switch, several desired functions can be manipulated. Another variation includes separate buttons on the camera head to increase or decrease the camera gain level. With this arrangement, the first button can operate the video printer, the VCR, and additional components. An infrared remote control is required for all components to make the buttons operable. Another camera with two buttons on the camera head can control any two components. This system has cables running from the CCU (camera box) to two selected components, the video printer and VCR, or to the video printer and the still video recorder. With this system, infrared remote control is not required. Another camera feature is field-replaceable camera cables. Since most camera problems occur in the camera cable, replacing cables at the hospital rather than sending a camera out for repair saves time and expense.

Camera Equipment

The first medical camera (Circon Corporation), which was developed in 1972, had three tubes and weighed 18 pounds. It used a fiberoptic image guide to transfer a microscopic image to the camera that transferred the image to a video monitor. In 1973, a single-tube camera was designed weighing 3.8 pounds (Figure 3-72). Although the weight was

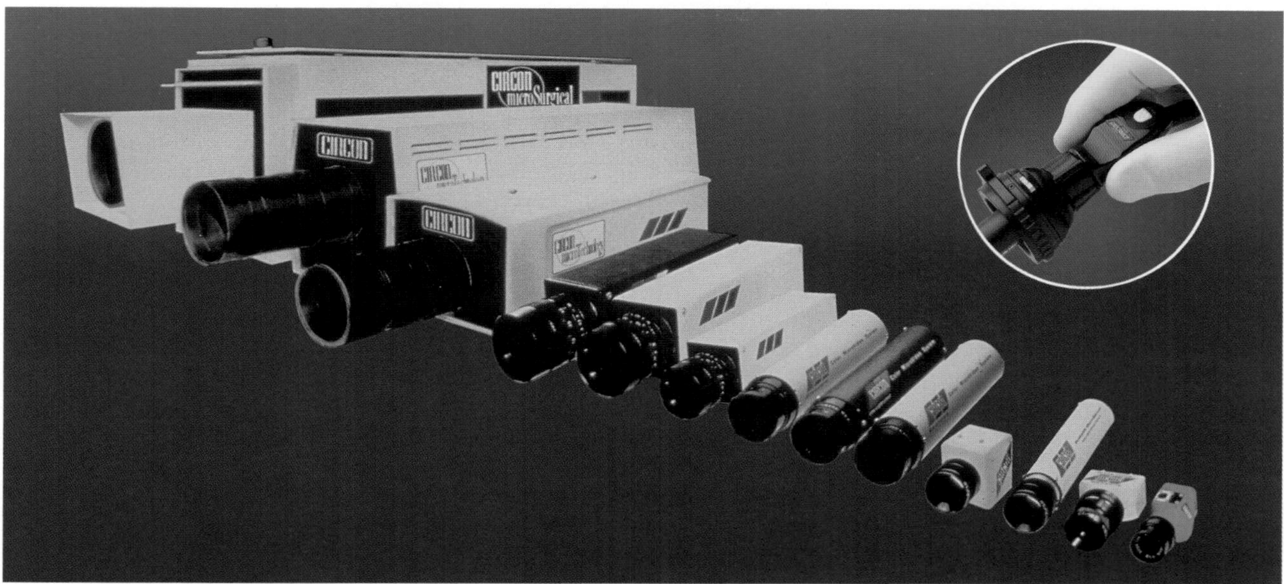

Figure 3-72. The decrease in size of video cameras over the years is illustrated. The inset shows a contemporary camera head.

reduced, the camera remained heavy and counterweights were needed. This camera was attached directly to the endoscope without using a fiberoptic image guide. The single 1-inch tube had a specially striped filter to produce a full-color picture. Video camera manufacturers continued to make improvements in size, weight, and image quality. In 1975, a camera weighing 1.25 pounds was developed, and in the following year, a low-light feature enabled it to be 10 times more light-sensitive. In 1980, a new 6-ounce camera was small enough to be held in the palm of the surgeon's hand. It produced excellent color separation and image resolution (Figure 3-73). Another milestone was achieved 2 years later with the first solid-state CCD camera. This camera weighed 3 ounces, and with the change from tubes to solid-state CCD sensors, two major achievements were accomplished. First, the camera could be disinfected in solutions so that there was no need to "bag the camera." Second, the colors produced by solid-state construction were more reliable than were colors produced by tube cameras.

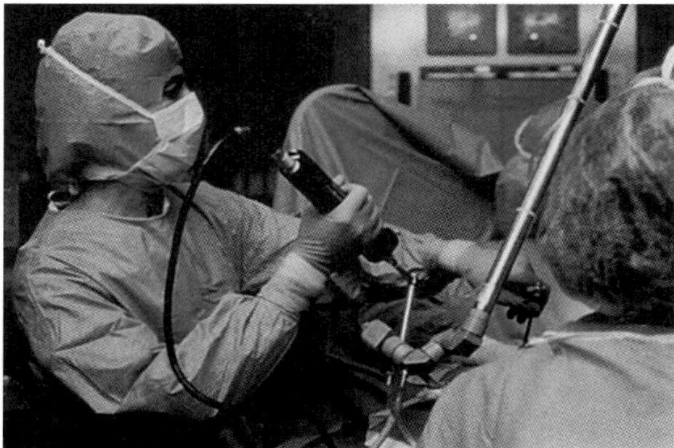

Figure 3-73. Camran Nezhat doing videolaparoscopy in early 1980.

Since 1982, all surgical camera manufacturers have switched to solid-state construction. Developments include low lux levels (enhancing the quality of the image in low-light situations), buttons on the cameras to start and stop VCRs, field-replaceable camera cables, increased lines of resolution [S-Video and RGB signal output as opposed to National Television Systems Committee (NTSC)]. Cameras also became more durable. The technologies of the 1990s added digitally processed signals, 3-chip cameras, and chip-on-a-stick to surgical video.

Basic Video Information

Within the camera is a CCD that "sees" an optical image through the lens and converts it into an electrical image. A CCD is composed of rows of tiny picture elements called pixels. Each pixel can sense red, green, or blue light to produce color. The more pixels, the better the picture.

An image is sent through camera cables to the CCU to the monitor input. The monitor converts the electrical image to the original optical image seen by the human eye. The electrical image also is directed to components other than the monitor after leaving the CCU. It is relayed by a cable to a VCR from the VCR to a printer and on to a monitor.

Scanning Formats

Video information is scanned to generate a signal frequency. The scanning is done at a rate of 525 lines per frame; there are 30 frames per second of video information. This scanning rate is like a television broadcast standardized by the National Television Systems Committee. NTSC scanning rates are used in the United States, Canada, Japan, South America, and Asia. Russia and France use a different scanning rate called Secam. PAL, a third type of scanning rate, is used in other European nations. These scanning rates are not compatible with NTSC standards. Videotapes made in the United States must be converted before they can be viewed in countries with non-NTSC scanning rates. The process of converting one scanning rate to another is expensive. When the NTSC scanning rates were created, technicians used a limited bandwidth to send the video signal to color and light information simultaneously. The format of the NTSC signal is called a composite signal. There are inherent problems with this method of transference because a camera first processes color and light separately and then combines the two to create a signal. Cross-talk is a signal noise that generates grainy images with soft edges and causes colors to be less consistent. The signal-to-noise ratio is a measurement that differentiates between video noise (cross-talk) and useful video information. The higher the signal-to-noise ratio, the better the detail at the edge and the better the total image. Signal noise is measured in decibels. A quick way to evaluate noise is not to allow any light to reach the camera chip. With the absence of picture information, the image contains only noise. Another way to see picture noise is to adjust the camera to place color bars on the monitor screen. One selects first an NTSC signal, then a Y/C signal, and finally an RGB signal. One looks at the edge of each bar color and notes that movement from NTSC to Y/C to RGB makes the edges progressively sharper because NTSC has the most noise and RGB has the least. Specifications (lines of resolution, pixels, signal-to-noise ratios) set the parameters of the video components, but one should always test the monitor.

The second format, called a component signal, carries the color and light separately. There is less cross-talk so that pictures generated by component signals have sharper edges and truer colors than do pictures generated by composite signals. The Y/C format and NTSC format carry the video signal in a single cable. Y/C (Y stands for light brightness, and C refers to color) is the name for the format. SVHS and Super VHS are tape formats that accept this type of signal.

The third format, RGB, is also a component signal. Video information is separated into four signals: red, green, blue, and a timing signal. Each signal carries its own light. Separation occurs in the camera head and is done electrically. Since the colors and light are separate, this format requires less electronic processing. There are four separate cables from the camera box. A monitor that accepts RGB input is needed. Although these monitors are more expensive, they have higher resolution capabilities. Thus, of the three signal-carrying formats, the first format, NTSC, is the least desirable. The second and third formats carry much clearer signals with less noise.

Resolution

The clarity and detail of the video image depend on the number of horizontal lines of resolution, which are detected by the number of distinct vertical lines seen in a picture. Resolution is set forth by the camera's pixel count and by a formula used to achieve the resolution number. No resolution number can be higher than the pixel count. Each line of resolution is composed of pixels, and the more pixels per line, the better the image. Another way to understand the pixel effect is to compare a large-screen television with a small (13-inch) monitor. Smaller monitors have a sharper, crisper image, especially at the edges of an image, because pixels are placed closer together on a small screen. The ability of the video system to carry and process signals, the components that transmit signals, and the resolution numbers of the monitor together determine the ultimate picture quality. The industry standard is to measure horizontal resolution using 75 percent of the chip. However, some manufacturers have been known to use 100 percent of the chip, resulting in a higher resolution number.

The Camera Box (CCU)

The most common features include a color bar button and a white balance button. Some CCUs have manual and automatic white balance features. The most important feature for the CCU is to provide an automatic shutter, because it adjusts each pixel's exposure time up to 1/15,000 of a second. The circuit can react to varying light conditions as fast as the human eye can. An electronic shutter is essential for a surgical videocamera.

The Monitor and Accessories

The sizes of the screens vary from 8 to 20 inches. Smaller monitors provide a better picture, and a product with at least 600 lines of resolution is preferable. It should accept all three video formats (NTSC, Y/C, and RGB). When purchasing a VCR, you will want to have Y/C inputs and outputs, which some consumer models do not have. Y/C-type VCRs will be called SVHS VCRs.

The video printer is an excellent method for recording and documenting the findings. Video prints can fit easily into a patient's chart. Another component is a 35-mm slide-making system that can produce 35-mm slides from any standard video signal and is designed to work with video printers. These systems make 35-mm slides more quickly and efficiently than the traditional method of fastening a 35-mm camera to the end of an endoscope. With 500 lines of resolution, it also produces high-quality images.

Equipment Problems and Troubleshooting

After the video system is moved to the operating room, plug it in and test the components. Plug in the camera, note the image, put color bars on the monitor screen, and evaluate the accuracy of the colors. Look at the monitor, check the buttons, turn on the light source, and check the light cord for damaged light bundles. Look through the scope before it is hooked up and illuminated because light hides defects. Hold the scope with the distal end pointed at a normal ceiling light and then look through the eyepiece. Is the scope clear? Check both the distal end and the eyepiece for cracks or other visible damage. If you follow this routine, unexpected events can be reduced in frequency.

If a problem with the image occurs during an operation, check the scope initially, then the light cord, and then the camera. If the picture is poor, check the color and light level to search for the cause. If there is no picture, be certain that the light source is turned on. If this does not solve the problem, detach the camera from the scope and focus it on an object in the room. If the picture is good, the camera is functioning properly and the scope or the light cord is at fault. When the picture is poor, the camera could be defective or the lens could be fogged; change a button on the CCU, or a new camera may be required. A methodical piece-by-piece examination of the components makes it easier to locate the fault so that it can be fixed or replaced.

Robotics

Efforts to improve surgical efficiency have led to the development of robotically assisted laparoscopic procedures. The Animated Endoscopic System for Optimal Positioning (AESOP) has been designed for the purpose of holding and maneuvering the laparoscope under the direct control of the surgeon. The elimination of the camera holder allows the two doctors to do complex laparoscopic operations faster than they could without the robotic arm. This technology also may allow the surgeon to carry out some procedures without the aid of an assistant. The AESOP system can be activated by voice or by foot and hand control. For 50 patients undergoing routine gynecologic endoscopic procedures, the operating time using voice control was compared with that using foot or hand control. The voice control worked more efficiently and faster than did hand or foot control.[31] In a comparison of the findings of five studies evaluating the need for a human camera holder assistant, the robotic man outperformed the human camera holder, and reduced laparoscopic operating time, resulting in efficiency and cost savings.[32]

Operating Room Setup

An organized and well-equipped operating room is essential for successful laparoscopy.[33] The surgical team and the operating room staff should be familiar with the instruments and their functions. Each instrument is inspected periodically. Scissors, graspers, trocars, trocar sleeves, and the like, are checked for loose or broken tips even if the same instruments were used during a previous procedure. Before a new instrument is used, it is tested by the surgeon. While the total cost of operative laparoscopy is decreased by the shortened hospital stay and recovery, the cost of the operating room is higher for operative laparoscopy because of the higher cost of instruments and the longer operating time.

Position of Equipment

Equipment positioning (Figure 3-74) varies according to the surgeon's preference. The following arrangements are suggested.

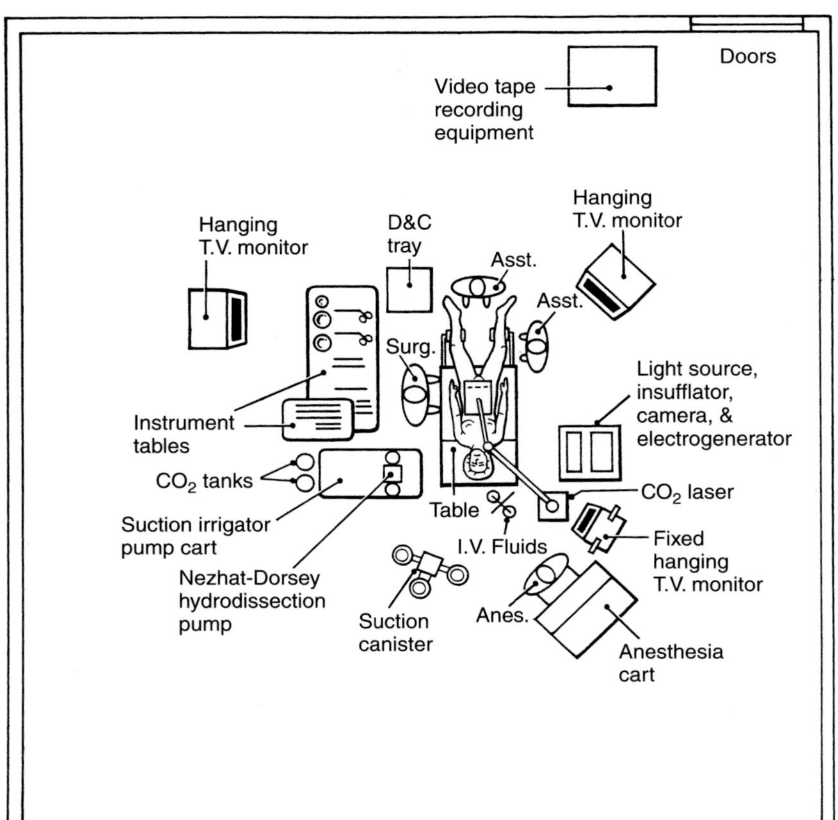

Figure 3-74. Positions of patient, assistants, surgeon, and equipment.

Operating Tables

Before the patient is brought to the operating room, the operating tables are set.

1. Mayo stand 1 contains a dilation and curettage setup with instruments for video-augmented hysteroscopy (videohysteroscopy). Included are a long-bladed weighted speculum, a double-or single-toothed tenaculum, dilators, a uterine sound, a small Kervokian curette, a uterine manipulator, Raytec (Baxter Healthcare, Deerfield, IL), telfa, and a Foley catheter. The videohysteroscopy equipment includes a Circon (Circon-ACMI, Santa Barbara, CA) or a Storz (Karl Storz, Culver City, CA) diagnostic and operative hysteroscope along with its appropriate scissors and grasper. An adaptive sleeve is available for passing a scissor, grasper, or the fiber laser when it is used in the uterus. For more complicated procedures such as resection of an intrauterine leiomyoma and endometrial ablation, electrosurgical wire loops and roller balls (Circon, Karl Storz) are added.
2. The back table is positioned behind the surgeon and next to the first assistant. The table contains a Veress needle, a scalpel, an Allis clamp, an 11-mm trocar and sleeve, a 10-mm laparoscope, a fiberoptic light cord, 5.5-mm secondary trocars and sleeves, a suction-irrigator probe (American Hydro-Surgical Instruments) with irrigation and suction tubing, tubing for the CO_2 insufflator with a CO_2 connector, atraumatic grasping forceps with teeth, bipolar forceps with cord, aspirating needles each with a 60-mL syringe, and telfa and Raytec (Baxter Healthcare). A small amount of dilute vasopressin (Pitressin) is made available (one ampule in 100 mL of bacteriostatic sterile water). This solution (1 to 2 mL) is injected through the laparoscopic needle before the removal of a large fibroid or endometrioma to reduce bleeding. Vicryl suture (3-0) on a cutting needle for closing the primary trocar site and 1.5-inch steristrips to be used with Mastisol (Ferndale Laboratories, Inc., Ferndale, MI), eye pads, and 3M tape for dressing care are placed on the back table.
3. Mayo stand 2 is positioned so that the surgeon and first assistant can reach the endoscopic scissors and grasping forceps with and without teeth.

Hydrodissection Pump

The Nezhat-Dorsey hydrodissection pump provides pressure during hydrodissection and is located behind the surgeon on a cart or specially designed stand. The plastic tubing is connected to the pump, brought to the operative field, and attached to the suction-irrigator probe.

Light Sources, Insufflator, and Electrogenerator

Other items kept on the side of the room opposite the surgeon include a storage table that holds the insufflator, electrosurgical equipment, camera boxes, and light sources. This equipment is stored in a specially designed stand opposite the surgeon and close to the patient, toward her head. This cart is placed so that it does not interfere with the assistants' position and does not obstruct the surgeon's view of the insufflator and light source. The camera is covered with a sterile cover, connected to the camera box, brought to the operative field, and attached to the laparoscope. Video cabinets are manufactured with removable backs, making adjustment of the machines easy.

Video Monitors

Video monitors should be positioned within view of the surgeon and the two assistants; one assistant stands between the patient's legs, and the other one is opposite the surgeon. Three video monitors provide adequate views for the surgeon, the assistants, and other observers. The monitor provides the surgeon's view of the operative site and should be set for maximal clarity and true color transmission. The video monitors can be fixed to the ceiling, placed on a portable stand, or attached to a mobile stand with an articulating arm. The monitors are positioned for optimal viewing from any area in the operating room and are pushed from the operative area at the end of the day.

Video Recording

Depending on the surgeon's preference, one or two VCRs are located in the room. Two are recommended if a videotape of the procedure will be provided for the patient or referring physician. The recorders are stored in a cabinet near a wall and are wired to the camera box. When surgery is not in progress, the cabinet is locked to prevent damage and tampering. For those who videotape procedures for educational purposes, a Beta recorder is recommended and kept in the same cabinet.

Lasers and Laser Equipment

Three different lasers are available in the operating room: a CO_2 laser (with a coupler), an argon or potassium titanyl phosphate (KTP) laser, and a neodymium-yttrium aluminum garnet (Nd:YAG) laser. They are used through the operative channel of the laparoscope or a suprapubic trocar. The CO_2 laser is on the patient's side, opposite the surgeon. The articulating arm is extended appropriately so that it does not weigh too heavily on the surgeon's hand. YAG and argon lasers are used less frequently than is the CO_2 laser and are located behind the first assistant, who stands between the patient's legs. This allows laser fibers to be passed from the back table through the second puncture site. Appropriate electrical outlets and special water connections are necessary when one uses fiber lasers. Typically, an outlet supplying a 220-V 30-A circuit is required. The YAG laser can be either three-phase or single-phase and air- or water-cooled, depending on the peak wattage required for a particular procedure. The CO_2 laser can be operated from a 100-V circuit supplied by any standard electrical outlet. Individually wrapped sterile fibers are kept with the fiber lasers, each with its own cleaver for sharpening fiber tips. Since the fibers break easily, they are handled carefully and checked repeatedly. Safety precautions are followed strictly when one is using lasers. One risk of fiber-equipped lasers that does not exist with a CO_2 laser is the possibility of fiber breakage in or outside the patient's abdomen. In the CO_2 laser, the beam is transmitted through and reflected by mirrors contained in the articulating arm. When fiber lasers are used, the appropriate tinted eye protection is worn by both the patient and the staff. Regular glasses can be worn when one is using the CO_2 laser but are not necessary during videolaseroscopy. The patient's eyes are covered with moistened eye pads when the CO_2 is used and with the appropriate tinted goggles when other lasers are used.

Preparation and Termination of the Procedure

All the setup tables are brought close to the operating table, and both the hysteroscope and the laparoscope are connected to the light sources and cameras. After they are checked and functioning, they are placed over the patient. After the videohysteroscopy is completed and as the laparoscopic portion begins, the first Mayo stand is moved out of the way and the surgeon moves to the side of the patient for the laparoscopy.

The anesthesiologist covers the patient's eyes with moistened 4 × 4 pads when the laser is used and places a foam pad over her neck to protect her if lightweight camera equipment is placed on the sterile field during the procedure.

When the procedure is completed, instruments are handled carefully so that laparoscopes and other delicate equipment are not damaged. The disposable equipment is discarded, and the reusable instruments are given to the circulating nurses for cleaning. Care is taken to ensure that reusable instruments are not mixed with disposables and inadvertently thrown out.

The patient's abdomen is washed thoroughly, and her legs are lowered. Although the patient is not fully alert, she often can hear conversation as she is being extubated and while awakening. A professional demeanor is maintained, and conversation is limited.

Managed Health Care

New endoscopic procedures are done with increasing frequency, and so hospitals need more video equipment to keep up with demand, and purchases must justify their cost. As medical services move from a large hospital-based facility to smaller community-based surgical centers, patients residing 2 hours from the main hospital could have a knee arthroscopy or laparoscopy done closer to home. The leading edge of technology includes three-dimensional (3-D) equipment, virtual reality, and HDTV. HDTV can expand the scanning rate from 525 lines of resolution to 1100 or 1200 lines per frame, and the quality of current pictures will more than double. One challenge is to reduce the cost to make it affordable for hospitals.

With virtual reality, a 3-D computer image is presented to the user through liquid crystal glasses. This technique is used in the United States by public institutions such as the Central Intelligence Agency and by architects so that clients can "see" a building inside and out before its construction. In a way, this is similar to a surgeon's use of virtual reality, but cost continues to be a major obstacle. The 3-D technology attempts to provide depth to the image that is not available with monocular endoscopic systems. The increased perception of depth of field enables the surgeon to locate instruments in relation to tissues and organs. These systems rely on special optical devices.

References

1. Nezhat F, Nezhat C, Silfen SO. Videolaseroscopy for oophorectomy. *Am J Obstet Gynecol* 1991; 165:1323.
2. Hurd WW, Diamond MP. There's a hole in my bucket: The cost of disposable instruments. *Fertil Steril* 1997; 67:13.
3. DesCoteaux JG, Tye L, Poulin EC. Reuse of disposable laparoscopic instruments: Cost analysis. *Can J Surg* 1996; 39:133.
4. DesCoteaux JG, Blackmore K, Parsons L. A prospective comparison of the costs of reusable and limited-reuse laparoscopic instruments. *Can J Surg* 1998; 41:136.
5. DesCoteaux JG, Poulin EC, Lortie M, et al. Reuse of disposable laparoscopic instruments: A study of related surgical complications. *Can J Surg* 1995; 38:497.
6. Schaer GN, Koechli OR, Haller U. Single-use versus reusable laparoscopic surgical instruments: A comparative cost analysis. *Am J Obstet Gynecol* 1995; 173:1812.
7. Nezhat C, Bess O, Admon D, et al. Hospital cost comparison between abdominal, vaginal, and laparoscopy-assisted vaginal hysterectomy. *Obstet Gynecol* 1994; 83:713.
8. Dorsey JH, Holtz PM, Griffiths RI, et al. Costs and charges associated with three alternative techniques of hysterectomy. *N Engl J Med* 1996; 335:476.
9. Wolf JS Jr. Laparoscopic access with a visualizing trocar. *Tech Urol* 1997; 3:34.
10. Kaali SG. Establishment of primary port without insertion of a sharp trocar. *J Am Assoc Gynecol Laparosc* 1998; 5:193.
11. Schaller G, Kuenkel M, Manegold BC. The optical "Veress-needle"—initial puncture with a minioptic. *Endosc Surg Allied Technol* 1995; 3:55.
12. Boike GM, Miller CE, Spiritos NM, et al. Incisional bowel herniations after operative laparoscopy: A series of nineteen cases and review of the literature. *Am J Obstet Gynecol* 1995; 172:1726.
13. Moore SS, Green CR, Wang FL, et al. The role of irrigation in the development of hypothermia during laparoscopic surgery. *Am J Obstet Gynecol* 1997; 176:598.
14. Nezhat C, Nezhat F, Silfen SO. Laparoscopic hysterectomy and bilateral salpingo-oophorectomy using multifire GIA surgical stapler. *J Gynecol Surg* 1990; 6:287.
15. Nezhat C, Nezhat F, Bess O, et al. Injuries associated with the use of a linear stapler

during operative laparoscopy: Review of diagnosis, management, and prevention. *J Gynecol Surg* 1993; 9:145.

16. Carter JE, McCarus SD. Laparoscopic myomectomy: Time and cost analysis of power vs. manual morcellation. *J Reprod Med*, 1997; 42:383.
17. Mecke H, Wallas F, Brocker A, Gertz HP. Pelviscopic myoma enucleation: Technique, limits, complications. *Geburtshilfe Frauenheilkd* 1995; 55:374.
18. Mettler L, Semm K, Lehmann-Willenbrock L, et al. Comparative evaluation of classical intrafascial-supracervical hysterectomy (CISH) with transuterine mucosal resection as performed by pelviscopy and laparotomy—our first 200 cases. *Surg Endosc* 1995; 9:418.
19. Kresch AJ, Lyons TL, Westland AB, et al. Laparoscopic supracervical hysterectomy with a new disposable morcellator. *J Am Assoc Gynecol Laparosc* 1998; 5:203.
20. Lobe TE, Schropp KP, Joyner R, et al. The suitability of automatic tissue morcellation for the endoscopic removal of large specimens in pediatric surgery. *J Pediatr Surg* 1994; 29:232.
21. Hasson HM. Ovarian surgery, in Sanfilippo JS, Levine RL, eds., *Operative Gynecologic Endoscopy*. New York, Springer-Verlag, 1989.
22. Valtchev KL, Papsin FR. A new uterine mobilizer for laparoscopy: Its use in 518 patients. *Am J Obstet Gynecol* 1977; 127:738.
23. Koh CH. A new technique and system for simplifying total laparoscopic hysterectomy. *J Am Assoc Gynecol Laparosc* 1998; 5:187.
24. Airan MC, Sandor J. A simple subcutaneous tissue closure device for laparoscopic procedure. *Min Invas Ther Allies Technol* 1996; 5:35.
25. Carter JE. A new technique of fascial closure for laparoscopic incisions. *J Laparosc Surg* 1994; 4:143.
26. Bezzi M, Silecchia G, De Leo A, et al. Laparoscopic and intraoperative ultrasound. *Eur J Radiol* 1998; suppl 2:14.
27. Nezhat F, Nezhat C, Nezhat CH, et al. Use of laparoscopic ultrasonography to detect ovarian remnants. *J Ultrasound Med* 1996; 15:487.
28. Hurst BS, Tucker KE, Awoniyi CA, Schlaff WD. Endoscopic ultrasound. A new instrument for laparoscopic surgery. *J Reprod Med* 1996; 41:67.
29. Weston, PV. A new clinch knot. *Obstet Gynecol* 1991; 78:144.
30. Clarke HC. Laparoscopy—new instruments for suturing and ligation. *Fertil Steril* 1972; 23:274.
31. Dunlap KD, Wanzwe L. Is the robotic arm a cost effective surgical tool? *American Opertaing Room Nurses J* 1998; 68:265.
32. Mettler L, Ibrahim M, Jonar W. One year experience working with the aid of a robotic assistant (the voice controlled optic holder, AESOP) in gynecological endoscopic surgery. *Hum Reprod* 1998; 13:2748.
33. Berguer R, Rab GT, Abu-Ghaida H, et al. A comparison of surgeon's posture during laparoscopic and open surgical procedures. *Surg Endosc* 1997; 11:139.
34. Nezhat C, et al. Reduce fatigue and discomfort: Tips to improve operating room set-up. *Laparosc Surg Update* 1997; 5:97.

4

Lasers in Endoscopic Surgery

Often called "the light that heals," the surgical laser was described in 1969 by Fox.[1] In 1979, Bruhat and associates[2] and Tadir and colleagues[3] used the CO_2 laser in laparoscopic gynecologic operations.[2–6] Nezhat and coworkers[7,8] coined the term *videolaseroscopy*. Although lasers have not replaced the scalpel or electrosurgery, they play an important role in selected gynecologic operations. In this chapter, the relevant physics of the various lasers and their clinical applications are reviewed.

Physical Properties

Laser is an acronym for *l*ight *a*mplification by *s*timulated *e*mission of *r*adiation. A laser is a device that produces and amplifies light energy to create intense, coherent electromagnetic radiation. Unlike the ionizing radiation of x-rays and gamma rays that results from nuclear destruction, the energy emitted by laser results from the release of photons. This process occurs when stimulated electrons circling their nuclei return from their "excited" (E2) state to their "resting" (E1) state (E2 − E1 = photon) (Figure 4-1). When they interact with tissue, these intermediate-energy photons induce molecular vibration, break chemical bonds, and create heat. Although laser light is powerful and penetrating, it is neither mutagenic nor carcinogenic, with the exception of ultraviolet lasers (krypton-fluoride excimer laser). Each lasing substance has a unique atomic or molecular structure with its characteristic electron orbits. The wavelength and frequency of emitted photons are unique and uniform for each substance [CO_2, potassium titanyl phosphate (KTP), argon, etc.] (Figure 4-2). Laser light is monochromatic, consisting of a single wavelength that cannot be separated into other components. Regular light can be separated into the colors of the spectrum as it passes through a prism. When all the light waves are in phase with each other, they are coherent. The light is collimated when all waves are parallel. Lasers are focused precisely by lenses into a very small spot because the light waves of lasers have the same length, are in phase with each other, and always run parallel. They can develop a high power density (Figure 4-3, A and B).

Power Density

The amount of power delivered by lasers is measured in watts. It is adjusted at various settings by turning the power dial on the machine. The penetrating power of the laser ascertained by the power density depends mostly on the diameter of the laser beam affecting the tissue. The power density is related directly to the wattage but inversely related to the square of the spot size. This relationship is illustrated by the following formula:

$$\text{Power density (W/cm}^2) = \frac{\text{W} \times 100}{\text{Spot diameter}^2\ \text{(mm)}}$$

As a laser beam strikes tissue, the cells at the site of impact are heated rapidly and are vaporized, ablated, or coagulated, depending on the power density. Power densities less than 200 W/cm^2 result in surface heating and serosal contraction. Such lower-power densities are used to coagulate superficial endometriosis on bowel serosa or evert the ampullary stoma during salpingostomy. Power densities between 1200 and 4000 W/cm^2 result in

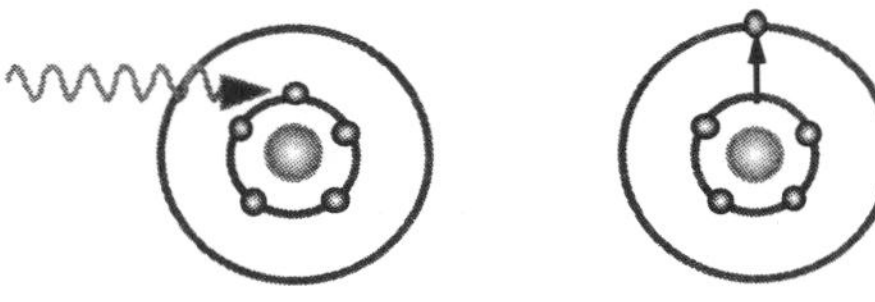

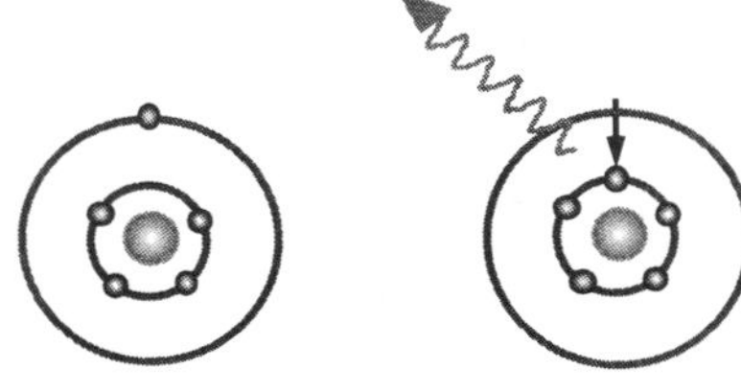

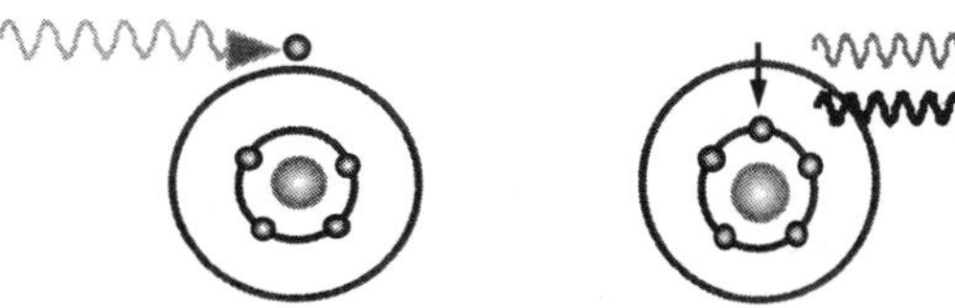

Figure 4-1. Laser energy results from the release of photons when electrons return from their "excited" phase to their "resting" phase during stimulated emission.

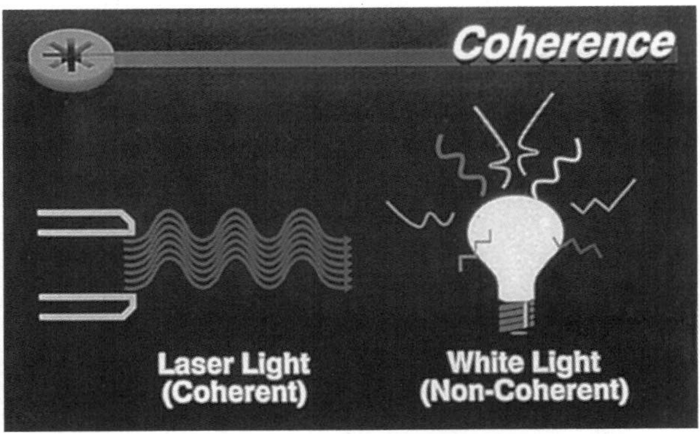

A

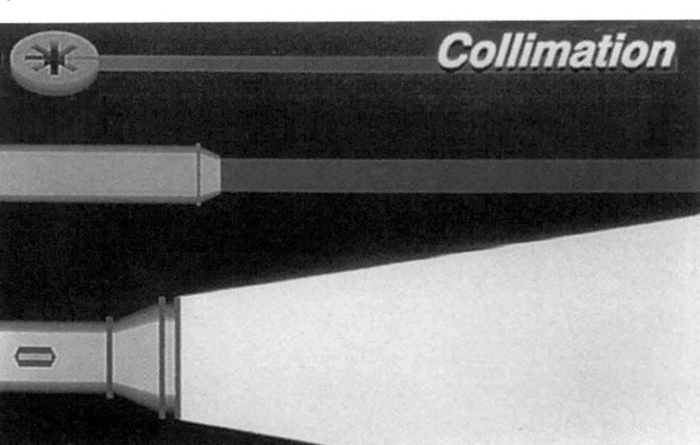

B

Figure 4-3. **A.** Laser light waves are the same length (coherent), unlike white light (noncoherent). **B.** Laser light waves are collimated and are focused by lenses into a very precise spot.

wide vaporization and less hemostasis. Power densities greater than 4000 W/cm^2 result in rapid, narrow vaporization with minimal coagulation or thermal damage.

Although these general guidelines for power densities and tissue effects were developed for the CO_2 laser,[9] they are applied to electrosurgery, radiosurgery, and other types of lasers.

Tissue Effects

The other major determinants of tissue effects include the degree to which each laser is absorbed, refracted, or reflected by the impacted tissue. For

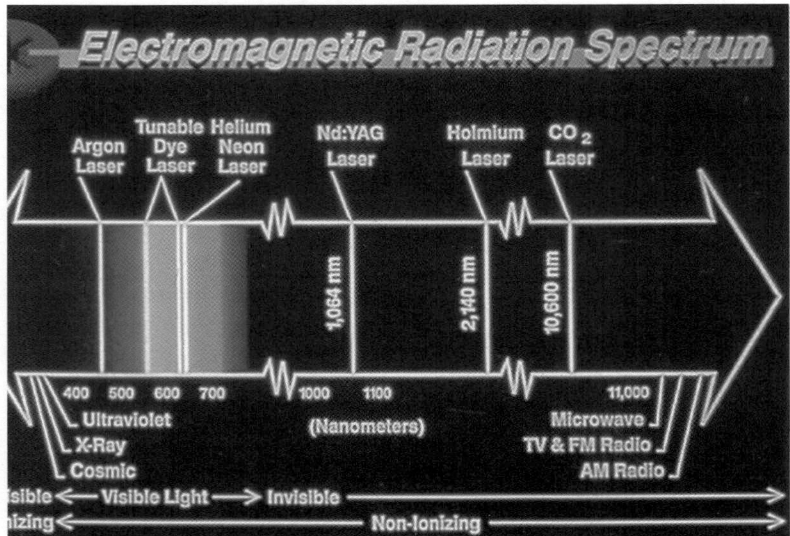

Figure 4-2. Laser light is unique and uniform, unlike regular light, which is divided into the colors of the spectrum.

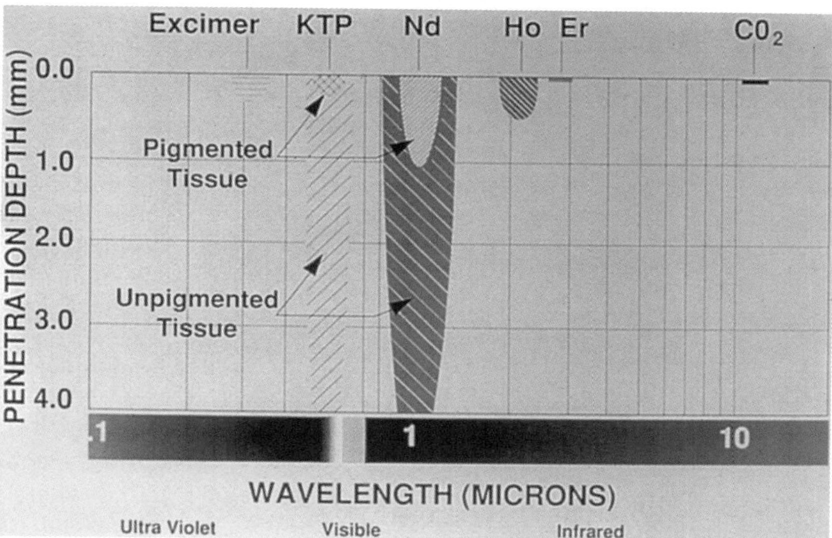

Figure 4-4. Argon, KTP, and Nd : YAG lasers are absorbed by pigmented tissues containing hemoglobin and pass through water and clear tissues.

example, the CO_2 laser is not color-dependent and is absorbed by water. Since tissue is mostly water, all tissues despite their color will absorb laser energy, boil, and vaporize immediately. Argon, KTP, and neodymium: yttrium aluminum garnet (Nd:YAG) lasers are absorbed by pigmented tissues that contain hemoglobin but are not absorbed. They penetrate deeply through water and clear tissues (Figure 4-4) and vaporize tissue less efficiently.[5] These lasers are better for coagulating bleeding esophageal varices[10] and ablating pigmented tissue such as endometrium[11] and vascular tumors.[12] Regular or silica fibers that are similar to the commercial fibers widely used in communications technology can deliver laser with practically no loss of the energy introduced. Such lasers have been applied to coagulate bleeding vessels on the retina without affecting the clear structures in front of it. The lasers commonly used in gynecologic procedures, their physical properties, and their tissue effects are listed in Table 4-1.

Laser Components

The basic components of lasers consist of a pumping system, the lasing medium, the optical cavity, and the operating system. The pumping system is the power source that energizes the atoms or molecules of the lasing medium to higher energy states. The ultimate power source of all lasers is the electrical outlet, which either stimulates the lasing medium directly or induces electrochemical reactions. The energy is pumped into the lasing medium to stimulate its electrons to higher energy levels.

The lasing medium consists of a selected assembly of atoms, molecules, or ions that are distributed in a solid crystal matrix (ruby, Nd:YAG), a gas (CO_2, helium-neon), or a liquid (organic dye lasers). Each lasing substance has a unique atomic or molecular structure with characteristic electron orbits and energy levels.

The optical cavity (resonator cavity) consists of a tube with parallel mirrors on either side that

TABLE 4-1. Physical Properties and Characteristics of Surgical Lasers

Type of Laser	CO_2	Argon	KTP	Nd:YAG
Wavelength (μm)	10.6	0.458–0.515	0.532	1.064
Color	Mid-infrared	Blue-green	Green	Near infrared
Delivery	Air or endoguide	Fiber	Fiber	Fiber
Absorption	All tissues and fluid	Color-dependent	Color-dependent	Color-dependent
Pass through fluids	No	Yes	Yes	Yes
Cutting	Excellent	Good	Good	Good
Coagulation	Fair	Good	Good	Excellent

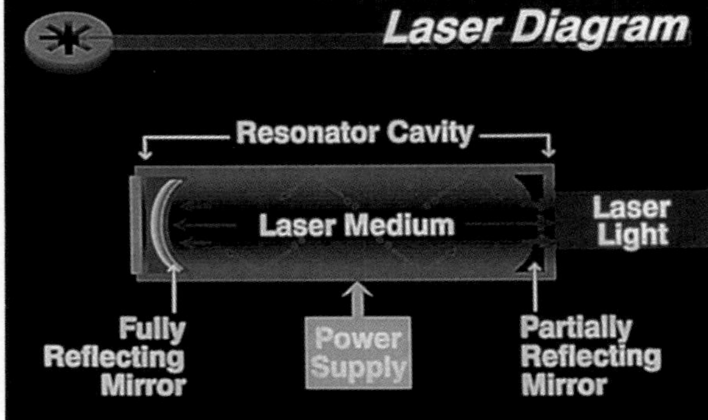

Figure 4-5. The resonator cavity of a laser consists of one reflective mirror and one partially reflective mirror to reflect the photons. This produces stimulated emission and lets coherent and collimated photons escape, creating the laser energy.

allow continuous reflection of photons back and forth in all directions as they strike other excited atoms to effect "stimulated emission of radiation" (Figure 4-5). At one end of the optical cavity, the mirror is partially reflective to allow the escape of photons that are in phase (coherent) and are traveling in the same parallel direction (collimated). As the photons repeatedly are reflected back and forth between the parallel mirrors of the optical cavity, the intensity of the laser beam inside the cavity builds. The small portion of the beam that is transmitted through the partially reflective mirror provides the laser energy for surgery.

Laser Energy

The operating system controls the delivery of laser energy to the tissue. It determines the power in watts and the mode in which the laser is delivered from the unit. Power is adjusted by the power control knob. The mode of delivery of laser energy is continuous, pulsed, superpulsed, or ultrapulsed. In the continuous mode, the laser energy is delivered to the tissue without interruption since the control pedal remains depressed. The pulsed mode is in single or repeated pulses (Figure 4-6). With single pulses, the operating system releases one burst of energy for a specified interval (range, 0.05 to 0.5 second) with every depression of the pedal. To discharge a second laser pulse, the pedal is released and depressed again. The single-pulse mode produces a controlled, precise penetration of the laser beam. It is used by surgeons to ablate endometriosis over the bowel to avoid perforating it and on the pelvic side wall to avoid perforating the blood vessels and ureter. The repeat-pulse mode delivers intermittent bursts of the laser beam of predetermined width and intervals (number of pulses per second), since the pedal remains depressed.

The superpulse mode of the CO_2 laser releases rapid pulses at short intervals alternating with refractory short periods when the laser energy is not delivered. During the pulse, the peak power is high (up to 10 times the continuous output). Through the release of "bursts" of peak power, the power density is increased fourfold or more over the

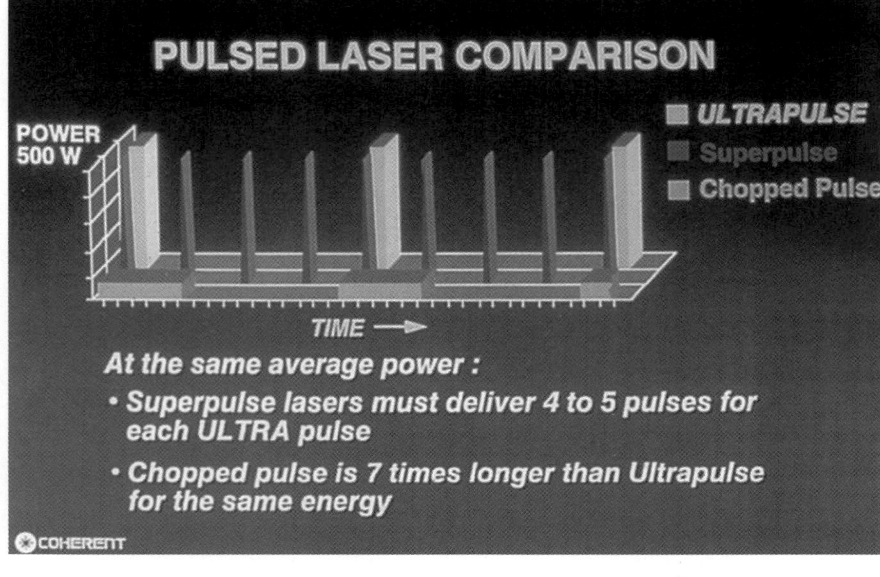

Figure 4-6. Comparison of ultrapulse, superpulse, and chopped pulse modes.

average obtainable with a continuous mode. The refractory periods between pulses of laser output allow heat dissipation and prevent heat buildup in adjacent tissue, reducing thermal injury. Use of the superpulse mode results in precise and rapid vaporization with decreased tissue desiccation, carbonization, thermal injury, and smoke plume. Although the same tissue effects can be obtained by using the continuous mode, this usually is impractical. The continuous mode is delivered in a small spot with high power density, and the resulting rapid tissue vaporization is difficult to control. The benefit of the superpulse mode is that it allows the use of the high power density necessary for tissue vaporization and minimal thermal damage at a controlled rate of delivery. Baggish and Elbakry[13] found in animal studies that pulse durations between 0.6 and 0.2 millisecond, at rates below 700 pulses per second, allow effective ablation with minimal thermal injury. For the superpulse mode, it is recommended that the pulse duration be less than 0.6 millisecond and the frequency be approximately 300 pulses per second. Superpulse lasers can be effective when used with spot sizes smaller than 0.75 mm. With larger spot sizes, increasing tissue desiccation, carbonization, and thermal injury will more likely occur. The superpulse mode cannot sustain the high power density long enough in a single pulse to vaporize all the tissue exposed to the larger spot. In endoscopy, the full advantages of the superpulse mode cannot be obtained, because the spot sizes are too large (typically 1.0 to 1.5 mm).

Ultrapulse mode for the CO_2 laser was introduced by Coherent Inc.[14] and delivers pulses with the highest power density available for laparoscopy. These high power densities are desirable whenever thermal tissue injury should be reduced and the coagulation effects of the laser are not important. The ultrapulse mode displays both the average power output of the laser and the energy delivered in each pulse (Figure 4-7). The pulse energy is related to the peak power in the pulse and the pulse duration. It determines the amount of tissue each pulse can vaporize. High pulse energy means that the laser can sustain high peak power long enough to vaporize all the tissue exposed by a larger spot. The ultrapulse mode delivers up to five times more energy per pulse than does the conventional superpulse mode. This feature allows clean tissue vaporization with decreased tissue desiccation, carbonization, and thermal injury. For example, 200 mJ per pulse can ablate spot sizes up to 2.5 mm. The ultrapulse mode provides separate controls for adjusting pulse energy and average power, allowing the surgeon to control the laser–tissue response at different operating speeds (Figure 4-8). By lowering the pulse energy, the surgeon can increase hemostasis by increasing the amount of thermal injury. The pulse energy reaching the tissue remains constant at different average power settings. The ultrapulse mode can produce char-free tissue ablation at slow working speeds with low average power and at rapid working speeds with high average power. This feature gives the surgeon a new level of control.

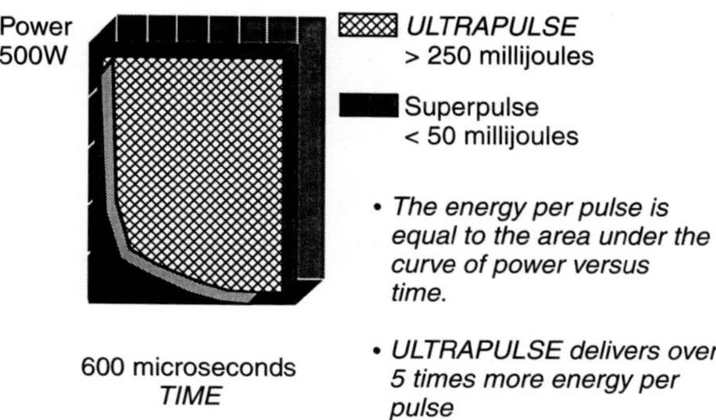

Figure 4-7. Pulse energy, ultrapulse, and superpulse modes are compared.

A problem associated with delivery of the CO_2 laser through the operating channel of the laparoscope is thermal blooming. When it is used through the operative channel of the laparoscope, the CO_2 laser energy is absorbed by the CO_2 insufflation gas in the channel (Figure 4-9A). This causes the CO_2 laser spot size to increase and reduces the transmitted energy by up to 30 to 60% at high power settings (Figure 4-9B). The "blooming effect" at high power settings (20 to 100 W) can provide effective coagulation. However, the larger spot size decreases precision and results in more

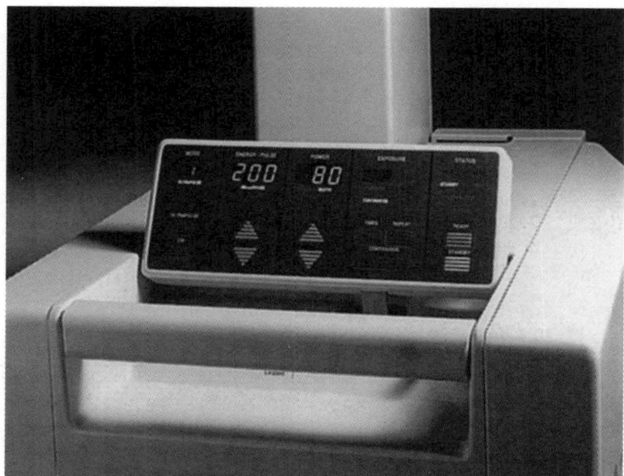

Figure 4-8. Control panel for ultrapulse mode.

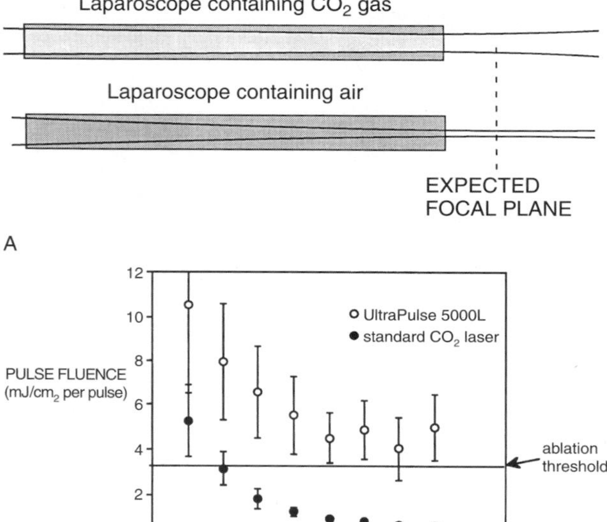

Figure 4-9. **A.** When used in the laparoscope, the CO_2 insufflation gas in the chamber absorbs the CO_2 laser energy and is heated, causing the "thermal blooming" effect. **B.** The increase in spot size reduces transmitted energy up to 30 to 60% at high power settings.

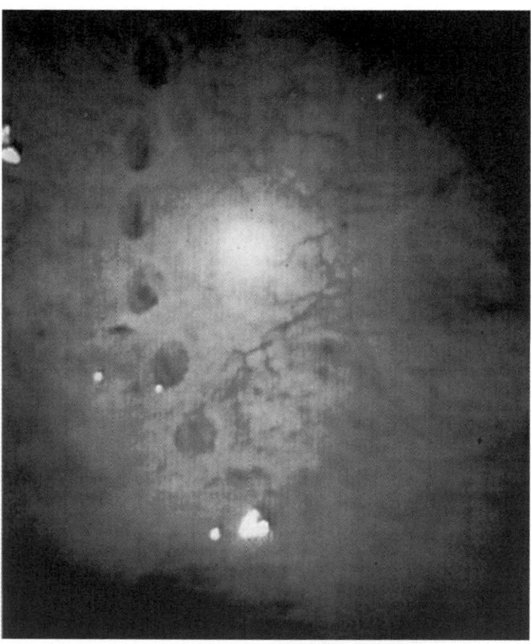

Figure 4-10. The new ultrapulse laser eliminates the thermal blooming effect and side effects such as the formation of charred tissue.

carbonization and thermal damage. The new ultrapulse laser eliminates the "thermal blooming" problem. This laser uses the carbon-13 isotope in the laser gas mix instead of the carbon-12 isotope used in conventional CO_2 lasers and CO_2 insufflation gas. No noticeable effect on tissue attributable to distortion or power loss from absorption in the insufflation gas has been noted. The surgeon can work with the least formation of charred tissue (Figure 4-10).

One study compared the tissue effects of a standard laser (Ultrapulse 5000) with those of a new design (Ultrapulse 5000L) that utilizes a different carbon isotope (carbon 13) on the rat uterine horn. When CO_2 was used as the insufflating gas, the Ultrapulse 5000L laser was associated with significantly deeper lesions compared with the Ultrapulse 5000 system.[15] The width of total injury and the thermal damage zone were significantly smaller with the former laser. The adverse effects on the CO_2 laser beam and the resultant altered tissue effects that occur in a regular CO_2 environment are avoided with the use of the Ultrapulse 5000L or an air environment. Clinical studies also suggest that the isotopic $^{13}CO_2$ laser for laparoscopic evaporation can be more efficient than other modalities in treating infertile women with minimal to mild endometriosis in terms of pregnancy rates.[16]

Delivery Systems

The CO_2 laser beam leaves the optical resonator and is delivered to the end of an articulated arm by several specially coated mirrors that are aligned to preserve the pattern and power of the beam as it leaves the generator (Figure 4-11). Since the CO_2 laser beam is invisible, a visible, low-power helium neon (He:Ne) laser beam is provided as an aiming beam. At the output of the arm, the CO_2

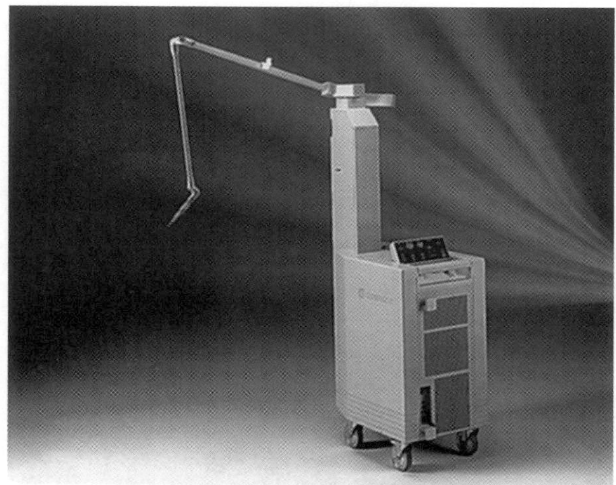

Figure 4-11. The CO_2 laser generator and articulated arm.

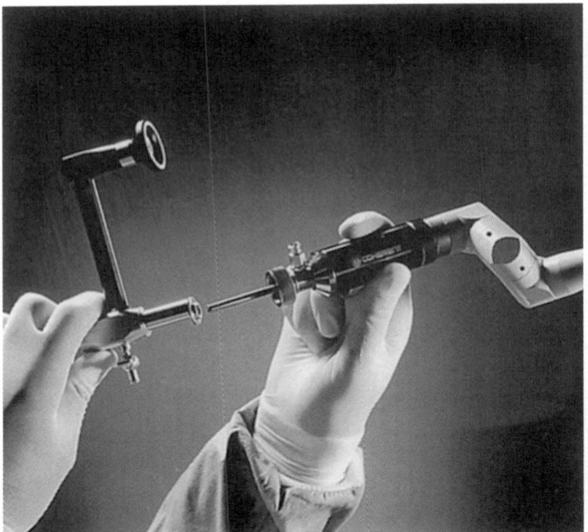

Figure 4-12. The coupling lens is assembled between the arm of the laser and the laparoscope.

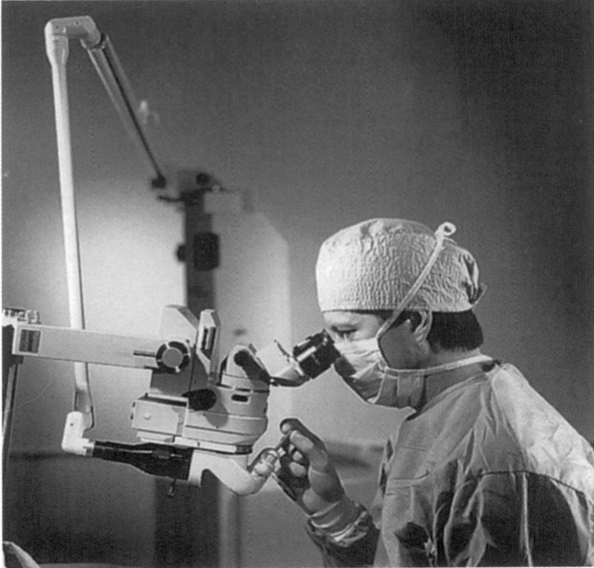

Figure 4-13. A laser coupler with a multiple lens system allows the surgeon to focus and defocus the laser beam by turning a knob on the coupler.

laser and the He:Ne beams are composed of parallel waves that need to be focused to increase power density. Coupling lenses of various focal lengths are used to focus the beams at the end of the hand-held probe or laparoscope. One type of coupling lens is a fixed lens that easily is assembled between the arm of the laser and the laparoscope (Figure 4-12). Its focal length is set at 28 cm if the laser is delivered through the operating channel of the laparoscope; it is set at 18 cm if the laser is delivered through a second puncture site to focus at the end of the shorter accessory trocar. In laparoscopic procedures, the focal point is usually 2.0 cm from the tip of the laparoscope.

The Coupler System

Instead of a fixed lens, laser couplers can have a multiple lens system with variable focal lengths, allowing the surgeon to focus and defocus the laser beam and change the spot size by turning a knob on the coupler (Figure 4-13). This system allows the spot size to vary 0.5 and 2.0 mm in diameter.

The quality of the CO_2 laser output depends on the proper alignment of the directing mirrors in the articulated arm of the laser, the quality and performance of the coupling lens, and the integrity of the operative channel of the laparoscope. A disturbance in any of these systems results in poor beam alignment and loss of laser power. Manufacturers continually improve the design and stability of the laser, articulated arm, and laparoscope coupling system. Laparoscope couplers such as the Coherent-Nezhat laparoscope coupler eliminate a major source of alignment error by aligning the laser beam directly with the operating channel of the laparoscope. Rigid wave guides have been developed to guide the focused laser beam from the articulated arm through the operative channel of the laparoscope or through a second puncture site. The beam exits the wave guide in perfect focus and close to the tissue. Rigid wave guides are composed of ceramics with a low index of refraction so that high power densities are transmitted with less than a 10% power loss. A purge of continuous carbon dioxide of up to 1000 mL/min flows down the wave guide channel to keep it cool and clear of smoke. This carbon dioxide serves as an additional source of insufflation to replace the gas evacuated with suctioning of the smoke.

Fiber Delivery System

The availability of fiber delivery systems is a major advantage of the argon, KTP and Nd:YAG lasers. These quartz fibers are flexible, light, and thin. They can be delivered at a greater distance from the laser generator than is the case with the CO_2 laser, which needs to be close to the operative field because of its short articulated arm. The laser beam is at maximal focus at the tip of the fiber, which delivers the laser with or without contact with the tissue. When the diameter of the fiber or the distance between the fiber and the impacted tissue is varied, the power density of argon and KTP lasers may be adjusted to vaporize, ablate, or coagulate. The Nd:YAG laser can be modified with sapphire tips to effect coagulation or vaporization.

Fiberoptics

Besides providing a delivery system for the laser beam, fiberoptics will be used in the future to monitor laser surgery. Sensor data can be returned to console computers for an analysis of tissue effects through the same fiberoptic bundles that are used to deliver the beam. This type of back-and-forth transmission of light is commonplace in the communications industry and can make laser application in surgery safer and more useful. Thermal sensing feedback devices, as well as acoustic and shock-wave sensing detectors, using fiberoptic two-way transmission are under development. Spectroscopic diagnosis using laser-induced fluorescence spectra at multiple excitation wavelengths has been employed in vivo for diagnosing cervical intraepithelial neoplasia (CIN).[17] The use of similar fluorescence markers may aid future laparoscopic macroscopic observation of small nodules of endometriosis or metastatic ovarian cancer.[18]

Lasers in Gynecology

The major lasers used in surgery are the CO_2, argon, KTP-532, and Nd:YAG. New types of lasers include the holmium:YAG (Ho:YAG) laser. It has been used for ovarian wedge resection and has been found to be a fiberoptic-compatible hemostatic laser that causes fewer adhesions than do scalpel, electrosurgery, Nd:YAG, Er:YAG, and continuous CO_2 lasers.[19] The pulsed Ho:YAG laser (wavelength, 2100 nm) is effective for endoscopic treatment of urinary[20] and biliary[21] calculi. The mechanism of action of the Ho:YAG laser is the generation of a gas plasma at the stone–fluid interface, causing a shock wave. The VersaPulse combination holmium:YAG/Nd:YAG laser (Coherent Inc.) is effective and versatile in the treatment of urolithiasis.[22] Holmium lasers are used for resection of the prostate, using a standard 550-μm end-firing fiber.[23] The most fascinating use so far of the Ho:YAG laser is for direct myocardial revascularization (DMR). This technique, either surgical or catheter-based, uses lasers to create channels between ischemic myocardium and the left ventricular cavity to improve perfusion and decrease angina.[24] This technique can be used to deliver medication to damaged tissue. Candidates include patients with chronic, severe, refractory angina and those who are unable to undergo conventional surgical revascularization or angioplasty because remaining conduits or acceptable target vessels are lacking. Although the mechanism of action of DMR is not known, several theories have been proposed, including laser-induced triggering of neovascularization and neural destruction.[25]

The erbium (Er):YAG laser, with its pulsed 2.94-μm radiation and maximal water absorption, is a new versatile instrument for microsurgical applications. It has been introduced for laser resurfacing of the facial skin.[26] The U.S. Food and Drug Administration cleared the Er:YAG to be used as a dental drill for caries removal and cavity preparation.[27] A flexible wave guide has been developed for Er:YAG laser radiation delivery.[28]

Developmental work involves the use of the krypton lasers, excimer lasers, tunable optical parametric oscillator laser systems, ultrashort pulsed lasers, free electron lasers, and tunable lasers that may have surgical applications in the future.

Carbon Dioxide Laser

The carbon dioxide laser was the first laser used in gynecology. The CO_2 laser emits photons with a wavelength of 10.6-μm that is within the infrared portion of the electromagnetic spectrum. Since it cannot be seen, it is delivered with the visible He:Ne laser serving as the aiming beam. The CO_2 laser has high power density and efficiency and is ideal for cutting and vaporizing. It is absorbed by nonreflective solids and liquids, is not dependent on the color of tissue for absorption, and is not scattered from the target point. The impact of the laser is limited to the target tissue, sparing adjacent tissue layers. The CO_2 laser cannot be delivered through fluids and is a poor coagulator. It can be delivered quite efficiently by a few types of hollow flexible plastic wave guides used as replacements for arms and external applicators.[29,30] The wave guide delivery system offers a fair alternative to reflective mirrors. When the output wattage or the diameter of the laser spot is varied, a large range of power densities is available with the CO_2 laser. Low power densities are used for the cervix and myomas where hemostasis is important and thermal damage is not a major concern. High power densities are preferred for reconstructive adnexal operations in which thermal damage must be reduced.

The most effective use of the CO_2 laser beam is through the operative channel of the laparoscope as a "long knife"; the beam does not obstruct the view and works well for delicate dissections. The CO_2 laser is stopped by water as a backstop. This characteristic of the CO_2 laser gives it high precision for dissection in sensitive areas such as the bowel, bladder, ureter, and blood vessels. The low morbidity and absence of mortality in more than 6000 advanced operative laparoscopic procedures is attributed in part to this characteristic.

When it is used in a laparotomy, the CO_2 laser is delivered with a hand-held probe or is attached to the operating microscope. The former method has the advantage of a shorter focal distance and a smaller spot size, resulting in greater power density. Greater power density produces higher penetrating power and less thermal damage to the adjoining normal tissue. The hand-held probe is subject to hand tremor and less accurate beam delivery. Attaching the laser to the microscope increases precision because of the magnification and the absence of hand tremor; as a result of the longer focal length, the spot size is larger. With more precise lasers, high power density is achievable through the laparoscope.

Lasers Delivered by Fibers

The argon and KTP-532 lasers are similar in their characteristics and clinical applications. They have similar wavelengths of 0.458 to 0.515 and 0.532-μm, respectively. Both release a visible green light that travels through clear fluids and is absorbed by darkly pigmented tissue. They are delivered through flexible fibers, making them suitable for endoscopic use. Since they are not absorbed by clear fluids or unpigmented tissue, these lasers are ideal for coagulation for ablation of peritoneal endometriosis in which tissue coagulation is effected without disrupting the normal tissue. The argon laser is available in two models, 5 W and 16 W, for abdominal and pelvic operations. The more powerful model is preferred for reconstructive operations and ablation of endometriosis. This model requires high electrical current energy, three phases, and more than 200 V at 60 A. The laser fibers range in size from 300 to 600-μm in diameter. They are introduced through the small channels of the operating laparoscope or ancillary trocars and steered toward the target with special bridges. The laser beam is focused at the tip of the fiber. As the distance from the tissue is increased, the spot size increases (the beam diffuses) and the power density diminishes. Besides protective goggles for the specific laser wavelength through the laparoscope, the operator can cover the eyepiece of the laparoscope with the "monoshutter," an electronically triggered eyepiece that attaches to the laparoscope and interposes a protective filter between the operator's eye and the laparoscope when the laser is fired. The monoshutter is used with video cameras for video surgery and documentation.

Nd : YAG laser

The Nd : YAG laser is a crystal laser with an infrared wavelength of 1.064-μm in the near infrared spectrum. This laser is invisible, highly color dependent, and transmitted through fibers and clear fluids. It penetrates deeply into tissue (~1.6 cm), an advantage in coagulating tumors, hemorrhaging ulcers, and endometrial ablation. Although it is an excellent coagulator, the Nd : YAG laser cuts poorly unless it is used with sapphire tips. The sapphire tips completely absorb the laser energy, reaching very high temperatures, resulting in a "hot tip" for cutting. This is not a good choice for reconstructive operations because of the large amount of scatter and excessive thermal damage to tissue.

Tissue Welding

Laser tissue welding is a technologic innovation that is beginning to move from the theoretical laboratory environment to the reality of clinical application.[31] Significant advances have been made with the development of exogenous chromophobe-containing solders.[31] Successful tissue approximation can be done using low-power laser energy combined with human albumin solder.[32] The combination of 1.32-μm laser light and 50% human albumin solder has been shown to create a deep tissue weld that results in higher acute repair tensile strength. This may allow a deep to superficial closure of wounds, resulting in an optimal method of acute closure for full-thickness wounds.[32,33]

Collagen solid-matrix patches have been used as a biologic solder in laser tissue welding. They were compared with an albumin liquid solder for the repair of arteriotomies in an in vitro porcine model. Although the solder and the patches yielded similar acute weld strengths, the solid-matrix patches facilitated the welding process and provided consistently strong welds.[34]

Laser welding, fibrin glue, and a mechanical suturing device (Endo-Stitch) were evaluated as alternatives to standard laparoscopic suturing with a free needle.[35] All the alternative laparoscopic ureteral closure methods compared favorably with standard free-needle suturing.

Tissue welding using human albumin solders may be improved by including growth factors such as exogenous bioactivation agents. Another approach to improving the efficacy of laser welding has been based on developing feedback and endpoint measurement techniques. For instance, an optical closed-loop temperature feedback control has been studied in rat femoral artery anastomoses with regard to improved patency, aneurysm rate, and histologically proved limited thermal damage. Temperature-controlled 1.9-μm laser soldering with optical feedback was found to improve the outcome in microvascular anastomosis by reducing transmural thermal injury caused by variations in surgical technique.[36]

Summary

Lasers, with some exceptions, do not touch tissue. The depth of the incision is controlled by the power density and the amount of time the laser is focused on one spot. This "action at a distance" allows for greater accessibility to the target tissue and perhaps less tissue trauma. Each laser has unique properties and tissue effects determined by wavelength and tissue absorption. If one varies the power density or mode of delivery (sapphire tips, fiber diameter, etc.), desired tissue effects such as ablation, coagulation, and vaporization can be achieved.

References

1. Fox G. The use of laser radiation as a surgical "light knife." *J Surg Res* 1969; 9:199.
2. Bruhat H, Mage C, Manhes M. Use of the CO_2 laser via laparoscopy, in Kaplan I, ed., *Laser Surgery III. Proceedings of the Third International Society for Laser Surgery*. Tel Aviv: Ot-Paz, 1979.
3. Tadir Y, Ovadia J, Zuckerman Z, et al. Laparoscopic application of the CO_2 laser, in *Proceedings of the 4th Congress of International Society for Laser Surgery*. Tokyo: Japanese Society for Laser Medicine, 1981.
4. Nezhat C, Crowgey S, Garrison C. Surgical treatment of endometriosis via laser laparoscopy. *Fertil Steril* 1986; 6:778.
5. Luciano AA, Frishman GN, Kratka SA, et al. A comparative analysis of adhesion reduction, tissue effects and incising characteristics of electrosurgery, CO_2 laser and Nd-Yag laser at operative laparoscopy: An animal study. *J Laparoendosc Surg* 1992; 2:287.
6. Nezhat C, Winer WK, Nezhat F. A comparison of the CO_2, argon, and KTP/532 laser in the videolaseroscopic treatment of endometriosis. *Colposc Gynecol Laser Surg* 1988; 4:41.
7. Nezhat C. Videolaseroscopy: A new modality for the treatment of endometriosis and other diseases of reproductive organs. *Colposc Gynecol Laser Surg* 1986; 2:221.
8. Nezhat C, Crowgey S, Nezhat F. Videolaseroscopy for the treatment of endometriosis associated with infertility. *Fertil Steril* 1989; 512:23.
9. Martin DC. Tissue effects of lasers. *Semin Reprod Endocrinol* 1991; 9:118.
10. Puliafito C. *Lasers in Surgery and Medicine: Principles and Practice*. New York: Wiley-Liss, 1996.
11. Keye W, Hansen LW, Astin M, et al. Argon laser therapy of endometriosis: A review of 92 consecutive patients. *Fertil Steril* 1987; 47:208.
12. Joffe SN, Brackett KA, Sankar MY, et al. Resection of the liver with Nd:Yag laser. *Surg Gynecol Obstet* 1986; 163:437.
13. Baggish MS, Elbakry MM. Comparison of electronic superpulsed and continuous wave CO_2 laser on the rabbit uterine horn. *Fertil Steril* 1986; 45:20.
14. Nezhat C, Nezhat F. Laparoscopic surgery with a new tuned high-energy pulsed CO_2 laser. *J Gynecol Surg* 1992; 8:251.
15. Yarali H, Gomel V, Koop D, Jetha N. A new type of CO_2 laser avoids power density loss due to absorption and the blooming effect by the CO_2 gas environment. *Hum Reprod* 1996; 11:677.
16. Chang FH, Chou HH, Soong YK, et al. Efficacy of isotopic $13CO_2$ laser laparoscopic evaporation in the treatment of infertile patients with minimal and mild endometriosis: A life table cumulative pregnancy rates study. *J Am Assoc Gynecol Laparosc* 1997; 4:219.
17. Ramanujam N, Mitchell MF, Mahadevan A, et al. Spectroscopic diagnosis of cervical intraepithelial neoplasia (CIN) in vivo using laser-induced fluorescence spectra at multiple excitation wavelengths. *Lasers Surg Med* 1996; 19:63.
18. Hornung R, Major AL, McHale M, et al. In vivo detection of metastatic ovarian cancer by means of 5-aminolevulinic acid-induced fluorescence in a rat model. *J Am Assoc Gynecol Laparosc* 1998; 5:141.

19. Bhatta N, Isaacson K, Flotte T, et al. Injury and adhesion formation following ovarian wedge resection with different thermal surgical modalities. *Lasers Surg Med* 1993; 13:344.
20. White MD, Moran ME, Calvano CJ, et al. Evaluation of retropulsion caused by holmium:YAG laser with various power settings and fibers. *J Endourol* 1998; 12:183.
21. Das AK, Chiura A, Conlin MJ, et al. Treatment of biliary calculi using holmium: yttrium aluminum garnet laser. *Gastrointest Endosc* 1998; 48:207.
22. Gould DL. Holmium : YAG laser and its use in the treatment of urolithiasis: Our first 160 cases. *J Endourol* 1998; 12:23.
23. Matsuoka K, Iida S, Tomiyasu K, et al. Holmium laser resection of the prostate. *J Endourol* 1998; 12:279.
24. Kornowski R, Hong MK, Leon MB. Current perspectives on direct myocardial revascularization. *Am J Cardiol* 1998; 81:44.
25. Mueller XM, Tevaearai HH, Genton CY, et al. Transmyocardial laser revascularisation in acutely ischaemic myocardium. *Eur J Cardiothorac Surg* 1998; 13:170.
26. Perez MI, Bank DE, Silvers D. Skin resurfacing of the face with the Erbium:YAG laser. *Dermatol Surg* 1998; 24:653.
27. Pelagalli J, Gimbel CB, Hansen RT, et al. Investigational study of the use of Er:YAG laser versus dental drill for caries removal and cavity preparation—phase I. *J Clin Laser Med Surg* 1977; 15:109.
28. Gannot I, Schrunder S, Dror J, et al. Flexible waveguides for Er-YAG laser radiation delivery. *IEEE Trans Biomed Eng* 1995; 42:967.
29. Gannot I, Dror J, Calderon S, et al. Flexible waveguides for IR laser radiation and surgery applications. *Lasers Surg Med* 1994; 14:184.
30. Gannot I, Inberg A, Oxman M, et al. Current status of flexible waveguides for infrared laser radiation transmission. *IEEE J Select Topics Quantum Electron* 1996; 880.
31. Scherr DS, Poppas DP. Laser tissue welding. *Urol Clin North Am* 1998; 25:123.
32. Wright EJ, Poppas DP. Effect of laser wavelength and protein solder concentration on acute tissue repair using laser welding: Initial results in a canine ureter Model. *Tech Urol* 1997; 3:176.
33. Massicotte JM, Stewart RB, Poppas DP. Effects of endogenous absorption in human albumin solder for acute laser wound closure. *Lasers Surg Med* 1998; 23:18.
34. Small W 4th, Heredia NJ, Maitland DJ, et al. Dye-enhanced protein solders and patches in laser-assisted tissue welding. *J Clin Laser Med Surg* 1997; 15:205.
35. Wolf JS Jr, Soble JJ, Nakada SY, et al. Comparison of fibrin glue, laser weld, and mechanical suturing device for the laparoscopic closure of ureterotomy in a porcine model. *J Urol* 1997; 157:1487.
36. Pohl D, Bass LS, Stewart R, Chiu DT. Effect of optical temperature feedback control on patency in laser-soldered microvascular anastomosis. *J Reconstr Microsurg* 1998; 14:23.

5

Electrosurgery

Electrosurgery was used initially during laparoscopy for tubal sterilization. A gynecologist can apply the basic principles of microsurgery and electrosurgery during laparoscopy to reconstruct fallopian tubes, resect ovarian cysts, or ablate endometriosis. If it is used incorrectly, serious complications can occur.[1] A survey of electrosurgical complications and surgical techniques during laparoscopy by the American College of Surgeons revealed that 18 percent of the 506 surgeons polled had noted an electrosurgical burn to a patient during laparoscopy.[2] Electrosurgery provides surgeons with options such as types of waveform, wattage, unipolar and bipolar systems, and various electrodes. The proper equipment and knowledge of electrosurgical principles are requirements for the safe use of electrosurgery. This chapter reviews the basic principles and clinical applications of electrosurgery.

Basic Terminology

Electrical energy results from the flow of electrons or current. *Ampere* (A) is the rate at which electrons flow; *volt* (V) is the unit of force (pressure) that drives electrons; *ohm* (Ω) is tissue resistance to the electrons; *watt* (W) is the amount of work produced. A current of 1 A is produced by 1 V applied across a resistance of 1 Ω (Table 5-1). A high impedance (resistance) of tissue to electron flow generates heat that boils (vaporizes) or denatures (coagulates) tissue. Wattage, the amount of work produced by the electron flow (current), is equal to volts multiplied by amperes. Voltage is measured by the electrosurgical generator, and resistance is measured in ohms in the tissue. It ranges from 100 to 1000 ohms and changes during the use of electrosurgery. With tissue coagulation, water evaporates from cells and results in tissue desiccation, leading to progressively increased resistance until current no longer flows. At this point, if a higher voltage is applied, the electrical energy seeks other outlets and sparking occurs. Under normal circumstances, a pressure of 15,000 V or more is required to cause sparking, that is, push electrons 1 cm in room air.[3,4] This is above the maximal voltage (peak to peak voltage) of 1200 V produced by the high-frequency electrogenerators currently recommended for laparoscopy by the U.S. Food and Drug Administration. With these generators, when the tissue resistance exceeds the driving force of 1200 V, flow stops provided that the desiccated tissue is not in contact with bowel, blood vessels, or ureter.

With direct current, electron flow is unidirectional, while the flow of electrons with alternating current is changing direction, increasing to a maximum in one direction. Then it drops to zero and increases to the maximum in the other direction, resulting in a waveform (Figure 5-1). The frequency with which the current changes direction (oscillation) is measured in hertz (Hz). Normal household current is 60 Hz, and nerves and muscles are stimulated by frequencies below 10,000 Hz. With electrosurgery, the alternating current must be converted into a higher frequency to avoid unwanted neuromuscular stimulation by a "step-up" transformer to increase the voltage and frequency (oscillation) of the electric circuit to between 500,000 and 4,000,000 Hz (Figure 5-2).

TABLE 5-1. Definitions of Electrical Terms

Term	Unit	Description
Current	Ampere (A)	Volume of electron flow per second
Voltage	Volt (V)	Force (pressure) driving the current
Resistance	Ohm (Ω)	Resistance (impedance) to flow
Power	Watt (W)	Amount of work produced by the flow

Since these frequencies are within the AM radio frequency range, the term *radiofrequency surgery* is used.

Types of Waveforms

Different electrical waveforms produce different tissue effects (Figure 5-3). A cutting current is a continuous high-frequency flow of electrons delivered from one peak polarity to the opposite peak without pausing at the zero polarity in the middle. Electrons are delivered constantly to tissue without interruption. Pure cutting, undamped current cuts through tissue by exploding the cells at their boiling point of 100°C (vaporization) without elevating tissue temperature to high levels, thus avoiding unintended thermal damage. It is similar to the superpulse delivery mode of the CO_2 laser. A coagulating or dampening current results when peak polarity alternates with zero polarity. Bursts of rapidly increasing current interrupted by intervals without current result in denaturation and dehydration with hemostasis and charring but no cutting. Many generators provide a blended current that combines undamped and damped waveforms where there is a continuous but altering waveform that will simultaneously cut and coagulate.

Unipolar and Bipolar Systems

In a unipolar system, current flows from the small electrode to the tissue being cut or coagulated, through the patient, and to a return electrode monitor (REM) attached to the buttock or leg. As the electrical energy spreads, the current density is diffused and the tissue under the return electrode is not heated. A situation that inadvertently concentrates electron flow results in tissue damage and is caused by an incompletely applied REM. Electrical injuries at the ground pad are avoided by employing generators with REMs. These circuits monitor the electrical contact between the pad and the skin, and if they are inadequate, the electrosurgical unit is deactivated.

A bipolar system does not require a REM, as only the small amount of tissue between the two

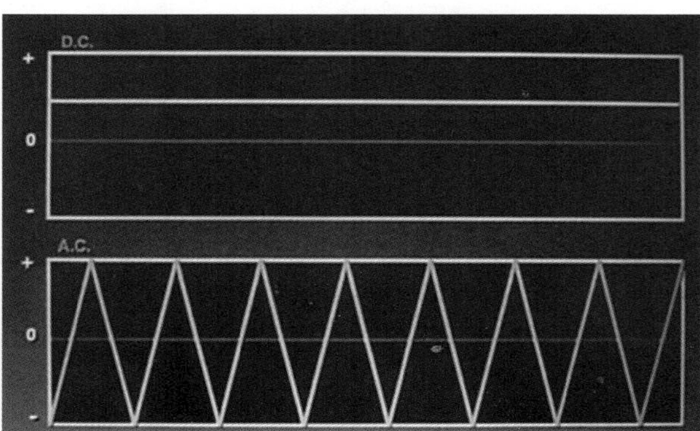

Figure 5-1. Current is either unidirectional (direct) or alternating.

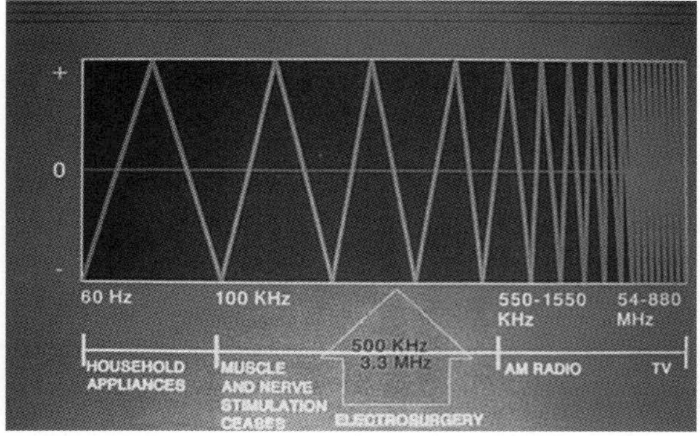

Figure 5-2. The frequency spectrum illustrates the variations in alternating current from household appliances to a television, with electrosurgery at the midpoint.

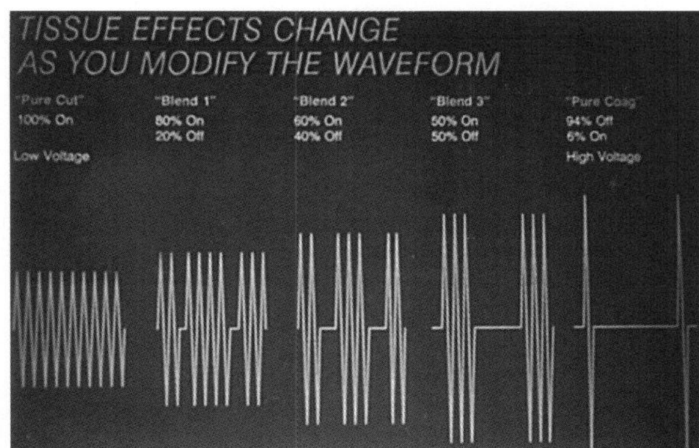

Figure 5-3. This diagram shows various modes of delivering electrical energy to tissue. At a fixed power setting, the voltage increases as the current flow interval decreases. The cutting current delivers the lowest voltage, is the least penetrating, and inflicts the least thermal damage.

electrodes is included in the circuit. With these forceps, one prong of the forceps is the active electrode and the other is the return electrode. Some heat is transmitted to the surrounding tissue. Bipolar coagulation requires that the tissue being coagulated be surrounded by the forceps, making the instrument more difficult to use with retracted vessels. Grasping tissue can coapt the walls of vessels before the current is passed, helping to seal the vessels. Bipolar current desiccates but does not cut tissue. As with unipolar systems, the tissue to be coagulated must not be in contact with other organs to avoid unintended thermal injury. During laparoscopy, the focus is on the target tissue and the tendency is to ignore vital structures that may be in physical (electrical) contact with the electrode. Bipolar forceps are safer than monopolar instruments. At present, bipolar current is used mainly for coagulation and desiccation, and its application is being incorporated rapidly into general operative laparoscopy.[5] Bipolar forceps will be capable of cutting and vaporizing tissue. A bipolar cutting forceps that includes a 5-mm version can function in both the locked mode and the manual mode. It provides effective bipolar coagulation and scalpel division of thick tissue with good hemostasis.[6]

The bipolar scissors is a safe device for laparoscopic tissue dissection and compares favorably with monopolar scissors.[7] Based on animal studies, the bipolar scissors cuts as well as does the monopolar scissors and causes less thermal injury.[8] These scissors offer safety advantages and equivalent or better performance compared with monopolar scissors in laparoscopic operations.

A feedback-controlled electrothermal sealer can apply a precise amount of energy and physical pressure and allows a brief cooling-down phase in compression.[9] In experimental animals and fresh abattoir vessels, it produced a distinctive translucent seal of partially denatured protein that could be transected after a single application. These seals have bursting strengths comparable to those of clips and ligatures and resist dislodgment because they are intrinsic to the vessel wall structure.[9] A commercial system utilizing this approach is available (Ligature Vessel Sealing System, Valleylab Inc., Boulder, CO) and includes a single-use laparoscopic instrument and a reusable gynecologic instrument for open procedures. This system allows fusion of the collagen in vessel walls to create a permanent seal without relying on a proximal thrombus. The seal that is created can withstand more than three times normal systolic pressure. It can be used with confidence on vessels up to 7 mm and causes minimal thermal spread and no charring. Visual assurance of a successful seal is given by tissue translucence that indicates no blood flow.

Capacitive Coupling

A capacitor is defined as two conductors separated by an insulator. During operative laparoscopy, the passage of electrosurgical energy into the abdomen requires a capacitor. The active electrode (a conductor) is surrounded by insulation (a nonconductor) that often is passed through a metal (conductive) cannula, creating a capacitor. A capacitor induces an electrical current into the metal cannula through the process of capacitance.

The phenomenon of capacitively coupled current consists of the inducement of currents through the intact insulation of active electrodes to the surrounding cannulas or instruments. Activating the generator in an open circuit increases the probability that capacitance will occur, and when the outer conductor (metal cannula or instrument) is isolated from the abdominal wall by a plastic nonconductor, the possibility for injury is increased. The smaller the cannula (5 mm compared to 10 mm) and the longer the active electrode, the greater the potential for capacitance. This capacitively coupled current wants to complete the circuit by finding a pathway to the patient return electrode. The electrical charge is stored in the metal cannula until the generator is deactivated or a pathway to complete the circuit presents itself. The amount of electrical energy induced through capacitance onto the metal cannula is dependent on whether the generator is started in an open circuit, in which case maximal voltage is created. Conversely, capacitance is small if the generator is begun in a closed circuit. As the active electrode touches or approaches the target tissue, the generator's output travels through the target tissue to the patient return electrode. Voltages remain lower, and the amount of capacitance remains low. Since cutting current uses less voltage, the amount of capacitively induced current is lower, and this waveform thus is used for vaporization and desiccation. High-voltage coagulation current is reserved for fulguration.

The cannula and trocar used influence the amount of capacitance produced and whether that capacitance can be dispersed. All metal is appropriate because capacitively induced currents are dispersed safely through the low current density provided by the abdominal wall. The surface area is adequate to dissipate any current buildup on the cannula without producing heat.

An all-plastic cannula system also is safe. When such a system is used, capacitance is eliminated. Instead of two conductors separated by a nonconductor, the conductive active electrode is covered by nonconductive insulation surrounded by the nonconductive cannula, and a capacitor no longer exists.

Capacitive coupling occurs when electrical energy is transferred from an insulated active electrode to nearby conductive material. A suction-irrigator serves as an effective capacitor (Figure 5-4). The electrical energy from the "insulated" electrode transfers to the surrounding suction-irrigator cannula. If the cannula is inserted through a metal trocar, the transferred energy disperses through the skin to the REM without causing injury. If the cannula is inserted through a plastic, nonconductive trocar, the transferred energy is not dispersed and thermal injury becomes possible. The capacitive effect is avoided by using metal (conductive) trocar sleeves or the electroshield monitor system. That system measures and shunts all capacitively coupled current back to the generator's return plate, avoiding transmission through the cannula to biologic tissue. If the electroshield cannot handle the capacitively coupled current, it automatically shuts off the generator.

Besides capacitive coupling, unintended electrical injuries result from direct coupling or insulation failure. Direct coupling of current refers to the unintended contact of the energized active electrode with another metal instrument or object within the abdomen. It occurs if the active electrode touches other metal instruments within the abdomen; energy is transferred to the second instrument, injuring tissue with which it comes in contact. For example, if the active electrode touches the laparoscope, the laparoscope can burn bowel or other juxtaposed organs. To avoid thermal damage from direct coupling, one should never energize the electrode until it is in full view and in contact with the intended target. Three potential problems arise from direct coupling of current. Metal-to-metal sparking causes unwanted heat production. Sparking to metal clips, for example, could cause necrosis of underlying tissue; clips fall off the vessels as the tissue begins to slough. Metal-to-metal sparking causes frequency demodulation that is noticed as neuromuscular stimulation of surrounding muscles. Metal-to-metal sparking causes current to flow to unintended sites. If the laparoscope is insulated from the abdominal wall by a plastic collar, the current is forced to find another point of exit from the laparoscope to complete the circuit. As in insulation failure, the determining factor regarding the amount of tissue damage (if any) is the amount of current density present. A large point of contact has low current density, and no tissue damage is expected. If the laparoscope touches a small amount of tissue, high current density occurs and tissue damage is possible. To avoid direct coupling,

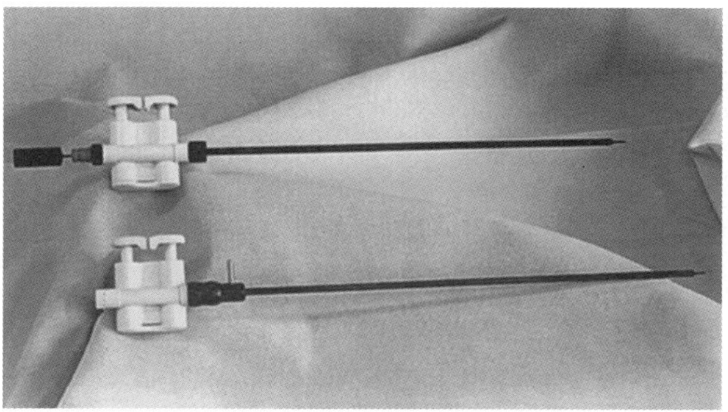

Figure 5-4. An electrode within a suction-irrigator cannula is an effective capacitor. When energized, the electrode induces an electromagnetic field along the entire length of the surrounding cannula. If the cannula is inserted through a nonconductive trocar sleeve, the coupled energy discharges to adjacent tissue, causing electrical burns.

one should never start the electrosurgical generator while the active electrode is touching or near another piece of metal.

Insulation Failure

Insulation failure occurs if the insulation shield of the electrode is compromised from wear, poor handling, or mechanical accidents. In a controlled laboratory setting, the passage of capacitive current across the insulated portion of unipolar 5-mm laparoscopic instruments was assessed for its ability to cause damage to biologic tissues. The results revealed that modulated (coagulating) current at power settings as low as 20 to 25 W led to the passage of current across the insulated portion of some laparoscopic instruments with thin insulation and accompanying thermal damage to tissue and instrument insulation.[10] Defective insulation that is too small to be recognized can deliver the full current of the generator to unintended tissue at the end of the electrode. The defect could be on the shaft of the electrode contained within the trocar sleeve. Some new disposable unipolar instruments can have small defects.

Insulation failure results from damage to the insulation by breaks or holes caused by reprocessing, repeated use, or high-voltage coagulation current. Breaks in the insulation provide an alternative pathway for the current to leave the electrode as it completes the circuit to the REM. The current completes the circuit by jumping from the electrode, through the insulation break, to adjacent tissue, and the current density can be high enough to produce tissue damage. This problem can occur outside the surgeon's field of vision and go undetected. It usually occurs when the surgeon selects the coagulation current because this current has a high voltage, sometimes more than 10,000 V can be avoided. Insulation failure by not starting the generator until the active electrode is near or touching the target tissue. This suggests an open circuit situation, and the high impedance created by the open circuit is interpreted by the generator as a need for maximal voltage to complete the circuit. While in an open circuit, if the insulation of the active electrode is touching tissue, the voltage is high enough to create a hole through the insulation. The surgeon has no way of controlling the current density of this exit point.

The insulation should be inspected carefully for small cracks and defects before use. The voltage in the cut waveform is preferable to coagulate when it is in the desiccation mode (direct electrode contact with tissue). As a result of the lower voltages, the cutting current is less likely to create holes in the insulation. The surgeon should make sure the generator can complete the circuit through the target tissue.

Clinical Applications

Electrosurgery is used to cut (vaporize) or coagulate tissue deeply (desiccate) or superficially (fulgurate). The cutting waveform is characterized by high frequency and a low-voltage sine wave (Figure 5-3). A needle electrode yields very high current density and generates intense intracellular heat, causing the water to boil and vaporize the cell. The vaporization has a cooling effect that prevents thermal damage to adjacent tissue and heat transfer to deeper tissue. Activation of the electrode before touching the tissue produces a plume of vapor between the electrode and the tissue, resulting in cutting with the least thermal damage (Figure 5-5). For adhesiolysis or for vaporization of endometriosis on the ovaries or bladder reflection, cutting current is used with a small needle electrode just before the target tissue is contacted.

Desiccation is effective for coagulating tissue and is achieved with electrodes used with a high frequency and low voltage with nonmodulated current. The extent of lateral damage observed with desiccation is reproduced in depth (Figure 5-6). Coaptive coagulation involves clamping a bleeding vessel with

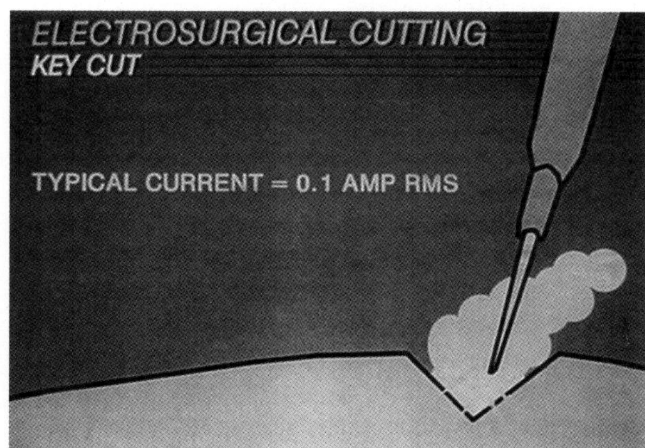

Figure 5-5. Activation of the electrode before it touches the tissue produces a plume of vapor between the electrode and the tissue, resulting in cutting with the least thermal damage.

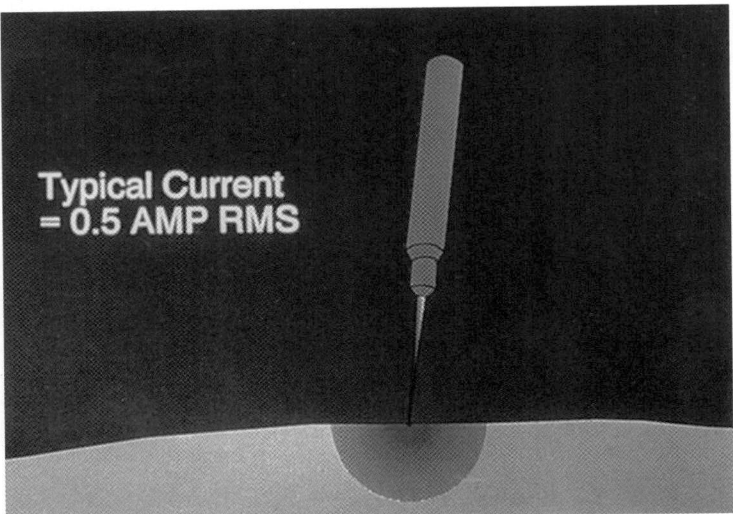

Figure 5-6. The extent of lateral damage observed with desiccation is reproduced in depth.

a conductive clamp and applying cutting current to coagulate and promote a collagen weld. The ammeter of the electrogenerator is used to detect the end of desiccation and provide assurance of hemostasis. The flowmeter measures the flow of electrons as they pass through the tissue contained between the electrodes. Its intensity depends on the resistance of the tissue in the field of the forceps. Excessive heating or inadequate hemostasis is seen with this device. Observation of the tissue before it becomes charred and decreasing the pneumoperitoneum after transection of vessels confirm hemostasis.

Fulguration is superficial coagulation of small capillaries usually over a large surface area, as in the ovarian capsule after cystectomy or in a uterine defect after a myomectomy. An electrode is activated with modulated current and placed over the bleeding area without touching it (Figure 5-7). This type of current requires a high peak-to-peak voltage and produces intermittent sparks of electricity that strike the bleeding tissue, causing superficial coagulation. The sparks lose some of their energy as they travel through the air, but deeper desiccation is produced if the tissue is touched by the electrode. With fulguration, the risk of stray current from capacitive coupling or insulation failure is increased.

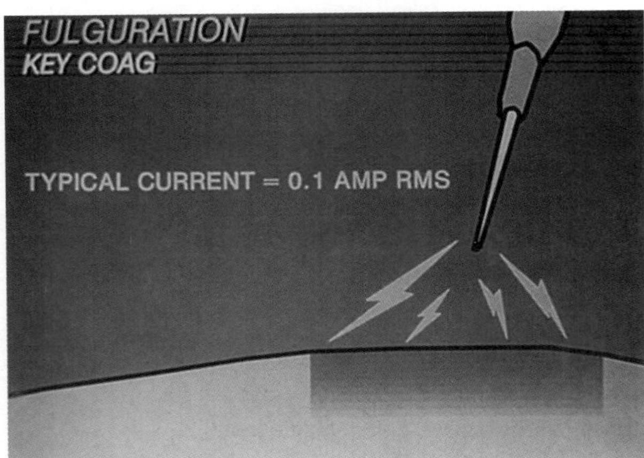

Figure 5-7. An electrode activated with coagulating current is placed over the bleeding area without touching it.

Laparoscopic Ultrasonic Surgery

Ultrasonic surgery involves the rapid mechanical vibration of a metal surgical tip. The vibrating tip is put in contact with tissue and causes cellular collapse through the process of cavitation. Because the tissue is hit repeatedly by the vibrating tip, cavitation occurs as intracellular pressures change rapidly.[11] Ultimately, the pressure differentials become so great that cellular implosions occur. It was not until the mid-1970s that a full-powered ultrasonic surgical aspirator known as the Cavitational Ultrasonic Surgical Aspirator (CUSA) found acceptance among neurosurgeons for the removal of intracranial tumors. CUSA has found favor among surgical and gynecologic oncologists and surgeons who use minimally invasive techniques.

CUSA consists of a console that regulates the amplitude or intensity, an operative handpiece connected to the console, and a foot pedal to start the system. The functional end of the handpiece consists of a hollow titanium tip that moves in and out (longitudinally) of the tissue at 23,000 cycles per second. This action fragments and removes tissue within a 1 to 2-cm radius of the vibrating tip. The amplitude setting on the console corresponds to the excursion of the tip into the tissue and the depth of tissue disruption. A setting of 1 produces cellular fragmentation to a depth of 30 μm, at 5 to a depth of 150 μm, and at 10 to a depth of 300 μm. The operative field is irrigated continuously with normal saline through the functioning tip. This reduces the heat produced by the vibrating tip and suspends the fragments of tissue to allow aspiration through the hollow tip. Tissue specimens are collected in a filter trap and can be sent for cytopathologic and histopathologic examination. CUSA simultaneously fragments, irrigates, and aspirates through the functional tip. All three activities are controlled from the front of the console.

Ultrasonic surgery provides the surgeon with the unique ability to selectively remove or fragment unwanted tissue while sparing vital structures. Highly precise tissue dissection is possible. Actual skeletonization of vital structures is achieved. Vibrating tips selectively fragment and remove through aspiration high-water-content tissue and spare high-collagen-content tissue such as blood vessels, nerves, and ductal structures. This selectivity is described by the rate at which different tissues are fragmented. High-water-content tissue is fragmented more easily and rapidly than is denser tissue. The selectivity of the ultrasonic aspirator provides visual and tactile reactions. Structures can be seen and felt as they present themselves within the surgical field. When differing amounts of pressure are applied gently, the tip can fragment unwanted tissue from vital structures without the risk of perforation or damage to the underlying structures.

Ultrasonic surgical aspiration is not hemostatic. In recent years, electrosurgical capabilities have been added to the tip. Electrosurgical cutting and coagulation currents are administered from the vibrating tip. The combination of rapid, selective ultrasonic tissue dissection with electrosurgical cutting and coagulation provides a synergistic effect. The combination affords increased performance and flexibility, with the added advantage of hemostatic control. With the introduction of a handpiece, ultrasonic dissection is possible with a 31.2-cm extended laparoscopic device attached to a standard autoclavable CUSA handpiece. The laparoscopic tip is used with the electrosurgical accessory. Laparoscopic tips are available as hook electrodes and coagulating shears that fit through 5-mm or 10-mm trocar cannulas.[4]

Since CUSA allows selective tissue dissection without the use of heat, it can provide precise tissue dissection with minimal trauma to the surrounding tissues. If hemostasis is needed, the built-in electrosurgical energy source is started. Laparoscopic ultrasonic dissection gives the surgeon improved observation (no plume or monitor interference) and reduced intraoperative blood loss.

The use of an ultrasonic vibrating scalpel in a rat model was associated with more tissue injury than occurred with a regular scalpel, but it did not cause more adhesions.[12] The authors of a prospective, randomized study in rabbits concluded that the ultrasonic scalpel at level 3 was not different from either the CO_2 laser or electrosurgery in terms of hemostatic properties, coagulation necrosis, and the formation of adhesions.[13]

Safe Use of Electrosurgery

Passing electrosurgical energy through cannulas and long insulated active electrodes changes the physics surrounding the use of high-frequency electrosurgical energy. The potential hazards presented by this environment are avoided through an understanding of recommended practices. The potential problems include insulation failure, direct coupling of current, and capacitively coupled energy. The new technology of active electrode monitoring (AEM) may eliminate stray currents generated by insulation failure and capacitative coupling.[14]

One should follow the guidelines listed below:

1. Always test the equipment before use and select bipolar equipment if possible.
2. Inspect all insulation for defects.
3. Avoid metal-to-metal sparking (direct coupling). Do not energize the active electrode until it is touching or near the target tissue.
4. Use the cut waveform whenever possible. The cutting current uses lower voltages and reduces the likelihood of creating holes in the insulation. Low-voltage waveforms reduce the amount of capacitively coupled current produced.
5. Avoid open current by energizing the active electrode only if it is touching or near the target tissue. Capacitance is low during closed circuit activation with defective insulation.
6. Use either all metal or all plastic for the operative channel.

7. Use the lowest power setting to achieve the desired results. A lower power setting (for both cutting and coagulation) reduces the likelihood of insulation failure, capacitance, and injury.

References

1. Levy BS, Soderstrom RM, Dail DH. Bowel injury during laparoscopy: Gross anatomy and histology. *J Reprod Med* 1985; 30:168.
2. Tucker RD. Laparoscopic electrosurgical injuries: Survey results and their implications. *Surg Laparosc Endosc* 1995; 5:311.
3. Soderstrom RM. Preventing adhesions—electrosurgery: Advantages and disadvantages, in DiZerega GS, Malinak LR, Diamond MP, Linsky, CB eds., *Progress in Clinical and Biological Research*. New York: Wiley-Liss, 1990.
4. Soderstrom RM. Electrosurgery's advantages and disadvantages. *Contemp Ob/Gyn* 1990; 35:35.
5. McKernan JB, Stuto A, Champion JK. New application of bipolar coagulation in laparoscopic surgery. *Surg Laparosc Endosc*1996; 6:335.
6. Schultz LS, Poppe K. Using 5-mm bipolar cutting forceps: A new multifunctional instrument. *J Laparoendosc Adv Surg Tech* 1997; 7:375.
7. Edelman DS, Unger SW. Bipolar versus monopolar cautery scissors for laparoscopic cholecystectomy: A randomized, prospective study. *Surg Laparosc Endosc* 1995; 5:459.
8. Baggish MS, Tucker RD. Tissue actions of bipolar scissors compared with monopolar devices. *Fertil Steril* 1995; 63:422.
9. Kennedy JS, Stranahan PL, Taylor KD, Chandler JG. High-burst-strength, feedback-controlled bipolar vessel sealing. *Surg Endosc* 1998; 12:876.
10. Grosskinsky CM, Hulka JF. Unipolar electrosurgery in operative laparoscopy: Capacitance as a potential source of injury. *J Reprod Med* 1995; 40:549.
11. McCarus SD. Physiologic mechanism of the ultrasonically activated scalpel. *J Am Assoc Gynecol Laparoscop* 1996; 3:601.
12. Tulandi T, Chan KL, Arseneau J. Histopathological and adhesion formation after incision using ultrasonic vibrating scalpel and regular scalpel in the rat. *Fertil Steril* 1994; 61:548.
13. Schemmel M, Haefner HK, Selvaggi SM, et al. Comparison of the ultrasonic scalpel to CO_2 laser and electrosurgery in terms of tissue injury and adhesion formation in a rabbit model. *Fertil Steril* 1997; 67:382.
14. Vancaille TG. Active electrode monitoring: How to prevent unintentional thermal injury associated with monopolar electrosurgery at laparoscopy. *Surg Endosc* 1998; 12:1009.

SECTION III

6

Anesthesia

Women who undergo operative gynecologic laparoscopy are usually young and healthy. However, the benefits of reduced postoperative morbidity, shorter hospital stay, and earlier return to normal activity encourage the use of minimally invasive surgery in more elderly and less healthy patients. The cardiovascular, respiratory, and endocrine changes generated by laparoscopic operations, which are tolerated easily by young, healthy women, are a concern in elderly patients and those with preexisting disease.

Pathophysiology of Laparoscopy

The use of pneumoperitoneum and the Trendelenburg position during laparoscopy introduces particular concerns for anesthesiologists.

Hemodynamic Effects

Hemodynamic changes during laparoscopy are summarized in Table 6-1. After CO_2 insufflation to an intraabdominal pressure greater than 10 mm Hg, cardiac output falls 25 to 35 percent, arterial pressure increases, and both systemic and pulmonary vascular resistance increase.[1,2] The fall in cardiac output is related to reduced flow in the inferior vena cava, pooling of blood in the legs, and the increase in systemic vascular resistance (SVR) (Figure 6-1).[3] SVR increases because of an increase in the vascular resistance of intraabdominal organs and increasing venous resistance. The Trendelenburg position increases preload, pulmonary capillary wedge pressure (PCWP), and pulmonary artery pressure (PAP) while returning afterload toward normal.[2,4] Pneumoperitoneum is associated with a 75 percent reduction in the glomerular filtration rate and a 50 percent reduction in urine output.[5]

These hemodynamic changes have been compared to those of chronic heart failure.[6] Endocrine responses to laparoscopy do not appear to differ from those seen with other surgery.[7,8] Increases in circulating catecholamines, cortisol, renin, and aldosterone are similar to those seen in open surgery. Vagal stimulation resulting in bradycardia and bradyarrhythmias can be provoked by mechanical distention of the peritoneum[9] or manipulation of pelvic organs.[10] The operation should be interrupted while an anticholinergic (atropine or glycopyrrolate) is administered and the level of anesthesia is deepened.

Ventilatory Effects

Pneumoperitoneum causes a cephalad shift in the diaphragm, stiffens the lower chest wall, and restricts lung expansion. There is an increase in peak inspiratory pressure (PIP) and a decrease in compliance.[11–13] These changes are accentuated in the Trendelenburg position as the abdominal contents rest against the diaphragm.[15] Ventilatory changes are summarized in Table 6-2.

Mechanical ventilation may become difficult in obese or in the patients with lung disease because of high inspiratory pressures. Pneumoperitoneum has been shown to shift the carina cephalad sufficiently to result in endobronchial intubation in some patients.[16] Increased PIP and decreased SaO_2 result.

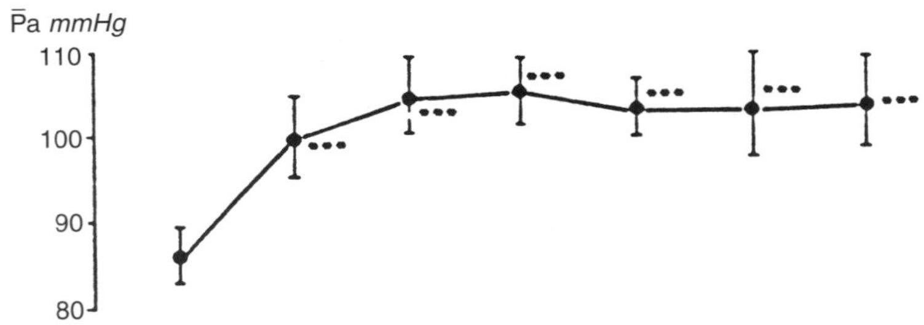

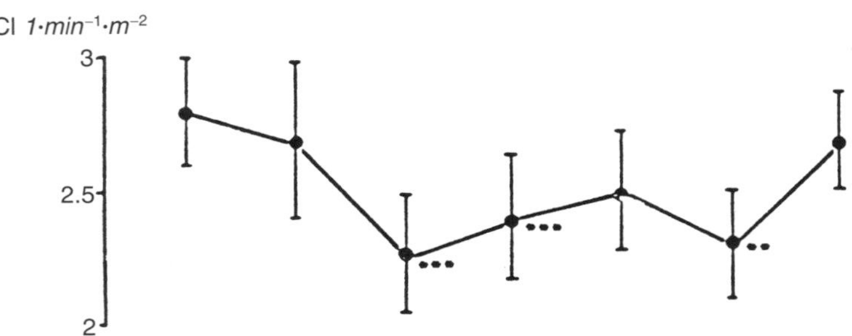

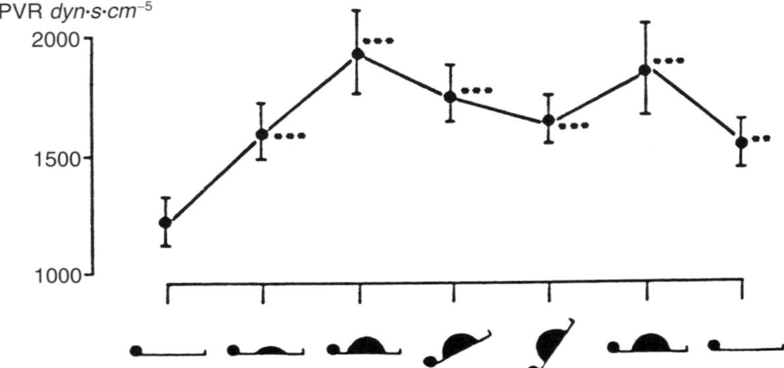

Figure 6-1. The effect of position and pneumoperitoneum on cardiovascular measurements.

After positioning of the patient, endotracheal tube placement should be rechecked by auscultation.

CO_2 is used commonly to provide a pneumoperitoneum. As CO_2 is absorbed from the peritoneal cavity, the CO_2 load increases over the first 20 minutes of pneumoperitoneum before reaching a plateau about 25 percent above preinsufflation values.[17,18] CO_2 absorption probably is limited by reduced peritoneal perfusion, which in turn is caused by increased intraabdominal pressure. An increase in minute ventilation of about 30 percent has been shown to maintain a normal $PetCO_2$.[12,18] Increasing respiratory rate rather than tidal volume tends to minimize the rise in peak inspiratory pressure.

TABLE 6-1. Hemodynamic Changes During Laparoscopy

Cardiac output	↓
Venous return	↓
Systemic vascular resistance	↑
Pulmonary vascular resistance	↑
Mean arterial pressure	↑
Central venous pressure	↑
Pulmonary artery pressure	↑
Heart rate	→

↓ decreased; ↑ increased; → no change

TABLE 6-2. Ventilatory Changes During Laparoscopy

Peak inspiratory pressure	↑
Intrathoracic pressure	↑
Vital capacity	↓
Functional residual capacity	↓
Compliance	↓
Physiologic dead space	↑
$PaCO_2$	↑
PaO_2	→

↑ increased; ↓ decreased; → no change

Investigations of arterioalveolar and CO_2 partial pressure differences have not shown a consistent change, but the differences may increase over time in prolonged operations.[13,14,17] $PetCO_2$ therefore may not be a reliable measure of $PaCO_2$, particularly in prolonged procedures or in patients with underlying lung disease.[13,14] Subcutaneous emphysema with CO_2 produces a severe rise in $PaCO_2$ that may prove difficult to control in spite of large increases in minute volume.

Intraoperative Complications

CO_2 Embolism

CO_2 embolism is a rare but potentially fatal event.[19] It occurs most commonly during initial insufflation of gas as a result of inadvertent insertion of the trocar or Veress needle into a vessel or abdominal organ. The severity of the response depends on the volume of gas entering the circulation and the speed of entrainment. Small CO_2 emboli appear to follow a more benign and transient course than do air emboli because of the high solubility of CO_2 in blood and tissues and the large buffering capacity of blood, which leads to rapid elimination.[19] The lethal dose of CO_2 is about five times that of air (25 mL/kg for CO_2 and 5 mL/kg for air) in dogs.[20] The expansion of an air embolus caused by diffusion of nitrous oxide into the bubble of air does not occur with CO_2 emboli because CO_2 has a solubility similar to that of N_2O. Unlike air, CO_2 does not cause bronchospasm. Large volumes of gas injected under pressure, however, can cause an "air lock" in the vena cava or right atrium, causing sudden cardiovascular collapse.[19] Paradoxical embolus occurs when gas passes through a patent foramen ovale into the systemic circulation, driven by high right atrial pressures.[2] About 25 percent of normal individuals have a probe patent foramen ovale. Transesophageal echo and esophageal or precordial Doppler probes are the most sensitive detectors of CO_2 emboli. However, the low incidence of this complication during laparoscopy does not justify their routine use. Capnography is the most sensitive detector of CO_2 embolism normally in use during laparoscopy. In case reports, capnography showed an initial small sharp rise in $ETCO_2$ with a subsequent fall caused by an increase in dead space in the lung.[21,22] SpO_2 and mean arterial pressure (MAP) fall, with the magnitude of the fall depending on the size of the embolus. Bradycardia occurs, and a characteristic "mill wheel" murmur may be heard. The alveolar-arterial CO_2 difference will increase. Treatment involves stopping insufflation, releasing the pneumoperitoneum immediately, and giving 100 percent oxygen. Turning the patient head down on the left side is recommended to remove the gas bubble from the outflow tract of the right heart. Cardiopulmonary resuscitation should be instituted as necessary. Aspiration of gas through a central venous pressure (CVP) line can be attempted. Cardiopulmonary bypass has been used successfully after a massive embolus.[22]

Pneumothorax, Pneumomediastinum, and Subcutaneous Emphysema

Although pneumothorax is a complication that is more commonly associated with upper abdominal laparoscopy, it has been reported during gynecologic procedures.[23,24] A congenital diaphragmatic defect may allow peritoneal gas to pass into the pleural cavity. An increase in PIP, a fall in SpO_2, and decreased breath sounds on one side point to the diagnosis, which should be confirmed by chest x-ray. The laparoscopist may be able to show abnormal motion of one hemidiaphragm. Falling MAP and SpO_2 suggest the presence of a tension pneumothorax that requires immediate decompression. In the absence of tension, unless there is a pulmonary cause (such as a ruptured bulla), pneumothorax resolves spontaneously after 30 to 60 minutes in the recovery period. If the patient is stable, Joris[25] suggests conservative intraoperative management. Chest tube drainage should be avoided during the operation because it will make it difficult to maintain the pneumoperitoneum. Increasing FiO_2, the addition of 5 cm of positive end-expiratory pressure (PEEP), and reduction of intraabdominal pressure will maintain oxygenation and allow the operation to be completed expeditiously.[26]

Subcutaneous emphysema can accompany pneumothorax or occur in isolation. An abrupt and severe rise in $ETCO_2$ is characteristic. It requires a higher than normal increase in minute ventilation for control. A reduction in electrocardiographic (ECG) voltage associated with subcutaneous emphysema has been reported.[27] Involvement of the neck can cause airway compression. If swelling of the neck is noted, delayed extubation is advisable until the swelling resolves. The possibility of pneumothorax and pneumomediastinum always should be considered when surgical emphysema is present. Surgical emphysema resolves over several hours. Explanation and reassurance may be necessary for the patient in the postoperative care unit.

Nerve Injury

The common peroneal and sciatic nerves are at risk for injury during laparoscopy because of the lithotomy position. Femoral neuropathy has been reported.[28] The brachial plexus can be injured by pressure or stretching from shoulder restraints, especially in the steep Trendelenburg position. Meticulous care is necessary when positioning the patient to minimize the risk of injuring these vulnerable nerves. Lower limb compartment syndrome has complicated prolonged operations done in the lithotomy position.[29,30]

Fluid Balance

A patient who has undergone a preoperative bowel preparation and a prolonged fast may be dehydrated on arrival in the operating room. Intraoperative blood loss is difficult to assess because of dilution in large volumes of irrigation fluid. Pulmonary edema has been described after the absorption of intraabdominal irrigating fluid, resulting in dyspnea and hypoxemia in the recovery room.[31] Maintaining a careful record of irrigating fluid balance intraoperatively will alert the anesthesiologist when large deficits are accumulating. A small dose of furosemide may be necessary to restore fluid balance.

Heat Loss

Postoperative hypothermia has been associated with an increased incidence of wound infection and prolonged hospital stay after laparotomy.[32] Shivering can increase oxygen consumption as much as 400 percent.[33] Peritoneal gas insufflation and the use of large volumes of peritoneal irrigation predispose a patient to hypothermia during laparoscopy.[34] Warming of irrigation fluids and the use of a forced-air warming blanket reduce the incidence of the undesirable postoperative effects of hypothermia.

Anesthesia for Laparoscopy

Preoperative Evaluation

The aims of the preoperative assessment are to identify problems that might cause perioperative morbidity, evaluate and stabilize any associated medical problems, and provide an opportunity to discuss the anesthesia plan with the patient. The importance of the preoperative visit in allaying anxiety has been shown.[35] Necessary laboratory investigations can be arranged. The value of obtaining routine preoperative laboratory investigations in all patients has been questioned.[36,37] For gynecologic patients, a hematocrit should be obtained in case of anemia. Other tests, such as an electrolyte analysis and a pregnancy test, are done as indicated by the history and physical examination. In asymptomatic patients without risk factors, a chest x-ray and ECG are unnecessary. Autologous blood donation can be arranged preoperatively in appropriate patients.

Preinduction Medication

Premedication is used to provide anxiolysis and possibly amnesia. Many patients are anxious about their operations. A small dose (1 to 2 mg) of the short-acting benzodiazepine midazolam allays anxiety without contributing to postoperative sedation. Other aims of premedication include emesis prophylaxis and acid aspiration prophylaxis. In susceptible patients, transdermal scopolamine is an effective adjunct to antiemetic medication given intraoperatively. It must be given at least 8 hours preoperatively to be effective.[38] In patients at risk for regurgitation of gastric contents, preoperative administration of a nonparticulate antacid increases gastric pH. Metoclopramide and H_2 receptor blockers are given to reduce gastric volume and acidity.

Choice of Anesthesia

Although regional and local anesthesia have been used successfully for laparoscopy, they are suitable only for brief procedures, such as tubal ligation, in motivated patients. Operative gynecologic laparoscopy necessitates optimal surgical conditions; steep Trendelenburg positioning, muscle relaxation, a large pneumoperitoneum, and multiple incisions all make general anesthesia the safest and most comfortable choice. Similarly, although the laryngeal mask airway has been used for laparoscopy, endotracheal intubation protects the airway from aspiration of gastric contents and facilitates the delivery of increased minute ventilation in the presence of increased airway pressures.[39]

Propofol is a useful induction agent for outpatients because of its antiemetic action and superior quality of wake-up.[40] After the administration of the muscle relaxant, care must be taken during mask ventilation not to inflate the stomach with gas. Once the endotracheal tube is secured, an orogastric tube is passed for aspiration of gastric contents. The choice of muscle relaxant is unimportant, although mivacurium has the advantage of a rapid offset of action, permitting deep relaxation during the operation while potentially avoiding the need for subsequent reversal agents. Balanced anesthesia with oxygen-enriched air, an inhalational agent, a muscle relaxant, and a short-acting narcotic such as fentanyl is suitable. Intraabdominal pressure can be kept as low as possible by controlled ventilation, maintaining muscle relaxation and a relatively deep plane of anesthesia. Nitrous oxide often is avoided during laparoscopy, although its role in producing bowel distention remains controversial. There is a lack of conclusive evidence for a difference in operating conditions or bowel distention with or without nitrous oxide.[41]

Continuous intraoperative monitoring should include pulse oximetry, ECG, $ETCO_2$, blood pressure, temperature, muscle relaxation, minute ventilation, and airway pressure. American Society of Anesthesiologists Physical Status class 3 and 4 patients may require invasive hemodynamic monitoring.

Recovery from Anesthesia

Postoperative Nausea and Vomiting

Nausea with or without vomiting is a common postoperative occurrence and is distressing to patients. The incidence of postoperative nausea and vomiting (PONV) overall is about 30 percent; after laparoscopy, it is about 50 percent.[42] Intractable nausea and vomiting occur in about 0.1 percent of all postoperative patients. Women are more likely to experience PONV than are men, and the incidence is higher in younger patients. Surgery during the first 8 days of the menstrual cycle increases PONV threefold, suggesting that the timing of surgery in this susceptible group can have a significant effect on patient comfort.[42,43] The use of prophylactic antiemetic medication is justified in laparoscopy because of this high probability of PONV. The optimal prophylactic regimen remains a matter of debate.[44,45] Given the complex causes of vomiting, it seems likely that the use of a combination of medications will produce better results than will one alone.

Dropridol is a butyrophenone with prolonged action. Given in small doses (10 μg/kg), it is effective with less risk of side effects associate with higher doses (drowsiness, hypotension, dysphoria, extrapyramidal effects).

Metoclopramide is a gastrokinetic agent that increases lower esophageal sphincter tone. It has antiserotoninergic and antidopaminergic effects. The selective 5HT3 antagonists ondansetron and dolasetron are effective in both prophylaxis and treatment of nausea and vomiting. Their side effects include headache and dizziness.

Pain Management

Postoperative pain occurs in the abdomen, shoulders, and back. Shoulder pain, presumably from phrenic nerve stimulation, tends to become more significant on the second postoperative day.[46] Its severity correlates with the size of the residual gas bubble and can be reduced by the use of a gas drain.[47] Many studies have examined the effect of nonsteroidal anti-inflammatory drugs (NSAIDs) on pain after laparoscopy. The intensity and duration of pain relief are improved by adding ketorolac to a short-acting opioid, but NSAIDs alone provide inadequate pain relief. Various local anesthetic techniques have been used, including infiltration of the abdominal wounds and rectus sheath block.[48] A combination of narcotics, local anesthesia, and an NSAID may offer the best relief.

References

1. Johansen G, Anderson M, Juhl B. The effect of general anesthesia on the hemodynamic events during laparoscopy with CO_2 insufflation. *Acta Anaesthesiol Scand* 1989; 33:132.
2. Hirvonen EA, Nuutinen LS, Kauko M. Hemodynamic changes due to Trendelenburg positioning and pneumoperitoneum during laparoscopic hysterectomy. *Acta Anaesthesiol Scand* 1995; 39:949.
3. Ivankovich AD, Miletich DJ, Albrecht RF, et al. Cardiovascular effects of intraperitoneal insufflation with carbon dioxide and nitrous oxide in the dog. *Anesthesiology* 1975; 42:281.
4. Odeburg S, Ljungqvist O, Svenberg T, et al. Haemodynamic effects of pneumoperitoneum and the influence of posture during anaesthesia for laparoscopic surgery. *Acta Anaesthesiol Scand* 1994; 38:276.

5. Harman PK, Kron IL, McLachlan HD. Elevated intra-abdominal pressure and renal function. *Ann Surg* 1982; 196:594.
6. Struthers AD, Cuschieri A. Cardiovascular consequences of laparoscopic surgery. *Lancet* 1998; 352:568.
7. Hirvonen EA, Nuutinen LS, Vuolteenaho O. Hormonal responses and cardiac filling pressures in head up or head down position and pneumoperitoneum in patients undergoing operative laparoscopy. *Br J Anaesth* 1997; 78:128.
8. Joris J, Cigarini I, Legrand M, et al. Metabolic and respiratory changes after cholecystectomy performed via laparotomy or laparoscopy. *Br J Anaesth* 1992; 69:341.
9. Carmichael DE. Laparoscopy—cardiac considerations. *Fertil Steril* 1971; 22:69.
10. Sprung J. Recurrent complete heart block in a healthy patient during laparoscopic electrocauterization of the fallopian tube. *Anesthesiology* 1998; 88:1401.
11. Bardoczky GI, Engelman E, Levarlet M, Simon P. Ventilatory effects of pneumoperitoneum monitored with continuous spirometry. *Anesthesia* 1993; 49:309.
12. Hirvonen EA, Nuutinen LS, Kauko M. Ventilatory effects, blood gas changes, and oxygen consumption during laparoscopic hysterectomy. *Anesth Analg* 1995; 80:961.
13. Monk TG, Weldon BC, Lemon D. Alterations in pulmonary function during laparoscopic surgery [abstract]. *Anesth Analg* 1994; 76:S274.
14. Wahba RWM, Mamazza J. Ventilatory requirements during laparoscopic cholecystectomy. *Can J Anaesth* 1993; 40:206.
15. Oikkonen M, Tallgren M. Changes in respiratory compliance at laparoscopy: Measurements using sidestream spirometry. *Can J Anaesth* 1995; 42:495.
16. Lobato EB, Paige GB, Brown MM, et al. Pneumoperitoneum as a risk factor for endobrochial intubation during laparoscopic gynecologic surgery. *Anesth Analg* 1998; 86:301.
17. Puri GD, Singh H. Ventilatory effects of laparoscopy under general anaesthesia. *Br J Anaesth* 1992; 68:211.
18. Tan PL, Lee TL, Tweed WA. Carbon dioxide absorption and gas exchange during pelvic laparoscopy. *Can J Anaesth* 1992; 39:677.
19. Wahba RW, Tessler MJ, Kleiman SJ. Acute ventilatory complications during laparoscopic upper abdominal surgery. *Can J Anaesth* 1995; 43:77.
20. Graff TD, Arbegast NR, Philips OC, et al. Gas embolism: A comparative study of air and carbon dioxide as embolic agents in the systemic venous system. *Am J Obstet Gynecol* 1959; 78:259.
21. Shulman D, Aronson HB. Capnography in the early diagnosis of carbon dioxide embolism during laparoscopy. *Can J Anaesth* 1984; 31:31.
22. Diakun TA. Carbon dioxide embolism: Successful resuscitation with cardiopulmonary bypass. *Anesthesiology* 1991; 74:1151.
23. Batra MS, Driscoll JJ, Coburn WA, Marks MM. Evanescent nitrous oxide pneumothorax after laparoscopy. *Anesth Analg* 1983; 62:1121.
24. Perko G, Fernandes A. Subcutaneous emphysema and pneumothorax during laparoscopy for ectopic pregnancy removal. *Acta Anaesthesiol Scand* 1997; 41:792.
25. Joris JL. Anesthetic management of laparoscopy in Miller RD, ed., *Anesthesia*, 4th ed. New York: Churchill Livingstone, 1994.
26. Chiche JD, Joris J, Lamy M. PEEP for treatment of intra-operative pneumothorax during laparoscopic fundoplication. *Br J Anaesth* 1994; 72:A38.
27. Yogosakaran N. Laparoscopy, surgical emphysema and ECG voltage. *Anaesthesia* 1992; 47:720.
28. Gombar KK, Gombar S, Singh B, et al. Femoral neuropathy: A complication of the lithotomy position. *Reg Anaesth* 1992; 17:306.
29. Lydon JC, Spielman FJ. Bilateral compartment syndrome following prolonged surgery in the lithotomy position. *Anesthesiology* 1984; 60:236.
30. Montgomery CJ, Ready LB. Epidural opioid analgesia does not obscure diagnosis of compartment syndrome resulting from prolonged lithotomy position. *Anesthesiology* 1991; 75:541.
31. Healzer JM, Nezhat C, Brodsky JB, et al. Pulmonary edema after absorbing crystalloid irrigating fluid during laparoscopy. *Anesth Analg* 1994; 78:1207.
32. Kurz A, Sessler DI, Lenhardt R. Peri-operative normothermia to reduce the incidence of surgical wound infection and shorter hospitalization. *N Engl J Med* 1996; 334:1209.
33. Bay J, Nunn JF, Prys-Roberts C. Factors influencing arterial pO_2 during recovery from anesthesia. *Br J Anaesth* 1968; 40:398.
34. Moore SS, Green CR, Wang FL, et al. The role of irrigation in the development of

hypothermia during laparoscopic surgery. *Am J Obstet Gyn* 1997; 176:598.
35. Egbert LD, Battit GE, Turndorf H, Beecher HK. The value of the preoperative visit by an anesthetist: A study of doctor patient rapport. *JAMA* 1963; 185:553.
36. Narr BJ, Hanson TR, Warner M. Preoperative laboratory screening in healthy Mayo patients: Cost effective elimination of tests and unchanged outcomes. *Mayo Clin Proc* 1991; 66:155.
37. Roizen MF, Cohn S. Preoperative evaluation for elective surgery—what laboratory tests are needed? *Adv Anesth* 1993; 10:25.
38. Bailey PL, Steisand JB, Pace NL, et al. Transdermal scopolamine reduces nausea and vomiting after outpatient laparoscopy. *Anesthesiology* 1990; 72:977.
39. Ho BY, Skinner HJ, Mahajan RP. Gastro-oesophageal reflux during day case gynaecological laparoscopy under positive pressure ventilation: Laryngeal mask vs. tracheal intubation. *Anaesthesia* 1998; 53:910.
40. De Grood RM, Habers JB, van Egmond J, Crul JF. Anesthesia for laparoscopy: A comparison of 5 techniques including propofol, etomidate, thiopentone and isoflurane. *Anaesthesia* 1987; 42:815.
41. Taylor E, Feinstein R, White PF, Sopor N. Anesthesia for laparoscopic cholecystectomy: Is nitrous oxide contra-indicated? *Anesthesiology* 1992; 76:541.
42. Beattie WS, Buckley DN, Forrest JB. The incidence of post operative nausea and vomiting in women undergoing laparoscopy is influenced by the day of menstrual cycle. *Can J Anaesth* 1991; 38:298.
43. Beattie WS, Lindblad T, Buckley DN, Forrest JB. Menstruation increases the risk of nausea and vomiting after laparoscopy. *Anesthesiology* 1993; 78:272.
44. Paxton LD, McCay AC, Mirakhur RK. Prevention of nausea and vomiting after day case gynecological laparoscopy. *Anaesthesia* 1995; 50:403.
45. Snaidach MS, Alberts MS. A comparison of the prophylactic anti-emetic effect of ondansetron and droperidol on patients undergoing gynecologic laparoscopy. *Anesth Analg* 1997; 85:797.
46. Alexander JI. Pain after laparoscopy. *Br J Anaesth* 1997; 79:369.
47. Alexander JI, Hull MGR. Abdominal pain after laparoscopy: The value of a gas drain. *Br J Obstet Gynaecol* 1987; 94:267.
48. Smith BE, Suchak M, Siggins D, Challands J. Rectus sheath block for diagnostic laparoscopy. *Anaesthesia* 1988; 43:947.

7

Laparoscopy

The modern era of laparoscopy began in 1954, when Palmer[1] reported the results of endoscopic procedures in 250 patients without sequelae. He produced a pneumoperitoneum with CO_2 at a rate of 300 to 500 mL/min and cautioned that the intraabdominal pressure should not exceed 25 mm Hg. The claimed advantages of laparoscopy over culdoscopy were a decreased chance of infection, a better view of the pelvis, improved access to the pelvic organs and cul-de-sac, and easier application of surgical techniques.

Although the basic principles of laparoscopy are the same, the instruments and the complexity of operative procedures have changed significantly since 1954. This chapter presents information for residents learning laparoscopic operations and clinicians who are updating their knowledge of operative laparoscopy.

Preoperative Evaluation

Advanced operative laparoscopy is a major intraabdominal procedure. Careful preoperative evaluation optimizes the operative outcome and decreases the incidence of injuries and complications. Preoperative consultations with surgeons in other disciplines (colorectal, urologic, oncologic) sometimes are necessary. The patient is informed about the possible outcome and results of the planned operation, possible complications, and the surgeon's experience in doing the particular procedure. The following preoperative workup is suggested:

1. History and physical
2. Complete blood count (CBC) with differential
3. Serum electrolytes
4. Urinalysis
5. Papanicolaou smear
6. Thrombin time, partial thrombin time, bleeding time
7. Transvaginal sonography (TVS)

In special situations an endometrial biopsy, cervical culture, hysterosalpingogram, barium enema, intravenous pyelogram, blood type and screen or type and cross-match, and bowel preparation are indicated.[2] Two bowel preparations are suggested (Tables 7-1 and 7-2).

Women who have had a previous laparotomy or have an adnexal mass, pelvic endometriosis, or adhesions are given instructions for the 1-day preparation. The 3-day regimen is used for a patient who may need an extensive laparoscopic procedure such as a bowel resection.

Patient Preparation and Position

The anesthesiology team and circulating nurses coordinate the patient's transfer onto the operating table. The operative site is cleansed and shaved preoperatively by an operating room (OR) nurse. Operating tables must be designed to provide a 25-degree Trendelenburg position. After the induction of endotracheal anesthesia, the patient's legs are placed in padded Allen stirrups to provide good support and proper position. Padding near the peroneal nerve is essential. To avoid nerve

TABLE 7-1. One-Day Bowel Preparation

1. Clear liquid the day before the operation
2. One gallon of Go-LYTELY consumed over 3 hours the evening before the laparoscopy or 45 mL of Fleet Phospho-Soda orally at bedtime
3. One Fleet enema at bedtime and in the morning
4. 1 g metronidazole (Flagyl) by mouth at 11 P.M.
5. 1 g cefoxitin one-half hour before the procedure (IV)

compression, no leg joint is extended more than 60 degrees. The buttocks must protrude a few centimeters from the edge of the table to allow uterine manipulation. The patient's arms are placed at the side, padded with foam troughs, and secured by a sheet. This allows the surgeon and assistants to stand unencumbered next to the patient. The anesthesiologist should have easy access to the patient's arm (Figure 7-1).

Once the patient is positioned, her abdomen, perineum, and vagina are prepared with a suitable bactericidal solution and a Foley catheter is inserted. She is draped to expose the abdomen and perineum, and a pelvic examination is done. Diagnostic hysteroscopy may be indicated for patients undergoing diagnostic and operative laparoscopy. After withdrawal of the hysteroscope, a uterine manipulator is inserted into the cervical os to manipulate the uterus and for chromopertubation. Rectal and vaginal probes can help separate the tissue planes of the cul-de-sac. The assistant can do a simultaneous rectal and vaginal examination for the same purpose. A sponge on a ring forceps is placed in the posterior fornix to outline the posterior cul-de-sac or anteriorly to identify the vesicouterine space. In patients who are suspected of having rectosigmoid endometriosis, a sigmoidoscopic examination is suggested. The rectum is insufflated to look for bubbles as they pass into the posterior cul-de-sac filled with irrigation fluid.[3]

TABLE 7-2. Three-Day Bowel Preparation

Day 1
100 mL Fleet Phospho-Soda by mouth at bedtime

Day 2
Clear liquid diet

Day 3
Clear liquid diet
10 mg prochlorperazine by mouth at noon
Begin drinking 1 gallon of Go-LYTELY at 2 P.M.
1 g neomycin by mouth at 6 P.M. and 11 P.M.
1 g erythromycin base by mouth at 6 P.M. and 11 P.M.
One Fleet enema at bedtime

Day of surgery
Two tap water enemas before reporting to the hospital

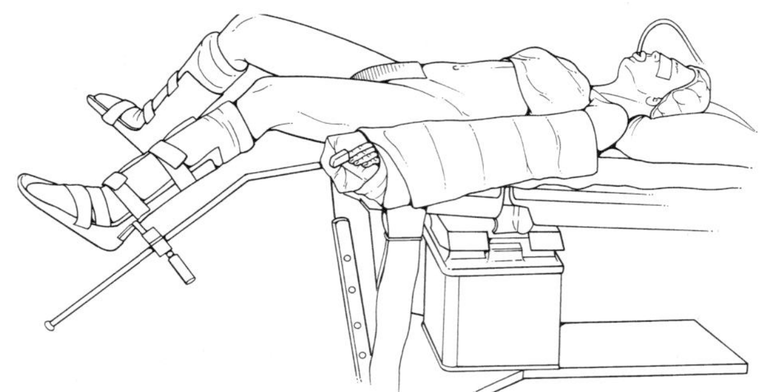

Figure 7-1. The patient is in a dorsolithotomy position, but the thighs are not flexed so that the suprapubic trocars may be maneuvered.

Placement of the Veress Needle

Insertion of the Veress needle, the primary trocar, and the secondary trocar is an important aspect of diagnostic and operative laparoscopy. Serious complications and injuries can occur during these procedures. The following factors increase the risk of injury:

1. Previous abdominal and pelvic operations
2. Body weight (whether patient is obese or very thin)
3. A large uterus and the presence of a large pelvic mass

The optimal location for the Veress needle and primary trocar is the umbilicus because the skin is attached to the fascial layer and anterior parietal peritoneum with no intervening subcutaneous fat or muscle (Figure 7-2). The transumbilical approach accounts for the shortest distance between the skin and the peritoneal cavity even in obese patients. These sites sometimes are modified. The primary trocar is inserted approximately 4 to 6 cm above the umbilicus in patients who have an enlarged uterus caused by a uterine leiomyoma or pregnancy or for para-aortic lymph node dissection.

Before the needle is inserted, a transverse or vertical cutaneous incision is made large enough to accommodate the primary trocar. A vertical umbilical incision provides better cosmetic results.[4] When one is incising the umbilicus, an Allis clamp

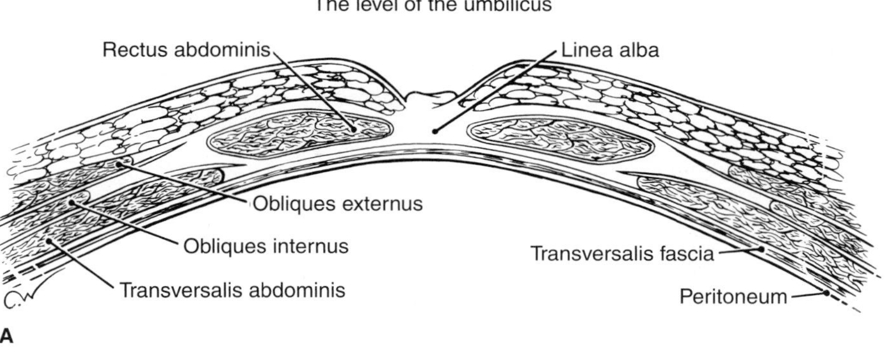

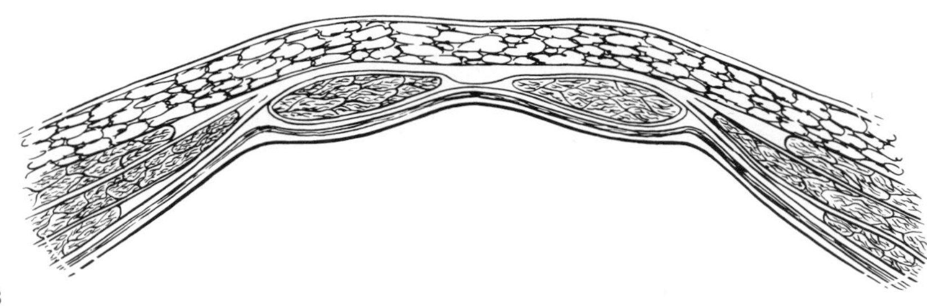

Figure 7-2. Transverse sections through the anterior abdominal wall. A. Immediately above the umbilicus. B. Below the arcuate line.

or skin hook is used to grasp and evert the base of the umbilicus, raising it from the abdominal structures.

One should check the patency of the needle before it is inserted. Traditionally, the angle of insertion is approximately 45 degrees for an infraumbilical placement while the patient is horizontal; a premature Trendelenburg position alters the usual landmarks (Figure 7-3). Transumbilical placement with a 90-degree angle of insertion is recommended after adequate training with this technique. Palpating the abdominal aorta and the sacral promontory is performed first. The patient is completely flat and the operating table is all the way down to maximize the surgeon's upper body control during insertion of the Veress needle (Figure 7-4). The Veress needle, held at the shaft, is directed toward the sacralpromontory (Figure 7-5). The surgeon and assistants apply countertraction by grasping the skin and fat on each side of the umbilicus with a towel clip (Figure 7-6).[5] In obese patients, a 90-degree angle is necessary initially to enter the peritoneal cavity. In thin individuals, vital structures are closer to the abdominal wall, so the surgeon makes certain that the abdominal wall is elevated and only a small portion of the needle is inserted into the abdominal cavity. That is rarely more than 2-3 cm of the Veress needle or trocar. A prospective study involving 97 women undergoing operative laparoscopy showed that the position of the aortic bifurcation is more likely to be caudal to the umbilicus in the Trendelenburg position, compared with the supine position regardless of body mass index.[6] Its presumed location can be misleading during Veress needle or primary cannula insertion. The physician must be careful to avoid major retroperitoneal vascular injury during this procedure.

Verification of Intraperitoneal Location

Failure to achieve and maintain a suitable pneumoperitoneum predisposes the patient to complications.

Hanging Drop Method

Correct needle placement is verified by the "hanging drop" technique. A drop of saline is placed on the hub of the Veress needle after insertion through the abdominal wall; lifting the abdominal wall establishes negative pressure within the abdomen, drawing the drop of fluid into the needle. Absence of this sign indicates improper placement of the Veress needle.

The Syringe Test

Alternatively, a 10-mL syringe with normal saline is attached to the Veress needle and aspiration

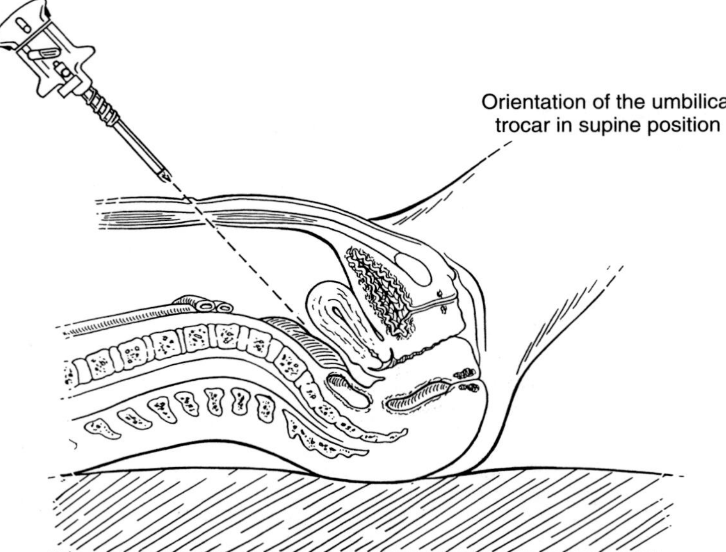

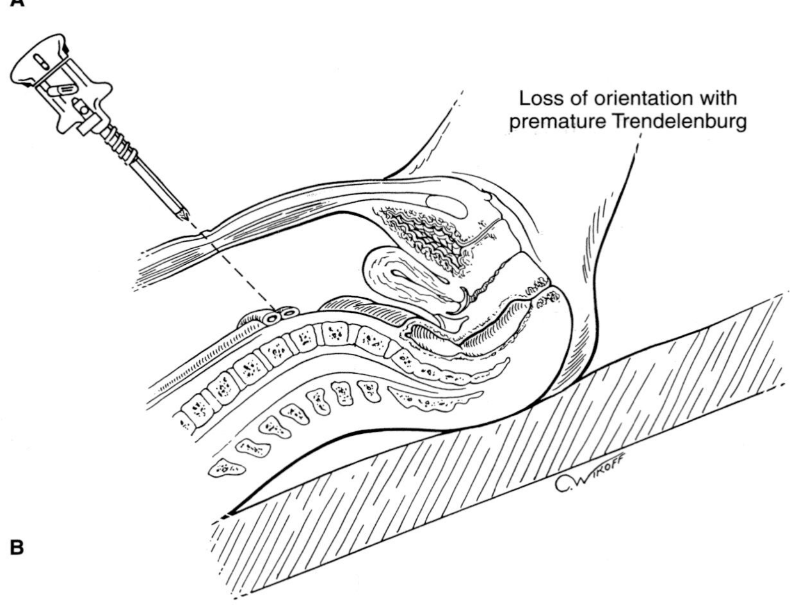

Figure 7-3. Angle of trocar insertion with operating table in flat **(A)** and Trendelenburg **(B)** positions.

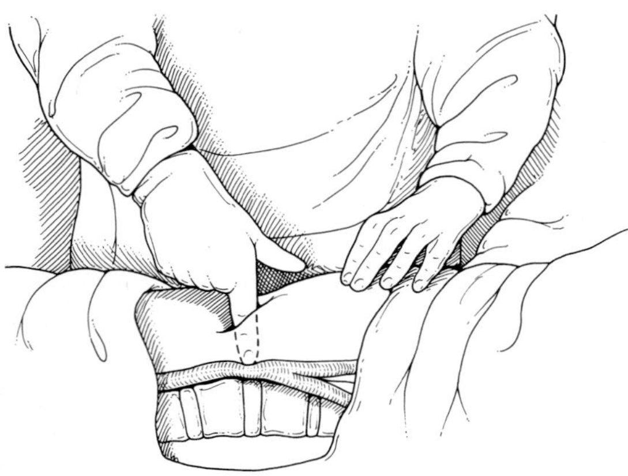

Figure 7-4. The aorta and sacral promontory are palpated.

verifies the absence of bowel contents or blood (Figure 7-7). The saline is injected into the peritoneal cavity, and if the needle placement is correct, the fluid cannot be withdrawn because it is dispersed intraperitoneally. If the needle is placed within adhesions or the preperitoneal space, the fluid usually is recovered by aspiration. If the needle has been placed intravascularly or in the intestine or bladder, characteristic contents are obtained. Additional methods of verifying proper placement of the Veress needle are summarized in Table 7-3. Once correct intraperitoneal placement of the Veress needle is assured, trocar-related injuries can be avoided by employing the technique of abdominal mapping before the insertion of the

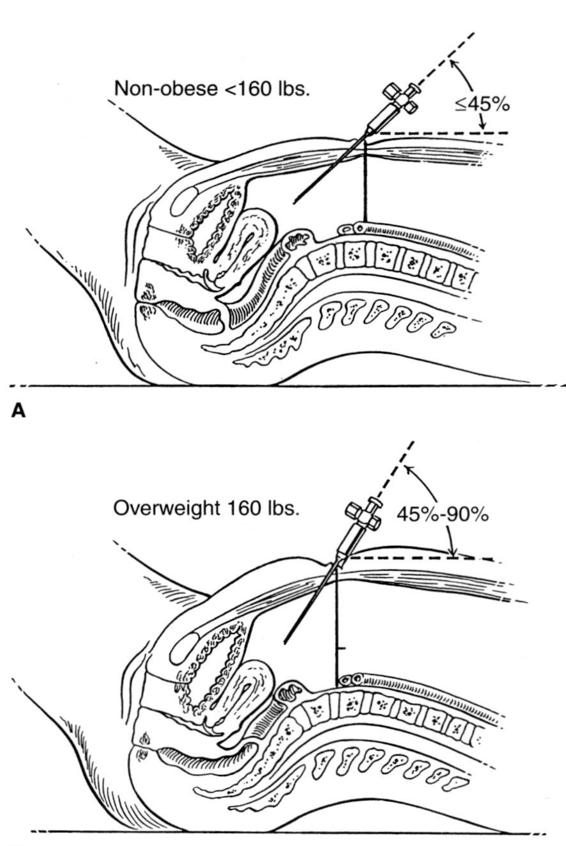

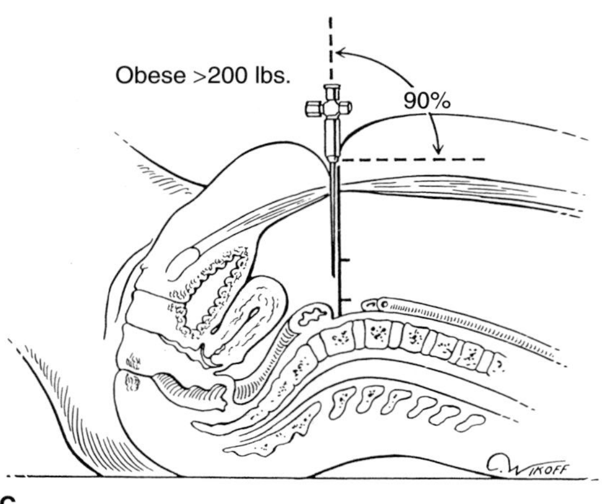

Figure 7-5. Note the anatomic location of the umbilicus and abdominal aorta in nonobese (A), overweight (B), and obese (C) patients.

initial trocar. Mapping of the abdomen at the site of the trocar placement requires an 18-gauge spinal needle attached to a syringe partially filled with saline. Pneumoperitoneum is maintained through the Veress needle by using low-flow insufflation with carbon dioxide gas. The needle is placed transabdominally into the peritoneal cavity at several points surrounding the proposed trocar

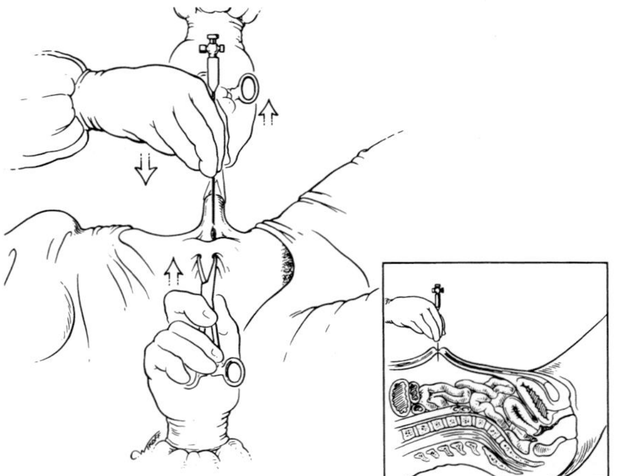

Figure 7-6. The Veress needle is grasped by the shaft and directed posteriorly at a 90° angle. Inset shows elevation of skin and subcutaneous tissue.

insertion site. Usually this is periumbilical. If the needle is placed in an area free of viscera or adhesions, bubbles of carbon dioxide gas should be seen rising through the fluid into the syringe. Mapping the abdomen will demonstrate the safest direction in which to place the primary trocar.

Alternative Sites for Insertion

Different sites can be used for insertion of the Veress needle (Figure 7-8), such as the left subcostal margin in the midclavicular line. This site is palpated and percussed to rule out splenomegaly or an insufflated stomach from a misplaced endotracheal tube. This site is useful especially in patients who have had multiple previous laparotomies. The transvaginal approach is used through the posterior cul-de-sac as long as there is no evidence of pelvic thickening or masses in the cul-de-sac and the uterus is mobile.[7] This technique is effective in patients who have developed preperitoneal emphysema from unsuccessful attempts to insert the needle through the umbilicus or other abdominal sites.

Another technique is the transabdominal route through the uterine fundus.[8,9] The fundus is pushed up against the abdominal wall by using the uterine manipulator. A needle is passed through all layers of the abdomen and into the uterine fundus. As the uterus is pulled away from the tip of the needle, intraabdominal placement is achieved. Alternatively, the Veress needle is inserted transcervically through the fundus into the abdominal cavity. These alternative methods have uncertain margins of safety. Puncture of the uterus with this technique can result in persistent low-grade bleed-

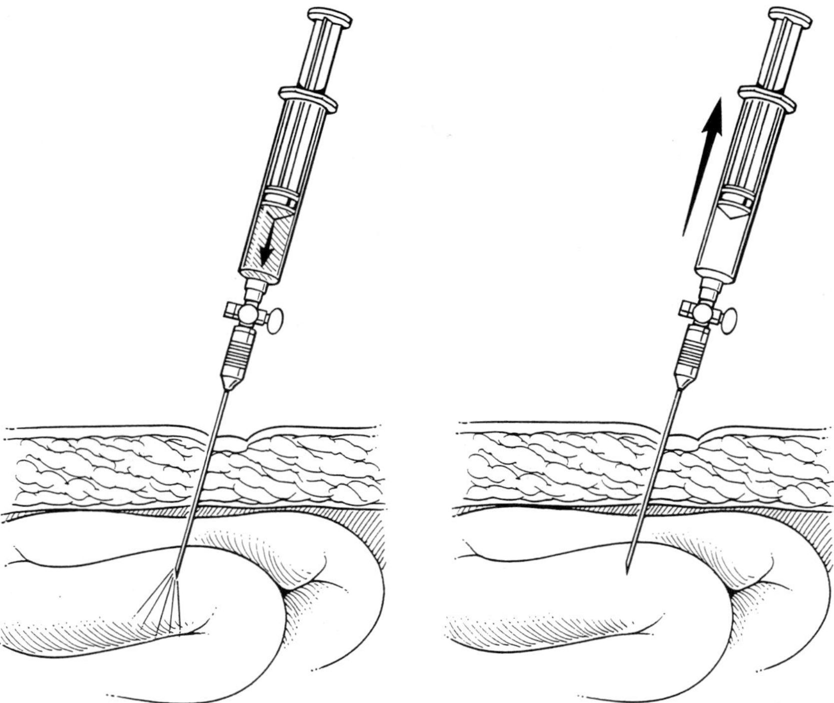

Figure 7-7. Syringe test helps determine that bowel or blood vessels are not adherent under the umbilicus before trocar insertion. A 10-mL syringe with 5 mL of normal saline is attached to the Veress needle, and aspiration verifies the absence of bowel contents or blood.

ing throughout the laparoscopy. Inadvertent perforation of the bladder, broad ligament perforation, and hemorrhage are possible. An intrauterine or intramyometrial position during insufflation can cause gas embolism. The technique is contraindicated if fundal adhesions are anticipated or chromopertubation is necessary.[10]

In an obese patient, proper placement of the Veress needle is difficult to achieve. If it is placed below instead of within the umbilicus at

TABLE 7-3. Tests to Confirm the Proper Position of the Veress Needle

1. Injection and aspiration of fluid through the Veress needle
2. Loss of liver dullness early in insufflation
3. Hanging drop test
4. An unimpeded arc of rotation of the needle to detect anterior abdominal wall adhesions
5. Sound of air entering Veress needle with elevation of the abdominal wall
6. Free flow of gas through the Veress needle
7. Observation of the fluctuation of pressure gauge needle with inspiratory and expiratory diaphragmatic motions

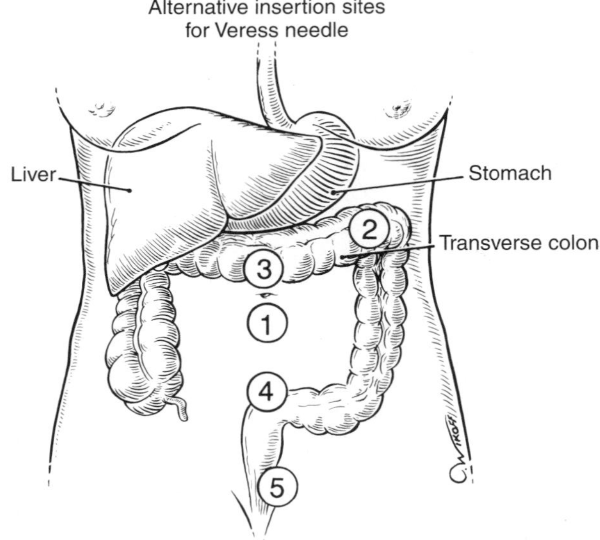

Figure 7-8. Alternative sites for Veress needle insertion. 1. Infra or intraumbilical. 2. Left upper quadrant, midclavicular. 3. Supraumbilical. 4. Midline suprapubic. 5. Transcervical through the uterine fundus or transvaginal through the posterior fornix into the abdominal cavity.

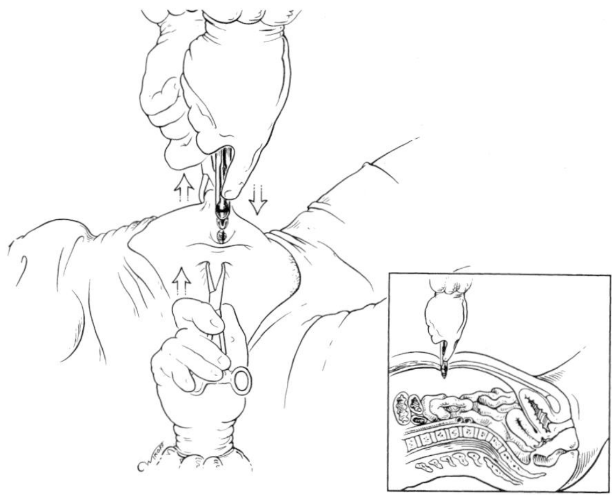

Figure 7-9. Countertraction is applied by grasping the lower abdomen; the surgeon inserts the trocar into the abdomen by palming it and using the index finger as a guard against sudden entry into the abdomen. Inset shows the portion of the trocar and intestines.

45 degrees to the abdominal wall, it can dissect into the preperitoneal space. It is preferable to insert the needle and trocar transumbilically and at 90 degrees, using towel clips for traction and abdominal wall elevation (Figure 7-9).[11]

A survey of the existing data on the rates of failure and complications for each of the available methods of creating pneumoperitoneum showed that no technique was superior. Laparoscopists should be familiar with at least two of these techniques.[12]

Pneumoperitoneum

A pneumoperitoneum is a prerequisite for laparoscopic observation and exposure to do intraperitoneal manipulations for endoscopic operations. Unless the surgeon is confident about the proper position of the Veress needle, the high flow is not used. The pressure recorded within the abdomen initially should be no greater than 9 or 10 mm Hg. If higher pressures are recorded, the needle has been placed improperly. The tip could be lodged in the omentum and can be dislodged by gently elevating and shaking the lower abdominal wall. If this maneuver fails, the needle hub is manipulated in a different direction because its distal hole could impinge on the anterior abdominal wall. If neither of these techniques relieves the increased recorded pressure, the Veress needle is removed and reinserted. Occasionally, while it is passing through the different layers of the abdomen, tissue lodges in the tip, obstructing the opening. Whenever the Veress needle is withdrawn because of high recorded pressures, the surgeon should check its patency.

After 1 L of CO_2 is insufflated, the surgeon percusses the right costal margin to check for loss of liver dullness. If liver dullness is detected, the Veress needle may be positioned improperly and is withdrawn and reinserted. The surgeon should use palpable abdominal distention and the pressure reading rather than the volume of gas insufflated because they more accurately reflect the adequacy of the pneumoperitoneum. After insertion of the trocars, the intraabdominal pressure should be preset between 12 and 16 mm Hg during the operative procedure. Higher pressures for long periods can cause subcutaneous emphysema.

Placement of the Primary Trocar

The sharp primary trocar is aimed toward the sacral promontory. Dull trocars require increased force during insertion, multiple insertions, and excessive instrument manipulation. The insertion of a disposable shielded trocar in the presence of a pneumoperitoneum requires half the force needed for the insertion of a reusable sharp trocar. The disposable trocar shield does not prevent injury completely.[13] Using these new devices can inflict injury because of the unexpected ease of their insertion. Numerous mesenteric, bowel, and vascular injuries have been reported with the use of disposable trocars.

A pneumoperitoneum reduces the proximity of the abdominal wall to the spine and the potential for damage to bowel and vessels.[14] Whether a pneumoperitoneum is associated with a lower incidence of trocar-related injuries is unproved.

Conventional Technique

The direction of trocar insertion, is 90 degrees to the abdominal wall plane toward the sacral promontory. Control of the laparoscopic trocar is essential as it penetrates each layer of the anterior abdominal wall. The trocar is inserted with the patient in a horizontal position because viscera tend to slide away from the advancing trocar. A premature Trendelenburg position does not prevent visceral injury even if significant adhesions are present. Altering the patient's position affects the surgeon's view of important landmarks such as the sacral promontory and sacral hollow. The major anatomic landmarks include the umbilicus located at the level of L3 and L4. The abdominal aorta bifurcates between L4 and L5 (Figure 7-4).

In a program for laparoscopic sterilization, Soderstrom and Butler[15] revealed that the complication rate was reduced 10-fold when a consistent operating format was used. Successful insertion depends on an adequate skin incision; trocars in good working condition (disposable trocars should be checked to be sure they are not locked); proper orientation of the trocar, sheath, and surgeon's hand; and control over the instrument's force and depth of insertion.

With all trocar insertions, the surgeon must hold the instrument properly with the patient in a supine position at the height of the surgeon's waist or slightly below it. The trocar and its sleeve are held with the index finger extended to the level of the maximal planned penetration to prevent the sharp trocar tip from thrusting too deeply. The trocar is palmed, and the dominant hand is used for this procedure. It is rotated in a semicircular fashion with its long axis as controlled, firm downward pressure is applied (Figure 7-9). As the trocar is advanced, the operator senses when the fascia is traversed; the force is reduced as the trocar is advanced slowly to enter the peritoneum. Disposable bullet tip trocars are preferable. A disposable shielded trocar has two advantages: a safety shield that snaps into position after the peritoneum is entered and a sharp instrument for each operation.

Direct Insertion

Trocar insertion without creating a pneumoperitoneum initially reduces the number of preliminary procedures, saving operative time and preventing potential complications. Direct insertion is a safe alternative to initially creating a pneumoperitoneum.[16–22,23] Nezhat and associates[16] compared the ease and safety of creating a pneumoperitoneum with those of direct insertion of either a reusable trocar or a disposable shielded trocar in 200 patients in a randomized, prospectively controlled study. Complications of 22%, 6%, and 0%, respectively, were observed. Although there were fewer complications from direct insertion, no differences were noted in the ease of insertion or the frequency of multiple attempts (Tables 7-4 and 7-5).

The technique is done by elevating the abdominal wall with towel clips applied close to the umbilicus. After the trocar is inserted into the peritoneal cavity, the laparoscope is introduced to verify its correct intraperitoneal placement. A pneumoperitoneum is created with high-flow insufflation. At our centers in Atlanta, Georgia, and Palo Alto, California, direct trocar insertion is used except in patients who have had multiple laparotomies. Since 1989, more than 4500 direct trocar insertions have been done without major complications.

In a randomized comparison of Veress needle and direct trocar insertion, Byron and Markenson[23] reported no major complications with either technique. Complications such as preperitoneal insufflation, failed entry, and needing more than three attempts to enter the peritoneal cavity were more common ($p < 0.05$) in the Veress needle group. Additionally, the mean times for doing the laparoscopic procedure using the direct insertion and Veress needle techniques were 15.3 and 19.6 minutes ($p < 0.01$), respectively, in 113 patients who underwent sterilization procedures.

TABLE 7-4. Comparison of Veress Needle and Direct Trocar Insertion

	Veress Needle ($n = 100$)	Direct Trocar Insertion ($n = 100$)
Complications	22	3
Two insertions required	20	20
Failed insertions	3	6

Open Laparoscopy

In 1971, Hasson[24] introduced the concept of open laparoscopy to eliminate the risks associated with insertion of the Veress needle and trocar. This technique involves direct trocar insertion through a small skin incision without prior pneumoperitoneum. Specially designed equipment consists of a cannula and trumpet valve fitted with a cone-shaped stainless-steel sleeve. A blunt obturator protrudes 1 cm from the tip of the cannula. The cone sleeve seals the peritoneal and fascial gap.

A small transverse, curved, or vertical incision is made at the umbilicus. Two Allis clamps, a knife handle with a small blade, a straight scissors, a tis-

TABLE 7-5. Comparison of Reusable and Disposable Trocars

	Reusable ($n = 50$)	Disposable ($n = 50$)
Complications	3	0
Two insertions required	10	10
Failed insertions	4	2

sue forceps with teeth, a right-angle skin hook, four S-shaped retractors, a needle holder, two curved Kocher clamps, and four small curved hemostats are needed. As the incision is made, Allis clamps or a self-retaining retractor is used to provide adequate exposure. Once the fascia is cut, a 1-cm incision is made in the peritoneum. One suture of 0 polydioxanone (Ethicon) is passed through each peritoneal edge and fascia and tagged. The corklike cannula carrying the blunt obturator is inserted through the opening into the peritoneal cavity. The obturator is withdrawn, and CO_2 is insufflated through the cannula, which is inserted as deep as required to prevent leakage. The previously placed sutures are used to fix the trocar sleeve so that the laparoscope can move freely within the abdominal cavity. At the end of the procedure, the abdominal wall is closed, using the previously placed sutures.

Open laparoscopy usually takes about 5 to 10 minutes longer than closed laparoscopy done by operators with comparable expertise. In more than 1000 consecutive operations done by Hasson,[24] the frequency of minor wound infection was 0.6% and that of small bowel injury was 0.1%. In a review of the laparoscopic complications, the open techniques reduced the incidence of failed procedures, inappropriate gas insufflation, gas embolism, bladder and pelvic kidney punctures, major vessel injuries, and postoperative herniations.[25]

In a survey conducted by Penfield,[26] intestinal laceration was the most serious complication of open laparoscopy, and most of those lacerations occurred during the early use of this technique. In 10,840 open laparoscopies attempted by 18 board-certified obstetricians/gynecologists, six bowel lacerations were reported, four were recognized and repaired, and two were not suspected until several days postoperatively.

To reduce the risk of bowel laceration, the surgeon should use a focus spotlight, work with an experienced assistant, make a vertical incision to facilitate exposure, grasp and elevate the fascia with small Kocher clamps, and cut between the clamps. A gynecologist who attempts open laparoscopy only in special situations will find that the procedure is slow and cumbersome because of difficulty in exposing and identifying each layer of the abdominal wall.

Accessory Trocars

Additional cannulas are needed through which various instruments are inserted into the abdomen for manipulation and operative procedures. Placement sites depend on the patient's anatomy, the contemplated procedure, and the surgeon's preference. For diagnostic purposes, an incision generally is made 4 to 5 cm above the symphysis pubis in the midline. This area, delineated by the two umbilical ligaments and the bladder dome, is safe and usually avascular.

For operative laparoscopy, two accessory trocars (5 mm) are placed 4 to 5 cm above the symphysis pubis at the outer border of the rectus muscle, 3 to 4 cm below the iliac crest, 2 to 3 cm lateral to the deep inferior epigastric vessels. These trocars are inserted under direct vision to lessen the risk of intraabdominal visceral, uterine, and vascular injury and to provide free access to the posterior cul-de-sac. Vascularization of the lower abdomen is provided by two vessels: the deep inferior epigastric originating from the external iliac artery and the superficial epigastric, a branch of the femoral artery. Transillumination helps identify the superficial vessels, but they are difficult to see in obese patients. The deep inferior epigastric vessels run lateral to the umbilical ligaments (Figure 7-10) and are seen intraperitoneally and identified easily. These vessels pass the round ligament, proceed to the anterior abdominal wall, and are seen above the peritoneum. To avoid injuring these vessels, the trocar is inserted medial or lateral to the umbilical ligaments by viewing the underside of the abdomen wall laparoscopically (Figure 7-11). Despite these precautions, aberrant vascular branches occasionally are traumatized, and the operator must be able to manage this type of injury.

To reduce the chance of trauma to the abdominal structures, the proposed site for the secondary

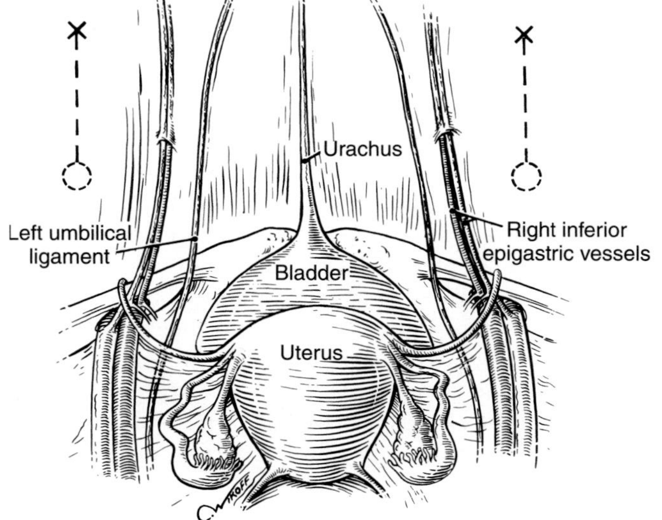

Figure 7-10. Deep inferior epigastric vessels run lateral to the umbilical ligaments.

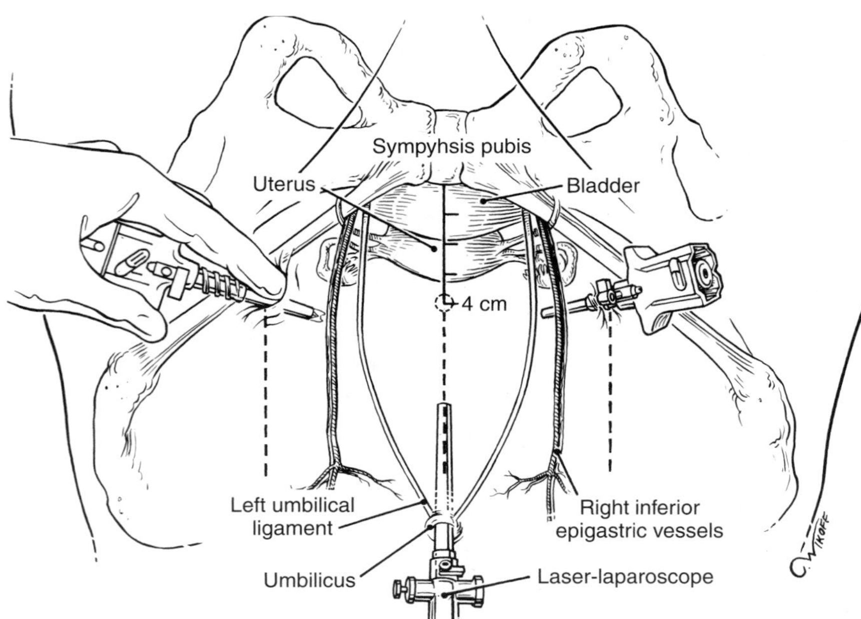

Figure 7-11. Accessory trocars are placed under direct vision to avoid injury to the inferior epigastric vessels and any organs that may be adherent to the pelvic side wall or the anterior abdominal wall. The trocar is inserted lateral to the left umbilical ligament, avoiding inferior epigastric vessels that are invariably lateral to umbilical ligaments.

puncture is indented by applying abdominal pressure with the index finger and observing the peritoneal surface with the laparoscope. Next, mapping of the potential sites for accessory trocar placement is done by advancing the tip of an 18-gauge needle attached to a syringe transabdominally through the peritoneum, revealing the exact course and placement of the accessory trocar. This allows optimal placement. These maneuvers are important, particularly in a patient with evidence of abdominal wall adhesions, and help ensure safe access.

The trocar, held with the index finger extended on the sheath to control the depth of penetration, is inserted through the skin, fat, and fascia. Further advancement is controlled under a laparoscopic view (Figure 7-11). The trocar is aimed toward the center of the abdomen and hollow of the sacrum. If it is aimed laterally, it can slide down the pelvic side wall without being seen through the laparoscope, resulting in injury to the iliac vessels. The accessory trocars are never inserted without laparoscopic observation of their indentation on the abdominal wall or before mapping the abdomen. When insertion of the trocars is viewed directly from the monitor, the surgeon should be sure the camera has not been rotated so that it shows the wrong view of the pelvis. Most laparoscopic procedures do not require more than two or three accessory trocars. Other sites of entry include the midpoint between the symphysis pubis and the umbilicus and McBurney's point.

Some accessory trocar sleeves are too long to allow free access to the pelvic structures and tend to slip out of the peritoneal cavity. The presence of trap valves can interfere with efficient instrument exchange, prevent the introduction and removal of suture material, and prevent the removal of tissue. Several accessory trocar sleeves either screw in or have an umbrella to secure them to the abdominal wall. Radially expanding trocars may reduce laparoscopic complications, lessen a surgeon's exposure to liability, and improve patient outcomes.[27] Two hundred twelve women underwent various laparoscopic procedures involving the placement of 541 radially expanding access cannulas, and no major complications occurred. One patient developed a postoperative mesenteric hematoma that was assumed to be secondary to a venous injury from the Veress needle. Despite the absence of fascial anchoring devices, only six (1%) cannulas slipped.

Accessory Sites

Examples of single accessory site procedures include tubal sterilization, aspiration of an ovarian cyst, and mild peritubal and periovarian adhesiolysis. The suction-irrigator probe is placed through a suprapubic trocar site. Two accessory sites are suggested for lysing peritubal and periovarian adhesions, doing a salpingectomy, removing an ectopic pregnancy, or excising moderate pelvic endometriosis. The suction-irrigator and one additional instrument are needed. Traction is required for these procedures. The suction-irrigator is used for manipulation and smoke evacuation. Bipolar forceps replace the grasping instruments if necessary to achieve hemostasis. For procedures requiring traction, hemostasis, and suturing almost simultaneously, three sites are necessary. Examples are salpingo-oophorectomy, hysterectomy, repair of an ovarian or uterine incisional defect, lysis of extensive abdominal or pelvic adhesions, myomectomy, and cystectomy. During oophorectomy, the infundibulopelvic ligament is grasped with forceps for traction. The assistant holds the grasping forceps, and the surgeon uses the bipolar electrocoagulator to desiccate the infundibulopelvic ligament. The forceps are removed and held by an assistant. The surgeon uses the suction-irrigator probe, and while the plume is suctioned, the CO_2 laser is used for excision. During reconstructive procedures, the operator can give the videolaparoscope to the assistant, freeing the operator's hands for applying traction and suturing. An assistant maintains traction with the grasping forceps as the surgeon uses the needle driver. As with other techniques, surgeons modify procedures as they gain experience.

Operative laparoscopy enables a physician to do complex, delicate procedures through small incisions, thus decreasing the patient's discomfort, morbidity, expense, and duration of convalescence.[28] Laparoscopy is a technique for accessing the patient's diseased organs and gives the surgeon an opportunity to remove abnormal tissue and reconstruct damaged organs.

High-Risk Patients

Body Habitus

Special considerations are required for obese patients because the trocar is inserted almost vertically. The distance between the sacral promontory and the trocar tip is relatively small, and there is a risk to the major vessels. In thin patients, it is safer to overdistend the abdomen with CO_2 before trocar insertion. The force required to introduce the trocar is less than anticipated because the fascia is thin and offers little resistance.

Bowel Distention

Bowel distention secondary to obstruction is a relative contraindication to laparoscopy. This condition may be iatrogenic, resulting from the placement of the Veress needle within the bowel lumen. The filling pressure of the small bowel is the same as that of the abdominal cavity because of the intestine's large capacity. The operator, unaware of the possibility of an "apparent" pneumoperitoneum, might lacerate the distended bowel during the insertion of the trocar.

Previous Laparotomy

In women who have had previous laparotomies, the underlying intraabdominal anatomy can be altered. Inflexible adhesive bridging between the intestine and the abdominal wall can nullify any protection from trocar injury afforded by elevating the abdominal wall, creating a pneumoperitoneum, using the Trendelenburg position, and maintaining intestinal mobility. In some patients, injury will occur to adherent omental vessels or directly to the bowel wall. The patients at the highest risk are those who have undergone major abdominal surgery, such as bowel resection, or an exploratory laparotomy for abdominal trauma or ovarian carcinoma.[5] Women who have had an uncomplicated abdominal operation are not at increased risk.

The association between intestinal and omental adhesions and injury to those structures during operative laparoscopy was evaluated in 360 patients who previously had undergone a variety of abdominal operations (Tables 7-6 through 7-8).[29]

The following approach is recommended.

1. Patients with prior midline incisions have more adhesions than do those with prior Pfannenstiel incisions.
2. Patients with multiple prior incisions do not have more adhesions than do those with a single prior incision.

TABLE 7-6. Patients by Type and Number of Incisions

Incision Type	No. Incisions						Total Patients
	1	2	3	4	5	6	
Pfannenstiel	180	51	19	4	4	0	258
Midline below umbilicus	55	18	9	4	0	1	87
Midline above umbilicus	10	2	1	2	0	0	15

TABLE 7-7. Incidence of Adhesions after Previous Laparotomy

Type of Incision	No.	Percent	Omental, %	Bowel, %
Pfannenstiel	258	72	23	4
Midline below umbilicus	87	24	46	9
Midline above umbilicus	15	4	40	27
Total	360	100		

3. The presence of adhesions does not have a linear correlation with increasing numbers of prior incisions.
4. Women with prior midline or Pfannenstiel incisions for gynecologic operations have more adhesions than do those who have undergone obstetric operations.
5. Patients with prior midline incisions for obstetric operations do not have more adhesions than do those with a prior Pfannenstiel incision for obstetric operations.

The following conditions were associated with severe adhesions:

1. Generalized peritonitis
2. Bowel resection after intestinal obstruction
3. Oncologic procedure with omentectomy
4. Previous radiation and intraperitoneal chemotherapy
5. Previous adhesions

During insertion of the primary trocar and entry into the abdominal cavity, intestinal injuries occurred in 21 (6%) instances (Table 7-9). Of these injuries, six were to the small bowel. Only one patient had a single incision; the remaining five had multiple incisions and complicated surgical histories. Two small bowel injuries occurred during open laparoscopy. In these two patients, the small bowel was attached to the anterior abdominal wall, directly under the umbilicus. It was entered during incision of the fascia that was attached to the intestine. With the exception of 32 patients in whom open laparoscopy was done, the closed technique with prior establishment of pneumoperitoneum was used. The use of open laparoscopy was based on the patients' surgical history (bowel resection, bowel obstruction, ovarian cancer surgery) and the surgeons' preoperative judgment.

TABLE 7-8 Patients by Clinical Indication and Incision Type

Incision Type	Gynecologic	Obstetric
Pfannenstiel	186	43
Midline above or below umbilicus	73	12
Total	259	55

The attachment of the bowel and omentum to the abdominal wall is primarily distal to the umbilicus (Figure 7-12A). If the insertion of the trocar is more vertical than oblique, the possibility of bowel injury is low if a disposable trocar with a shield is used. In patients who have had complicated abdominal operations (bowel resection, bowel obstruction, etc.), the bowel may be attached under, very close to, or occasionally above the umbilicus (Figure 7-12B).

In a subsequent study, the safety of direct trocar insertion was evaluated in 246 consecutive women with previous uncomplicated Pfannenstiel or midline incisions. All of them underwent bowel preparation and understood that laparotomy was possible. Trocar insertion was almost at a 90-degree angle while the operator and the assistant elevated the abdominal wall, lateral to the umbilicus. Fifty patients had omental adhesions, and 34 had bowel adhesions to the anterior abdominal wall. There were no small bowel injuries. There were five omental injuries; in one, the injury was associated with bleeding and was managed laparoscopically.

On the basis of these findings, it can be concluded that the incidence of subumbilical bowel adhesions and subsequent bowel injury is related to the indication for previous laparotomy rather than to the type or number of previous laparotomies. The incidence of bowel injuries during insertion of the primary trocar is low. The closed technique with or without prior establishment of a pneumoperitoneum is used in most instances without increasing the chance of bowel injury.

Special Techniques

Several procedures have been described to assess the anterior abdominal wall for intestinal adhesions. DeCherney[30] advocates using a small-gauge

TABLE 7-9. **Incidence of Injury—21/360 (6%)**

Type of Injury	Omental Hematoma (Closed Technique)		Omental Bleeding (Closed Technique)		Small Bowel Injury (Closed, 6; Open, 2)	
	Single	Multiple	Single	Multiple	Single	Multiple
Number	1	5	7	2	1	5
Percent	0.3	1.4	1.9	0.6	0.3	1.4

needle laparoscope 2 to 3 mm in diameter. The needle scope is inserted instead of the Veress needle under direct vision through the umbilical, preperitoneal, and subperitoneal structures. The Veress needle is inserted intraabdominally, and insufflation proceeds under direct observation.

Exploring the periumbilical area with an 18-gauge needle attached to a syringe after establishing the pneumoperitoneum (Figure 7-13) also is possible. If adhesions are detected by these techniques, the options include open laparoscopy and alternative sites of abdominal entry. The primary trocar is inserted in the midline between the xiphoid and the pubic symphysis provided that care is taken to remain at least 5 cm below the xiphoid and 5 cm above the pubic symphysis (Figure 7-8).[15] Although these techniques help detect periumbilical adhesions, they are not definitive and are time-consuming. Based on these observations, the following approach is recommended:

1. Patients who have had a previous laparotomy are allocated to noncomplicated and complicated groups.
2. One-day or 3-day bowel preparation is administered, based on the patient's history. All patients must understand that bowel injury is possible and must consent to a possible conversion of the procedure to laparotomy.
3. In the noncomplicated group, open or closed techniques are used. If the closed technique is used, a disposable trocar with a bullet shield is preferable. Trocar entry is controlled, and the placement angle is vertical rather than oblique (Figure 7-14). Either previous establishment of a pneumoperitoneum by a Veress needle or

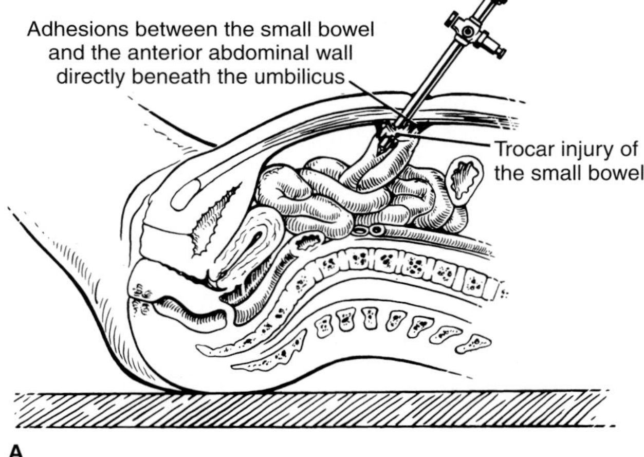

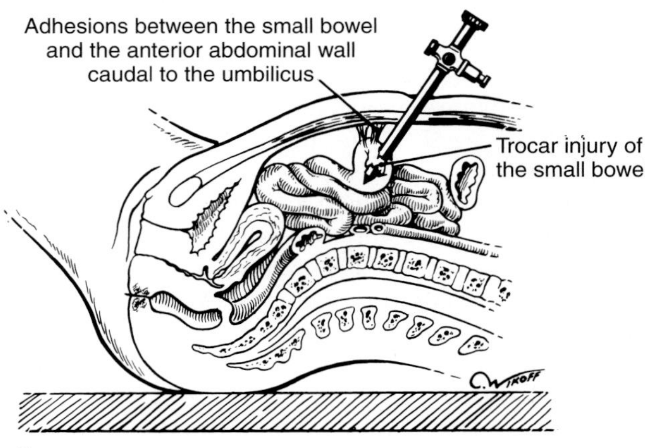

Figure 7-12. The bowel is attached to the anterior abdominal wall. **A.** The bowel is attached directly under the umbilicus. **B.** The attachment is below and distal to the umbilicus.

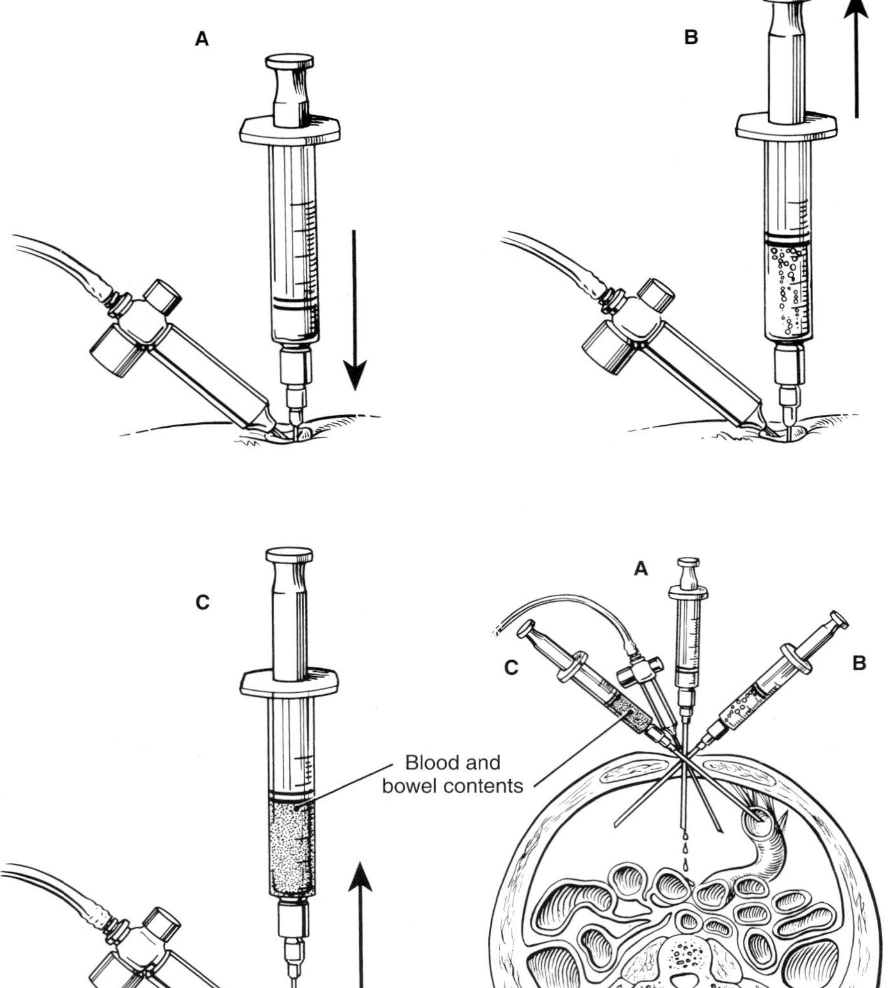

Figure 7-13. The abdomen is "mapped" by using an 18-gauge spinal needle around the Veress needle. A 20-gauge needle is inserted under negative pressure at several cardinal points of a 20-mm circle around the umbilicus. If blood or bowel content is aspirated instead of CO_2 gas at any of these points, alternative sites for trocar insertion should be chosen.

direct trocar insertion is used. If the Veress needle is used, the subumbilical area is searched for bowel adhesions before trocar insertion. If adhesions are suspected, other locations are explored until a safe area is detected and the trocar is inserted. In patients at risk for significant adhesions, a pneumoperitoneum is created by inserting the Veress needle trans-umbilically or in the left subcostal area in the midclavicular line after aspirating with a syringe to rule out bowel entry. The abdomen is insufflated with CO_2. The area is explored with a 20-gauge needle to inject saline (Figure 7-13). If no fluid is aspirated (the conditions are favorable), a 5-mm trocar is inserted and a 4-mm laparoscope is placed to observe the peritoneal cavity (Figure 7-14). If there is no intestinal injury, the 5-mm trocar is replaced with the 10-mm trocar. If intestinal entry occurs, the 5-mm trocar is left

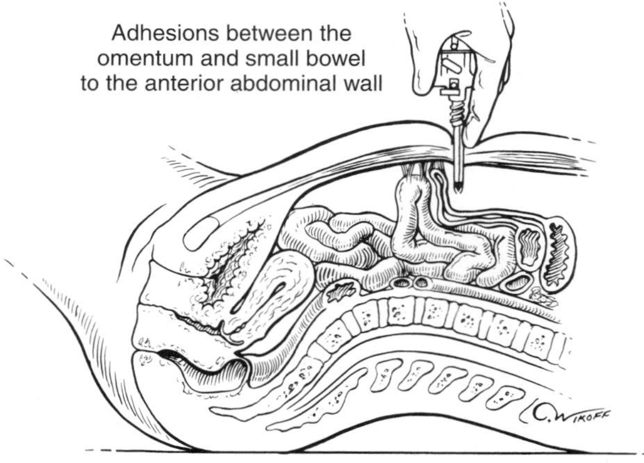

Figure 7-14. This patient had bowel adhesions from a previous laparotomy.

in place and a safe area is found to insert the 10-mm trocar and laparoscope. The loops of injured bowel are mobilized and repaired laparoscopically or through a minilaparotomy.[2] Since this approach was adopted, no bowel injuries have been observed resulting from trocar insertion in more than 700 patients with different types of laparotomies for different indications. Another instrument that can be helpful is the 2-mm microlaparoscope for initial intraabdominal evaluation. If the patient has undergone an adequate bowel preparation, an incidental bowel perforation can be managed conservatively after thorough and extensive irrigation of the abdominal cavity, unlike similar injuries caused by the 4-mm laparoscope.

4. For patients in the complicated group, a mapping technique is used to lessen the chance of sequelae. After insertion of the laparoscope, the abdominal wall with adherent bowel or omentum is explored. If the adhesions are severe and no clear space for accessory trocar insertion is seen, the abdominal wall is observed through the laparoscope and gentle external compression is done, marking areas that seem free of adhesions. Before inserting the trocar, the surgeon should simulate its track with a 21-gauge spinal needle. If this identifies a clear path, the trocar is introduced next to the needle, or the needle is removed and the trocar is introduced. An advantage of first inserting the 21-gauge needle is its small diameter because the injury incurred does not require repair. As the needle's placement is seen, there is little risk of missing a visceral injury. The insertion of the needle through the skin of the abdominal wall is easy, and so the surgeon can control the needle precisely and prevent any deviation from the present course.

Pelvic Exploration

The initial phase of laparoscopy is done to assess the extent of disease, document it with photographs or video recordings, and identify anatomic landmarks. The characteristics of the bladder, ureters, colon, rectum, uterosacral ligaments, and major blood vessels are noted (Figure 7-15). The appendix is inspected for endometriosis. The upper abdomen, including the abdominal

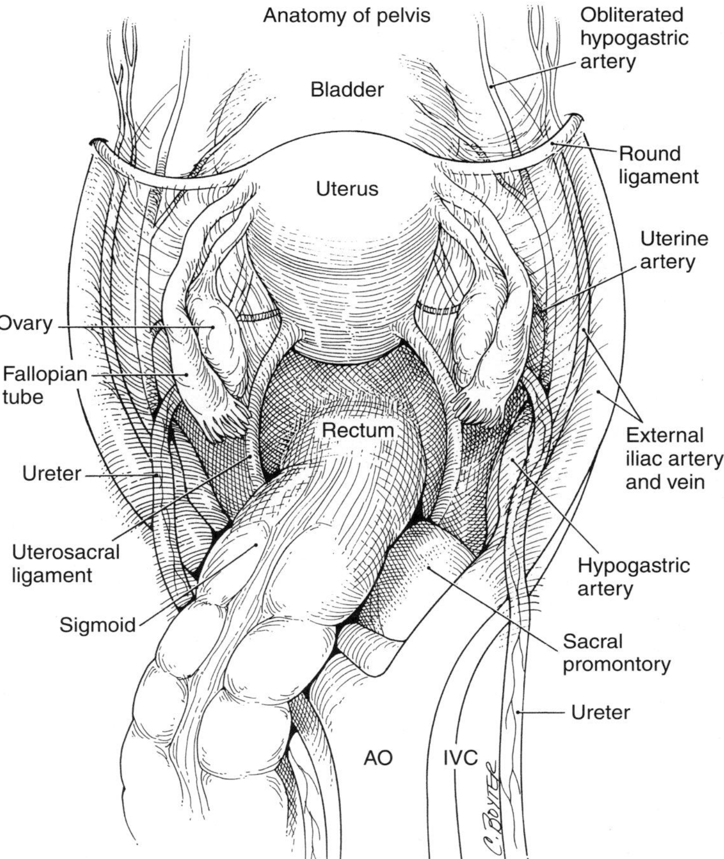

Figure 7-15. Panoramic view of the lower abdomen and pelvis.

walls, liver, gallbladder, and diaphragm, is examined for any abnormality that could contribute to the patient's symptoms. As the laparoscope is turned toward the left, the intestine is evaluated, and then the laparoscope is returned to view the pelvic cavity. The omentum and intestines are examined to confirm that they were not injured during insertion of the Veress needle and trocar.

After the posterior cul-de-sac is filled with irrigation fluid, the right adnexa are assessed. The fimbria are lifted, and the posterior aspect of the ovary and the ovarian fossa are evaluated. The ureter is seen, and its direction is traced from the pelvic brim to the bladder. The uterus is anteverted, and the uterosacral ligaments, posterior cul-de-sac, and rectum are examined. The patient is placed in a 30-degree Trendelenburg position to allow the surgeon to push the small bowel into the upper abdomen to aid in viewing the posterior cul-de-sac (Figure 7-16). The rectosigmoid colon and its folds are evaluated, and after the rectosigmoid colon is pushed laterally, the left and right pararectal areas are examined. The left ovary and tube are evaluated. In the presence of extensive adhesions, this technique is modified. The gynecologist ascertains the approximate location of the normal structures, assesses the type of adhesion, plans the procedure, and decides whether the procedure is to be done by laparoscopy or laparotomy. This decision depends on the abnormalities, the time needed to correct them, and the surgeon's experience.

End of the Operation

Chromopertubation is done in all infertility patients intraoperatively. The patient's position is changed from Trendelenburg to horizontal to allow

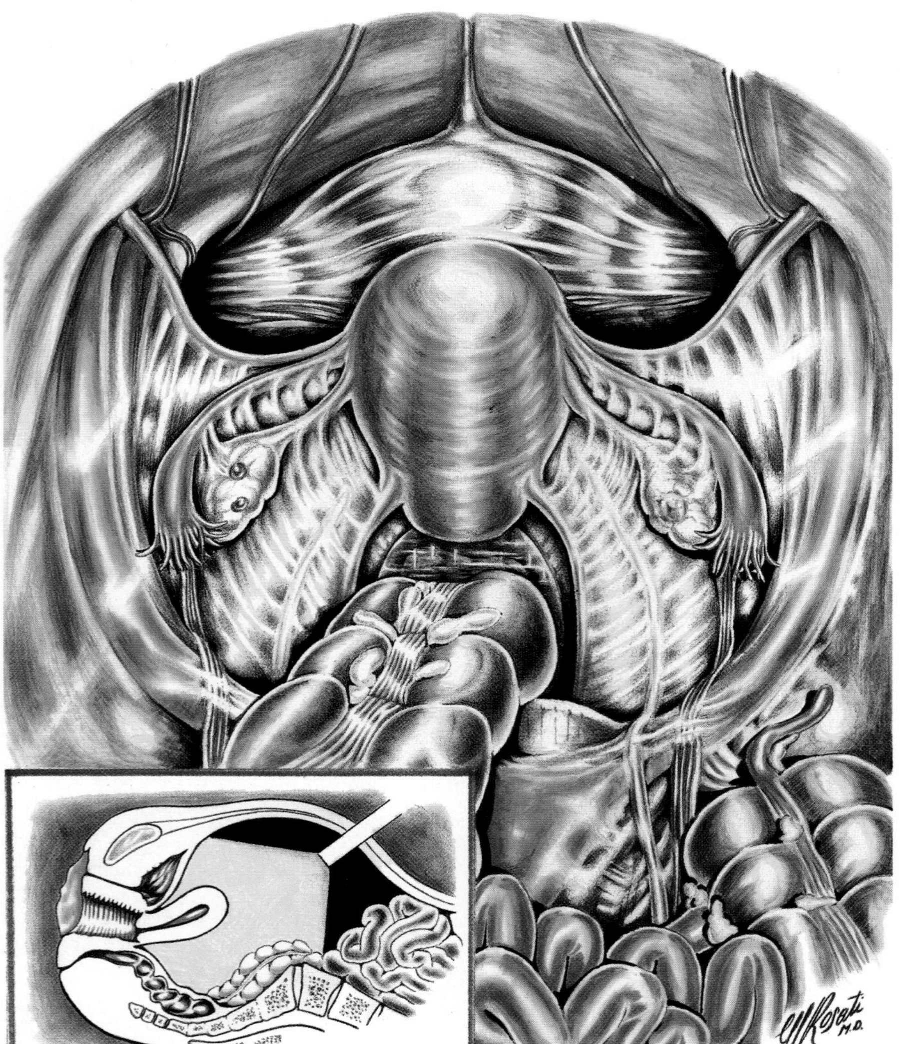

Figure 7-16. The patient is placed in a Trendelenburg position. Inset shows the elevation of the pelvis.

fluid from the upper abdomen to collect in the pelvic cavity. The entire peritoneal cavity is irrigated copiously with isotonic fluid, usually lactated Ringer's, solution and inspected for blood clots, pieces of adhesions, cyst wall, endometriosis implants, and bleeding. Bleeding points are identified and coagulated with bipolar forceps. Since the intraabdominal pressure created by the pneumoperitoneum can tamponade bleeding from small vessels, the gas is evacuated temporarily and the operative sites are inspected for bleeding before the abdominal cavity is reinsufflated. The presence of clear irrigating fluid confirms adequate hemostasis. The procedure is concluded by evacuating the CO_2 from the abdomen.

Release of Pneumoperitoneum

The CO_2 used to distend the abdomen is evacuated to reduce postoperative shoulder pain caused by gas trapped under the diaphragm. The patient is put in a straight, supine position as the gas escapes from the umbilical and suprapubic trocars. Suprapubic trocars are removed under low pneumoperitoneal pressure to search for possible inferior epigastric vessel injury. The umbilical trocar is removed, and the skin incisions are inspected for bleeding. Except for patients in whom Interceed (Ethicon) is applied, 300 to 400 mL of lactated Ringer's solution is left in the abdominal cavity to aid in displacing the gas and possibly to decrease postoperative adhesions.[31] Since this procedure has been instituted, the prevalence of postoperative shoulder pain has decreased.

Closure of Incisions

The trocar incisions are closed using steristrips or inverted subcutaneous 4-0 polyglactin (Ethicon) sutures. Incisions made for trocars larger than 5 mm are closed in layers, especially in older or thin women because failure to close the fascia has been associated with small bowel strangulation and hernia. Several instruments, including the J-needle and the Carter-Thomason needle (Figure 7-17), have been developed to allow for fascial and peritoneal closure of the trocar site incisions under direct observation.

Postoperative Care

Patients are provided with postoperative instructions before the operation to prepare them for the postoperative experience. The gynecologist sees the patient in the outpatient extended recovery room to explain the operative findings and the expected postoperative course. Before discharge, patients are given prescriptions for pain medications (usually Tylenol with codeine) as needed and routine postoperative instructions. Outpatient nurses or office nurses contact the patient 1 or 2 days postoperatively to answer additional questions and monitor her recovery. If a patient complains of pain, fever, or bowel or bladder symptoms, she is examined promptly. Patients routinely are seen 1 to 6 weeks postoperatively. Most women return to normal activity within 1 week. The time required for full recovery is between 1 and 3 weeks, depending on the extent of the operation.

Common Postoperative Complaints

Nausea and vomiting most likely are related to intraabdominal CO_2 and the narcotics frequently used perioperatively. Usually these symptoms respond to parenteral antiemetic medication, but patients occasionally are admitted overnight for continued care. Shoulder pain referred from the collection of CO_2 under the diaphragm is the most common complaint and generally resolves within 48 hours. Resting on the abdomen with pillows under it is helpful. Elevating the lower pelvis also will alleviate this pain.

Occasionally a patient develops hypotension unrelated to blood loss. These patients are cured promptly after a bolus of intravenous fluid is given.

Postoperative incisional pain is usually mild and is managed by using a heating pad and analgesics. A randomized, double-blinded trial of preemptive analgesia in laparoscopy patients concluded that the administration of bupivicaine before laparoscopy results in decreased postoperative pain compared with the popular practice of infiltrating bupivicaine at the time of incision closure.[32] Patients who undergo extensive intraabdominal procedures can have severe visceral pain. Narcotic or nonsteroidal anti-inflammatory agents are needed in addition to a heating pad. Persistent pain for more than a few hours after release from the hospital requires that the patient be examined.

When large amounts of isotonic fluid are left in the abdomen, the patient tends to drain pinkish fluid through the abdominal puncture wounds. This ceases within 24 to 48 hours. Reassurance allays the patient's concern.

To become proficient with operative laparoscopy, a gynecologist must understand the learning curve and begin with simple procedures before gradually advancing to more complicated ones. Complications can occur during the simplest procedures. The primary steps are exposure (by iden-

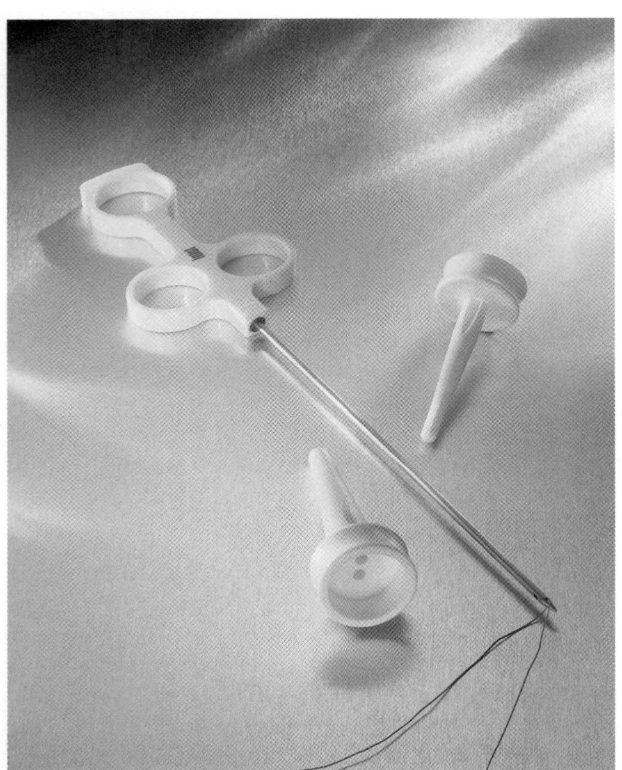

A

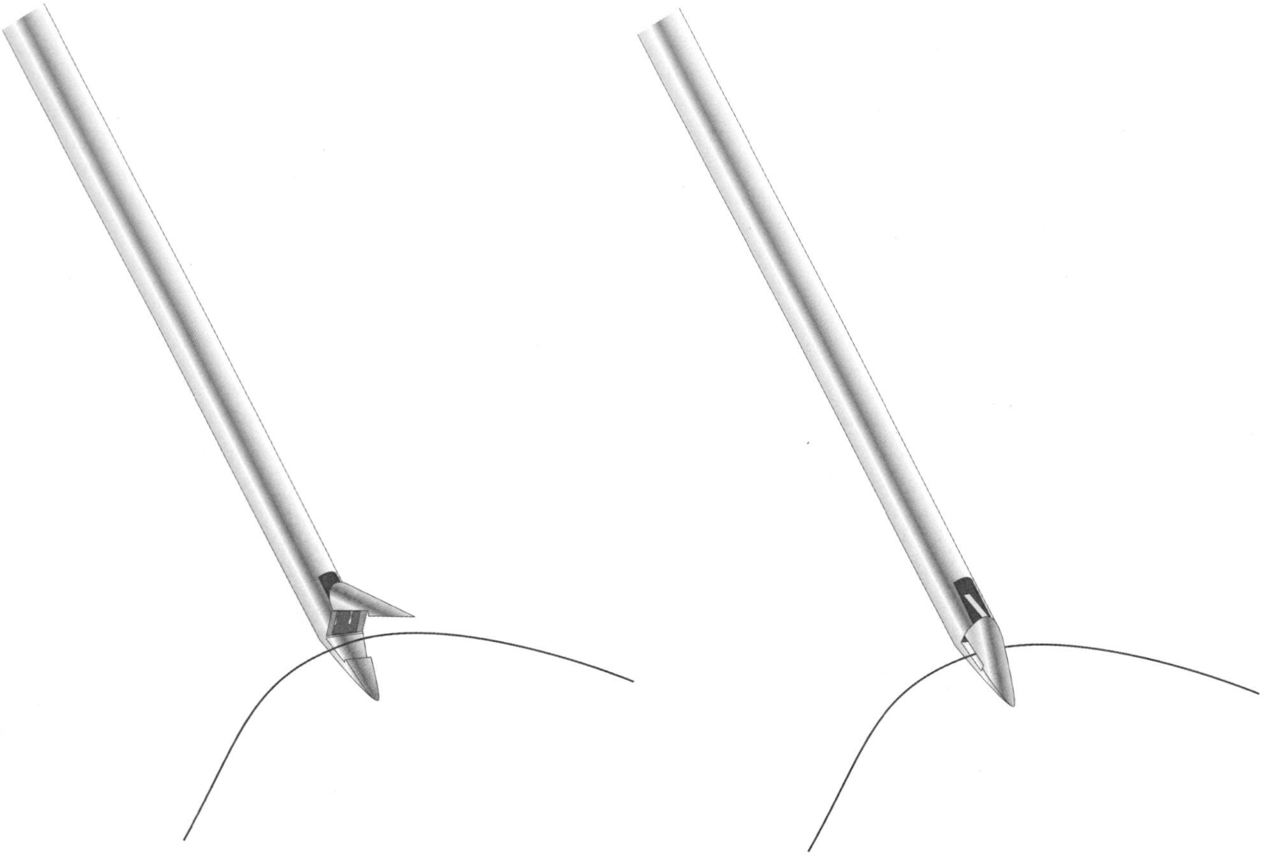

Figure 7-17. The Carter-Thomason needle. The system allows the passage of suture through soft tissue and then retrieval from a separate entry with the same device. **A.** The CloseSure Procedure Kit contains the Carter-Thomason suture passer and the Pilot suturing guides. **B.** A stepdown from the distal to proximal segment of the jaws allows the distal tip to close completely with the suture in the proximal stepdown segment. **C.** Suture passer is used to push suture material through the pilot guide, fascia, muscle, and peritoneum and into the abdomen. The suture is dropped, and the suture passer is removed. **D.** Suture passer is pushed through opposite side of the Pilot guide and used to pick up the suture. **E.** Suture passer is removed, pulling the suture through the peritoneum, muscle, fascia, and guide. **F.** Guide is removed, and the suture is tied to complete the closure.

B

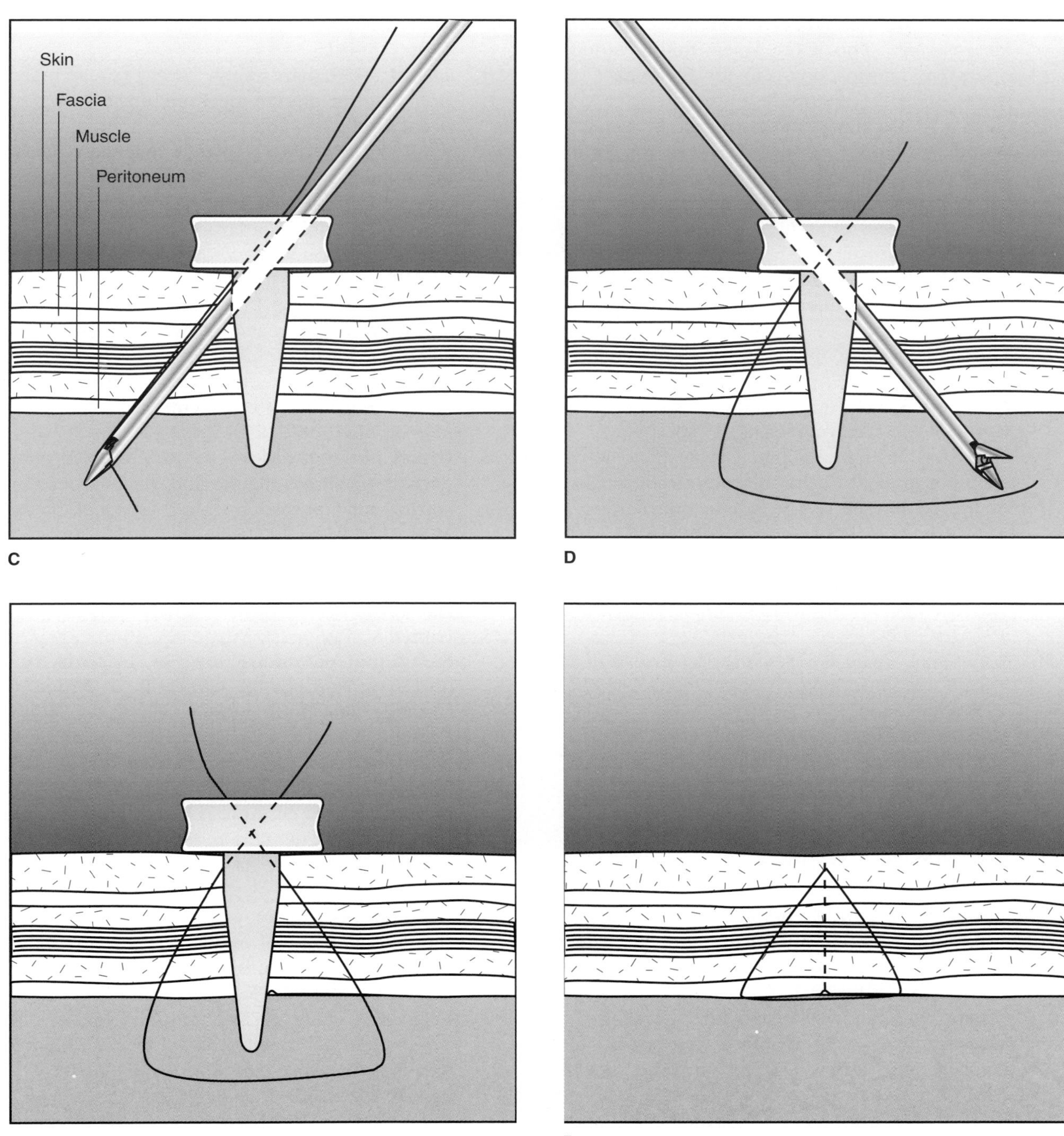

Figure 7-17.

tifying the anatomy and pathology), traction, and action (cutting, vaporization, hemostasis, or suturing). The gynecologist holds the videolaseroscope with the dominant hand. Most procedures require only one or two accessory instruments.

References

1. Palmer R: La coelioscopie gynecologique, ses possibilities et ses indications actuelles. *Semin Hop Paris* 1954; 30:4441.

2. Nezhat CR, Nezhat FR, Silfen SL. Videolaseroscopy: The CO_2 laser for advanced operative laparoscopy. *Obstet Gynecol Clin North Am* 1991; 18:585.
3. Nezhat C, Nezhat F, Pennington E. Laparoscopic treatment of infiltrative rectosigmoid colon and rectovaginal septum endometriosis by the technique of videolaseroscopy and the CO_2 laser. *Br J Obstet Gynaecol* 1992; 99:664.
4. East MC, Steele PRM. Laparoscopic incisions at the lower umbilical verge. *Br Med J* 1988; 296:753.
5. Loffer FD. Endoscopy in high risk patients, in Martin DC, ed., *Manual of Endoscopy*. Santa Fe Springs, CA: American Association of Gynecologic Laparoscopists, 1990.
6. Nezhat F, Brill AI, Nezhat CH, et al. Laparoscopic appraisal of the anatomic relationship of the umbilicus to the aortic bifurcation. *J Am Assoc Gynecol Laparosc* 1998; 5:135.
7. Neely MR, McWilliams R, Makhlouf HA. Laparoscopy: Routine pneumoperitoneum via the posterior fornix. *Obstet Gynecol* 1975; 45:459.
8. Wolfe WM, Pasic R. Transuterine insertion of Veress needle in laparoscopy. *Obstet Gynecol* 1990; 75:456.
9. Morgan HR. Laparoscopy: Induction of pneumoperitoneum via transfundal puncture. *Obstet Gynecol* 1979; 54:260.
10. Awadalla SG. Letter to the editor. *Obstet Gynecol* 1990; 76:314.
11. Loffer FD, Pent D. Laparoscopy in the obese patient. *Am J Obstet Gynecol* 1976; 125:104.
12. Rosen DM, Lam AM, Chapman M, et al. Methods of creating pneumoperitoneum: A review of techniques and complications. *Obstet Gynecol Surv* 1998; 53:167.
13. Corson SL, Batzer FR, Gocial B, Maislin C. Measurement of the force necessary for laparoscopic entry. *J Reprod Med* 1989; 34:282.
14. Phillips JM. *Laparoscopy*. Baltimore: Williams & Wilkins, 1977.
15. Soderstrom RM, Butler JC. A critical evaluation of complications in laparoscopy. *J Reprod Med* 1973; 10:245.
16. Nezhat FR, Silfen SL, Evans D, Nezhat C. Comparison of direct insertion of disposable and standard reusable laparoscopic trocars and previous pneumoperitoneum with veress needle. *Obstet Gynecol* 1991; 78:148.
17. Borgatta L, Gruss L, Barad D, Kaali SG. Direct trocar insertion versus Veress needle use for laparoscopic sterilization. *J Reprod Med* 1990; 35:891.
18. Jarrett JC. Laparoscopy: Direct trocar insertion without pneumoperitoneum. *Obstet Gynecol* 1990; 75:725.
19. Kaali SG, Bartfai G. Direct insertion of the laparoscopic trocar after an earlier laparotomy. *J Reprod Med* 1988; 33:739.
20. Saidi MH. Direct laparoscopy without prior pneumoperitoneum. *J Reprod Med* 1986; 31:684.
21. Copeland C, Wing R, Hulka JF. Direct trocar insertion at laparoscopy: An evaluation. *Obstet Gynecol* 1983; 62:655.
22. Dingfelder JR. Direct laparoscopic trocar insertion without prior pneumoperitoneum. *J Reprod Med* 1978; 21:45.
23. Byron JW, Markenson GA. Randomized comparison of Veress needle and direct trocar insertion for laparoscopy. *Surg Gynecol Obstet* 1993; 177:259.
24. Hasson HM. Open laparoscopy versus closed laparoscopy: A comparison of complication rates. *Adv Plan Parent* 1978; 13:41.
25. Gomel V, Taylor PJ, Yuzpe AA, Rioux JE. The technique of endoscopy, in *Laparoscopy and Hysteroscopy in Gynecologic Practice*. Chicago: Year Book, 1986.
26. Penfield AJ. How to prevent complications of open laparoscopy. *J Reprod Med* 1985; 30:660.
27. Galen DI, Jacobson A, Weckstein LN, et al. Reduction of cannula-related laparoscopic complications using a radially expanding access device. *J Am Assoc Gynecol Laparosc* 1999; 6:79.
28. Luciano AA, Lowney J, Jacobs SL. Endoscopic treatment of endometriosis-associated infertility: Therapeutic, economic and social benefits. *J Reprod Med* 1992; 37:573.
29. Brill AI, Nezhat F, Nezhat CH, Nezhat CR. The incidence of adhesions after prior laparotomy: A laparoscopic appraisal. *Obstet Gynecol* 1995; 85:269.
30. DeCherney AH. Laparoscopy with unexpected viscous penetration, in Nichols DH, ed., *Clinical Problems, Injuries and Complications of Gynecologic Surgery*. Baltimore: Williams & Wilkins, 1988.
31. Pagidas K, Tulandi T. Effects of Ringer's lactate, Interceed (TC7) and Gore-Tex Surgical Membrane on postsurgical adhesion formation. *Fertil Steril* 1992; 57:199.
32. Ke RW, Portera SG, Bagous W, Lincoln SR. A randomized, double-blinded trial of preemptive analgesia in laparoscopy. *Obstet Gynecol* 1998; 92:972.

8

Office Microlaparoscopy

The technologic progress made since 1990 has been a major driving force behind the rapid acceptance of laparoscopy as an effective instrument for advanced surgery. Continuing innovation has resulted in an operative approach with a small-diameter laparoscope.

This new technique has been called microlaparoscopy,[1–5] minilaparoscopy,[6,7] office laparoscopy,[8,9] microendoscopy,[10] endoscopic microsurgery, needlescopic surgery, small-diameter laparoscopy,[11,12] and optical catheter laparoscopy.[9,13,14] The term *minilaparoscopy* has been used to describe a 1.2-mm laparoscope used for diagnostic purposes[7] and laparoscopic appendectomy with a single umbilical puncture.[15] The term *microlaparoscopy* was used previously to refer to 4-mm laparoscopes,[16] but at present it is reserved for scopes with a diameter less than 2 mm.

The Development of Microlaparoscopy

The pursuit of less invasive surgical means for diagnosis has led to the development of laparoscopes with a diameter smaller than 2 mm. Initially, 0.5- to 1.4-mm flexible fiberoptic scopes, constructed originally for vascular angioscopy or falloposcopy, were used.[2,17] However, these instruments resulted in low levels of light, a reduced field of view, and poor resolution.[13] New high-resolution fiberoptic lens technology has been incorporated into microlaparoscopes, offering better light transmission and a clearer image. Current microlaparoscopes provide an optical capacity similar to that of conventional laparoscopes.

Indications for Microlaparoscopy

Diagnosis

Despite advances in noninvasive diagnostic imaging modalities, the ability to diagnose pelvic and abdominal disease accurately often remains dependent on direct viewing of intraabdominal abnormalities. The need to rely on laparoscopy under general anesthesia, with its associated risks and costs, can lead to a delay in the diagnosis of patients with pelvic pain or infertility. The availability of an instrument that allows a physician to arrive rapidly at a definite diagnosis in the office or emergency room would be a great advance. Microlaparoscopy under local anesthesia, with its low associated morbidity and cost, may fulfill this important diagnostic need.

Microlaparoscopy provides prompt and accurate diagnosis in the emergency room.[16] It has been used successfully by general surgeons to diagnose hepatic disease and to perform liver biopsy.[18] Diagnostic laparoscopy under local anesthesia has been advocated for patients with suspected appendicitis and those who present with an atypical clinical picture or when conventional laboratory and imaging tests have been inconclusive.[19]

Similar diagnostic accuracy can be expected in patients with acute abdominal pain caused by a ruptured corpus luteum cyst, an ectopic pregnancy, pelvic inflammatory disease (PID), or torsion of the adnexa. Ectopic pregnancy has been detected accurately with sub-2-mm and 10-mm laparoscopes.[1,7] Surgical management can be replaced with conservative observation when the rupture of a tubal pregnancy is excluded by microlaparoscopy. The diagnostic accuracy of microlaparoscopy in comparison to laparoscopy with a standard 10-mm laparoscope has been demonstrated in patients with endometriosis and adnexal adhesions.[3,5,9]

The role of diagnostic microlaparoscopy can be extended beyond direct observation. Microbiologic cultures can be collected in patients with pelvic infectious disease, and tissue biopsies can be obtained to confirm endometriosis.[12]

Chronic Pelvic Pain

An advantage of microlaparoscopy for diagnostic purposes is the ability to communicate with a conscious woman during the procedure. Information can be obtained, under direct viewing, regarding sensitive intraabdominal areas. This technique, which is termed conscious pain mapping, is effective in women with chronic pelvic pain.[4] These women are asked to rate their pain during grasping with a word selection–weighted scale. The pain can be localized to a specific point, or it can be determined whether it is generalized throughout the pelvis or abdomen. If the patient experiences pain during local manipulation of the viscera, the pain is rated after direct application of 1% lidocaine. Utilizing microlaparoscopy, conscious pain mapping identified a focal source of pain in 3 of 11 patients with a history of chronic pelvic pain and identified generalized visceral hypersensitivity in most of the other patients. The procedure is tolerated acceptably, especially in patients undergoing infertility evaluation.

Conscious pain mapping with microlaparoscopy revealed the appendix as the source of chronic pelvic pain in two women.[20] They had microlaparoscopic appendectomies under local anesthesia.

Infertility

Microlaparoscopy allows the accurate diagnosis of tubal adhesions and the results of chromopertubation. The evaluation of the tubes can be improved by combining microlaparoscopy with falloposcopy.[17] Other conditions associated with infertility, such as endometriosis, also can be assessed. Microlaparoscopy can ascertain the feasibility of sterilization reversal or referral to in vitro fertilization and the efficacy of postoperative tuboplasty. Gamete intrafallopian transfer (GIFT) and zygote intrafallopian transfer (ZIFT) have been done under local anesthesia with conscious sedation.[21,22] The use of microlaparoscopic equipment may facilitate the performance of these procedures under sedation and contribute to their widespread acceptance in routine practice.

Oncology

Microlaparoscopy under local anesthesia is a safe and effective diagnostic procedure for evaluating the peritoneal cavity for office screening of early ovarian cancer. It is not clear who should be tested or when in the workup the procedure should be done.

Although the usefulness of second-look laparoscopy in the follow-up of ovarian cancer is debatable, high tolerance to the examination done under local anesthesia has been demonstrated.[23] Neoplasia was found and laparotomy was avoided in 35 (48.6%) of 72 explorations. The correlation between gross and microscopic findings was excellent. Nevertheless, there were 31% (4 of 13) false negatives in second-look laparotomy after laparoscopy. No complications occurred despite previous abdominal operations.

Microlaparoscopy may allow the more liberal use of safe and effective assessment after ovarian cancer treatment, including peritoneal biopsies. Childers and colleagues[8] used a 1.8-mm optical catheter to do office microlaparoscopy and biopsy for the evaluation of patients with intraperitoneal carcinomatosis. The diagnosis was confirmed by biopsy specimens in six of seven patients. Those authors were able to obtain sufficient tissue for histologic review and special immunohistochemical stains. Microlaparoscopy may play a role in the future in ascertaining the type of operation required in women who have an abdominal or pelvic mass. It can be used to obtain ascitic fluid for cytologic examination.

Operative Microlaparoscopy

Tubal ligation was one of the first operative applications of microlaparoscopy,[18,24] and the potential for cost savings in an outpatient or clinic setting is obvious.

Microlaparoscopic adhesiolysis is feasible with either lasers transmitted through small-diameter fiberoptic fibers or scissors. Coagulation of endometriosis has been done successfully with microlaparoscopy and fiberoptic lasers. Microlaparoscopic myolysis using neodymium-yttrium aluminum garnet (Nd:YAG) laser fibers has been reported.[6] Laparoscopic tubal ligation has been done for over two decades under local anesthesia.[25,26] The use of microlaparoscopes is more comfortable for patients during local anesthesia for sterilization.[27-29]

Monitoring Medical Treatment

Gynecologists provide many common treatments with only a limited ability to directly assess the patient's response. Microlaparoscopy allows sequential monitoring of the response to antibiotics given to patients with PID. The regression of endometriosis after medical treatment with hormone-suppressive drugs such as gonadotropin analogues can be examined. Other possibilities include the verification of the absorption of a tubal pregnancy after methotrexate administration.

Monitoring Surgical Treatment

The development of postoperative adhesions is a major concern. Postoperative microlaparoscopy can discover the degree of adhesion formation and offers a way to cut new or re-formed adhesions. The procedure can be repeated sequentially in infertility patients and those with chronic pelvic pain. Steege[29] did repeated clinic microlaparoscopy for the evaluation and treatment of postoperative pelvic adhesions. Through a Tenckhoff catheter placed in the umbilicus after lysis of adhesions at hysterectomy, he examined the pelvis twice a week for 2 weeks. Of the 32 attempts at second-look observation with an optical catheter, 26 (81.3%) were successful. Recurrent adhesions were detected and treated in only 1 of the 10 patients. No complications occurred in this series.

Microlaparoscopy may improve the safety of endoscopic operations. It can verify unequivocally the intraperitoneal position of the Veress needle before gas insufflation and eliminate preperitoneal insufflation or bowel perforation. In patients with known or suspected adhesions, the microlaparoscope inserted into the abdominal area, deemed most likely free of adhesions, can assist in safe placement of the conventional laparoscopic trocar. Microlaparoscopy allows monitoring during operative hysteroscopy, removal of a septum, myomectomy, or endometrial resection to lessen the risk of uterine perforation.

Contraindications

Many conditions previously considered contraindications for laparoscopy currently are accepted as indications. For instance, despite concerns regarding the possible spread of malignancy, laparoscopy is offered routinely to some patients who have pelvic cancer. However, their inability to withstand general anesthesia still limits the use of laparoscopy in some of those patients. Microlaparoscopy may allow the procedure in these patients. The successful use of a 4-mm microlaparoscope in patients with acute trauma illustrates these new possibilities.[16]

Relative contraindications to microlaparoscopy include patients who have had multiple abdominal adhesions or previous multiple surgical procedures, especially in conditions where the need for a laparotomy is likely. Obesity can preclude

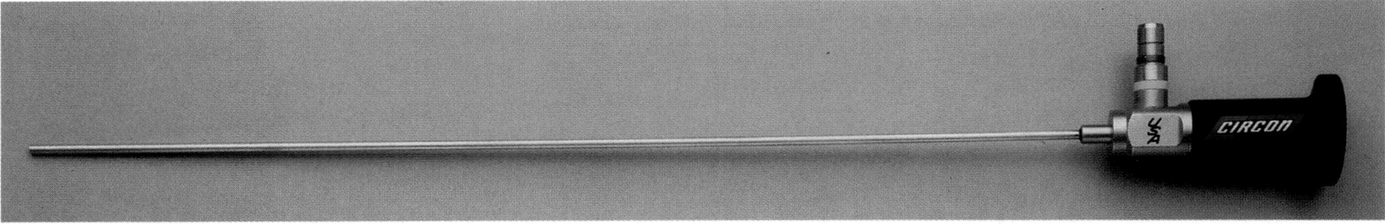

A

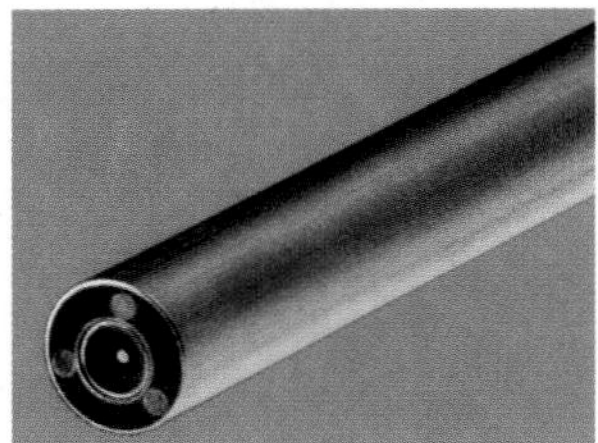

B

Figure 8-1. **A.** This microlaparoscope is a 2.7-mm reusable telescope (Medical Dynamics, Inc). **B.** The distal end.

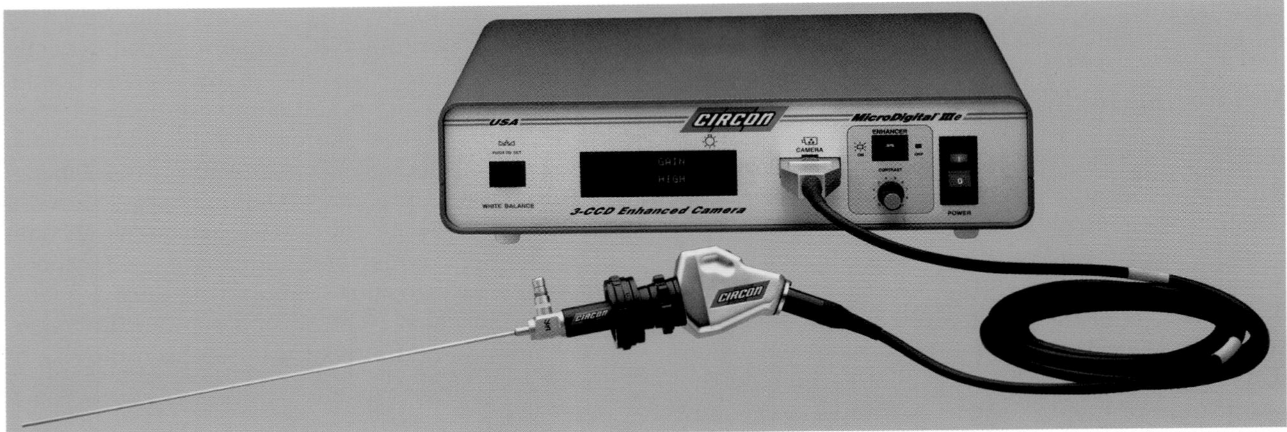

Figure 8-2. The MicroDigital enhanced image three-chip video camera is attached to the telescope.

microlaparoscopy under local anesthesia because the heavy abdominal wall may not be raised sufficiently by the limited volumes of gas. Some microlaparoscopes can be too short in obese patients since the optics require a relatively short distance between the tip of the scope and the observed organ. An enlarged uterus or a pregnancy beyond 12 weeks of gestation can make the insertion of a microlaparoscope and the examination of the pelvis technically more difficult. Any medical disability that limits the use of the deep Trendelenburg position makes both microlaparoscopy and laparoscopy inadvisable.

The Equipment

Microlaparoscopy is relatively new, and a gynecologist should evaluate several different microlaparoscopes before choosing a specific system. The quality of the image produced, the ease of use, and the surgeon's operating comfort are important. The cost of the system is influenced by the compatibility of the system with other available equipment at the operative site and the durability of the equipment. The effort associated with cleaning and sterilizing the instruments is another significant factor, especially in an office setting.

One of the first systems introduced was the Optical Catheter (Medical Dynamics, Inc., Englewood, CO). It consists of a 2.7-mm rigid tube containing a bundle of imaging fibers (Figure 8-1). This system includes its own video camera, monitor, and light source (Figure 8-2). It is inserted through a disposable Adair Veress needle. Although this was one of the earliest tested systems, the fact that it cannot be hooked directly to standard laparoscopic video cameras and light sources is a major limitation. It is easy to use but provides inferior images compared with other commercial microlaparoscopes.[30]

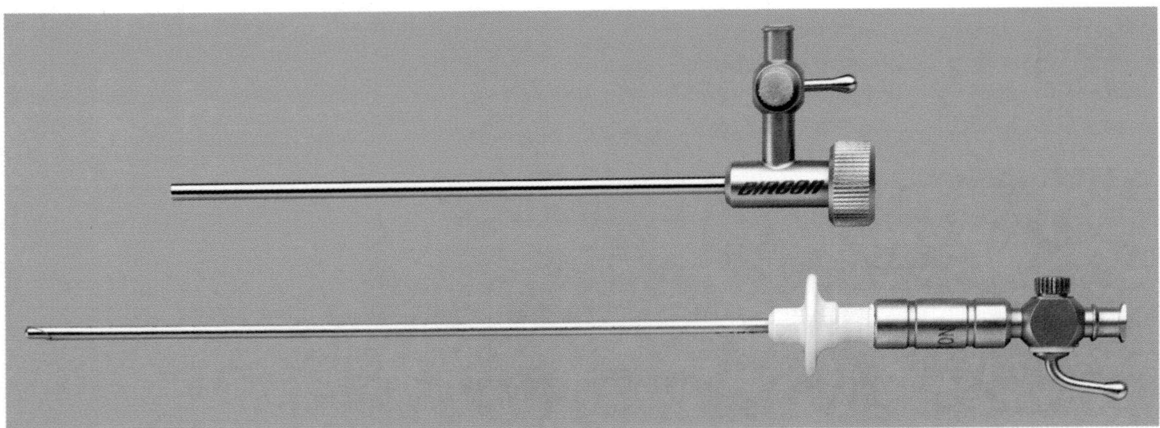

Figure 8-3. The 2.7-mm introducer is used with the microlaparoscope. Also seen is a 2.7-mm Veress needle.

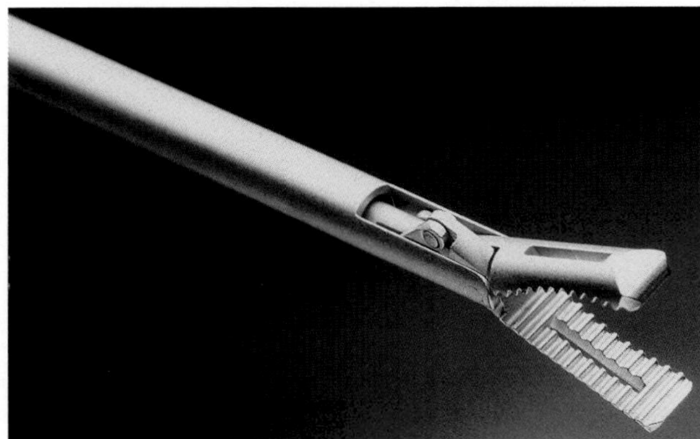

Figure 8-4. The microlaparoscopic grasping forceps.

Another system is the MicroLap (Imagyn Medical, Inc., Laguna Niguel, CA).[1,3–5,9,11,30] This reusable 2-mm telescope is 34.5 cm long and contains both imaging and light-carrying fiberoptic fibers in a semirigid stainless-steel outer jacket. It uses an introducer with an anchoring mechanism. It has a depth of field of 100 mm. The eyepiece can be attached to any type of laparoscope. A small nonrandomized comparative study suggested that this microendoscope offers a superior combination of field of vision, clinical adaptability, ease of operation, and operating cost.[31] The "Pixie" microlaparoscope (Origin Medical Systems, Inc., Palo Alto, CA) can be connected to a standard video camera and light source system (Figure 8-3). This microlaparoscope has a depth of field of 150 mm compared with about 25 mm for the Optical Catheter (Medical Dynamics, Inc.) and is placed through a disposable Adair Veress needle. The greater depth of field is similar to the field of conventional 5- to 10-mm diagnostic laparoscopes. Karl Storz (Culver City, CA) markets a 1.2-mm microlaparoscope, 13 cm long, with a 0-degree direction of view. It is placed through a reusable "optic pneumoperitoneum" Veress needle.[7]

The laparoscopes are inserted through plastic sheaths that remain in the abdominal wall after withdrawal of the Veress needle. The Adair Veress needle (Medical Dynamics, Inc.) is an 18-gauge laparoscopic insufflation needle. Like an angiocath, it is inserted through a 3-mm plastic sheath. The Adair Veress needle is connected to a gas extension tube, allowing gas insufflation. It has a diaphragm that allows the insertion of the optical catheter, retaining the pneumoperitoneum. Another microlaparoscope introducer device (Imagyn Medical, Inc., Laguna Niguel, CA) has a small unfoldable anchor at the distal end of the 2-mm trocar to prevent accidental dislodging after removal of the Veress needle. Additional equipment that is currently available includes sub-2.0-mm blunt probes, grasping forceps, scissors, and biopsy devices (Figures 8-4 and 8-5). Electrosurgical microinstruments, Endoloops, sutures, and fiber lasers [Nd:YAG and potassium titanyl phosphate (KTP)] also are obtainable in appropriate small diameters.

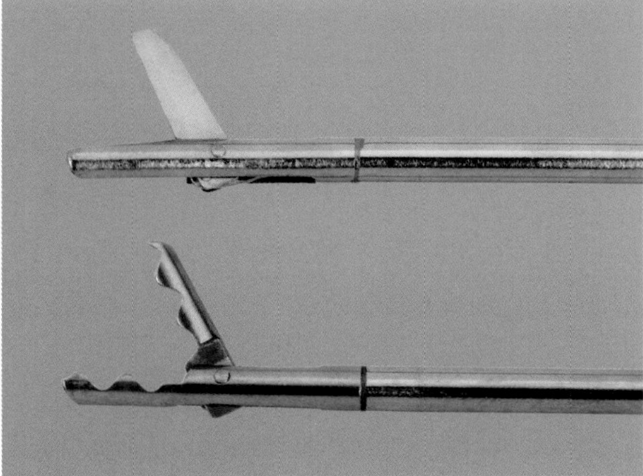

Figure 8-5. The straight scissors and another pair of grasping forceps.

Anesthesia

The patient is premedicated 1 to 4 hours preoperatively, usually with 10 to 20 mg of oral diazepam, for sedation.[31] Atropine 0.4 mg is advisable to prevent a vagal response. An intravenous line is started. The use of supplemental oxygen is recommended throughout the procedure, administered through a nasal cannula at 3 L/min.[21,24]

Local anesthesia is given at the sites of cannula insertion with a 5- to 20-mL injection of bupivicaine, lidocaine, or a mixture of the two. A paracervical block is created if there is a need for a uterine manipulator. It is important to anesthetize the abdominal layers, the cervix, and the vagina. The use of postoperative intraperitoneal subdiaphragmatic instillation of 0.5% lidocaine and 0.5% bupivicaine infiltration at cannula sites offers a detectable benefit to women undergoing diagnostic microlaparoscopy.[32] The temporary effect provides significant pain relief postoperatively for approximately 6 hours.

Continuous pulse oximetry and an electrocardiogram monitor the procedure. Blood pressure is measured every 5 to 10 minutes. Patients who need additional analgesia are given incremental intravenous doses of meperidine, fentanyl, diazepam, and midazolam. The operation is done in the office treatment room, where an emergency crash cart must be available.

Studies examining the respiratory, cardiac, and hemodynamic changes observed using local anesthesia suggest that with proper monitoring, these procedures can be done safely in an outpatient setting.[33–35] Patients undergoing laparoscopy under local anesthesia were found not to develop significant carbon dioxide retention or hypoxemia during the procedure. Despite the presence of underlying cardiovascular disease in half these patients, no serious cardiac arrhythmias were noted. No adverse effects on hemoglobin saturation or carbon dioxide exchange were noted in healthy women undergoing laparoscopy for tubal ligation in a non-operating-room setting with monitoring of ventilatory measurements, blood gas pH, blood pressure, and pulse. Laparoscopic tubal sterilization under intravenous conscious sedation is associated with minimal pain, a short recovery, and low anesthesia costs.[27,28,35,36]

The Technique

Microlaparoscopy can be carried out in an office treatment room or more commonly in a hospital minor procedure room. Adequate monitoring and resuscitation equipment are essential. Many gynecologists already have such a setting available in the office for minor operative procedures such as hysteroscopy. The patient receives oral diazepam about 1 hour preoperatively for sedation and empties her bladder. She is placed on the operating table in the dorsal lithotomy position in the 10- to 15-degree Trendelenburg position. A blood pressure cuff and a pulse oximeter are applied. A Hep-Lock needle (18- to 22-gauge) is inserted. If necessary, a paracervical block is created and a Cohen cannula is inserted for uterine manipulation. Bupivicaine or lidocaine (20 to 30 mL) is injected with a 25- to 27-gauge needle down through all the layers of the abdomen at the site for Veress needle insertion.

The procedure varies somewhat according to the specific system used, although the general principle deviates little from that of standard laparoscopy. It is advisable to do the first cases of microlaparoscopy in conjunction with standard laparoscopy to become acquainted with the scope and its placement. This approach also allows the gynecologist to compare the adequacy of the view obtained with a microlaparoscope and a conventional laparoscope. Placing the microlaparoscope in the midline, midway between the umbilicus and the symphysis, shortens the distance from the pelvic organs. The Veress needle used to insert the microlaparoscope is introduced into the abdomen at a 45-degree angle with the uterus held down by the intrauterine manipulator. The Veress needle is removed from its plastic sheath. The extension tube is connected to the CO_2 insufflator, and about 500 to 600 mL of gas is passed into the peritoneal cavity. Intraabdominal pressure is kept below 15 mm Hg. The small volume (500 to 600 mL) of gas insufflated minimizes patient discomfort and decreases vagal stimulation.

Experience has shown that pneumoperitoneum becomes unpleasant when CO_2 volume is over 3 L and intraperitoneal pressure exceeds 15 mm Hg. Hartmann solution can be instilled into the peritoneal cavity as a viewing medium. It causes little pain and irritation and allows good visibility. However, the fluid tends to become turbid from peritoneal debris and exudate that cannot be flushed through the 2-mm cannula. The time frame available for observation seems to be sufficient for most diagnostic purposes. Nitrous oxide may be superior to CO_2 because it is less irritating to the peritoneal surfaces, causes less concern if it is absorbed rapidly, and is of less physiologic consequence once absorbed.

When the Optical Catheter (Medical Dynamics, Inc., Englewood, CO) is used, an Adair Veress needle is inserted midway between the umbilicus and the symphysis. The needle is removed from its plastic sheath, and an extension tube is connected. The optical catheter is inserted.

With the MicroLap (Imagyn Medical, Inc., Laguna Niguel, CA), a 15-cm Veress needle is used to enter an introducer that fits snugly over it. The anchoring mechanism on the introducer allows for slight elevation of the abdominal wall. A second Adair Veress needle or a long spinal needle is inserted to allow manipulation and to do aspiration, culturing, and biopsies. A laser fiber can be passed through an ancillary 3-mm port, permitting vaporization of small endometrial implants and incision of some adhesions.

The patient is encouraged to watch the video monitor, and the findings are explained. She can cooperate and change the position of her hips to move the adnexa or cough and take a deep breath to reposition the bowel. At the end of the procedure, the gas is removed. Sterile adhesive strips are used to close the incision. The patient should be monitored for 15 to 45 minutes after diagnostic procedures.

Advantages

The ability to do microlaparoscopy under local anesthesia with minimal sedation and analgesia avoids the risks associated with general anesthesia (Table 8-1). It facilitates doing the procedure in outpatient facilities with less need for extensive monitoring and obviously reduces the cost. Microlaparoscopy minimizes some additional risks of conventional laparoscopy, including gas embolism and bowel perforation, because the tip of the Veress needle in the abdomen is seen immediately after insertion. Another benefit of microlaparoscopy is the small abdominal incision that obviously results in reduced local pain, less wound hematoma, and no visible scar. In addition, there is no risk of incisional hernia, and the need for repair of the puncture is eliminated. The use of local anesthesia, lower insufflation pressures, and lower gas volumes results in less discomfort and pain. This technique is associated with rapid recovery, a shorter hospital stay, and reduced costs. Office laparoscopy under local anesthesia was associated with an almost 80% reduction in billed charges, averaging $1700 rather than $7500 compared with hospital-based, operating room laparoscopy under general anesthesia. Feste[9] found in 36 patients that diagnostic laparoscopy under general anesthesia costs overall in the range of $5000 to $7000, while the charges for microlaparoscopy under local anesthesia, including the surgeon's fee and the cost of the treatment room and disposable equipment, should total about $1250.

Microlaparoscopy has a negligible learning curve even among surgeons less experienced in laparoscopic procedures. However, the gynecologist must adapt to the narrower field of view and the need to work closer to the observed organ.

TABLE 8-1. Advantages of Microlaparoscopy

Minimal sedation, less need for monitoring, facilitation of outpatient care, reduced costs
No risk of gas embolism; early detection of bowel perforation
Lower insufflation pressures leading to less patient discomfort
Small abdominal incision: reduced local pain, less wound hematoma, no risk of incisional hernia, elimination of the need for repair of puncture site, no visible scar
Rapid recovery; shorter hospitalization
Easy to master with minimal learning curve

Disadvantages

The limitations of microlaparoscopy are related to the features of the currently available optics (Table 8-2). These are characterized by a narrower field of view compared with conventional 5- and 10-mm scopes. The picture on the video monitor is about 40% smaller and more difficult to center on the target area, and more attempts are necessary to achieve an optimal focus. The visual field of sub-2-mm compared with 5-mm laparoscopes was estimated to be at 1-mm resolution 1.5 to 3.0 cm and 14 cm, respectively, and at "clinical" resolution 4 to 7 cm and 35 cm, respectively.[30] It requires time to adapt to the use of these scopes. The light intensity during minilaparoscopy is reduced compared with conventional laparoscopy because of the small diameter of the fiberoptic telescope. The tip of the microlaparoscope has to be placed closer to the observed organ to obtain accurate resolution because the length of the microlaparoscope can result in unacceptable image resolution, especially with infraumbilical insertion.

Other difficulties are related to the lack of effective small-diameter accessory instruments. Lack of suction and irrigation probes limits the ability to do peritoneal lavage. Evacuation of vapor and smoke tends to be inefficient and impairs the view. Similarly, it is difficult to secure hemostasis with the available small-diameter electrosurgical equipment. Other technical limitations of microlaparoscopy include the inability to use non-fiber-guided lasers such as the CO_2 laser. Many of the technical limitations will be solved with the introduction of a wider array of improved sub-2-mm-diameter surgical instruments. Some inherent problems associated with sole reliance on small-diameter ports are difficult to solve, such as the removal of bulky tissues from the abdomen.

A significant concern with microlaparoscopy is the fragile nature of most of the available equipment. This requires extra caution in handling,

TABLE 8-2. Disadvantages of Microlaparoscopy

Narrower field of view
Vapor and smoke impair view
Limited peritoneal lavage
Difficult to secure hemostasis
Difficult to remove bulky tissues
Some surgical instruments not available with sub-2-mm diameter
Certain operative procedures require deeper sedation

cleaning, and sterilizing microendoscopes and other small-diameter instruments. The cost savings of microlaparoscopy compared with conventional laparoscopy are obvious. They are attributed to doing the procedure in a non-operating-room setting and not using general anesthesia. Several expenses must be considered in establishing an office-based microlaparoscopy system. The initial capital expenses of microlaparoscopy equipment have been estimated to range between $13,000 and $19,000.[30] Additional costs include the price of the introducer, especially if a disposable one is used. Some microlaparoscopy systems require a backup system, as the video and light sources are not adaptable to other 5- or 10-mm laparoscopes. Labor and sterilization costs and the durability of the system must be taken into account. Some manufacturers limit the warranty to only five procedures, and microlaparoscopes break easily. The need for monitoring and resuscitation equipment must be considered if that equipment is not available in the procedure room. The number of patients undergoing microlaparoscopy will decide whether the physician should equip his or her office with the necessary equipment.

Future

Technologic improvements will include versatile microinstruments such as miniature ultrasonographic probes for intraabdominal imaging. Other expected developments include optical catheters that integrate an infrared laser and a Doppler unit, producing an endoscope that not only provides an image but simultaneously can do measurements. Direct assessment of multiple tissue characteristics may become possible, such as blood flow, pressure, temperature, and oxygen saturation. Further information on tissue characteristics may be obtained from direct spectroscopic analysis, identifying structures that lie beyond the visible organ surface. The use of markers can locate endometriosis or detect cancer within the abdominal cavity. Such markers may include fluorescent material and even genetic probes.

The widespread application of microlaparoscopy is going to be influenced by the availability of small-diameter cheaper, more durable, and easier to sterilize endoscopes. The new microlaparoscopes may be steerable and have an operating channel. Further miniaturization of the fibers is likely to increase the safety and convenience of the procedure. Better light sources and optic fibers will enhance image quality.

New applications may include amnioscopy for the evaluation of fetal anatomy, as an extension of routine amniocenteses, tubal sterilization procedures, laser evaporation of myomas, and presacral nerve ablation.

Summary

Microlaparoscopy is comparable to conventional 10-mm laparoscopy for diagnostic purposes. The ability to do abdominal interventions under minimal sedation with microlaparoscopy will depend on further technologic advances in small-diameter equipment. Microlaparoscopy has the potential to change the way diagnostic evaluation is done in the acute hospital setting. Office microlaparoscopy requires new equipment and a staff adequately trained in administering and monitoring anesthesia.

References

1. Haeusler G, Lehner R, Hanzal E, Kainz C. Diagnostic accuracy of 2 mm microlaparoscopy. *Acta Obstet Gynecol Scand* 1996; 75:672.
2. Risquez F, Peenehouat G, Fernandez R, et al. Microlaparoscopy: A preliminary report. *Hum Reprod* 1993; 8:1701.
3. Downing BG, Wood C. Initial experience with a new microlaparoscope 2-mm in external diameter. *Aust NZ J Obstet Gynaecol* 1995; 35:202.
4. Palter SF, Olive DL. Office microlaparoscopy under local anesthesia for chronic pelvic pain. *J Am Assoc Gynecol Laparosc* 1996; 3:359.
5. Faber BM, Coddington CC III. Microlaparoscopy: A comparative study of diagnostic accuracy. *Fertil Steril* 1997; 67:952.
6. Dorsey JH, Tabb CR. Mini-laparoscopy and fiber-optic lasers. *Obstet Gynecol Clin North Am* 1991; 18:613.
7. Barisic D, van der Ven H, Prietl G, Strelec M. The diagnostic accuracy of a 1.2 mm minilaparoscope. *Gynecol Endosc* 1996; 5:283.
8. Childers JM, Hatch KD, Surwit EA. Office laparoscopy and biopsy for evaluation of patients with intraperitoneal carcinomatosis using a new optical catheter. *Gynecol Oncol* 1992; 47:337.
9. Feste JR. Use of optical catheters for diagnostic office laparoscopy. *J Reprod Med* 1996; 41:307.

10. Van der Wat J. Microendoscopy in the operating room. *Gynecol Endosc* 1997; 6:265.
11. Bauer O, Kupker W, Felberbaum R, et al. Small-diameter laparoscopy using a microlaparoscope. *J Assist Reprod Genet* 1996; 13:298.
12. Karabacak O, Tiras MB, Taner MZ, et al. Small diameter versus conventional laparoscopy: A prospective, self-controlled study. *Hum Reprod* 1997; 12:2399.
13. Grochmal SA. Gynaecological applications of optical catheters (microhysteroscopy and microlaparoscopy), in Grochmal SA, ed., *Minimal Access Gynecology.* Oxford, UK: Radcliffe, 1995.
14. Feste JR. Outpatient diagnostic laparoscopy using the optical catheter. *Contemp Ob/Gyn* 1995:54.
15. Pelosi MA, Pelosi MA 3d. Laparoscopic appendectomy using a single umbilical puncture (mini-laparoscopy). *J Reprod Med* 1992; 37:588.
16. Berci G. Elective and emergent laparoscopy. *World J Surg* 1993; 17:8.
17. Dunphy BC. Office falloposcopic assessment in proximal tubal occlusive disease. *Fertil Steril* 1994; 61:168.
18. Schwaitzberg SD. Use of microlaparoscopy in dagnostic procedures: A case report. *Surg Laparosc Endosc* 1995; 5:407.
19. Kuster GG, Gilvoy SB. The role of laparoscopy in the diagnosis of acute appendicitis. *Am Surg* 1992; 58:627.
20. Almeida OD Jr, Val-Gallas JM, Rizk B. Appendectomy under local anaesthesia following conscious pain mapping with microlaparoscopy. *Hum Reprod* 1998; 13:588.
21. Milki AA, Tazuke SI. Office laparoscopy under local anesthesia for gamete intrafallopian transfer: Technique and tolerance. *Fertil Steril* 1997; 68:128.
22. Waterstone JJ, Bolton VN, Wren M, Parsons JH. Laparoscopic zygote intrafallopian transfer using augmented local anesthesia. *Fertil Steril* 1992; 57:442.
23. Marti-Vicente A, Sainz S, Soriano G, et al. Usefulness of laparoscopy as a second-look method in neoplasms of the ovary. *Rev Esp Enferm Dig* 1990; 77:275.
24. Penfield AJ. Laparoscopic sterilization under local anesthesia. *Am J Obstet Gynecol* 1974; 119:733.
25. Alexander GD, Goldrath M, Brown EM, et al. Outpatient laparoscopic sterilization under local anesthesia. *Am J Obstet Gynecol* 1973; 116:106.
26. Risquez F, Pennehout G, McCorvey R, et al. Diagnostic and operative microlaparoscopy: A preliminary multicentre report. *Hum Reprod* 1997; 12:1645.
27. Hibbert ML, Buller JL, Seymour SD, et al. A microlaparoscopic technique for Pomeroy tubal ligation. *Obstet Gynecol* 1997; 90:249.
28. DeQuattro N, Hibbert M, Buller J, et al. Microlaparoscopic tubal ligation under local anesthesia. *J Am Assoc Gynecol Laparosc* 1998; 5:55.
29. Steege JE. Repeated clinic laparoscopy for the treatment of pelvic adhesions: A pilot study. *Obstet Gynecol* 1994; 83:276.
30. Fuller PN. Microendoscopy surgery: A comparison of four microendoscopes and a review of the literature. *Am J Obstet Gynecol* 1996; 174:1757.
31. Almieda OD, Val-Galls JM, Browning JL. A protocol for conscious sedation in microlaparoscopy. *J Am Assoc Gynecol Laparosc* 1997; 4:591.
32. Zullo F, Pellicano M, Cappiello F, et al. Pain control after microlaparoscopy. *J Am Assoc Gynecol Laparosc* 1998; 5:161.
33. Groover JR, Bierfeld JL. Cardiac arrhythmias during peritoneoscopy under local anestheia. *Dig Dis* 1976; 21:465.
34. Brown DR, Fishburne JI, Robertson VO, Hulka JF. Ventilatory and blood gas changes during laparoscopy with local anesthesia. *J Obstet Gynecol* 1976; 124:741.
35. Diamant M, Benumof JL, Saidman LJ, et al. Laparoscopic sterilization with local anesthesia: Complications and blood-gas changes. *Anesth Analg* 1977; 56:335.
36. Bordahl PE, Raeder JV, Nordentoft J, et al. Laparoscopic sterilization under local or general anesthesia: A randomized study. *Obstet Gynecol* 1993; 81:131.
37. Molloy D. The diagnostic accuracy of a microlaparoscope. *J Am Assoc Gynecol Laparosc* 1995; 2:203.

SECTION IV

9

Laparoscopic Adhesiolysis

Peritoneal adhesions can cause intestinal obstruction, pelvic pain, and infertility.[1–3] Intraabdominal adhesions between the abdominal scar and the underlying viscera are a common consequence of laparotomy. Patients undergoing laparoscopy after a previous laparotomy should be considered at risk for the presence of adhesions between the old scar and the bowel and omentum. Patients with midline abdominal incisions had more adhesions (58 of 102) than did those with Pfannenstiel incisions (70 of 258). Patients with midline incisions done for gynecologic indications had more adhesions (109 of 259) than did patients with any abdominal incision made for obstetric indications (12 of 55). The presence of adhesions in patients with previous obstetric operations was not affected by the type of incision. Adhesions to the bowel were more common after midline incisions above the umbilicus. Twenty-one women had direct injury to adherent omentum and bowel during the laparoscopic procedure.[4]

Caspi and associates[2] reported an inverse relation between the severity of pelvic adhesions and pregnancy rates. After adhesiolysis, pregnancy rates vary according to the extent of adnexal damage and, to a lesser degree, the severity of the adhesions.[2,3,5,6]

Since the development of postoperative adhesions is a major factor in deciding the outcome of fertility-promoting operative procedures, gynecologists should understand the mechanism of their formation, use optimal techniques for adhesiolysis, and apply agents or devices to reduce their development.

Formation of Adhesions

Normal fibrinolytic activity usually prevents fibrinous attachments (fibrinous exudate) for 72 to 96 hours after injury. Mesothelial repair occurs within 5 days of trauma. A single cell layer of mesothelium covers the injured raw area, replacing the fibrinous exudate. However, if the fibrinolytic activity of the peritoneum is suppressed, fibroblasts will migrate, proliferate, and form fibrous adhesions with collagen deposition and vascular proliferation.[1] The factors that suppress fibrinolytic activity and promote the formation of postoperative adhesions are listed in Table 9-1.

Microsurgery includes the use of magnification, gentle handling of tissues, constant irrigation, meticulous hemostasis, the use of microsurgical instruments, the use of fine nonreactive sutures, and precise approximation of tissue. Fertility-promoting operations done by laparotomy often are followed by re-formation of adhesions[7] and the development of new adhesions even when proper microsurgical techniques are applied.[8] Reformation of adhesions is found at 37 to 72% of operative sites,[7,8] and 51% of patients develop new adhesions after reproductive procedures by laparotomy.[8]

Several animal and clinical studies compared the formation of postoperative adhesions after fertility-promoting operations by laparoscopy and laparotomy. With few exceptions, operative laparoscopy resulted in the development of fewer re-formed and new adhesions.[5,9–12] These results are consistent with the observations made a century ago by Von

TABLE 9-1. Predisposing Factors for Adhesions

Ischemia
Drying of serosal surfaces
Excessive suturing
Omental patches
Traction of peritoneum
Blood clots retained in peritoneal cavity
Prolonged operations
Adnexal trauma
Infection

Dembrowski[13] and later confirmed by Ellis.[16] They reported that uncomplicated peritoneal injuries, such as those likely to occur at operative laparoscopy, heal without the development of adhesions (Table 9-2).

Decreased adhesion formation after laparoscopic procedures has been attributed to the reduced presence of foreign bodies within the peritoneum that tend to stimulate more numerous and dense adhesions.[18] Laparoscopic operations may lead to fewer adhesions because tissue trauma distant from the site of adhesions increases their formation. The type of injury to the peritoneum can control the formation of intraabdominal adhesions. The potential to form adhesions is significantly higher in visceral than in parietal peritoneal lesions.[19] Transperitoneal laparoscopy did not increase adhesions compared with extraperitoneal laparotomy in an animal model.[20] The transperitoneal laparoscopy approach also induced fewer adhesions than did transperitoneal laparotomy. A presumed advantage of the extraperitoneal approach is the avoidance of adhesions because the peritoneum is not entered and direct contact with intraabdominal structures is avoided.

TABLE 9-2. Historical Perspective

Author	Year	Contribution
Von Dembrowski[13]	1898	Peritoneal defects in dogs heal mostly without adhesions.
DeRenzi and Boeri[14]	1903	Ischemia is a major factor in the formation of adhesions.
Thomas[15]	1950	Oversewing serosal defects increases rather than decreases adhesions.
Ellis[16]	1971	Excision of parietal peritoneum from rats healed without adhesions in 52 of 58 experiments. “Meticulous” repair of peritoneal defects in 16 of 19 experiments resulted in fibrous adhesions.
Ryan et al[17]	1971	The combination of tissue drying and bleeding is a major promoter of adhesions.

When the peritoneum is dissected from the abdominal wall, it is partially devascularized, leading to scars and potential adhesions. Dissection of the peritoneum from the overlying abdominal wall in a murine model can cause intraabdominal adhesions. The totally extraperitoneal approach may not avoid the risk of intraabdominal adhesions.[21]

Laparoscopic procedures result in fewer adhesions than do laparotomy procedures, but adhesions can develop even after laparoscopy. To minimize the formation of adhesions, good surgical technique involves the basic principles of microsurgery, liberal irrigation of the abdominal cavity, and instillation of a large amount of lactated Ringer’s solution at the completion of the procedure.[22] Alternatively, an early second-look laparoscopy after laparoscopy can be useful for assessing the degree of postoperative adhesions, allow technically easy adhesiolysis, and result in lower adhesion scores, as shown by third-look procedures.[23]

The Value of Adjuvants

Although microsurgical techniques and operative laparoscopy can reduce the formation of adhesions, the benefit derived from various adjuvants remains controversial despite their widespread use. The most commonly used pharmacologic agents are listed in Table 9-3, but they lack the efficacy and safety required for general acceptance. Steroids and antihistamines are used infrequently because of their questionable efficacy and potential adverse effects, such as delayed wound healing and the risk of wound dehiscence.[24] Hyskon (Medisan Pharmaceuticals Inc., Parsippany, NJ), a high-molecular-weight form of dextran, is absorbed from the peritoneal cavity over 7 to 10 days. Its osmotic effect draws fluid into the peritoneal cavity to float

TABLE 9-3. Adjuvants to Prevent Adhesions

Adjuvant	Mechanism of Action
1. Corticosteroids/ antihistamines	Inhibit fibroblast migration, stabilize lysosomal membranes, decrease vascular permeability, and antagonize effects of histamine
2. Antibiotics	Reduce risk of infections
3. Nonsteroidal anti-inflammatory drugs	Decrease foreign body reaction
4. Dextran 70 (Hyskon)	Effects hydroflotation of peritoneal organs by drawing fluid into the peritoneal cavity and reducing adherence between peritoneal structures
5. Surgical membranes	Separate interposing peritoneal surfaces

mobile peritoneal organs, reducing adherence between intraperitoneal structures. Some studies in animals[25] and humans[25,26] have shown reduced postoperative adhesions, but inconsistent results suggest limited efficacy. In addition, there have been reports of allergic reactions,[27,28] infections, and complications of fluid overload. Preliminary studies have demonstrated that a cross-linked hyaluronan solution (ACP gel) holds promise as a novel resorbable biomaterial for the reduction of postoperative adhesions after laparoscopy.[29]

Barrier methods using absorbable surgical membranes are more effective because they separate peritoneal surfaces and prevent fibrous bands from binding different structures.

Interceed (Johnson & Johnson Medical, Somerville, NJ) is an absorbable adhesion barrier made of oxidized regenerated cellulose. Evidence has shown that Interceed is safe and effective in reducing the incidence of postoperative adhesions in patients undergoing various laparoscopic operations.[30] It has been postulated that it may compete for the macrophage scavenger receptor because of its polyanionic nature. Results from in vitro studies suggest that the interaction of Interceed with macrophages with scavenger receptors results in decreased secretion of matrix components, inflammatory mediators, and cellular growth factors. Thus, Interceed cellulose may function as a biologic barrier in preventing adhesions.[31] In two multicenter clinical studies,[32,33] Interceed was placed on only one pelvic side wall at the conclusion of the operation although both areas had been treated for comparable disease. At a second-look laparoscopy, fewer adhesions re-formed on the side treated with Interceed, although postoperative adhesions were not eliminated completely. Haney and Doty[34] applied Interceed in the abdominal cavity of normal mice. They found peritoneal injury and new adhesions between the abdominal peritoneum and the intraabdominal viscera. Pagidas and Tulandi[35] found that Interceed was not effective in decreasing postoperative adhesions in rats. Fewer adhesions were found in animals treated with Gore-Tex and lactated Ringer's solution than in control and Interceed-treated animals.[35] In the rabbit model, Interceed reduced the incidence and score of postoperative ovarian adhesions and improved the reproductive outcome.[36] Azziz[37] observed in a prospective, randomized trial involving 134 patients undergoing adhesiolysis by standard microsurgical techniques at laparotomy that 90% benefited from the use of Interceed.

Randomized prospective studies showed a significant reduction in the formation of postoperatve adhesions after laparoscopic ovarian operations,[38,39] myomectomy,[40] and surgical treatment of endometriosis.[41] Fixation of Interceed by placing 6/0 vicryl sutures[42] and the addition of heparin[43] did not enhance the adhesion-reducing capacity. The efficacy of this absorbable barrier is limited to situations where the traumatized area can be covered completely. Effective application is limited by technical difficulties, including the need for hemostasis and removal of excess peritoneal fluid.[30]

Another barrier material is an expanded polytetrafluoroethylene (PTFE, Gore-Tex Surgical Membrane, W.L. Gore & Associates, Inc., Flagstaff, AZ). This material is a nonabsorbable, nonreactive surgical membrane that has been used to repair and reconstruct the pericardium and peritoneum.[44] Animal studies by Boyers and associates[45] revealed that the Gore-Tex surgical membrane was effective in reducing primary adhesions after pelvic operations. Gore-Tex membrane was applied over the raw surface of the peritoneal wall or uterus after adhesiolysis or myomectomy by laparotomy. At second-look laparoscopy, when the surgical membrane was removed, the mean postoperative adhesion score had been reduced from 10.13 ± 0.35 to 0.75 ± 2.12 ($p < 0.001$).[45] The Gore-Tex surgical membrane can reduce postmyomectomy adhesions.[46] At laparoscopy, 15 of 27 incisions covered with PTFE (55.6%) and only 2 of 27 uncovered sites (7.4%) were completely free of adhesions. A randomized, prospective cross-over study in nonhuman primates found that the Gore-Tex surgical membrane was better than Interceed with respect to the size of the adhesion area, tenacity, and vascularity, with a significant improvement in the total adhesion score.[47] These results were confirmed in a multicenter, nonblinded randomized clinical trial that enrolled 32 women with bilateral pelvic side wall adhesions undergoing reconstructive pelvic operations and second-look laparoscopy. Expanded PTFE was associated with fewer postsurgical adhesions to the pelvic side wall compared with Interceed.[48]

The Gore-Tex surgical membrane can be used laparoscopically.[48] It is easy to introduce and position over a peritoneal defect, since its handling properties do not diminish with wetting. Fixation is secured with laparoscopic staples.[49] Removal of the PTFE barrier at early second-look laparoscopy 11 days after myomectomy was not associated with adhesions.[50]

Other commercially available bioresorbable films consisting of various polyethylene glycol 6000 and polylactic acid block copolymers, including REPEL (Life Medical Sciences, Edison, NJ) and Seprafilm (Genzyme, Cambridge, MA), were effective in reducing adhesion development and reformation in rabbits.[51]

Barrier methods using either absorbable Interceed or nonabsorbable Gore-Tex are safe and relatively effective in the reduction of postoperative adhesions. There is no substitute for careful surgical technique, but some patients are predisposed to form adhesions.

A 0.5% ferric hyaluronate gel called Intergel was introduced as a new adjuvant therapy for in the prevention of adhesions. Intergel Adhesion Prevention Solution is a single-use, sterile, nonpyrogenic 0.5% ferric hyaluronate gel. This amber-colored aqueous gel of sodium hyaluronate has been ionically cross-linked with ferric ions and adjusted to isotonicity with sodium chloride. It is packaged in a bellows-type container designed to deliver 300 mL of INTERGEL solution.

INTERGEL solution functions by providing a viscous, lubricated coating on the peritoneal surfaces, minimizing tissue apposition during the critical period of fibrin formation and mesothelial regeneration. Lymphatic drainage appears to be the major elimination pathway for intraperitoneally administered INTERGEL solution. The elimination half-life ($t_{1/2}$) of INTERGEL solution in humans has been estimated from animal studies to be approximately 51 hours. The 300-mL INTERGEL solution instillation is expected to clear from the peritoneal cavity in 5 to 7 days.

INTERGEL solution has been shown to be easy to use in a multicenter, international study and to reduce the number, severity, and extent of postoperative adhesions after laparotomy.

The minimum standard AFS score of the right and left adnexa was ($p < 0.05$) lower in the INTERGEL solution group than in the lactated Ringer's solution group. The mean modified AFS score for 24 sites throughout the peritoneal cavity was ($p < 0.05$) lower in the INTERGEL solution group than in the lactated Ringer's solution group.

The proportion of sites with postsurgical adhesions was ($p < 0.05$) lower in the INTERGEL solution group than in the lactated Ringer's solution group. Almost twice as many INTERGEL solution–treated patients were totally adhesion-free at second-look compared to control patients (mAFS score = 0). The severity and extent of postsurgical adhesions were ($p < 0.05$) lower in the INTERGEL solution group than they were in the lactated Ringer's solution group. De novo and reformed adhesions were ($p < 0.05$) reduced in the INTERGEL solution group compared with the lactated Ringer's solution group.

The reduction in adhesions was observed whether all 24 sites, only the general surgical sites, or only the pelvic sites were considered. The reduction in adhesions was observed regardless of the presence or absence of endometriosis, the use of sutures, the method of adhesiolysis, or the surgical procedure, including myomectomy, adhesiolysis, and tubal and ovarian surgery.

The safety profile (adverse event incidence rates and clinical laboratory test results) of patients treated with INTERGEL solution was comparable to that of patients treated with lactated Ringer's solution.

In conclusion, INTERGEL Adhesion Prevention Solution provides a new, clinically proven intraperitioneal surgical therapy for the reduction of adhesions that is both broad in coverage and easy to use.[52]

Laparoscopic Adhesiolysis

To do laparoscopic adhesiolysis adequately, three or four abdominal punctures are required: the infraumbilical incision for the operative laparoscope and two to three lower, lateral suprapubic punctures about 4 cm below the level of the iliac crests (Figure 9-1). Through the lateral trocar, on the side

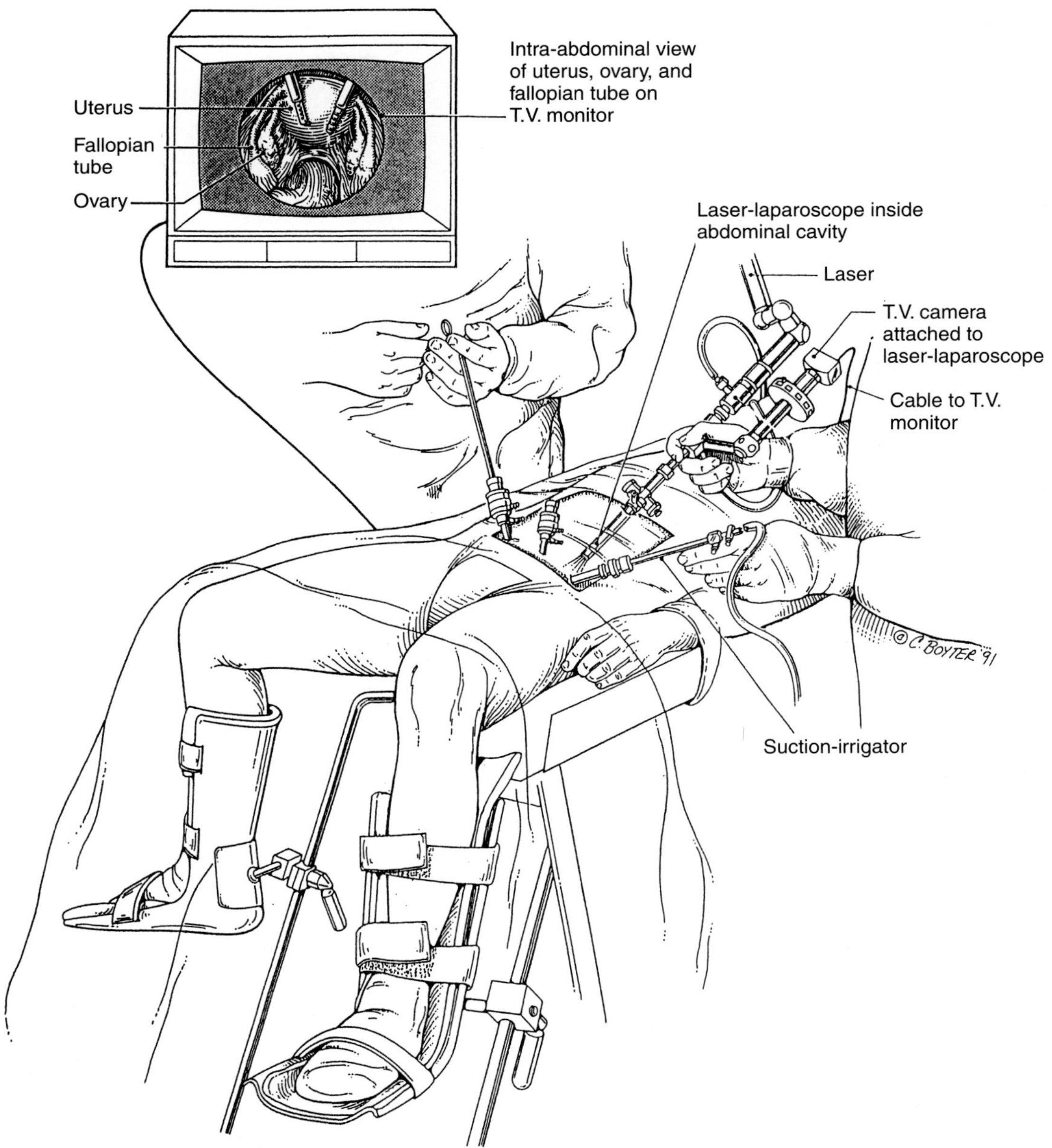

Figure 9-1. Suprapubic punctures are made to introduce the suction-irrigator probe and grasping forceps.

of the assistant, an atraumatic grasping forceps is inserted to hold the adhesion or involved organ, stretch it, and identify its boundaries and avascular planes. The opposite trocar, on the side of the primary surgeon, is used for microscissors or the suction-irrigator probe. That probe can serve as a manipulator or backstop when the CO_2 laser is used (Figure 9-2).

Adhesions are cut close to the affected organ at both ends and, if possible, removed from the abdomen. Vascular adhesions are coagulated with lasers or microelectrodes. When scissors are used, filmy and avascular adhesions are stretched and then cut (Figures 9-3 and 9-4). Thick, vascular adhesions must be coagulated before being cut (Figures 9-5 and 9-6).

Intestinal adhesions are severed first, followed by periovarian adhesions and peritubal adhesions. This approach allows progressive exposure of the pelvic structures. Once the intestines are freed from adjacent structures, they are pushed gently cephalad. Adherent ovaries are freed from the

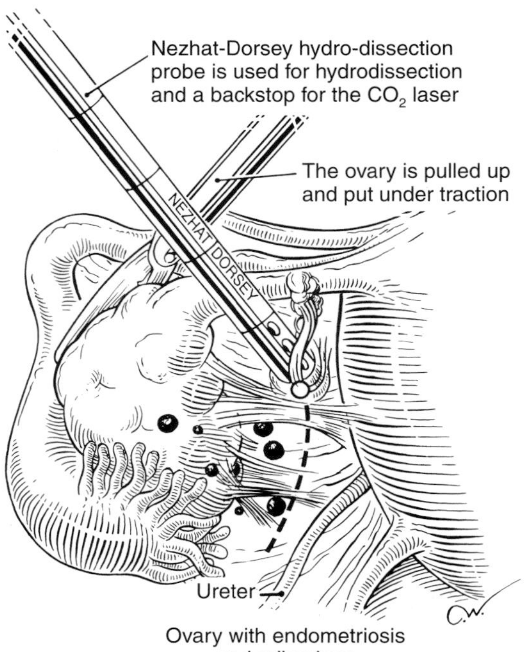

Figure 9-2. The left ovary is grasped and put under traction. The suction-irrigator is used for a backstop, and the adhesions are cut using the CO_2 laser.

pelvic side wall, broad ligament, tubes, and uterus. Grasping forceps are essential for applying traction to the ovary, tube, intestines, or abdominal wall so that a plane of dissection can be identified.

Bleeding areas are coagulated with the laser or a bipolar electrocoagulator. Whenever possible, either the adhesions or the ovarian ligaments are grasped instead of the ovarian cortex to reduce trauma. Once the ovaries are lifted from the cul-de-sac and mobilized, the peritubal adhesions are removed.

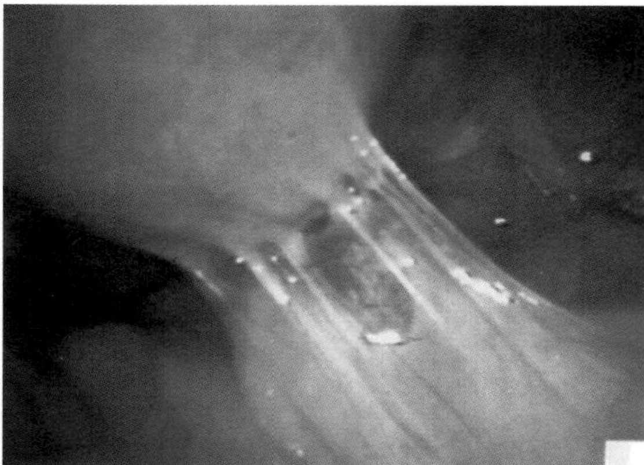

Figure 9-3. Avascular adhesions between the uterus and the omentum are put under stretch before dissection with scissors.

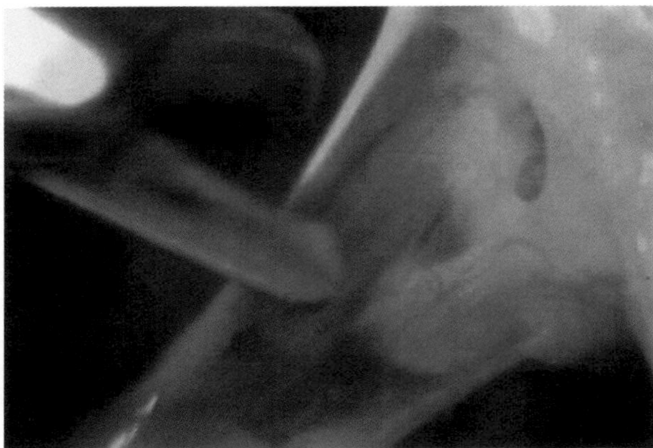

Figure 9-4. Avascular adhesions are dissected with scissors.

Adhesions can be coagulated effectively and incised with a CO_2 laser, superpulse (40 W) laser, ultrapulse (20 to 80 W and 25 to 200 mJ), fiber laser (15 to 25 W), or microelectrode (15 to 20 W, cutting mode). When there are dense adhesions among different organs (bowel, uterus, ovaries, pelvic side wall, and anterior abdominal wall), hydrodissection with the suction-irrigator probe is useful to create tissue planes before dissection.

Since an intestinal injury can occur during enterolysis, patients with a history of previous laparotomies or severe endometriosis should undergo a preoperative bowel preparation. Inadvertent enterorrhaphy can be repaired with the use of a one-layer closure of 0 polyglactin (Vicryl, Ethicon) or an Endoloop. Details for such repairs are found in Chapt. 12.

Once the pelvic structures are freed and hemostasis is achieved, the cul-de-sac is filled with lactated Ringer's solution and the adnexa are allowed to float in the clear fluid (Figure 9-7).[53]

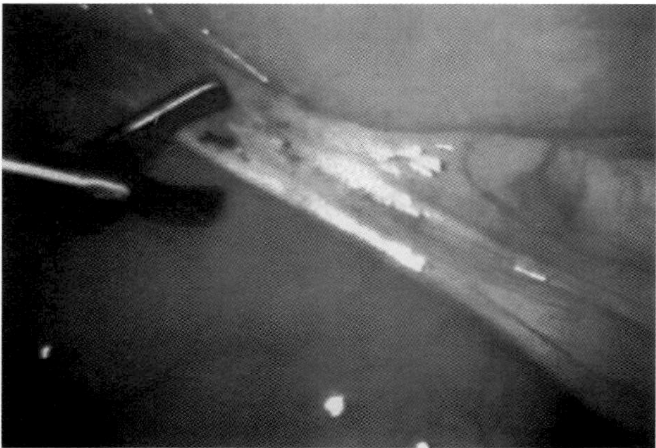

Figure 9-5. Thick, vascular adhesions are coagulated before dissection.

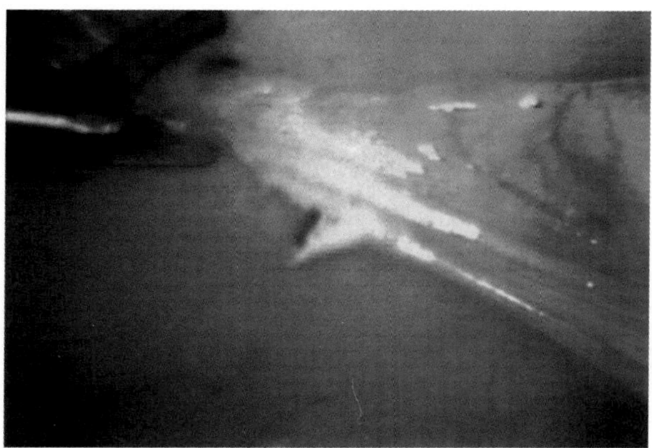

Figure 9-6. A coagulated vascular adhesion is cut with scissors.

Filmy adhesions that are difficult to identify on the surface of the ovary become visible as they float from the ovarian cortex. These adhesions are grasped with the forceps, cut, and removed from their attachments, using laparoscopic microscissors. They are filmy and avascular, and so coagulation is not required.

Agglutinated fimbrial folds are caused by fine avascular adhesions. As the fimbrial folds float and disperse in the fluid, the adhesions become visible; they are grasped, stretched, and sharply cut with fine scissors or an ultrapulse laser. The laser beam (other than ultrapulse) delivered through the laparoscope is at least 1 mm in diameter and is too wide for these narrow bands of adhesions. Thermal damage can occur with electrosurgery and the fiber laser (neodymium-yttrium aluminum garnet, potassium titanyl phosphate, or argon). For delicate microscopic procedures of fimbriolysis and salpingo-ovariolysis, the microscissors or ultrapulse laser is preferable.

Conclusion

Although significant progress has been made toward understanding the development of postoperative adhesions and their prevention, adjuvants and microsurgery have not eliminated them. Operative laparoscopy may be more effective than laparotomy in reducing their formation and should be the first procedure in their management.

References

1. DiZerega GSD, Holtz G. Cause and prevention of postsurgical pelvic adhesions, in Osofsky H, ed., *Advances in Clinical Obstetrics and Gynecology*. Baltimore: Williams & Wilkins, 1982.
2. Caspi E, Halperin Y, Bukovski I. The importance of periadnexal adhesions in tubal reconstruction surgery for infertility. *Fertil Steril* 1979; 31:296.
3. Hulka JF. Adnexal adhesions: A prognostic staging and classification system based on a five year survey of fertility surgery results at Chapel Hill, North Carolina. *Am J Obstet Gynecol* 1982; 144:141.

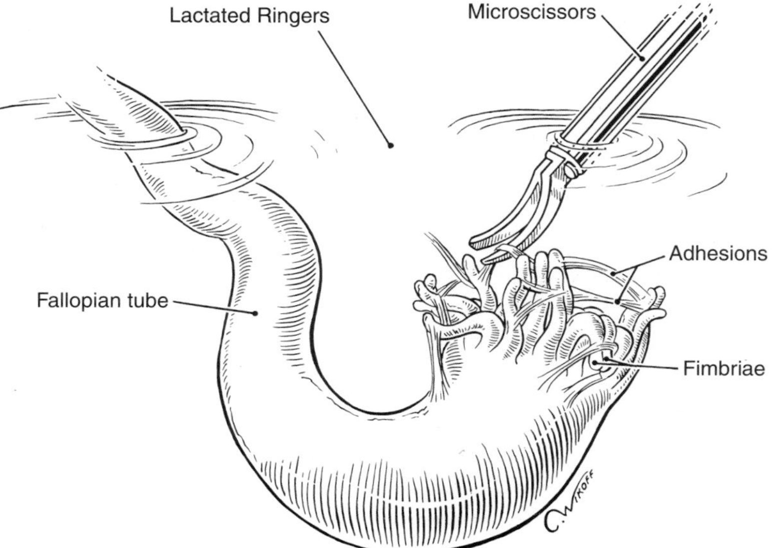

Figure 9-7. Hydroflotation of the tube and fimbria is used to detect and remove filmy adhesions.

4. Brill AI, Nezhat F, Nezhat CH, Nezhat C. The incidence of adhesions after prior laparotomy: A laparoscopic appraisal. *Obstet Gynecol* 1995; 85:269.
5. Nezhat C, Metzger MD, Nezhat F, et al. Adhesion formation following reproductive surgery by videolaseroscopy. *Fertil Steril* 1990; 53:1008.
6. Donnez J, Casanas-Roux F. Prognostic factors of fimbrial surgery. *Fertil Steril* 1986; 45:778.
7. Trimbos-Kemper TCM, Trimbos JB, van Hall EV. Adhesion formation after tubal surgery: Results of the 8 day laparoscopy in 188 patients. *Fertil Steril* 1985; 43:395.
8. Gomel V, McComb P. Microsurgery in gynecology, in Silver JS, ed., *Microsurgery*. Baltimore: Williams & Wilkins, 1979.
9. Luciano AA, Maier DB, Koch E, et al. A comparative study of postoperative adhesions following laser surgery by laparoscopy versus laparotomy in the rabbit model. *Obstet Gynecol* 1989; 4:220.
10. Operative Laparoscopy Study Group. Postoperative adhesion development after operative laparoscopy: Evaluation at early second-look procedures. *Fertil Steril* 1991; 55:700.
11. Lundorff P, Hahlin M, Kallfelt B, et al. Adhesion formation after laparoscopic surgery in tubal pregnancy: A randomized trial versus laparotomy. *Fertil Steril* 1991; 55:911.
12. Schippers E, Tittel A, Ottinger A, Schumpelick V. Laparoscopy versus laparotomy: Comparison of adhesion-formation after bowel resection in a canine model. *Dig Surg* 1998; 15:145.
13. Von Dembrowski T. Ueber die ursachen der peritoneum ashasionennach cirugischen: Eiugriffen mit rucksieht auf die frage des ileus nach laparotomien. *Arch Klin Chir* 1898; 37:745.
14. DeRenzi E, Boeri G. Das Hetz als Schutzorgan. *Bed Klin Wochenschr* 1903; 40:773.
15. Thomas JW. Continued hyaluronidase on the formation of intraperitoneal adhesion in rats. *Proc Soc Exp Biol Med* 1950;74:497.
16. Ellis H. The cause and prevention of postoperative intraperitoneal adhesions. *Surg Gynecol Obstet* 1971; 133:497.
17. Ryan GB, Groberty J, Majino G. Postoperative peritoneal adhesions: A study of the mechanisms. *Am J Pathol* 1971; 675:117.
18. Garrard CL, Clements RH, Nanney L, et al. Adhesion formation is reduced after laparoscopic surgery. *Surg Endosc* 1999; 13:10.
19. Wallwiener D, Meyer A, Bastert G. Adhesion formation of the parietal and visceral peritoneum: An explanation for the controversy on the use of autologous and alloplastic barriers? *Fertil Steril* 1998; 69:132.
20. Chen MD, Teigen GA, Reynolds HT, et al. Laparoscopy versus laparotomy: An evaluation of adhesion formation after pelvic and paraaortic lymphadenectomy in a porcine model. *Am J Obstet Gynecol* 1998; 178:499.
21. Halverson AL, Barrett WL, Bhanot P, et al. Intraabdominal adhesion formation after preperitoneal dissection in the murine model. *Surg Endosc* 1999; 13:14.
22. Tulandi T. How can we avoid adhesions after laparoscopic surgery? *Curr Opin Obstet Gynecol* 1997; 9:239.
23. Ugur M, Turan C, Mungan T, et al. Laparoscopy for adhesion prevention following myomectomy. *Int J Gynaecol Obstet* 1996; 53:145.
24. Jansen BPS. Failure of intraperitoneal adjuncts to improve the outcome of pelvic operations in young women. *Am J Obstet Gynecol* 1983; 153:363.
25. Luciano AA, Hauser KS, Benda J. Evaluation of commonly used adjuvants in the prevention of postoperative adhesions. *Am J Obstet Gynecol* 1983; 146:88.
26. Rosenberg SM, Board JA. High-molecular-weight dextran in human fertility surgery. *Am J Obstet Gynecol* 1984; 148:380.
27. DiZerega GS. Reduction of postoperative pelvic adhesions with intraperitoneal 32% dextran 70: A prospective randomized clinical trial. *Fertil Steril* 1983; 40:612.
28. Borten M, Seibert CP, Taymor ML. Recurrent anaphylactic reaction to intraperitoneal dextran 75 used for prevention of postsurgical adhesions. *Obstet Gynecol* 1983; 61:755.
29. De Iaco PA, Stefanetti M, Pressato D, et al. A novel hyaluronan-based gel in laparoscopic adhesion prevention: Preclinical evaluation in an animal model. *Fertil Steril* 1998; 69: 318.
30. Larsson B. Efficacy of Interceed in adhesion prevention in gynecologic surgery: A review of 13 clinical studies. *J Reprod Med* 1996; 41:27.
31. Reddy S, Santanam N, Reddy PP, et al. Interaction of Interceed oxidized regenerated cellulose with macrophages: A potential mechanism by which Interceed may prevent adhesions. *Am J Obstet Gynecol* 1997; 177:1315.

32. Interceed (TC7) Barrier Adhesion Study Group. Prevention of postsurgical adhesions by Interceed (TC7), an absorbable adhesion barrier: A prospective randomized multicenter clinical study. *Fertil Steril* 1989; 51:933.
33. The Obstetrics and Gynecology Adhesion Prevention Committee. Use of Interceed (TC7) absorbable adhesion barrier to reduce postoperative adhesion reformation in infertility and endometriosis surgery. *Obstet Gynecol* 1992; 79:518.
34. Haney AF, Doty E. Murine peritoneal injury and de novo adhesion formation caused by oxidized-regenerated cellulose (Interceed [TC7]) but not expanded polytetrafluoroethylene (Gore-Tex Surgical membrane). *Fertil Steril* 1992; 57:202.
35. Pagidas K, Tulandi T. Effects of Ringer's lactate, Interceed (TC7) and Gore-Tex surgical membrane on PST surgical adhesion formation. *Fertil Steril* 1992; 57:199.
36. Marana R, Catalano GF, Caruana P, et al. Postoperative adhesion formation and reproductive outcome using Interceed after ovarian surgery: A randomized trial in the rabbit model. *Hum Reprod* 1997; 12:1935.
37. Azziz R. Microsurgery alone or with INTERCEED Absorbable Adhesion Barrier for pelvic sidewall adhesion re-formation: The INTERCEED (TC7) Adhesion Barrier Study Group II. *Surg Gynecol Obstet* 1993; 177:135.
38. Franklin RR. Reduction of ovarian adhe sions by the use of Interceed: Ovarian Adhesion Study Group. *Obstet Gynecol* 1995; 86:335.
39. Keckstein J, Ulrich U, Sasse V, et al. Reduction of postoperative adhesion formation after laparoscopic ovarian cystectomy. *Hum Reprod* 1996; 11:579.
40. Mais V, Ajossa S, Piras B, et al. Prevention of de-novo adhesion formation after laparoscopic myomectomy: A randomized trial to evaluate the effectiveness of an oxidized regenerated cellulose absorbable barrier. *Hum Reprod* 1995; 10:3133.
41. Mais V, Ajossa S, Marongiu D, et al. Reduction of adhesion reformation after laparoscopic endometriosis surgery: A randomized trial with an oxidized regenerated cellulose absorbable barrier. *Obstet Gynecol* 1995; 86:512.
42. Ramsewak S, Narayansingh G, Bassaw K, et al. Fixation of Interceed does not improve its efficacy against adhesion formation in rats. *Clin Exp Obstet Gynecol* 1996; 23:147.
43. Bulletti C, Polli V, Negrini V, et al. Adhesion formation after laparoscopic myomectomy. *J Am Assoc Gynecol Laparosc* 1996; 3:533.
44. Minale C, Nikol S, Hollweg G, et al. Clinical experience with expanded polytetrafluoroethylene Gore-Tex surgical membrane for pericardial closure: A study of 110 cases. *J Cardiac Surg* 1988; 3:193.
45. Boyers SP, Diamond MP, DeCherney AH. Reduction of postoperative pelvis adhesions in the rabbit with Gore-Tex surgical membrane. *Fertil Steril* 1988; 49:1066.
46. The Myomectomy Adhesion Multicenter Study Group. An expanded polytetrafluoroethylene barrier (Gore-Tex Surgical Membrane) reduces post-myomectomy adhesion formation. *Fertil Steril* 1995; 63:491.
47. Haney AF. Removal of surgical barriers of expanded polytetrafluoroethylene at second-look laparoscopy was not associated with adhesion formation. *Fertil Steril* 1997; 68:721.
48. Crain J, Curole D, Hill G, et al. Laparoscopic implant of Gore-Tex surgical membrane. *J Am Assoc Gynecol Laparosc* 1995; 2:417.
49. The Surgical Membrane Study Group. Prophylaxis of pelvic sidewall adhesions with Gore-Tex surgical membrane: A multicenter clinical investigation. *Fertil Steril* 1992; 57:921.
50. Haney AF. Removal of surgical barriers of expanded polytetrafluoroethylene at second-look laparoscopy was not associated with adhesion formation. *Fertil Steril* 1997; 68:721.
51. Rodgers K, Cohn D, Hotovely A, et al. Evaluation of polyethylene glycol/polylactic acid films in the prevention of adhesions in the rabbit adhesion formation and reformation sidewall models. *Fertil Steril* 1998; 69:403.
52. Johns DA: Clinical Evaluation of Intergel Adhesion Prevention Solution for the Reduction of Adhesions Following Peritoneal Cavity Surgery. D. Alan. Johns. Texas Healthcare, Fort Worth, Texas, and the Intergel International Adhesion Study Group. Conjoint Annual Meeting, Sept. 1999, Canada. ASRM/CFAS p. S57(O-144).
53. Nezhat F, Winer WK, Nezhat C. Fimbrioscopy and salpingoscopy in patients with minimal to moderate pelvic endometriosis. 1990; 75:15.

10

Ovarian Cysts

Evolving technology has made it possible to treat most persistent ovarian cysts laparoscopically. However, these operations must be done judiciously. Although the role of laparoscopy in the management of malignancy is expanding, laparotomy remains the procedure of choice when ovarian malignancy is encountered or strongly suspected.

Introduction

One to 2% of women develop ovarian cancer during their lifetimes, and when the disease is detected, two-thirds of them are in stage III or stage IV.[1] During laparoscopy, ovarian cancer can be discovered so that immediate laparotomy and appropriate staging are possible. Laparotomy is required for optimal surgical therapy, and postoperative radiotherapy or chemotherapy is instituted as needed. A recent study suggested that a delay between laparoscopy and laparotomy may affect the distribution of disease stage adversely.[2] Whenever a malignant tumor has been missed at laparoscopy, restaging is required and should be considered an oncologic emergency.[3] Given the reduced morbidity, patient disability, and cost, having an oncologist available facilitates the safe treatment of adnexal masses by operative laparoscopy. Conversion from the laparoscopic approach rarely is required.[4]

A serious concern is that an ovarian cyst assumed to be benign subsequently is proved to be a stage I ovarian carcinoma. Even careful laparoscopic examination can underestimate early-stage ovarian cancer or borderline tumors.[5,6] If contents spill during their aspiration or with an ovarian cystectomy, the stage is upgraded from IA to IC. The risks associated with spillage of cystic contents[7] have been evaluated. In a multivariate analysis of stage I epithelial ovarian cancer, the factors that influenced the rate of relapse in 519 patients were the tumor grade, the presence of dense adhesions, and a large volume of ascites. Intraoperative spillage at laparotomy showed no adverse effect on the prognosis of stage I ovarian cancer.[8] The survival of women with borderline tumors who were managed initially by cystectomy, with or without spillage, was not decreased, and there was no evidence of disseminated disease an average of 7.5 years after diagnosis.[9] The laparoscopic approach to borderline ovarian tumors is possible in early-stage disease but is associated with a high risk of recurrence after cystectomy.[10]

The risk of spread remains questionable in patients who have the appropriate operation. In two large studies, the incidence of ovarian malignancy in patients with a known adnexal mass was between 1.2%[11] and 0.3%.[12] The results of a 1991 survey of the members of the American Association of Gynecologic Laparoscopists (AAGL) showed that laparoscopic excision of unsuspected invasive ovarian cancer was uncommon. Only 53 instances were reported among 13,739 laparoscopic ovarian cystectomies, an incidence of 0.4%.[13] Similar results were found in a countrywide survey undertaken in Austria, which included 16,601 laparoscopies on adnexal masses. Ovarian tumors subsequently were found to be malignant in 108 cases (0.65%).[14]

A laparotomy is mandatory to ensure optimal staging and treatment in cases of malignancy. A survey of gynecologic oncologists revealed 12 borderline ovarian tumors and 30 invasive ovarian cancers initially managed by laparoscopic excision.[15] Most patients did not have a staging laparotomy for weeks after the cancer was found. These patients did not have careful preoperative screening, and appropriate surgical treatment was delayed.

Preoperative Evaluation

Laparoscopic treatment of adnexal masses depends on the patient's age, a pelvic examination, sonographic images, and serum markers.

Physical Examination

A large, solid, fixed or irregular adnexal mass accompanied by ascites is suspicious for malignancy (Table 10-1). Cul-de-sac nodularity, ascites, cystic adnexal structures, and fixed adnexa occur with both endometriosis and ovarian malignancy.

Ultrasound

Transvaginal ultrasound is the primary imaging modality for evaluating adnexal masses.[16] Cystic, unilocular, unilateral masses less than 10 cm with regular borders are probably benign. Malignant ovarian cysts are associated with irregular borders, a size greater than 10 cm with papillations, solid areas, thick septa (>2 mm), ascites, and a matted bowel. Using ultrasonographic criteria, accurate predictions of benign masses were made in 96% of patients.[16,17] Nezhat and coworkers[12] found that none of the four malignant cysts in their series had any ultrasound criteria for malignancy. However, laparoscopic diagnosis of adnexal masses that are suspicious at ultrasound prevents many laparotomies for the treatment of benign masses.[18]

The role of ultrasound screening in detecting ovarian cancer in asymptomatic women is still questionable. A systematic review of prospective screening studies found that the sensitivity of ultrasound screening at 1 year was around 100% (95% Confidence Interval (CI) 54% to 100%).[19] However, false-positive rates ranged between 1.2 and 2.5% for gray scale ultrasound, between 0.3 and 0.7% for ultrasound with color Doppler, and between 0.1 and 0.6% for CA-125 measurement followed by ultrasound screening. This implies that in an annual screening of a population with an incidence of 40 per 100,000, with no cancers missed, between 2.5 and 60 women would be operated upon for every primary ovarian cancer detected.

Functional cysts gradually regress or resolve spontaneously or with hormonal suppressive therapy within 8 weeks (Figure 10-1). Persistent cysts that are functional or hemorrhagic on ultrasound should be removed.

Serum Markers

CA-125 is a tumor-associated antigen that is used to detect the nature of an ovarian cyst (Tables 10-2 and 10-3). Levels below 35 U/mL are associated with benign tumors, but the sensitivity and specificity vary. The presence of other benign conditions can elevate CA-125 levels. In 80% of premenopausal women, elevated CA-125 levels were associated with pregnancy, endometriosis, fibroids, adenomyosis, cystic teratomas, and acute or chronic salpingitis. Only 50% of patients with stage I ovarian cancers had elevated CA-125 levels, compared with 90% of women with stage II.[20]

In 70 women with a history of endometriosis, serum CA-125 concentrations were not correlated with the persistence or resolution of ovarian cysts.[21]

Cyst Aspiration

Cytologic examination of the cystic fluid does not provide an accurate diagnosis in many patients.[22] Ten to 65% of aspirates were interpreted as benign when malignancy was present.[12,23,24] In a review, the accuracy of transvaginal and transrectal fine needle aspiration and ultrasound-guided punctures of ovarian cysts was disappointing.[25] The false-negative rate was especially high for nonfollicular cystic lesions.[26] This procedure is not suggested for treatment because of the high rate of recurrence.[27–29]

In a study, 278 women with simple ovarian cysts were allocated randomly to either simple observation or ultrasound-guided fine needle aspiration. The rate of resolution was 46% with aspiration and 45% with observation. The authors concluded that expectant management for up to 6 months does not cause risks for the patients and that aspiration does not provide better results than does simple observation.[30]

Sonographically guided therapeutic aspiration of symptomatic ovarian cysts may alleviate symptoms.[31] However, this procedure, although more rapid than extirpation, can be associated with abscess formation.[32]

Computed Tomography and Magnetic Resonance Imaging

The role of computed tomography (CT) and magnetic resonance imaging (MRI) relative to

TABLE 10-1. CA-125 Levels Correlated with Type of Cyst

					CA-125 Level U/mL		Ultrasonographic Characteristics of Cysts							
							Cystic		Semicystic		Solid		Other	
No. Patients	Cyst	No.	Size, cm	Age Range, years	Range	Mean	No.	%	No.	%	No.	%	No.	%
360	Endometrioma	162	2–5	16–54	>2–212	45.7	123	68.9	22	22.8	14	7.5	3	0.8
		179	6–10		2–195	28.7	115		54		10		—	
		19	11–25		5–237	48.2	10		6		3		—	
219	Functional	172	2–5	11–47	<2–135	15.7	98	58.0	40	25.1	6	3.7	28	13.2
		45	6–10		<2–53	11.2	28		14		2		1	
		2	11–12		6	6.0	1		1		—		—	
34	Simple	13	2–5	23–47	5–76	7.0	10	76.5	—	8.8	—	5.9	3	8.8
		19	6–10		2–195	31.5	14		3		2		—	
		2	11–12		—	—	2		—		—		—	
30	Benign cystic teratoma	16	2–5	17–44	<5–9	7.0	7	43.3	7	36.7	1	13.3	1	6.7
		12	6–10		5–29	14.9	6		3		2		1	
		2	11–14		12	12.0	—		1		1		—	
17	Serous	8	2–5	33–40	14–47	30.5	7	82.4	—	5.9	—	5.9	1	5.9
		7	6–10		10–42	23.7	6		1		—		—	
		2	11–15		47–51	49.0	1		—		1		—	
11	Mucinous	4	2–5	31–35	<5	<5.0	2	54.5	2	45.5	—	—	—	—
		5	6–10		<5–30	10.6	2		3		—		—	
		2	11–25		9–11	10.0	2		—		—		—	
17	Hydrosalpinges	16	5–10	26–45	<5–35	12.8	6	41.2	8	47.1	—	—	2	11.8
		1	11–12		<5	<5.0	1		—		—		—	
46	Miscellaneous	30	2–5	22–45	<5–135	27.4	19	67.4	2	6.5	—	4.3	9	21.7
		15	6–10		<5–10	5.5	11		1		2		1	
		1	11–17		36	36.0	1		—		—		—	

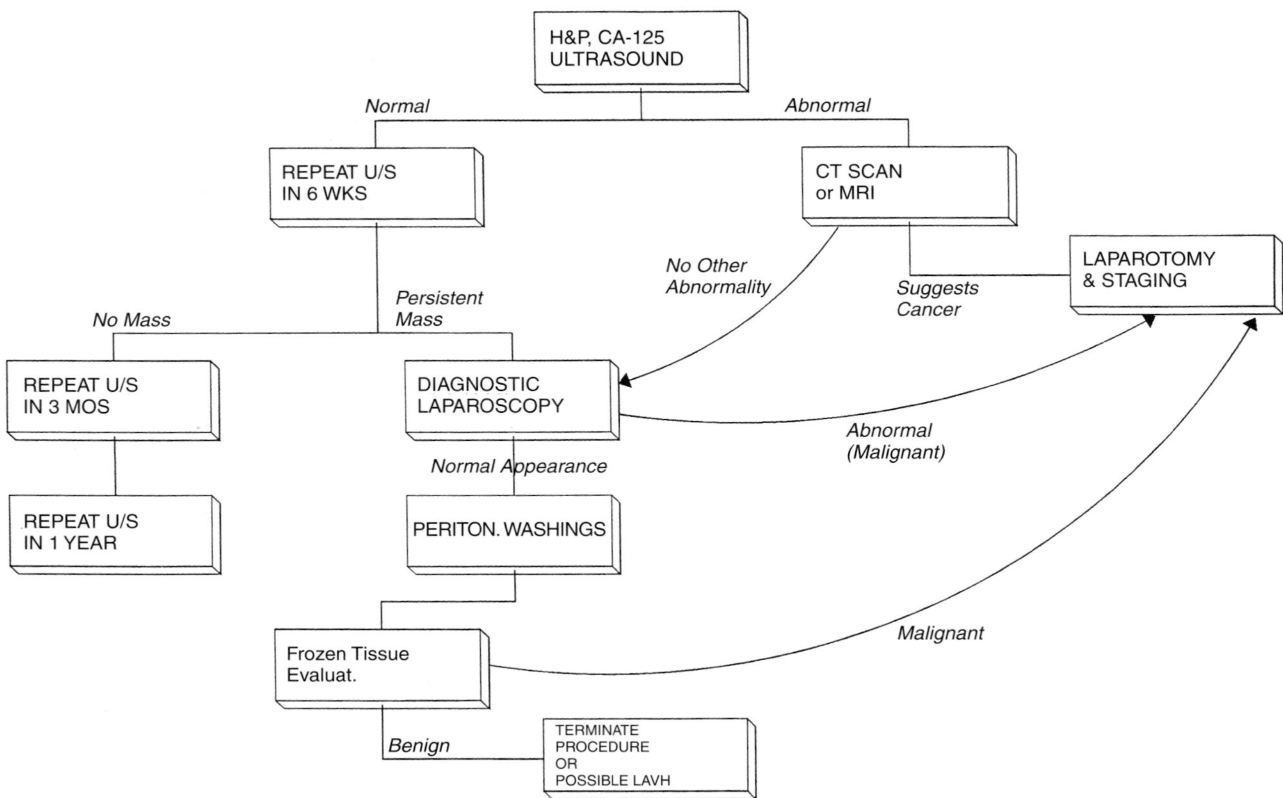

Figure 10-1. Evaluation of a postmenopausal ovarian cyst.

ultrasound in evaluating an ovarian cyst is evolving. The resolution characteristics of CT depend on differences in x-ray attenuation between calcium, water, fat, and air. Soft tissue differences are enhanced with intravenous contrast. MRI relies on differences in the hydrogen content of fat and water, magnetic relaxation time, and blood flow, ultimately resulting in additional soft tissue contrast. In one study, MRI had a sensitivity of 95% and a specificity of 88% in distinguishing malignant from benign lesions, while transvaginal ultrasound had 75% sensitivity and 98% specificity.[33] MRI and the T_2 signal intensity were useful for detecting the presence of endometriomas based on evaluating the density of the cyst fluid and its iron concentration.[34] Unenhanced and contrast-enhanced MRI was shown to maximize the discrimination between benign and malignant masses in patients with sonographically indeterminate ovarian lesions.[35]

TABLE 10-2. Findings at Laparoscopy in Four Women Who Had Ovarian Cancer

	Case 1 Serous Cystadenocarcinoma	Case 2 Endometrioid Low-Malignant-Potential Tumor	Case 3 Papillary Mucinous Cystadenocarcinoma	Case 4 Clear Cell Carcinoma
Patient age (y)	44	45	43	33
Stage	IIIC	IA	IIA	IA
Tumor size (cm)	7	3	13	6
Serum CA-125 level (U/mL)	N/A	7	17	2
Ultrasonographic finding	Septated semicystic	Cystic	Septated semicystic	Septated semicystic

TABLE 10-3. Malignant Potential of Ovarian Cysts by Physical Examination

Clinical Findings	Benign	Malignant
Size >7 cm	++	++
Size <7 cm	++	++
Unilateral	++++	+
Bilateral	++	++++
Cystic	++++	+
Solid	++	+++
Solid and cystic	+	++++
Mobile	++++	+
Fixed	+	++++
Irregular	+	++++
Smooth	++++	+
Ascites	+	++++
Cul-de-sac nodules	+	+++

+ = least probable; ++++ = most probable.

Serial turboFLASH (fast, low-angle shot) images with and without diffusion-perfusion (DP) gradients have been used to evaluate the contents of cystic ovarian lesions. When these images were used, the apparent diffusion coefficients were calculated within the cystic contents of these lesions. It was found that the diffusion-weighted MRI could be used to differentiate between the cystic contents of benign and malignant ovarian lesions.[36]

Meticulous pretreatment evaluation remains basic to the successful management of suspected ovarian masses. The additional expense of CT and MRI seem justified only in selected patients in whom further characterization of the adnexal mass may influence directly the type of management selected.[37,38]

Treatment

Medical Treatment

Oral contraceptives have been prescribed for some cystic adnexal masses (<6 cm) in reproductive-age women on the assumption that decreasing gonadotropin stimulation to a functional cyst will hasten its resolution. The results of one study[39] failed to report any benefit from ovarian suppressive therapy. However, the cysts were less than 5 cm, and the study included women who had received ovulation induction medication. Two additional randomized trials have since shown that although oral contraceptive therapy is very effective in the management of functional ovarian cysts, expectant management achieves similar success rates.[40,41]

A randomized study evaluated the effectiveness of various hormonal regimens in treating 70 women who had unilateral or bilateral ovarian cysts assumed to be physiologic (functional) and a history of endometriosis.[21] The patients were assigned randomly to one of the following groups: group I (control), no treatment; group II, oral contraceptives (35 μg ethinyl estradiol and 1 mg norethindrone); group III, oral contraceptives (50 μg ethinyl estradiol and 1 mg norethindrone); group IV, danazol 800 mg/day. Serum CA-125 concentrations were measured in 32 women. At 6 weeks of follow-up, complete resolution of cysts was found in group I, 12 of 18 (66.7%); group II, 5 of 9 (55.6%); group III, 8 of 14 (57.1%); and group IV, 7 of 13 (53.9%). Two of the 22 women with persistent cysts opted for 6 weeks of additional medical therapy and achieved complete resolution, 19 underwent laparoscopy, and 1 was lost to follow-up. All laparoscopic findings revealed benign masses. It was concluded that no statistically significant effect was found when hormonal treatment was compared with expectant management.[21]

Hormonal suppressive therapy can be prescribed during the follow-up of benign-appearing ovarian cysts, but there is little scientific evidence for its effectiveness compared with expectant management.

Recommended Approach

Attempts to remove ovarian cysts laparoscopically sometimes require conversion to laparotomy because cancer can be discovered and an immediate laparotomy then becomes necessary. Treatment of benign-appearing adnexal masses must follow a protocol of (1) cytologic examination of pelvic and cyst fluid, (2) frozen section of a biopsy specimen, and (3) removal of the mass for histologic examination. Aspirating a cyst and vaporizing or coagulating the capsule are not acceptable choices. The safe laparoscopic approach to ovarian cysts has been described by Mage and coworkers.[11] Those authors reported findings in 481 women (ages 9 to 88) who had ovarian cysts, including 96 functional cysts, 100 endometriomas, 100 serous cysts, 91 teratomas, 51 mucinous cysts, and 58 paraovarian cysts. Among these patients, 19 underwent laparotomy for confirmed or suspected malignancy based only on laparoscopic evaluation, and 10 of them were benign. Five ovarian cancers and four borderline tumors were found and handled immediately by laparotomy. Dense pelvic adhesions or cysts

TABLE 10-4. Sensitivity and Specificity of Diagnostic Tests

	Premenopausal		Postmenopausal	
	Sensitivity, %	Specificity, %	Sensitivity, %	Specificity, %
Specialist ultrasound	50	96	78	92
Clinical impression	17	92	68	85
CA-125	50	69	84	92

Source: Modified from Finkler N, Benacerrat B, Lavin F. Comparison of serum CA-125, clinical impression and ultrasound in the preoperative evaluation of ovarian masses. *Obstet Gynecol* 1988; 72:659.

larger than 10 cm were the indications for laparotomy in 42 women. Nezhat and colleagues[12] evaluated 1011 premenopausal women with ovarian cysts laparoscopically and found four ovarian cancers. Preoperative assessment included an initial pelvic exam, vaginal ultrasound, and the CA-125 level.[11] Three of the four unsuspected cancers were found on frozen or permanent sections of the cyst wall. One malignant tumor was 3 cm and grossly appeared to be an endometrioma; histologic examination revealed an endometrioid carcinoma (Table 10-4).[12] Preoperative examinations did not detect malignancy.

Although ovarian neoplasms can occur at any age, the risk of malignancy is highest during prepuberty and menopause. Ovarian activity is associated with an increased incidence of functional ovarian cysts and other benign pathologic conditions. These observations, combined with age differences in the sensitivity and specificity of clinical testing, have led to the following recommendations for evaluating and managing adnexal masses.

Although clinical examination and the results of the preoperative workup often indicate the benign or malignant nature of cysts, only histology can provide the absolute diagnosis. The benefits of doing frozen sections during laparoscopic management of organic ovarian cysts were investigated in 228 patients who underwent adnexectomy for an ovarian mass.[42] After the preoperative workup and the diagnostic phase of laparoscopy, 26 patients (11.4%) presented with suspected signs of malignancy restricted to the ovary. Those 26 patients underwent a laparoscopic adnexectomy with extraction of the excised tissues using an endoscopic bag, followed by frozen section. For all these patients, the results of the frozen section were that the lesion was benign. In every case, the definitive histologic results confirmed the frozen section findings. This strategy allowed the gynecologist to avoid laparotomy, especially in the nine postmenopausal patients whose adnexal masses appeared complex on ultrasound.

Malignancy is not the only concern in handling an ovarian cyst. If the risk of malignancy is relatively low, patients who wish to preserve their reproductive organs should have the least aggressive therapy. Preoperative evaluation should include a history and physical examination, pelvic ultrasound to evaluate both ovaries, possible hormonal suppressive therapy, and a blood sample to be held for baseline tumor marker status if the mass subsequently is malignant. In premenopausal women, besides ascertaining the characteristics of the adnexal mass, resection of ovarian tissue can cause adhesions and should be minimized (Table 10-5).

In postmenopausal women, the incidental finding of adnexal masses will increase with the more frequent application of diagnostic imaging. Although routine pelvic sonographic screening of asymptomatic postmenopausal women may find early ovarian cancer, the procedure is not cost-effective. Wolf and coworkers[43] screened 149 asymptomatic women more than 50 years of age and discovered cysts in 22 (14.8%), ranging in size from 0.4 to 4.7 cm. Two additional women had septated masses, but no ovarian cancers were detected. In a study that screened 5479 women age 45 or older, 6.1% had abnormal scans.[44] When the scans were repeated 2 to 8 weeks later, only 59% were persistently abnormal. Five ovarian

TABLE 10-5. Premenopausal Ovarian Cysts

Preoperative Evaluation	Intraoperative Evaluation
History and physical examination	Diagnostic laparoscopy
Transvaginal ultrasound	Peritoneal washing
Hormonal suppressive therapy if indicated	Cyst aspiration
Informed consent	Evaluation of the cyst
Draw blood and save for possible tumor marker	Possible frozen section
	Cystectomy or oophorectomy

cancers were found, two in the first screen and three in the follow-up screen; all were stage I.

The low prevalence of ovarian cancer in the population and its rate of progression may limit the potential cost-effectiveness of screening.[19] Current data do not seem to support the view that screening asymptomatic postmenopausal women who have a normal pelvic examination is justified. Although it is clear that ultrasound and multimodal screening can detect ovarian cancer in asymptomatic women, there is currently no evidence that screening improves the outcome for women in any risk group.

The preoperative evaluation for an ovarian cyst includes a history, pelvic examination, ultrasound, and serum CA-125. If any combinations of these tests are suggestive of malignancy, an abdominal and pelvic CT scan is done. If the scan shows malignancy (ascites, omental cake, etc.), the patient undergoes a staging laparotomy or chemotherapy. When the CT is negative, a laparoscopy is planned and consent is obtained for laparotomy. Preoperatively, the patient has a mechanical and antibiotic bowel preparation and a chest x-ray and signs the appropriate consent.

Intraoperative Therapy

Intraoperative evaluation includes cell washings from the pelvis and upper abdomen to be saved for evaluation if a malignancy is found. The upper abdomen and pelvis are explored and excrescences or suspicious areas are sampled and sent for frozen section.

After the pelvis and upper abdomen are examined, the cyst contents are aspirated. Once the capsule is opened, the interior of the capsule is examined and suspicious areas are biopsied, and then the tissue is sent for frozen section. The entire cyst capsule is removed to search for an early carcinoma that may escape gross detection.[12] Whether to do an oophorectomy or cystectomy depends on the patient's age and the characteristics of the mass.

Ovarian Cystectomy

An ideal ovarian cystectomy consists of the removal of the intact cyst with limited trauma to the residual ovarian tissue. Alternatively, the cyst fluid can be drained to minimize spillage and facilitate removal.

Three methods to manage ovarian cysts are drainage, excision, and thermal ablation or coagulation. When the cyst is excised, histopathologic examination is complete and the risk of recurrence is lessened. Aspiration is recommended for functional cysts detected laparoscopically and confirmed by frozen section. Postoperatively, hormonal suppressive therapy is advised. Since thermal ablation does not destroy the entire cyst wall and the underlying ovarian cortex can be damaged by the heat, excision is preferred.

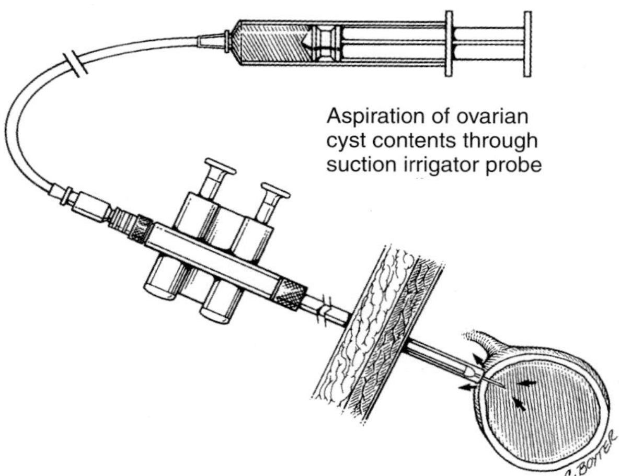

Figure 10-2. For pure cysts larger than 2 cm, an 18-gauge laparoscopic needle is passed through the suction-irrigator probe. While the cyst is stabilized with suction applied over the cyst wall, the needle is inserted into the cyst and the contents are aspirated.

Many cysts are ruptured during their manipulation despite the use of a delicate technique. The intact removal of a cyst >10 cm is difficult laparoscopically. Aspiration before removal of large cysts is practical. It is accomplished with an 18-gauge laparoscopic needle passed through the suction-irrigator probe while the cyst is stabilized with suction applied over the cyst. The needle is inserted into the cyst, and the contents are aspirated (Figure 10-2). The suction-irrigator system reduces the spillage by applying suction at the cannula. Alternatively, a suction-irrigator probe can be inserted into the cyst (Figure 10-3, inset). Another technique involves the passage of a 5-mm trocar and sleeve. The trocar is placed into the cyst and then removed, and then the suction-irrigator is inserted (Figure 10-3). This method works well for endometriomas and mucinous cystadenomas but is not advisable for benign teratomas that contain hair.

The aspirate is sent for cytologic examination, and the ovary is freed from adhesions to the lateral pelvic wall, uterus, or bowel. The cyst and pelvis are irrigated continuously, especially for benign cystic teratomas, mucinous cystadenomas, and endometriomas. The most dependent portion of the

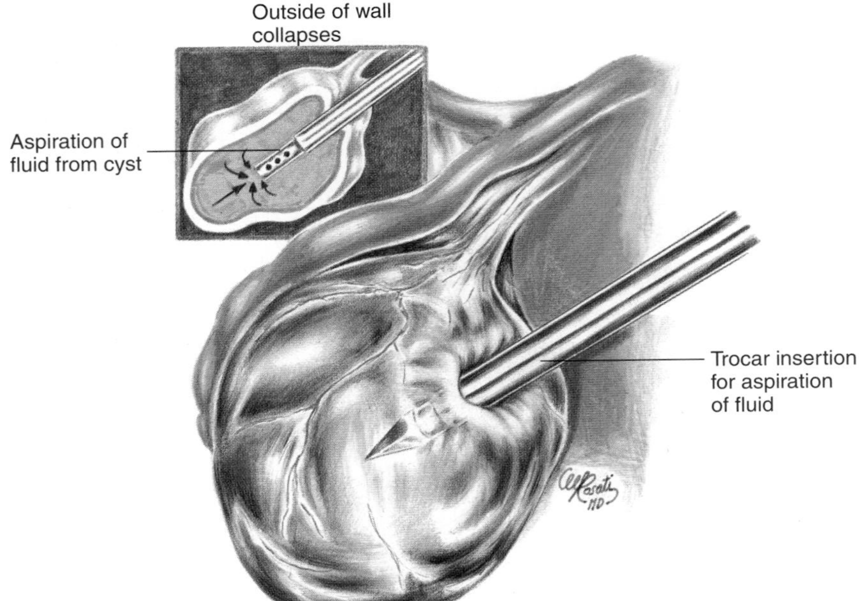

Figure 10-3. The trocar is placed into the cyst and then removed, and the suction irrigator (inset) is inserted. This method works well for endometriomas and mucinous cystadenomas but is not advisable for teratomas that contain hair. The aspirate is sent for cytologic examination. The cyst and pelvis are irrigated continuously.

cyst wall is opened, and the internal surface is inspected (Figure 10-4). If excrescences or papillae are found, a biopsy specimen is sent for frozen section (Figure 10-4, inset). Dilute vasopressin is injected between the capsule and the ovarian cortex to create a plane for hydrodissection and reduce oozing in the capsule (Figure 10-5A). The capsule is stripped from the ovarian stroma, using two grasping forceps and the suction-irrigator probe for traction and countertraction (Figure 10-5B). It is sent for histologic examination. The laser is used at low power (10 to 20 W continuous) to seal blood vessels at the base of the capsule and at higher power to vaporize small remnants of capsule. Bipolar forceps are used to control bleeding (Figure 10-5C).

Sometimes it is difficult to remove the capsule from the ovarian cortex, and so injecting dilute vasopressin between the capsule and the cortex facilitates the stripping procedure (Figure 10-6). If the cyst wall cannot be identified, the edge of the ovarian incision can be "freshened" with scissors, and the resulting clean edge reveals the different

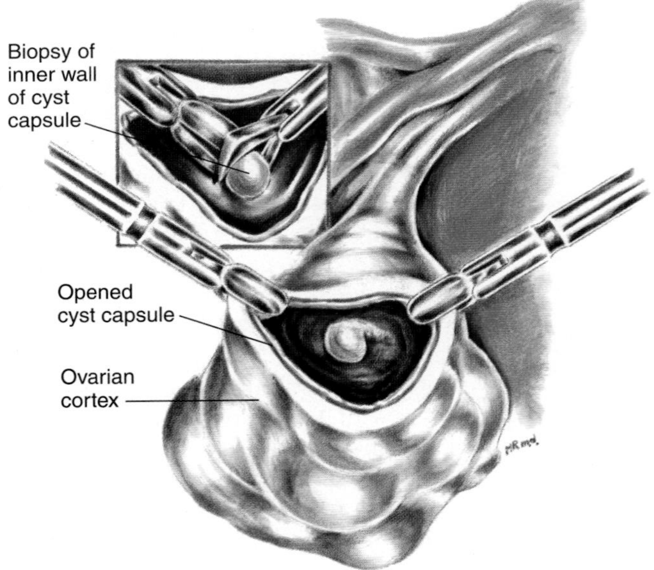

Figure 10-4. The most dependent portion of the cyst wall is opened, and the internal surface is inspected. If excrescences or papillomas are found, a biopsy specimen (inset) is taken and sent for frozen section. The ovarian cortex is held apart with graspers.

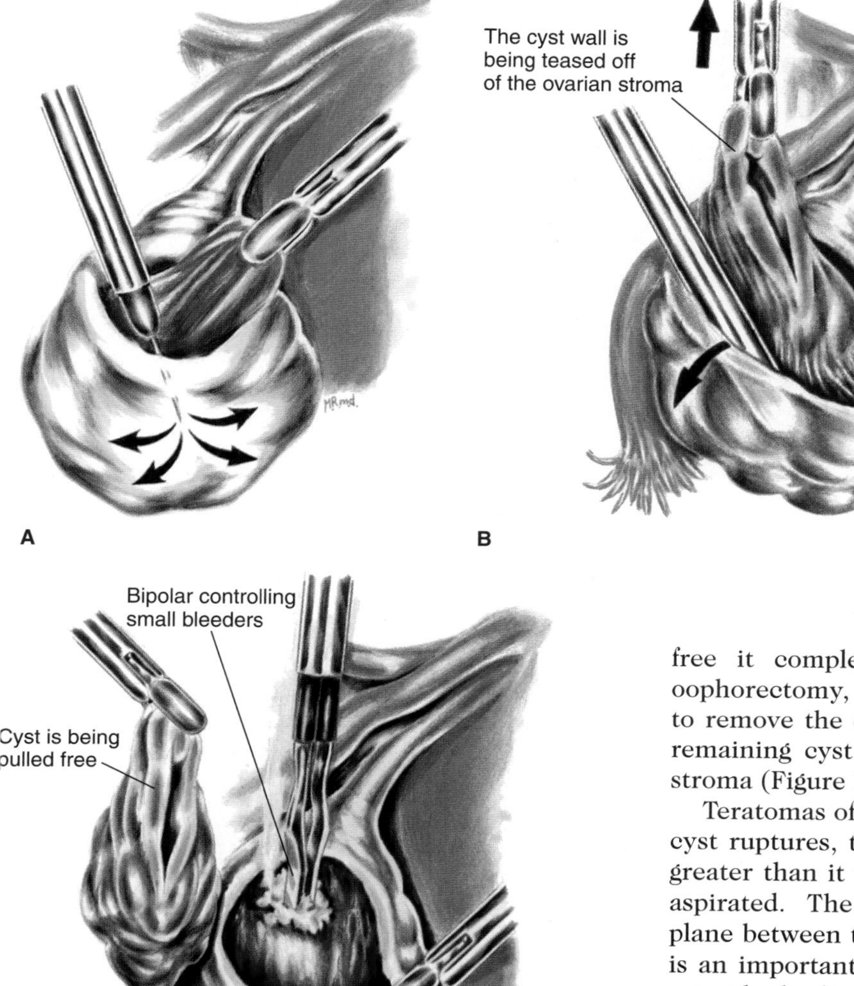

Figure 10-5. **A.** Dilute vasopressin is injected between the capsule and the ovarian cortex to create a plane for hydrodissection and to reduce oozing in the capsule. Sometimes it is difficult to separate the cyst wall from the ovarian cortex, and so this injection technique facilitates the stripping procedure. **B.** The capsule is stripped from the ovarian cortex by using two grasping forceps and the suction-irrigator probe for traction and countertraction. The specimen is sent for histologic examination. **C.** Bipolar forceps can be used to control bleeding.

structures. If this does not free the capsule, the base of the cyst is grasped, and traction is applied to the cyst with countertraction to the ovary. The entire cyst or portions of the wall may be adherent to the ovary, requiring sharp or laser dissection to free it completely. Large cysts require partial oophorectomy, using a high-power laser or scissors to remove the distorted portion of the ovary. The remaining cyst wall is stripped from the ovarian stroma (Figure 10-7).

Teratomas often can be excised intact, but if the cyst ruptures, the resulting contamination will be greater than it would if the cyst were opened and aspirated. The atraumatic development of the plane between the cyst wall and the ovarian tissue is an important first step that is accomplished by using hydrodissection. An 18- or 20-gauge needle is introduced through an accessory trocar sleeve, or a 7.5 inch spinal needle (American Hydro-Surgical Instruments) is inserted through the abdominal wall into the space between the cyst wall and the ovary. The plane is developed by using the suction-irrigator as a blunt probe. After removal of the cyst, the base of the capsule is irrigated and coagulation is achieved with a CO_2 laser or bipolar electrocoagulation. The edges of the ovarian cortex are connected with a low-power laser (10 to 20 W) or bipolar electrocoagulator. A grasping forceps helps merge the ovarian edges. If the ovarian edges overlap, the defect is left to heal without suturing because adhesions are more likely after the use of sutures (Table 10-6).[45] If the edges of the ovarian capsule do not meet, a low-power laser applied to the inner surface will invert them. In rare instances one or two fine absorbable monofilament sutures are needed to bring the ovarian edges together (Figure 10-8). Sutures are placed inside the ovary to decrease the formation of adhesions.

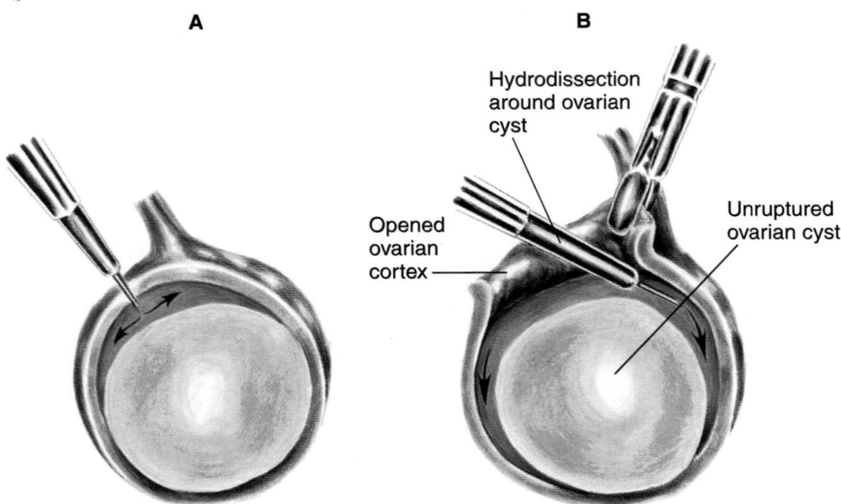

Figure 10-6. **A.** A 16- or 20-gauge needle is introduced through an accessory trocar sleeve into the space between the cyst wall and the ovarian cortex. **B.** A plane is developed, using the suction-irrigator as a blunt probe.

TABLE 10-6. Incidence of Adhesion Formation with and without Laparoscopic Ovarian Suturing

	Type of Cyst					Adhesions			
Suture	**Endometrioma**	**Benign Cystic Teratoma**	**Mucinous**	**Serous**	**Simple**	**None**	**Filmy/Minimal Vascularity**	**Dense/Non-vascular**	**Dense/Vascular**
No	27	4	2	1	2	11	22	2	1
Yes	19	6	0	2	4	5	6	15	5

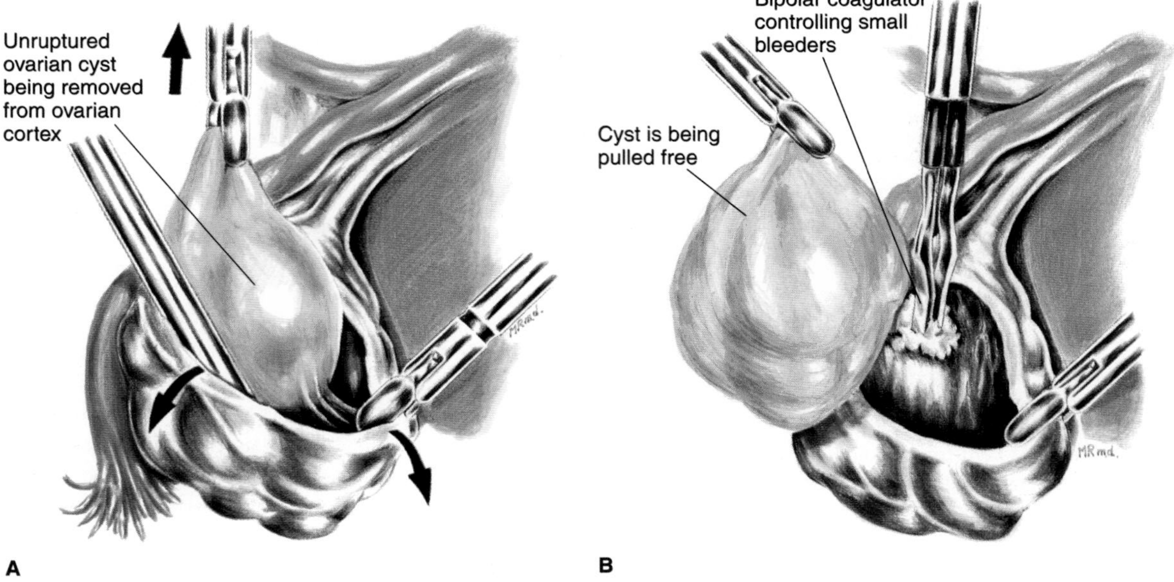

Figure 10-7. **A.** The unruptured ovarian cyst is removed from the ovarian cortex. Irrigation helps in the hydrodissection as the ovarian cortex is held with graspers for countertraction. **B.** As the cyst is enucleated, the base of the ovarian bed is coagulated with bipolar forceps to achieve hemostasis.

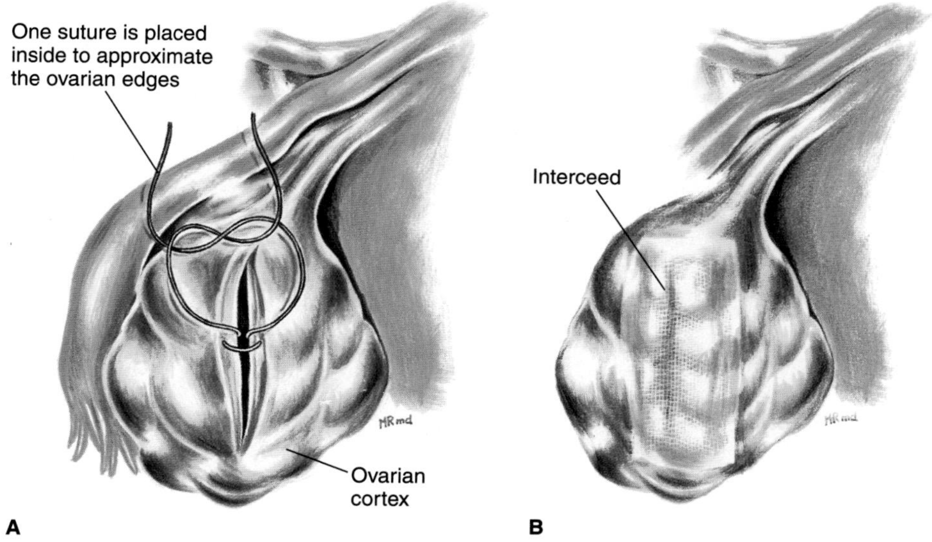

Figure 10-8. **A.** In some instances, one or two fine monofilament absorbable sutures are required to approximate the edges of the ovarian cortex. The sutures are placed inside the ovary to lessen the formation of adhesions. **B.** Interceed can be placed over the sutured site.

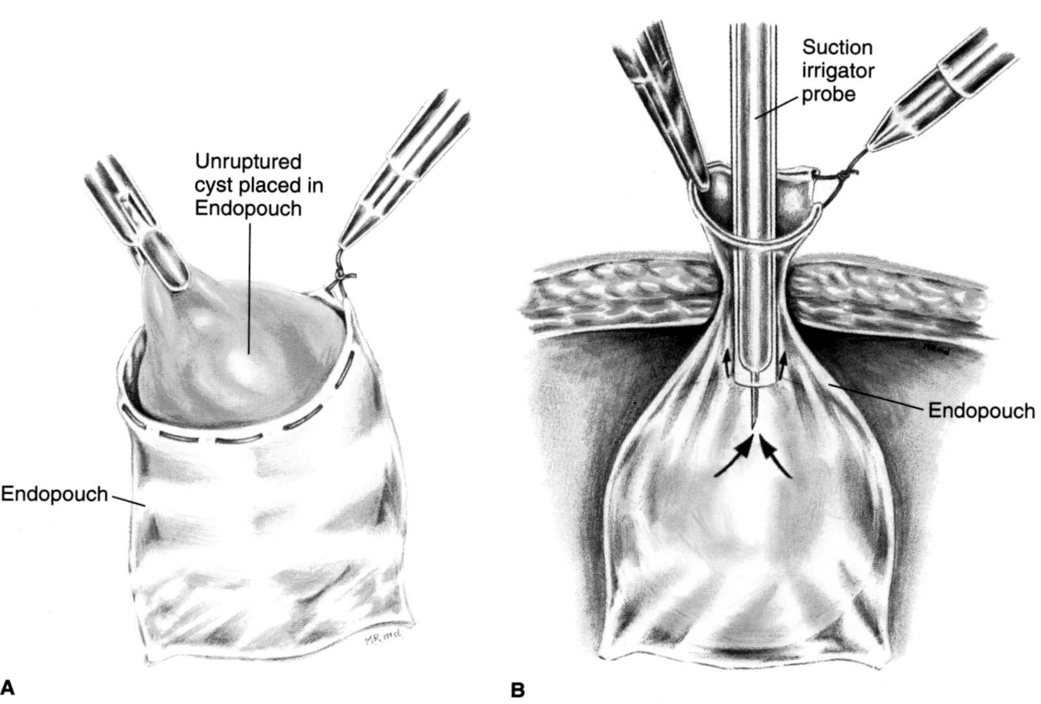

Figure 10-9. **A.** The unruptured cyst is placed in an Endopouch introduced into the pelvic cavity through a 10-mm trocar sleeve. **B.** The containment plastic bag is pulled to the level of the anterior abdominal wall. If the mass is cystic and too large to be pulled through the cannula, a suction-irrigator probe is used to aspirate the cystic fluid and reduce the size of the mass. If the excised tissue is solid, it can be cut into pieces or morcellated until the material can be pulled safely through a 10-mm trocar sleeve. Pulling the bag before the included tissue can be pulled through the sleeve can rupture the cyst and contaminate the anterior abdominal wall and peritoneal cavity.

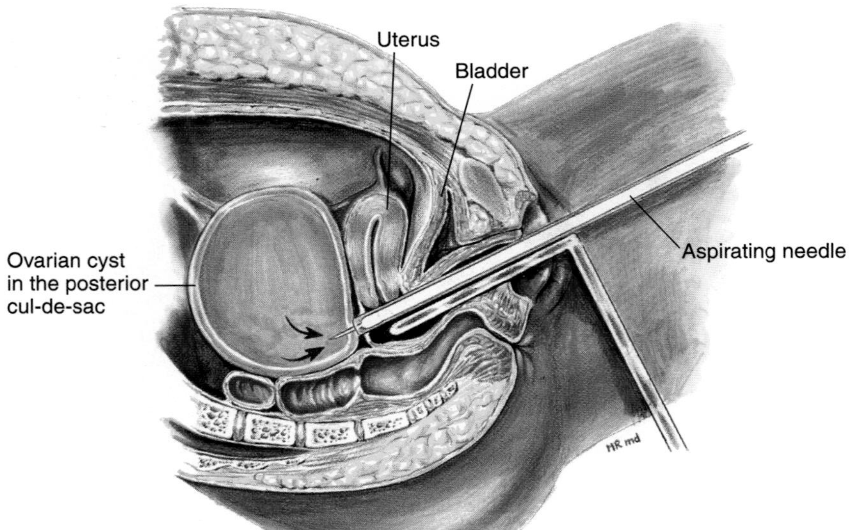

Figure 10-10. A colpotomy can be used to remove large pieces of myoma or cystic masses. The cystic mass is brought into the cul-de-sac and drained transvaginally. The culdotomy can be repaired either vaginally or laparoscopically. After the mass is removed, the pelvis is irrigated copiously and suctioned. Laparoscopic culdotomy has not been associated with significant pelvic adhesions.

Tissue can be removed from the abdominal cavity by using one of the following techniques.

1. *Containment bags*. Excised tissue is placed into a small plastic prepared bag introduced into the pelvis through a 10-mm trocar (Endobag, Ethicon). The tissue is placed in the bag, traction is applied to the bag, and, after the trocar sleeve is removed, it is pulled through a trocar incision to the anterior abdominal wall. The edges of the bag are pulled toward the anterior abdominal wall. Cystic contents are aspirated, and the deflated cyst is pulled out of the peritoneal cavity (Figure 10-9). A solid mass is morcellated inside the bag and removed. Attempting to pull the bag out of the abdomen before the cyst is collapsed or morcellated causes rupture of the bag and contamination of the abdominal cavity or anterior abdominal wall.
2. Through a colpotomy, large pieces of solid tissue such as myomas and cystic masses can be removed. Some cystic masses are so fragile and large that it is impossible to remove them intact through a colpotomy. The tumor mass is brought to the vaginal incision and drained transvaginally (Figure 10-10). After the mass is removed, the pelvic cavity is irrigated and suctioned. The colpotomy is repaired vaginally or laparoscopically. Nezhat and colleagues[46] found that colpotomy is not associated with significant postoperative adhesions.
3. With another technique, the cystic mass is brought to the surface of the abdominal incision, drained, and extracted similarly to the method for removal by colpotomy.

No tissue should be left in the pelvic cavity or on the abdominal wall. Implantation of ovarian tissue in the abdominal and pelvic cavity can cause an ovarian remnant syndrome.[47] Contamination of the anterior abdominal wall should be avoided, and if this happens, all tissue must be removed and the incision must be irrigated copiously. Abdominal wall metastasis has been reported after contamination of the wall during laparoscopy for ovarian cancer.[48]

Benign Cystic Teratomas

These germ cell tumors occur predominantly in young women. Laparoscopic removal can be technically difficult, but it can be done successfully. After laparoscopic excision and removal by a posterior colpotomy, normal ovaries and few adhesions were seen at a repeat laparoscopy.[49] If this is unsuccessful, one should go on to laparotomy to ensure complete excision of the tumor.

The suction-irrigator is placed in the cyst, the contents are aspirated, and the cavity is irrigated copiously. The interior of the cyst is inspected, and its lining is grasped and removed from the ovary. The lining is removed from the pelvis through a 10-mm accessory trocar, the operating channel of the laparoscope, a colpotomy, or an Endobag. The cyst wall is inspected and sent for frozen section. The pelvis is irrigated with lactated

Ringer's solution until all evidence of sebaceous material is removed because incomplete removal can cause peritonitis. During irrigation, the ovarian stroma is inspected to verify hemostasis. Bleeding areas are coagulated with a defocused laser or bipolar forceps.

The ability to prevent rupture and spillage of teratomas using this laparoscopic technique has been demonstrated, but this approach can be time-consuming and requires expert surgical technique.[50] During laparoscopic operative management, aquadissection compared with blunt dissection and scissors is associated with less intraoperative spillage, because with this method it is easier to avoid cyst rupture.[51]

For large teratomas (>8 cm); the ovary is placed in the cul-de-sac next to a colpotomy. Draining the cyst and removing its wall transvaginally lessen the risk of contamination and maintain a minimally invasive approach. The vagina is prepared with povidone-iodine (Betadine) before colpotomy.

Laparoscopically assisted vaginal removal of these cysts is an alternative to laparotomy when adnexal mobility is proven and vaginal extraction is feasible.[52] Laparoscopically assisted transvaginal ovarian cystectomy allows the removal of larger cystic teratomas. Less of a tendency to spill the contents and decreased operative time result compared with conventional laparoscopic cystectomy.[53]

The outcome of conservative laparoscopic treatment of these cysts removed from the abdominal cavity without and with an Endobag was studied in a prospective, randomized trial in Rome.[54] In the 55 women studied, 58 cysts (mean diameter, 5.6 ± 2.03 cm) were enucleated and removed at operative laparoscopy through a 10- to 12-mm cannula sleeve without intraoperative or postoperative complications. Mean operating time was 73 minutes. When cysts were removed with an Endobag, operating time was reduced over removal without the Endobag (63 versus 81 minutes, $p < 0.05$). Obvious spillage of contents occurred in 13 (43.3%) patients when the Endobag was not used but occurred in only 1 patient in the study group because the bag ruptured ($p < 0.05$). No signs or symptoms of peritonitis were observed in women with evident cystic spillage and patients in whom no bag was used when spillage was possible. It was concluded that removing cysts in an Endobag reduced both operating time and spillage. However, controlled intraperitoneal spillage of cyst contents did not increase postoperative morbidity as long as the peritoneal cavity was washed thoroughly. The observation that spillage of the contents of the cyst does not lead to complications was noted earlier and attributed to liberal irrigation of the peritoneal cavity.[55]

References

1. Benjamin I, Rubin SC. Initial surgical management of advanced epithelial ovarian cancer. *Cancer Invest* 1997; 15:270.
2. Lehner R, Wenzl R, Heinzl H, et al. Influence of delayed staging laparotomy after laparoscopic removal of ovarian masses later found malignant. *Obstet Gynecol* 1998; 92:967.
3. Canis M, Botchorishvili R, Kouyate S, et al. Surgical management of adnexal tumors. *Ann Chir* 1998; 52:234.
4. Hidlebaugh DA, Vulgaropulos S, Orr RK. Treating adnexal masses: Operative laparoscopy vs. laparotomy. *J Reprod Med* 1997; 42:551.
5. Guglielmina JN, Pennehouat G, Deval B, et al. Treatment of ovarian cysts by laparoscopy. *Contracept Fertil Sex* 1997; 25:218.
6. Malik E, Bohm W, Stoz F, et al. Laparoscopic management of ovarian tumors. *Surg Endosc* 1998; 12:1326.
7. Webb MJ, Decker DG, Mussey E, et al. Factors in influencing survival in stage I ovarian cancer. *Am J Obstet Gynecol* 1973; 116:222.
8. Dembo AJ, Davy M, Stenwick AE, et al. Prognostic factors in patients with stage I epithelial ovarian cancer. *Obstet Gynecol* 1990; 74:263.
9. Lim-Yan S, Cajigas H, Scully R. Ovarian cystectomy for serous borderline tumors: A follow-up study of 35 cases. *Obstet Gynecol* 1998; 72:775.
10. Darai E, Teboul J, Fauconnier A, et al. Management and outcome of borderline ovarian tumors incidentally discovered at or after laparoscopy. *Acta Obstet Gynecol Scand* 1998; 77:451.
11. Mage G, Canis M, Manhes H, et al. Laparoscopic management of adnexal cystic masses. *J Gynecol Surg* 1990; 6:71.
12. Nezhat C, Nezhat F, Welander CE, et al. Four ovarian cancers diagnosed during laparoscopic management of 1,011 adnexal masses. *Am J Obstet Gynecol* 1992; 167:790.
13. Hulka JF, Parker WH, Surrey M, et al. Management of ovarian masses: AAGL 1190 survey. *J Reprod Med* 1992; 37:599.

14. Wenzl R, Lehner R, Husslein P, Sevelda P. Laparoscopic surgery in cases of ovarian malignancies: An Austria-wide survey. *Gynecol Oncol* 1996; 63:57.
15. Maimon M, Seltzer V, Boyce J. Laparoscopic excision of ovarian neoplasms subsequently found to be malignant. *Obstet Gynecol* 1991; 77:653.
16. Herrmann U, Locher G, Goldhirsch A. Sonographic patterns of malignancy: Prediction of malignancy. *Obstet Gynecol* 1987; 69:777.
17. Granberg S, Norstrom A, Wikland M. Comparison of endovaginal ultrasound and cytological evaluations of cystic ovarian tumors. *J Ultrasound Med* 1991; 10:9.
18. Canis M, Pouly JL, Wattiez A, et al. Laparoscopic management of adnexal masses suspicious at ultrasound. *Obstet Gynecol* 1997; 89:679.
19. Bell R, Petticrew M, Sheldon T. The performance of screening tests for ovarian cancer: Results of a systematic review. *Br J Obstet Gynaecol* 1998; 105:1136.
20. Jacobs I, Bast R. The CA-125 tumor associated antigen: A review of the literature. *Hum Reprod* 1989; 4:1.
21. Nezhat CH, Nezhat F, Borhan S, et al. Is hormonal treatment efficacious in the management of ovarian cysts in women with histories of endometriosis? *Hum Reprod* 1996; 11:874.
22. DeCrespigny L, Robinson HP, Daboren RAM, et al. The "simple" cyst: Aspirate or operate? *Br J Obstet Gynecol* 1989; 96:1035.
23. Kjellgren RK. Ovarian cyst fenestration via laparoscopy. *J Reprod Med* 1978; 21:16.
24. Trope C: The preoperative diagnosis of malignancy of ovarian cysts. *Neoplasia* 1981; 28:117.
25. Hasson HM. Ovarian surgery, in Sanfilippo JS, Levine RL, eds., *Operative Gynecological Endoscopy*. New York: Springer-Verlag, 1989.
26. Mulvany NJ. Aspiration cytology of ovarian cysts and cystic neoplasms: A study of 235 aspirates. *Acta Cytol* 1996; 40:911.
27. Lipitz S, Seidman DS, Menczer J, et al. Recurrence rate after fluid aspiration from sonographically benign-appearing ovarian cysts. *J Reprod Med* 1992; 37:845.
28. Larsen JF, Pedersen OD, Gregerson E. Ovarian cyst fenestration via the laparoscope. *Acta Obstet Gynecol Scand* 1986; 65:529.
29. Marana R, Caruana P, Muzii L, et al. Operative laparoscopy for ovarian cysts: Excision vs. aspiration. *J Reprod Med* 1996; 41:435.
30. Zanetta G, Lissoni A, Torri V, et al. Role of puncture and aspiration in expectant management of simple ovarian cysts: A randomised study. *Br Med* 1996; 313:1110.
31. Troiano RN, Taylor KJ. Sonographically guided therapeutic aspiration of benign-appearing ovarian cysts and endometriomas. *AJR Am J Roentgenol* 1998; 171:1601.
32. Mikamo H, Kawazoe K, Sato Y, et al. Ovarian abscess caused by Peptostreptococcus magnus following transvaginal ultrasound-guided aspiration of ovarian endometrioma and fixation with pure ethanol. *Infect Dis Obstet Gynecol* 1998; 6:66.
33. Scoutt L, McCarthy SM, Lange R, et al. Evaluation of ovarian masses on MRI with ultrasound correlation. *Radiology* 1990; 177:242.
34. Takahashi K, Okada S, Okada M, et al. Magnetic resonance relaxation time in evaluating the cyst fluid characteristics of endometrioma. *Hum Reprod* 1996; 11:857.
35. Yamashita Y, Hatanaka Y, Torashima M, et al. Characterization of sonographically indeterminate ovarian tumors with MR imaging: A logistic regression analysis. *Acta Radiol* 1997; 38:572.
36. Moteki T, Ishizaka H. Evaluation of cystic ovarian lesions using apparent diffusion coefficient calculated from turboFLASH MR images. *Br J Radiol* 1998; 71:612.
37. Patel VH, Somers S. MR imaging of the female pelvis: Current perspectives and review of genital tract congenital anomalies, and benign and malignant diseases. *Crit Rev Diagn Imaging* 1997; 38:417.
38. Woodward PJ, Gilfeather M. Magnetic resonance imaging of the female pelvis. *Semin Ultrasound CT MR* 1998; 19:90.
39. Steinkampf MP, Hammond KR, Blackwell RE. Hormonal treatment of functional ovarian cysts: A randomized, prospective study. *Fertil Steril* 1990; 54:775.
40. Ben-Ami M, Geslevich Y, Battino S, et al. Management of functional ovarian cysts after induction of ovulation: A randomized prospective study. *Acta Obstet Gynecol Scand* 1993; 72:396.
41. Turan C, Zorlu CG, Ugur M, et al. Expectant management of functional ovarian cysts: An alternative to hormonal therapy. *Int J Gynaecol Obstet* 1994; 47:257.
42. Chapron C, Dubuisson JB, Kadoch O, et al. Laparoscopic management of organic ovarian cysts: Is there a place for frozen section diagnosis? *Hum Reprod* 1998; 13:324.

43. Wolf SL, Gosnik BB, Feldesman MR, et al. Prevalence of simple adnexal cysts in postmenopausal women. *Radiology* 1991; 180:65.
44. Campbell S, Goessens L, Goswamy R, et al. Real-time ultrasonography for the determination of ovarian morphology and volume: A possible early screening test for ovarian cancer. *Lancet* 1982; 1:415.
45. Nezhat C, Nezhat F. Postoperative adhesion formation after ovarian cystectomy with and without ovarian reconstruction. American Fertility Society Annual Meeting, Orlando, FL, October 21, 1991. (Abstract)
46. Nezhat F, Brill AI, Nezhat CH, et al. Adhesion formation after endoscopic posterior colpotomy. *J Reprod Med* 1993; 38:534.
47. Nezhat C, Nezhat F. Operative laparoscopy for the management of ovarian remnant syndrome. *Fertil Steril* 1992; 57:1003.
48. Gleeson NC, Nicosia SV, Mark JE, et al. Abdominal wall metastases from ovarian cancer after laparoscopy. *Am J Obstet Gynecol* 1993; 169:522.
49. Nezhat C, Winer W, Nezhat F. Laparoscopic removal of dermoid cysts. *Obstet Gynecol* 1989; 73:278.
50. Remorgida V, Magnasco A, Pizzorno V, Anserini P. Four year experience in laparoscopic dissection of intact ovarian dermoid cysts. *J Am Coll Surg* 1998; 187:519.
51. Luxman D, Cohen JR, David MP. Laparoscopic conservative removal of ovarian dermoid cysts. *J Am Assoc Gynecol Laparosc* 1996; 3:409.
52. Pardi G, Carminati R, Ferrari MM, et al. Laparoscopically assisted vaginal removal of ovarian dermoid cysts. *Obstet Gynecol* 1995; 85:129.
53. Teng FY, Muzsnai D, Perez R, et al. A comparative study of laparoscopy and colpotomy for the removal of ovarian dermoid cysts. *Obstet Gynecol* 1996; 87:1009.
54. Campo S, Garcea N. Laparoscopic conservative excision of ovarian dermoid cysts with and without an Eendobag. *J Am Assoc Gynecol Laparosc* 1998; 5:165.
55. Lin P, Falcone T, Tulandi T. Excision of ovarian dermoid cyst by laparoscopy and by laparotomy. *Am J Obstet Gynecol* 1995; 173:769.

11

Laparoscopic Operations on the Ovary

Although most benign ovarian tumors can be treated laparoscopically, observation of the adnexa enables a gynecologist to decide whether laparotomy is indicated.

Ovarian Biopsies

It is often difficult to immobilize the ovary because of its smooth surface and firm texture. The uterine-ovarian ligament can be grasped to lift and rotate it, or the ovary can be wedged against the pelvic side wall by using the flattened edges of open or closed forceps. Sometimes Morgagni peritubal cysts can be used as a handle or the uterus can be manipulated under the ovary to provide a shelf (Figure 11-1). Overly aggressive manipulation can cause lacerations in the capsule and result in bleeding from follicles or cysts.

A punch biopsy specimen of a lesion from the antimesenteric border of the ovary is sufficient for most purposes. Palmer biopsy forceps can take tissue without penetrating the vascular medulla,[1] although a small wedge resection yields the best histologic features of the ovarian stroma and cortex. Alternatively, tissue can be obtained by using toothed forceps and laparoscopic scissors or a laser (Figure 11-2). Bleeding is controlled with bipolar electrocoagulation; sutures should not be used so that postoperative adhesions can be minimized.[2]

Indications for Oophorectomy

In 1980, Semm[3] reported his experience with a laparoscopic approach to oophorectomy and salpingo-oophorectomy. Since then, several authors have described the efficacy and safety of these procedures using different techniques.[4–8] Laparoscopy may encourage ovarian conservation during hysterectomy and more conservative management of pain caused by adnexal disease. If necessary, oophorectomy can be done laparoscopically at a later date with a short hospital stay and recovery period. The indications for oophorectomy are as follows:

1. Persistent localized pain despite previous lysis of adhesions or treatment of endometriosis
2. Residual ovary syndrome
3. Dysgenetic gonads
4. Ovarian cysts >5 cm with ovarian damage or when spillage of cystic contents increases the likelihood of complications (cystic teratomas, mucinous cystadenomas, malignancy)
5. Unilateral tubo-ovarian abscess
6. Prophylactic therapy for advanced breast cancer
7. Early ovarian cancer in young women (stage I)

A uterine manipulator is inserted for traction and countertraction to aid in the exposure and manipulation of the ovary. The pelvis and especially the adnexa are inspected to plan the surgical approach. Before starting the procedure, it is important to observe the course of the ureter as it crosses the external iliac artery near the bifurcation of the common iliac artery at the pelvic brim. The left ureter can be more difficult to find because the base of the sigmoid mesocolon often covers it. If the ureter cannot be seen

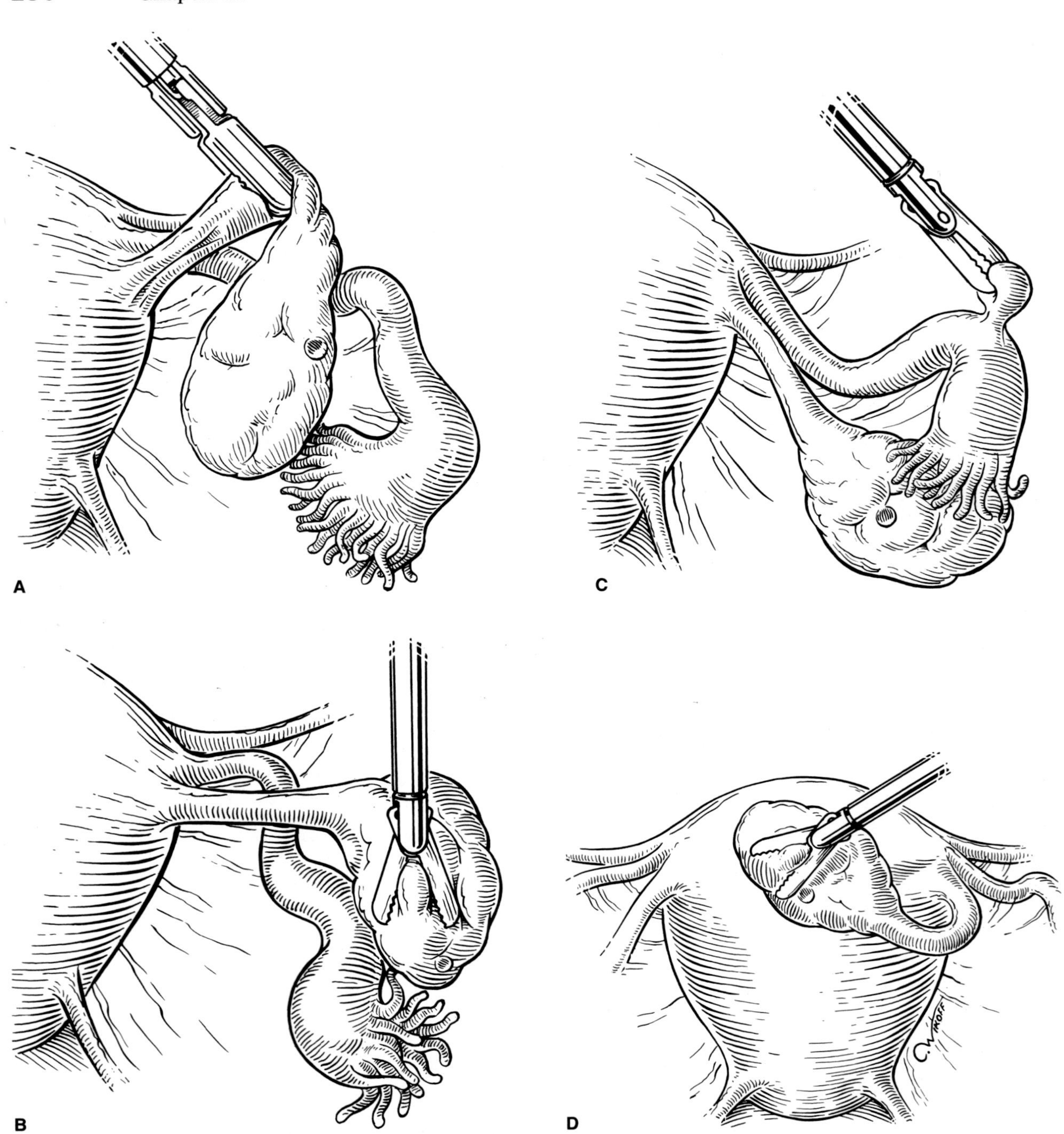

Figure 11-1. Different methods of immobilizing the ovary. **A.** Grasping the utero-ovarian ligament. **B.** Wedging the ovary against the pelvic side wall. **C.** Grasping tubal or ovarian inclusion cysts. **D.** Using the uterus as a platform.

through the intact peritoneum, it must be identified by retroperitoneal dissection. If the patient does not have a uterus, it is essential to insert a vaginal probe or sponge stick so that the surgeon can maintain orientation, particularly with procedures involving extensive adhesions. When anatomic landmarks are distorted by adhesions, endometriosis, or prior surgical extirpation, one should begin the procedure at the most normal area and work toward the more distorted parts of the operative field. The entire ovary must be removed to prevent ovarian remnant syndrome

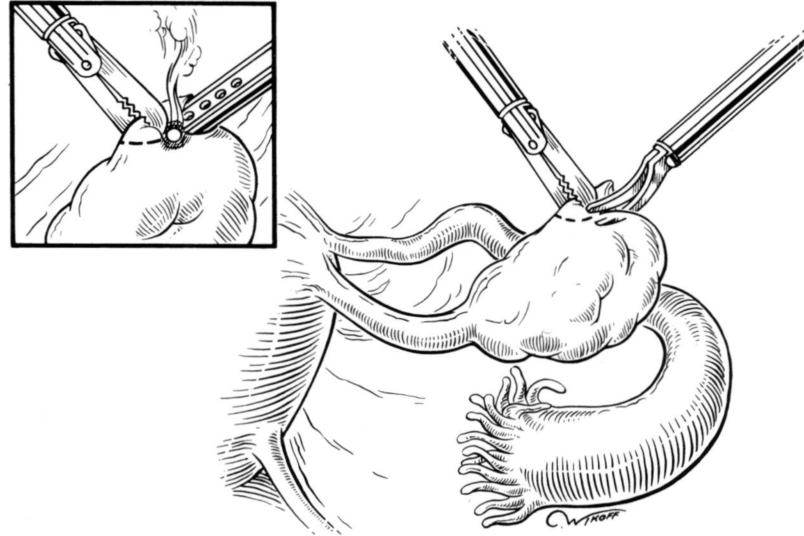

Figure 11-2. A small wedge biopsy specimen of the ovary is taken using a scissors or CO_2 laser (*inset*).

or tumor development in a dysgenetic gonad. At the conclusion, the operative field is inspected and clots are removed with a suction-irrigator or grasping forceps. Pedicles are inspected under water and with decreased pneumoperitoneum,[9] and hemostasis is obtained with bipolar electrocoagulation.

Oophorectomy and Salpingo-Oophorectomy

Management of the Infundibulopelvic Ligament

Three techniques have been described for managing the infundibulopelvic ligament: bipolar electrodesiccation, suture ligation with pretied sutures, and automatic stapling. Patient cost for the linear stapler is approximately $600 and $48 for each pretied ligature. There is no extra charge for bipolar electrocoagulation.

A bipolar forceps is preferable for hemostasis of the infundibulopelvic ligament.[4] Endoloop sutures cannot be applied in the presence of adhesions that distort the anatomy, and it is difficult to place Endoloop sutures on large pedicles such as the mesovarium and infundibulopelvic ligament even if the anatomy is normal. Once it is applied, the slipknot can loosen under the tension of the large pedicle, increasing the risk of intraoperative hemorrhage, or a piece of the ovary may be left in the pedicle, predisposing the patient to ovarian remnant syndrome.[10]

Aside from cost, there are several drawbacks to the stapling device. The instrument is bulky, and the operator must note its proximity to the ureter, bowel, and bladder. Adequate desiccation of tissue with bipolar forceps by monitoring the flow of electrons on an ammeter has been suggested before transecting the pedicles. Excessive desiccation creates friable tissue and increases thermal damage, and the tissue may adhere to the forceps. A self-limiting bipolar electrocoagulator (Valley Lab Force II series generator, Boulder, CO) provides controlled desiccation without charring the adjacent tissue. In this mode, the power peaks at 100 ohms instead of 300 to 500 ohms in typical generators. The power then "rolls off" to provide the desired surgical effect without excess drying, blanching, or destruction of tissue.

The mechanism of closure of large blood vessels with high-frequency electrocoagulation was described by Sigel and Dunn.[11] Electrocoagulation begins with shrinkage of the vessel wall resulting from the denaturation of tissue proteins combined with the melting of the carbohydrate tissue components and the dehydration of tissue fluids. The resulting coagulum formed by this melting and fusion of the vessel wall obliterates the lumen. The most successful closures are characterized by low levels of heating that end before char is formed, which preserve the inherent fibrillar structure of the connective tissue. Too much heating destroys the inherent fibrillar structure, forming a more amorphous coagulum that is poorly penetrated by fibroblasts and capillaries and characterized by an inflammatory-type reorganization and healing process that results in unsuccessful or weak closures. Further heating during electrocoagulation causes complete disintegration of the amorphous coagulum and carbonization.[11,12] Ammeters or flowmeters measure only the flow of current in relation to tissue resistance and have no value in assuring hemostasis. Pedicles are reinspected after the intraabdominal pressure has been lowered[9] because they can bleed again at the termination of a procedure once the hemostatic effects of the elevated abdominal pressures are lost.

The technique for oophorectomy is similar to that for salpingo-oophorectomy except that the tube must be protected from thermal damage. The procedure begins at the utero-ovarian ligament (Figure 11-3A). The pedicles are desiccated and cut.[4] The mesovarium is coagulated and cut into 2-cm bites, working from the uterine side to the fimbria until the ovary is removed (Figures 11-3, B,C, and D). The latter step may jeopardize the fallopian tube if the mesovarium is overdesiccated. In some circumstances, it may be preferable to sharply incise the individual leaves of the mesovarium if the distance between the tube and the ovary is small. The underlying vascular tissue can be coagulated and divided to allow excision of the remaining ovary. Laparoscopic oophorectomy causes less morbidity than does oophorectomy by laparotomy, and the patient's recovery is shorter.[4]

An ovary and tube minimally involved with adhesions or endometriosis are approached from the infundibulopelvic ligament or the utero-ovarian ligament. Filmy adhesions that limit the mobility of the ovary are lysed. Ovarian cysts are aspirated and deflated, making removal of the ovary easier. The adnexa are removed by beginning with the infundibulopelvic ligament. This approach is preferable if the uterus is to be removed or significant disease is found in the uterine-ovarian ligament, in patients with a prior hysterectomy, or if hemostasis of the ovarian vessels is necessary. The procedure begins with ureteral identification through the peritoneum as it enters the pelvic brim and travels parallel to the infundibulopelvic ligament.

The isthmic portion of the tube and the ovarian ligament are desiccated and cut (Figure 11-4). The ovary is held with a grasping forceps, and the infundibulopelvic ligament is put under traction by elevating it and pulling it medially. The infundibu-

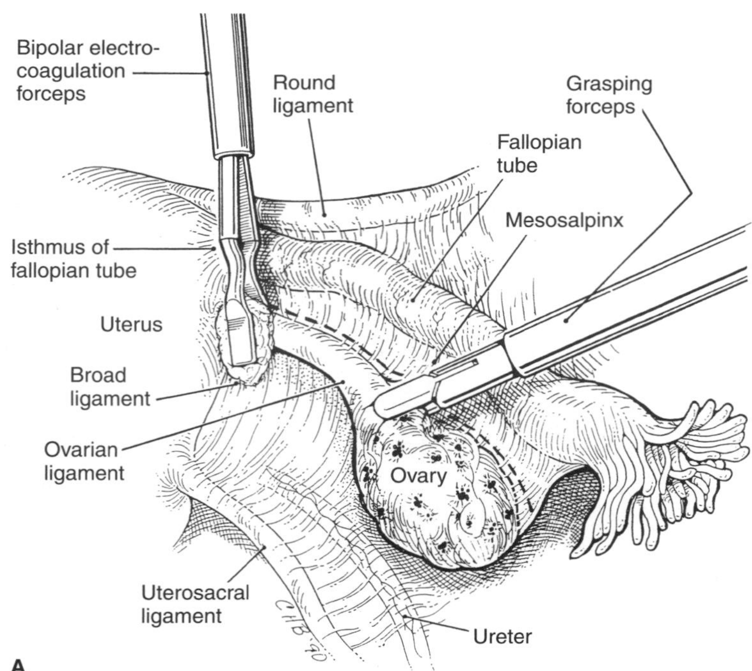

Figure 11-3. Oophorectomy is done by coagulating and cutting the mesovarium. **A.** The procedure starts from the utero-ovarian ligament.

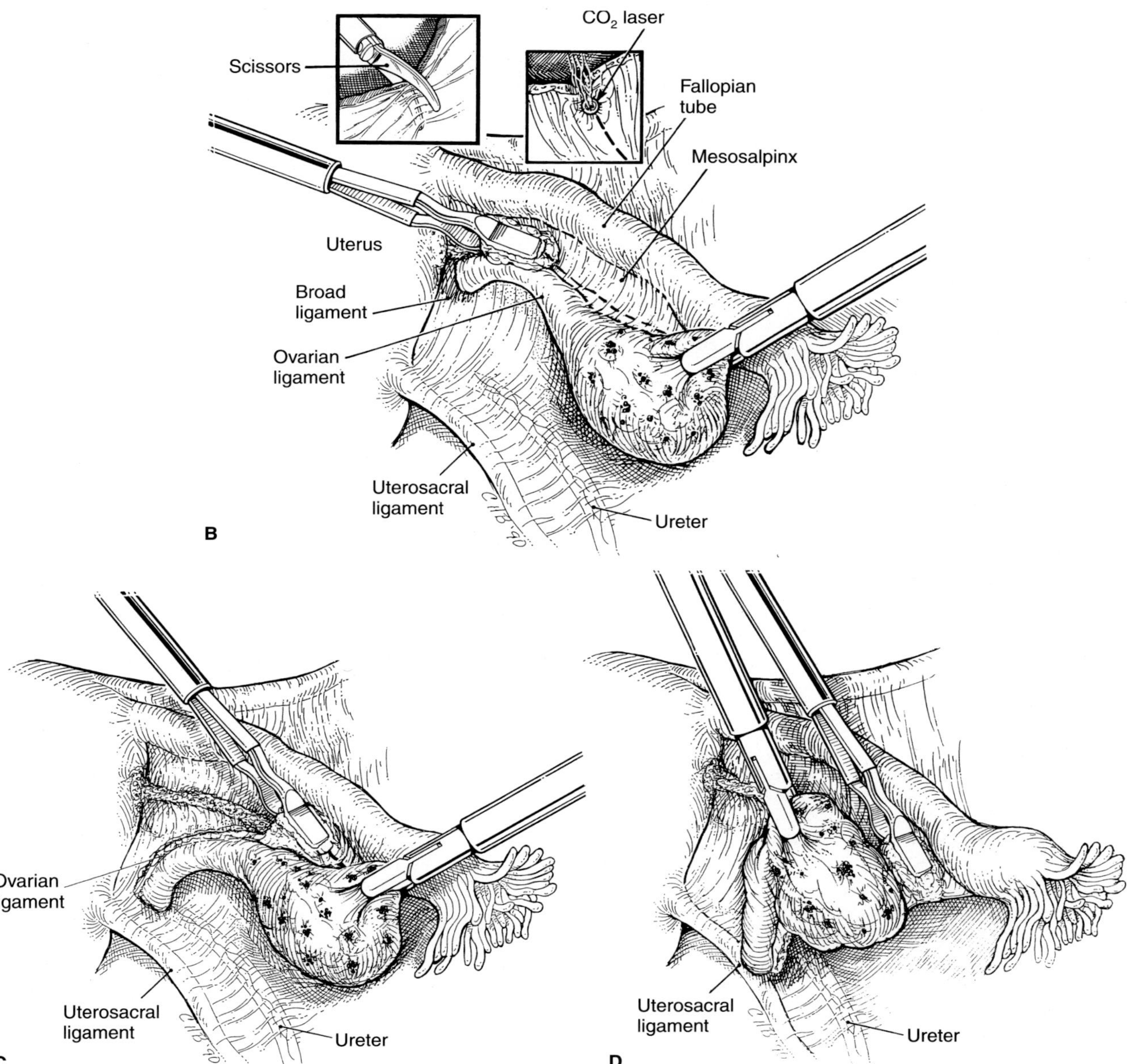

Figure 11-3. (*Continued*) **B, C,** and **D.** It continues toward the fimbria. Insets show the use of the scissors or a laser for a completing the reparation.

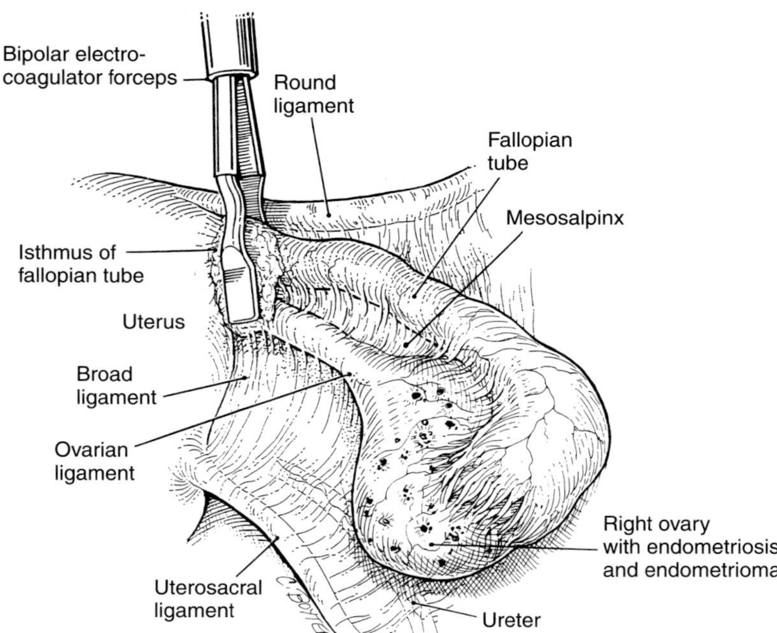

Figure 11-4. The procedure of salpingo-oophorectomy is begun by electrodesiccation and transection of the utero-ovarian ligament and the isthmic portion of the fallopian tube.

lopelvic ligament is desiccated with bipolar forceps and cut with a laser or scissors in 1- to 2-cm increments, working from lateral to medial until the adnexa are removed (Figures 11-5 through 11-8). To avoid damage to the lateral pelvic side wall, traction is used on the tube and ovary and excessive coagulation is avoided.

The Stapling Device

The laparoscopic linear stapling device used during gynecologic procedures is a modification of the stapling device used for bowel resection. The trocar site used to introduce the stapler is modified, depending on the specific adnexal disease. The

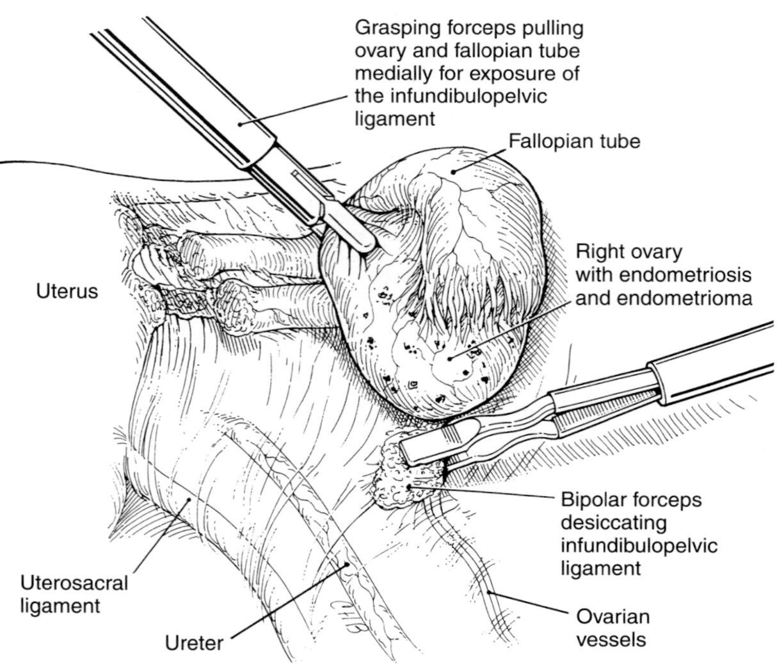

Figure 11-5. After identification of the ureter, the infundibulopelvic ligament is coagulated using a bipolar forceps, while gentle traction is applied to the adnexa.

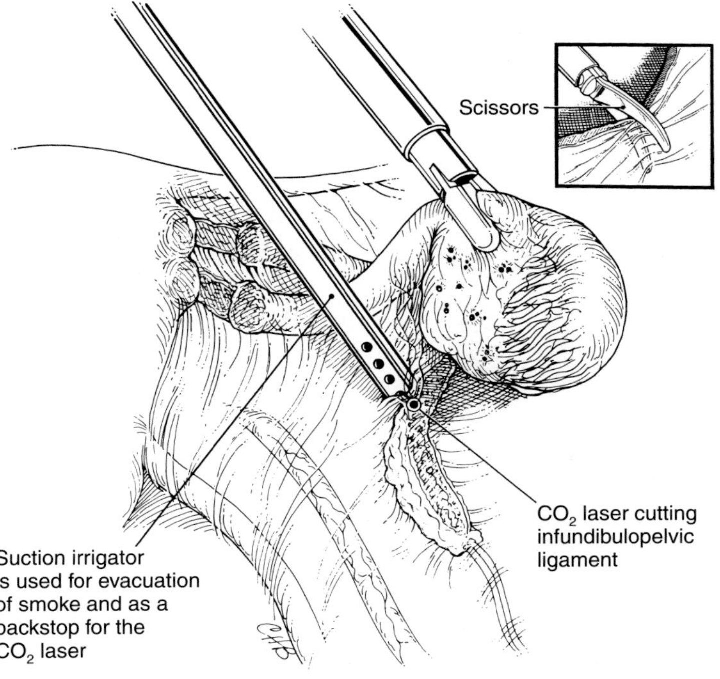

Figure 11-6. A laser or scissors (*inset*) is used to cut the coagulated infundibulopelvic ligament.

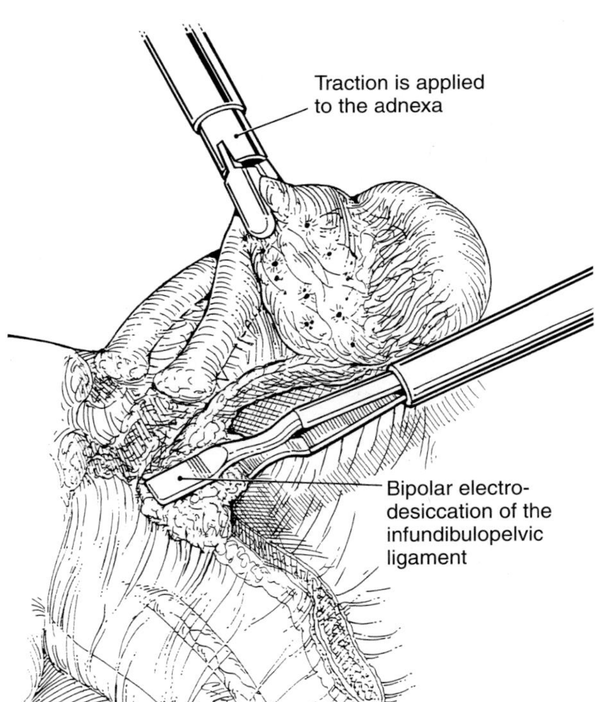

Figure 11-7. Coagulation and cutting of the infundibulopelvic ligament continue in 1- to 2-cm increments until it is removed completely.

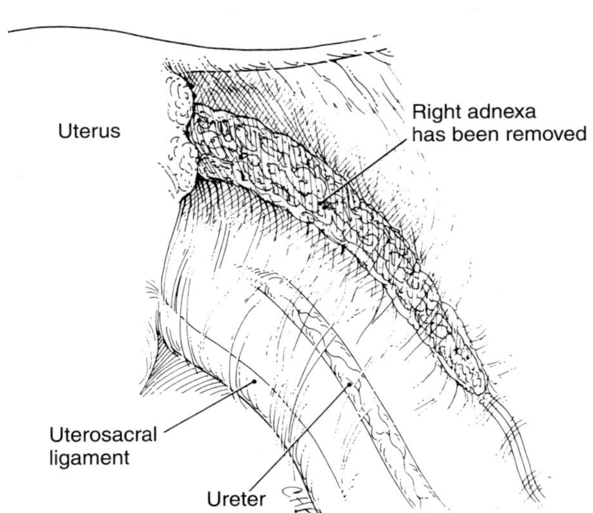

Figure 11-8. A view of the pelvic side wall after the adnexa is removed.

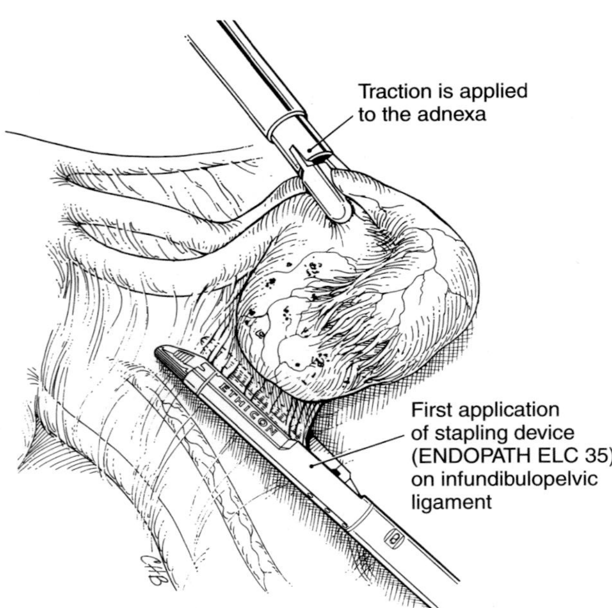

Figure 11-9. A right salpingo-oophorectomy is done using a stapling device. The tube and ovary are under traction as the Endopath ELC 35 is applied across the infundibulopelvic ligament.

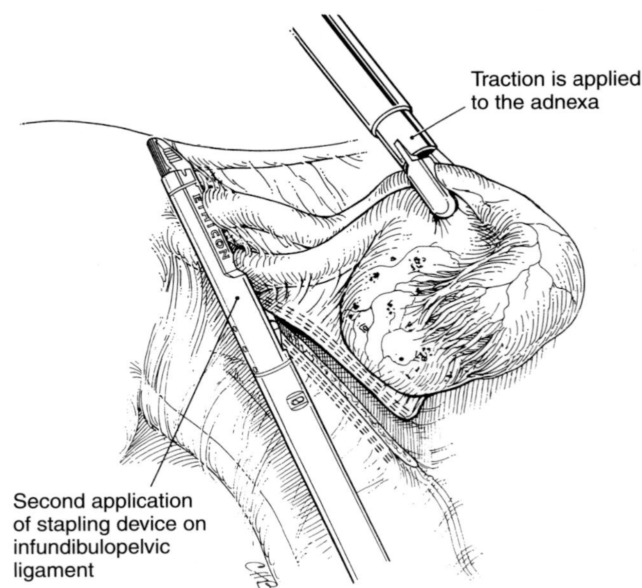

Figure 11-10. In most cases, the second application is necessary for complete removal of the adnexa.

trocar is introduced between the symphysis pubis and the umbilicus lateral to the rectus muscle and inferior epigastric vessels, although injury to inferior epigastric vessels is possible. At the end of the procedure, the fascia is closed to prevent a hernia. After the stapler is introduced, the adnexa are grasped with laparoscopic forceps and retracted medially and caudally to stretch and outline the infundibulopelvic ligament. The ligament is grasped and secured with the stapler (Figures 11-9 and 11-10). The stapler is not fired until the contained tissue is identified and the ureter's safety is assured. Once transected, the staple line is examined for placement and hemostasis (Figure 11-11). Usually one or two stapler applications are required for each adnexa.

The Endoligature

Pretied Endoloop sutures can be used in an oophorectomy or a salpingo-oophorectomy.[13] Periovarian adhesions are lysed, and the ovary is freed. If a cyst is present, it is aspirated so that manipulation will be easier. The mesovarium and ovarian ligament are electrodesiccated and dissected to facilitate placement of the Endoligature (Figure 11-12). The Endoloop (0 polydioxanone or polyglactin suture, Ethicon) is introduced into the abdominal cavity through the mid-suprapubic trocar sleeve. Using forceps, the ovary is pulled through the Endoloop (Figure 11-12). Atraumatic

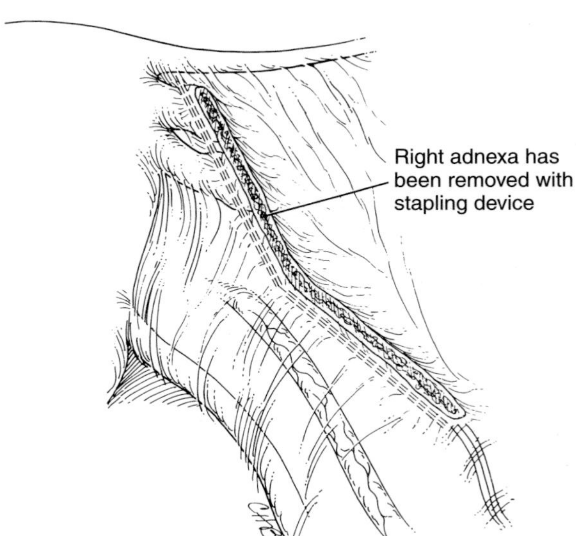

Figure 11-11. The pelvic side wall is seen after an adnexectomy with a stapling device.

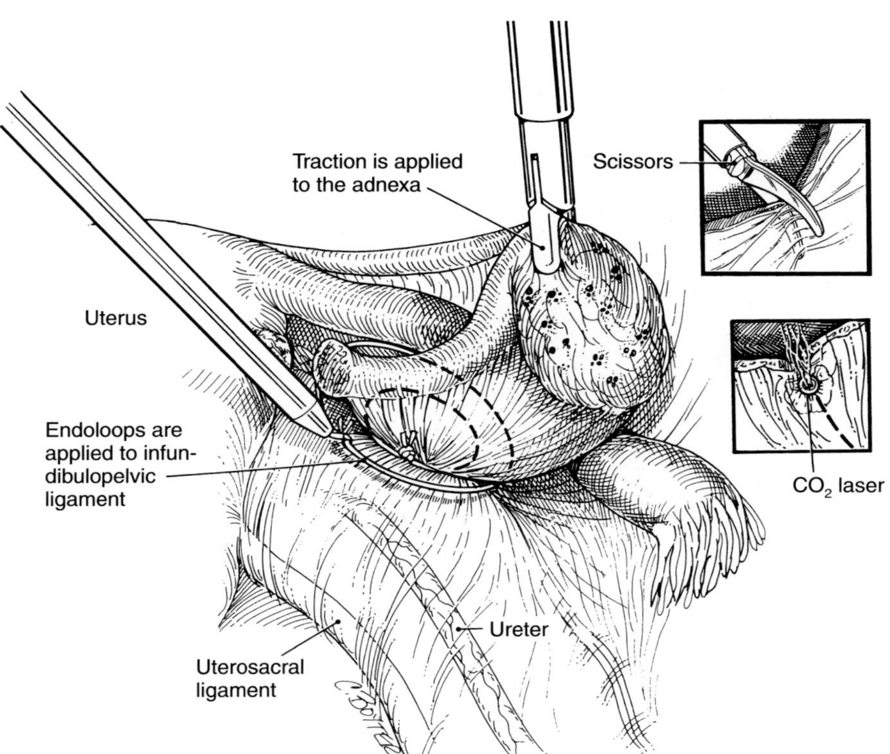

Figure 11-12. Oophorectomy is achieved with a partial Endoloop. After the ovarian ligament is coagulated and cut, two Endoloop sutures are passed over the ovary and mesovarium and tied beyond the ovarian tissue. Insets show the scissors (*top*) and laser (*bottom*) for the removal of the ligated mesovarium.

forceps are used to assist in placement. The suture is pushed onto the mesovarium while a knot pusher is used on the opposite side to place the slipknot at the most lateral position on the mesosalpinx and mesovarium. The suture is tightened as the ovary is pulled toward the midline, and the tube is retracted with the atraumatic forceps. A second and, if necessary, a third Endoloop are placed, each successively closer to the pelvic wall so that the mesovarian pedicle will be long. The mesovarium is transected with scissors. The pedicle is evaluated to confirm that the sutures have been placed beyond any ovarian tissue to avoid ovarian remnant syndrome (Figure 11-13).

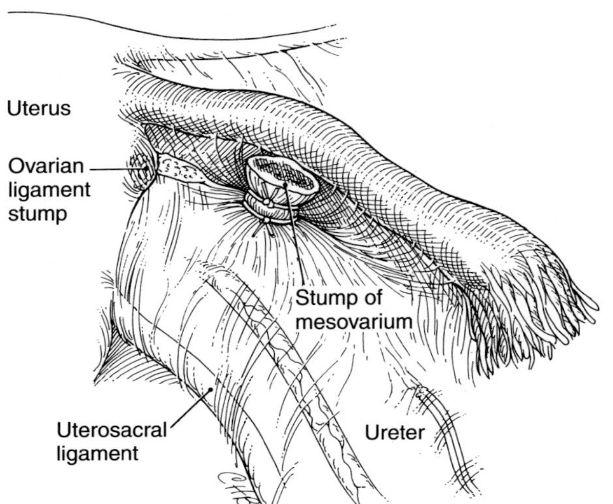

Figure 11-13. The right ovary is removed. An adequate stump should be left to prevent slippage of the ligature.

For salpingo-oophorectomy, an Endoloop is placed over the adnexa after the ovarian ligament and tubal isthmus have been electrocoagulated and cut. The ovary and tube are grasped with forceps and pulled contralaterally. Simultaneously, the atraumatic forceps are used to push the Endoloop laterally, ensuring that the ligature is placed as far lateral as possible on the infundibulopelvic ligament. One or two additional sutures are placed progressively closer to the pelvic wall (at least 1 cm below the infundibulopelvic ligament) so that the pedicle will be long enough to prevent the sutures from slipping (Figure 11-14). The adnexal pedicle is transected with scissors. The ureter is evaluated at the pelvic brim to confirm that it is not damaged (Figure 11-15).

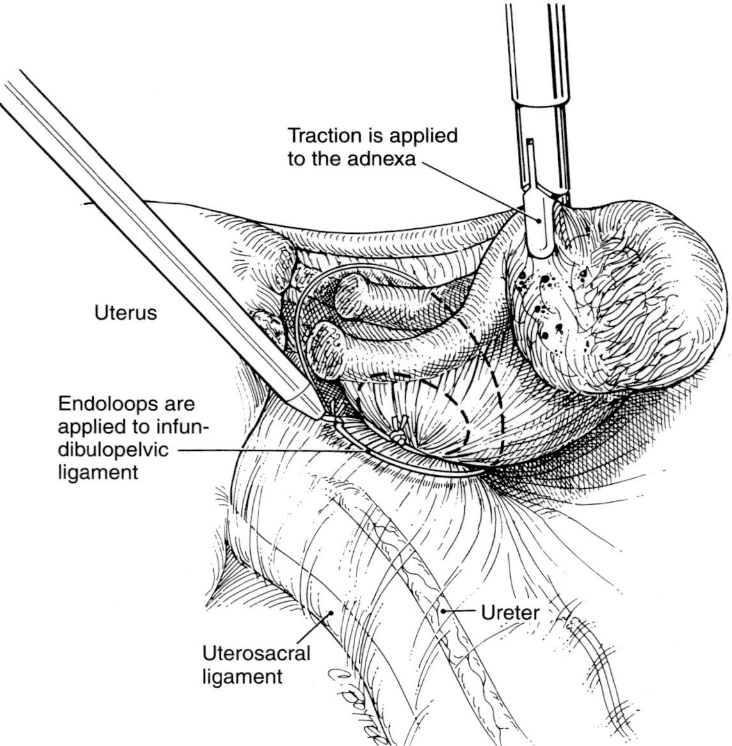

Figure 11-14. A right salpingo-oophorectomy is done using a pretied Endoligature. After the ovarian ligament and tubouterine junction are coagulated and cut, the Endoloop is passed over the tube, ovary, and infundibulopelvic ligament and tied. One to two additional sutures may be necessary.

Dysgenetic Gonads

Individuals with androgen insensitivity syndrome have a high risk (20 to 30%) of developing malignancy in their gonads.[14] Phenotypic females with the XY karyotype require gonadectomy to protect them from developing gonadoblastoma. These gonads present as streaks, and the boundaries between the gonadal tissue and the peritoneum are not always clear. Since there is a chance that some of the dysgenetic gonadal tissue will be missed, the peritoneal borders must be kept

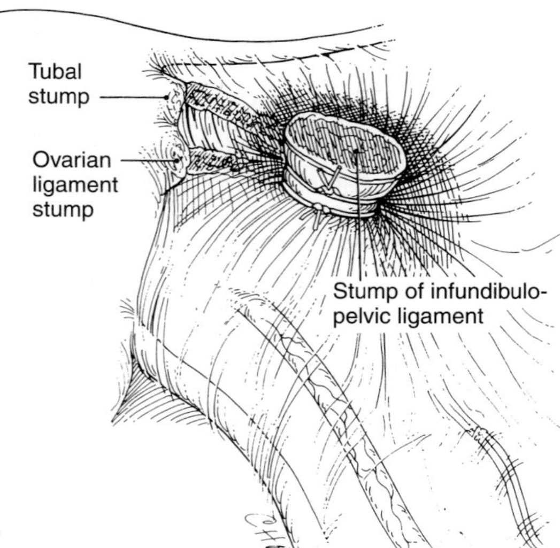

Figure 11-15. A view of the pelvic side wall after removal of the right adnexa.

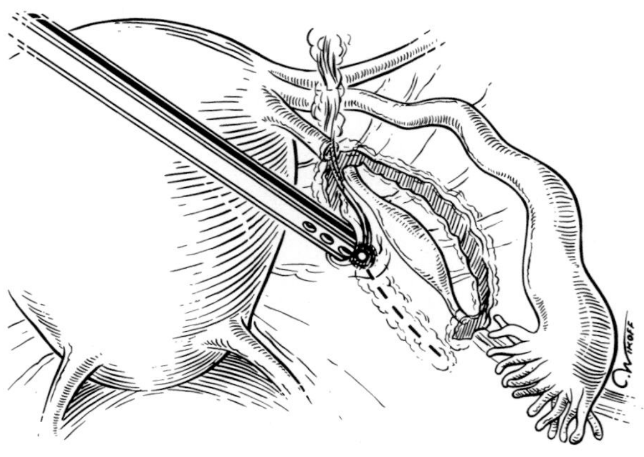

Figure 11-16. Excision of a streak ovary or dysgenetic gonad. The utero-ovarian and infundibulopelvic ligaments are electrocoagulated and cut. The mesovarium is incised with a CO_2 laser to free the tissue.

wide. The laparoscopic approach for gonadectomy has been used in patients with male pseudohermaphroditism, including patients with pure gonadal dysgenesis, testicular feminization, and mixed gonadal dysgenesis and dysgenetic male pseudohermaphroditism.[14–16]

The laparoscopic procedure for removing a dysgenetic gonad is similar to that for removing an ovary that is densely adherent to the pelvic side wall.[17,18] Both the utero-ovarian and infundibulopelvic ligaments are electrocoagulated and cut. The mesovarium above and below is incised with scissors or the CO_2 laser with hydrodissection (Figure 11-16). The loose areolar tissue immediately below the gonad is dissected away from the gonad.

Adherent Adnexa

Adhesions between the ovary and pelvic side wall, broad ligament, and bowel are lysed with the CO_2 laser or scissors until the ovary is freed. The ovary is grasped with a toothed forceps and elevated. It is put on stretch to create a plane between the ovary and the peritoneum. To avoid injury to ureters, blood vessels, and other underlying structures, the retroperitoneal area is entered and hydrodissection is carried out.[19] Using the suction-irrigator probe as a backstop, the adhesions are lysed close to the ovary. Removal of ovarian tissue may require excision of the peritoneum attached to the ovary.

The ovary may be enlarged, may be adherent to the pelvic side wall and broad ligament, or may contain endometriomas so that the surgeon may need to enter the retroperitoneal space (Figure 11-17). In this case, the ovary is removed by retroperitoneal dissection. After hydrodissection is done, an incision is made between the round and infundibulopelvic ligaments medial to the pelvic side wall (Figure 11-18). Blunt dissection, hydrodissection, and sharp dissection with the CO_2 laser are used to lyse adhesions and separate the adnexa and peri-

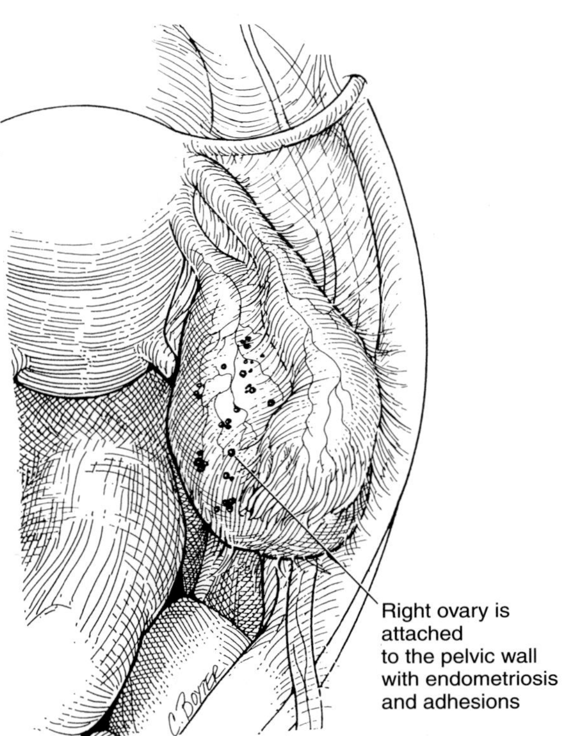

Figure 11-17. A large right endometrioma is attached to the pelvic side wall and ureter with fibrosis and adhesions.

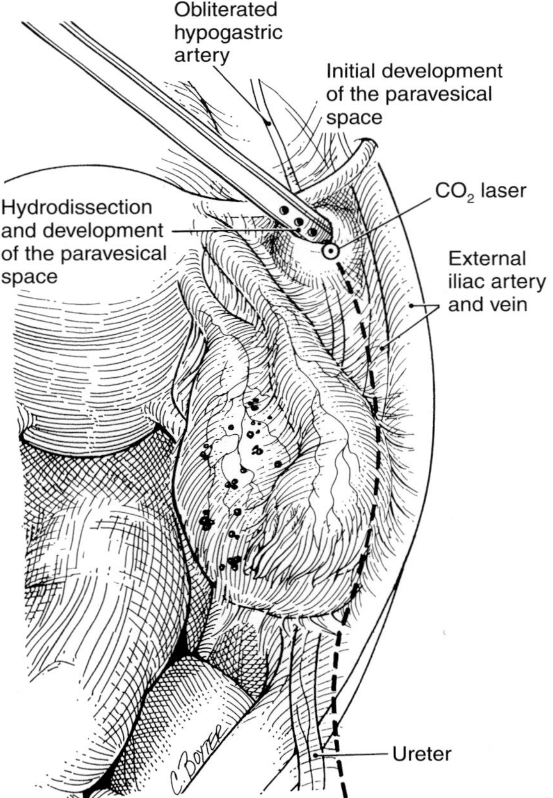

Figure 11-18. An incision is made with the CO_2 laser between the round ligament and the infundibulopelvic ligament to achieve an oophorectomy by retroperitoneal dissection. Hydrodissection and the suction-irrigator probe are used as a backstop for the laser.

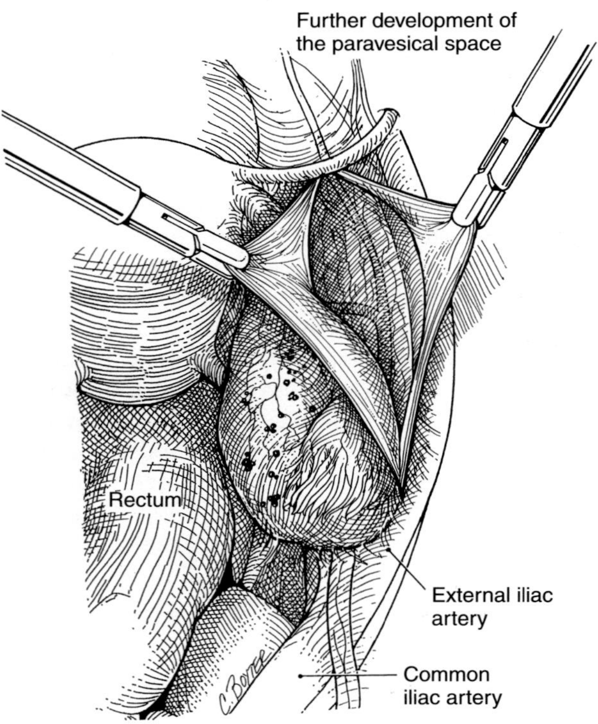

Figure 11-19. The peritoneum attached to the ovary is dissected medially from the retroperitoneal ureter and major pelvic side wall vessels.

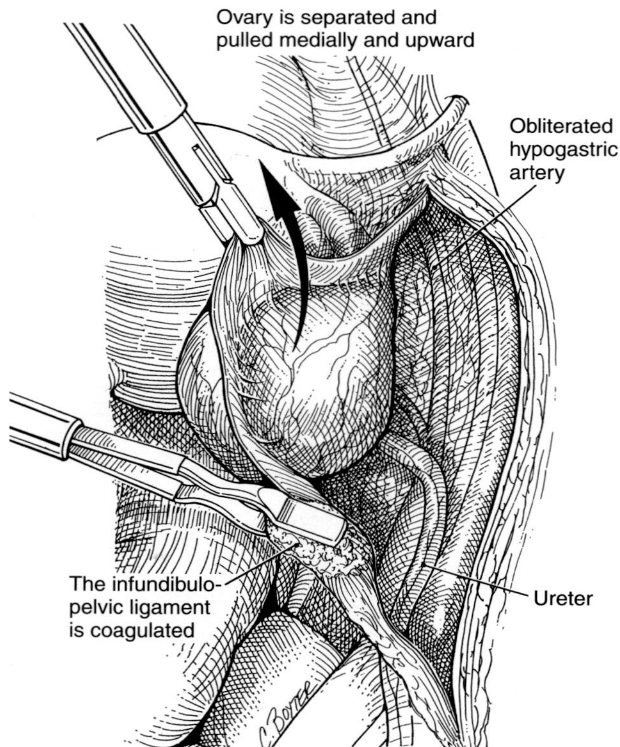

Figure 11-20. The adnexa are under traction, and the infundibulopelvic ligament is coagulated.

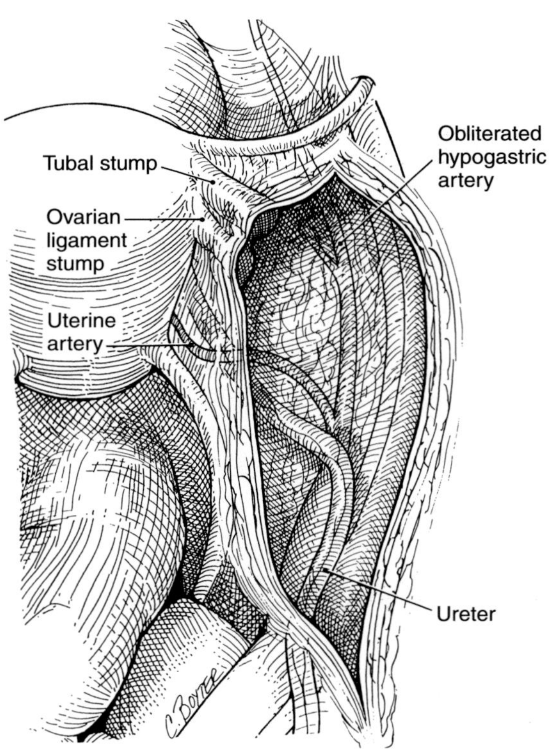

Figure 11-21. The pelvic side wall is observed after the right adnexa is removed with retroperitoneal dissection. The ureter and major retroperitoneal vessels can be seen.

toneum, ureter, and blood vessels (Figure 11-19). Hemostasis is achieved with bipolar forceps. After dissection of the pelvic side wall, the remaining infundibulopelvic ligament, the ovarian ligament, and the proximal portion of the tube are coagulated and cut (Figure 11-20). The ureter is dissected from the ovary, and the adnexa are removed (Figure 11-21).

Residual Ovary

In patients who have had a previous hysterectomy, many of the usual landmarks in the pelvis are absent and extensive adhesions may involve the left ovary and descending colon. Lysis of adhesions is carried out cautiously to avoid damaging the bowel. If the ureter cannot be identified, it is necessary to open the retroperitoneal space. A sponge stick placed in the vagina aids in orientation.

The ovary often is adherent to the vaginal cuff and is dissected from its attachment with scissors or the laser. The ureter is proximal to the lateral margins of the vaginal cuff, and its position can be altered from a previous operation. No ovarian fragments should remain on the pelvic side wall or vaginal cuff.

The ovary is immobilized with a grasping forceps and put on stretch, and the infundibulopelvic ligament is coagulated and transected in 1- to 2-cm increments until the ovary is removed. Depending on the pelvic anatomy, it is preferable to begin the oophorectomy from the infundibulopelvic ligament to improve the anatomic relationships.

The ovary is removed through an abdominal incision as was described above. If the ovary is large, it is cut into pieces. Colpotomy is done if the ovary is >5 cm. However, colpotomy remote from a hysterectomy is technically difficult and is associated with significant risks if the bladder and rectosigmoid colon are adherent to the vaginal cuff.

Removal of Tissue

Removal of the ovary can be difficult if it is more than 5 cm in diameter. It can be removed through a 10-mm trocar sleeve placed in a suprapubic puncture, pulling the sleeve and forceps together and bringing the tissue to the incision. A Kelly or Kocher clamp is used to grasp the tissue to remove it from the abdomen. Alternatively, a long clamp is inserted through the accessory trocar incision and the tissue is grasped under direct observation and pulled from the abdomen through the trocar incision. The tube and ovary can be divided with scissors, a morcellator, or a laser and removed through trocar sleeves if fragmentation is not contraindicated by the characteristics of the cyst. If an open laparoscopy is required, the ovary is removed through an enlarged umbilical incision or through the umbilical incision. After the ovary is removed, the pelvic cavity is irrigated and the pelvis is examined to assure hemostasis. For endometriomas and other cysts >5 cm, the tissue is removed by posterior colpotomy. The cul-de-sac is identified by placing a sponge stick in the vagina and applying pressure to the posterior fornix between the uterosacral ligaments. An incision is made between the uterosacral ligaments with a laser or unipolar knife electrode. Once the incision extends to the sponge stick, the ovary is brought to the incision and grasped vaginally with an Allis clamp. If a cyst is present, it is deflated with a large-bore needle or trocar while traction is applied to the ovary. As the ovary collapses, it is pulled into the vagina intact with minimal spillage of its contents. The colpotomy is closed vaginally or laparoscopically, using two to three sutures. Removal of the ovary and vaginal closure of the colpotomy are facilitated by placing the patient's legs in the position for a vaginal hysterectomy.

If it is necessary to avoid spillage of the cyst contents, the ovary is removed in a specially designed laparoscopic bag (Endopouch, Ethicon).[20] The bag is removed through a posterior colpotomy incision[21] or an extended suprapubic incision. When the ovary is large and cystic, the bag is brought to the suprapubic or posterior colpotomy, the cyst is drained, and the deflated contained cyst is pulled from the abdominal cavity.

Ovarian Wedge Resection

Stein and Leventhal[22] described enlarged polycystic ovaries with the clinical features of menstrual aberrations, obesity, and hyperandrogenism. Although polycystic ovarian disease (PCOD) has variable manifestations, its hallmark is chronic anovulation. It was believed that the enlarged ovaries cause the condition, and so ovarian wedge resection was advocated. As ovulation induction agents were unavailable, ovarian wedge resection represented a major breakthrough, with ovulation and pregnancy rates of 80% and 50%, respectively. However, many patients who were initially ovulatory reverted to the previous anovulatory state after several months.[23] Although most had appar-

TABLE 11-1. Results or Bilateral Ovarian Wedge Resection by Laparotomy

Authors	No. Patients	Medical Failure	Percent Ovulation	Percent Conception
Adashi et al[33]	90	Yes/no	64	48
Goldzieher and Green[56]	219	Yes/no	85	67
Buttram and Vaquero[57]	173	No	62	43
Lunde[58]	92	Yes	80	58
Hjortrup et al[59]	29	No	86	77
Ronnberg et al[60]	23	Yes	61	22

TABLE 11-2. Frequency of Adhesions after Wedge Resection by Laparotomy

Authors	No. Patients	Percent with Adhesions
Adashi et al[33]	7	100
Buttram and Vaquero[57]	40	100
Stein[61]	6	67
Weinstein and Polishuk[62]	19	42
Toaff et al[63]	7	100
Portuondo et al[64]	12	92
Total	91	85

ently normal ovulatory cycles, only 50% conceived (Table 11-1) because postoperative adhesions developed in many of these women (Table 11-2). The availability of ovulation-inducing medications in the 1960s and 1970s [clomiphene citrate (CC) and human menopausal gonadotropins (hMGs)] offered a nonsurgical approach to the treatment of anovulatory infertility that was safer than ovarian wedge resection. As a result, ovarian wedge resection was carried out rarely. CC therapy does not induce ovulation in all women. The alternative, hMG, is expensive, requires intensive monitoring, and can cause ovarian hyperstimulation. For clomiphene-resistant patients, laparoscopic techniques have many advantages over gonadotropin therapy, including serial repetitive ovulation events, no increased risk of ovarian hyperstimulation or multiple pregnancies, and a lower incidence of spontaneous abortion. These procedures are not the first-line treatment for anovulatory patients with polycystic ovarian syndrome (PCOS), for whom clomiphene citrate remains the primary therapy.[24]

Some endoscopists have accomplished ovarian wedge resections laparoscopically,[25] while others have reduced ovarian volume by taking multiple biopsies,[23,26] coagulating with monopolar current,[27–29] creating craters on the ovarian surface with lasers,[30,31] or puncturing the small cysts on the ovarian surface.[32] Broadly similar results have been obtained using biopsy, multielectrocoagulation, and laser surgery: >50% ovulation and a mean pregnancy rate of 50%.[24] Laparoscopic ovarian drilling appears to be associated with comparable rates of ovulation and conception (Table 11-3). Regardless of the method used to decrease ovarian mass, the hormonal changes observed with the laparoscopic procedures are similar to those observed after ovarian wedge resection by laparotomy.[24,34] Laparoscopic techniques offer cost savings and a lower risk of postoperative adhesions compared with wedge resection by laparotomy.[24] A disappointing finding is that the risk of postoperative adhesions is high (average, 30%) in women undergoing ovarian drilling (Table 11-4). While adhesions were less common after laparoscopic multiple biopsies, they were observed in about 90% of patients after resection by laparotomy, 30% after laparoscopic electrocoagulation, and 50% after laparoscopic laser vaporization.[34] The possible effect of applying an oxidized regenerated cellulose (Interceed) barrier on postoperative surfaces after laparoscopic electrosurgical treatment for polycystic ovarian syndrome was studied in a prospective, randomized controlled study.[35] After bilateral ovarian treatment, one ovary was chosen randomly to

TABLE 11-3. Results of Wedge Resection/Ovarian Drilling at Laparoscopy

Authors	No. Patients	Percent Ovulation	Percent Conception
Gjonnaess[23]	62	92	69
Kojima[25]	12	83	58
Campo et al[26]	12	45	41
Aakvag[27]	58	72	N/A
Kovacs et al[29]	10	70	30
Keckstein et al[30]	19	72	44
Daniell and Miller[31]	85	71	56
Greenblatt and Casper[65]	6	82	50
Armar et al[66]	21	81	50
Gjonnaess[67]	252	92	84
Campo et al[68]	23	56	56
Armar and Lachelin[69]	50	86	66
Gurgan et al[70]	40	70	50
Naether et al[71]	206	81	70

TABLE 11-4. Frequency for Postoperative Adhesions after Laparoscopic Ovarian Drilling

Authors	No. Patients	Percent with Adhesions
Portuondo et al[64]	24	0
Greenblatt and Casper[65]	6	100
Gurgan et al[72]	17	82
Dabirashrafi et al[73]	43	16
Naether and Fischer[74]	62	19
Naether et al[75]	26	27
Keckstein et al[76]	11	27

have Interceed applied to its surface, using a specially designed applicator, with the other ovary serving as a control. Periadnexal adhesions of significant extent and severity developed in 57% of the women and 38% of the adnexa. The incidence of adhesions on the Interceed-treated side was 43%, while on the control side it was 33%. In addition, the extent and severity of the adhesions appeared to be similar on the Interceed-treated and control sides. Larger numbers are required to ascertain statistically the effects of Interceed on prevention of adhesions after laparoscopic electrosurgical treatment of PCOS.

Theoretically, wedge resection and ovarian drilling work by reducing androgen production in the ovarian stroma. Appropriate patients are women who fail to ovulate after 3 to 4 months on clomiphene and do not respond to hMG. The procedure is achieved by using a 10-mm videolaparoscope coupled to a CO_2 laser. A 5-mm second puncture is placed suprapubically in the midline and is used for a suction-irrigator or grasping instrument. Associated pelvic abnormalities are corrected before ovarian coagulation. Each ovary is fixed in the anterior cul-de-sac or held by the utero-ovarian ligament during treatment. The ultrapulse (40 to 80 W, 25 to 200 mJ) or superpulse (25 to 40 W) CO_2 laser is used. All visible subcapsular follicles are vaporized and drained, and randomly placed 2- to 4-mm-diameter craters are made in the ovarian stroma (Figure 11-22). Each ovary is treated symmetrically, and cysts are vaporized. The ovaries are irrigated, and hemostasis is obtained with bipolar forceps.

A potassium titanyl phosphate, neodymium-yttrium aluminum garnet, or argon laser can be used also.[30,31] The fiber is threaded through the central channel of a special 5-mm dual-channel suction-irrigation probe. When the dual-channel probe is used, it is possible to suction the smoke from vaporization at the site of occurrence. Holes are drilled in the ovary in a manner similar to that described for the CO_2 laser.

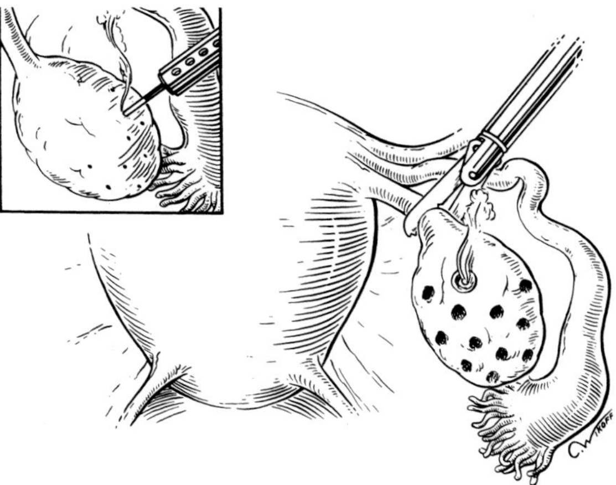

Figure 11-22. Ovarian drilling is used for PCOD. While the ovarian ligament is grasped and the ovary is held, multiple surface craters are created by the CO_2 laser, fiber laser, or needle electrode (inset).

Ovarian coagulation has been done using unipolar punch biopsy forceps[23] or a needle electrode.[26–28] The power setting for the monopolar current is 20 to 30 W in a cutting mode to minimize thermal damage, and the power is activated just before the ovary is touched. The ovary is penetrated in approximately 10 to 15 sites at a depth of 3 to 5 mm.

Ovarian Torsion

Adnexal torsion is a surgical emergency. When this is diagnosed early, the adnexa can be unwound.[36,37] However, the diagnosis often is delayed because of the inconsistent presenting symptoms and signs and intermittent pain. When the diagnosis is delayed, the adnexa become congested, ischemic, hemorrhagic, and necrotic.[38] Gynecologists have been taught to remove tissue that has undergone torsion and ischemia because of the risk of thrombotic embolism arising from the ovarian vein. Way[39] reported successful conservative management of adnexal torsion. The affected structure was straightened to assess the viability, and even ovaries that appeared infarcted at laparotomy regained normal color after untwisting. No complications related to the procedure were reported. Since adnexal torsion produces no pathognomonic clinical findings, laparoscopy is used for diagnosis and treatment. Prompt laparoscopic examination is essential, since delay is associated with gangrene.

A prospective, controlled follow-up study was designed to examine the effects of adnexal torsion on long-term ovarian histology and free radical scavenger (FRS) activity and subsequent viability after the detorsion of twisted ischemic adnexa. Adnexal torsion was created by twisting the adnexa three times and fixing on to the side wall or by applying vascular clips in cycling female rats at 70 days of age. After an ischemic period of 4 to 36 hours, the twisted adnexa were removed and fixed. In the second group of rats, after the above ischemic periods, the torsions were relieved by untwisting or removing the vascular clips. Then the animals were perfused for a week, and adnexa were extirpated. After both ischemia and reperfusion, the removed adnexa were examined histologically and tissue concentrations of glutathione peroxidase, superoxide dismutase, catalase, and glutathione were ascertained. Regardless of the ischemic time, all the twisted adnexa were black-bluish. Despite the gross ischemic-hemorrhagic features, histologic sections revealed negligible changes, with intact ovarian structure similar to that of controls in 4- to 24-hour groups. Although decreased compared with controls, the change in tissue concentrations of FRS was not significant in the 4- to 24-hour groups. Only the 36-hour group showed prominent congestion on all sections and a significant decrease in all FRS concentrations studied. While no long-term reperfusion injury was observed histologically in the 4- to 24-hour groups, the 36-hour group ended with adnexal necrosis. These findings support the importance of early diagnosis and conservative surgical management (detorsion) in adnexal torsion. Lack of histologic changes and unimpaired FRS metabolism are consistent with recent data showing that vascular compromise is caused by venous or lymphatic stasis in early torsion; adnexal integrity is not correlated with gross ischemic appearance, thus providing evidence of adnexal resistance against ischemia.[40]

The causes of ovarian or adnexal torsion are para-ovarian cysts, functional and pathologic ovarian cysts, ovarian hyperstimulation, tubal pregnancy, adhesions, and congenital malformation.[41,42] The ischemic structures are straightened gently with atraumatic forceps to avoid additional adnexal damage. In women with ovarian hyperstimulation, the functional cysts are drained before untwisting.[43] The abnormalities contributing

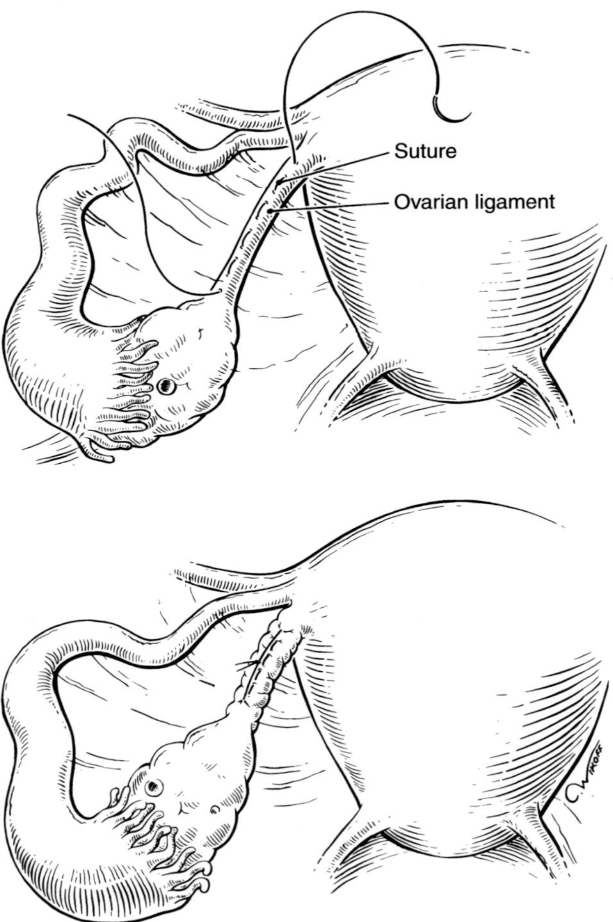

Figure 11-23. Ovarian suspension is achieved with a monofilament suture placed along the length of the utero-ovarian ligament and tied.

to torsion should be treated. One should shorten the utero-ovarian ligament if its length may have contributed to ovarian torsion. A running suture of monofilament material is placed along the length of the utero-ovarian ligament (Figure 11-23) and tied to shorten it, limiting ovarian mobility.

Mage and associates,[41] in a report of 35 patients, noted that 21 women showed no gross evidence of ischemia or mild changes, with immediate and complete recovery within 10 minutes of untwisting. In eight, the tube or ovary was dark red or black, but partial recovery was apparent after the pedicle was untwisted. Six had gangrenous adnexa that required salpingectomy or oophorectomy. The first two groups were managed conservatively; the third group underwent excision of the involved organ(s). The postoperative course in all patients was uneventful. Six of the eight women in the intermediate group underwent a second-look laparoscopy that showed complete recovery.

Ovarian Remnant Syndrome

In premenopausal women who have had a bilateral oophorectomy, a small piece of functional ovarian tissue can respond to hormonal stimulation with growth, cystic degeneration, or hemorrhage and produce pain.[44–46] In a rat model, Minke and colleagues[47] showed that devascularized ovarian tissue can reimplant on intact or denuded peritoneal surfaces and that the revascularized tissue can become functional as evidenced by follicle formation and vaginal cornification.

Ovarian remnants remain because of dense adhesions, and distorted anatomic relationships invariably worsen with subsequent operations. It is not unusual for these patients to have had previous attempts to excise an ovarian remnant. Removal of the ovarian remnant is preferred, although the reported incidence of complications with laparotomy ranges from 16 to 30%.[48] The challenge and complications are related to the presence of extensive pelvic and abdominal adhesions from multiple previous operations, endometriosis, pelvic inflammatory disease, or ovarian cysts.

Diagnosis is based on history and localization of pelvic pain. While some patients have cystic adnexal structures or ill-defined fixed masses, others have normal pelvic findings. Vaginal ultrasound can help locate the ovarian remnant.[49] Low or borderline levels of follicle-stimulating hormone in patients with documented bilateral oophorectomy are consistent with the presence of active ovarian tissue.[44] Hormonal suppression with oral contraceptives or a gonadotropin-releasing hormone agonist provides no relief in most patients.[10,50] CC or hMG is used to increase ovarian remnant size to confirm the diagnosis preoperatively or to aid in locating the tissue intraoperatively.[51] Laparoscopic ultrasonography is used to detect ovarian remnants in patients in whom the pelvic anatomy is distorted by multiple adhesions.[52]

Past reviews have considered laparoscopy ineffective in the management of ovarian remnant syndrome because of the presence of dense pelvic adhesions.[48] However, the absence of complications in a series of 22 patients attests to the feasibility of the laparoscopic approach.[10]

Attention should be focused on prevention. Factors associated with ovarian remnant syndrome are the use of Endoloops for laparoscopic oophorectomy, multiple operative procedures with incomplete removal of pelvic organs, densely adherent ovaries, and multiple ovarian cystectomies for functional cysts.[10] When pretied sutures are used for the infundibulopelvic ligament, they should be placed below the ovarian tissue. Electrocoagulation and transection of the infundibulopelvic ligament or the application of clips is preferred. When the ovary is adherent to the pelvic side wall, retroperitoneal hydrodissection, meticulous adhesiolysis, and removal of the peritoneum underlying the ovary are essential in achieving a laparoscopic oophorectomy (Figure 11-20). The need for restraint in managing functional cysts is underscored by the fact that some patients in the author's[10] series had only a corpus luteum resected at first laparotomy.

A preoperative bowel preparation of Go-LYTELY, enemas, and oral metronidazole are indicated. Anterior abdominal wall adhesions are probable after multiple laparotomies, and an open laparoscopy or mapping technique[53] is advisable. After all instruments are inserted, intraabdominal adhesions are lysed and the ovarian remnants are dissected. Extensive and careful retroperitoneal dissection is required to facilitate identification and removal of the ovarian remnant tissue.[54,55] The anatomy of the retroperitoneal space is identified when the ovarian remnant is adherent to the lateral pelvic wall. The space beneath the peritoneum is injected with lactated Ringer's solution, and the peritoneum is opened to the infundibulopelvic ligament or its remnant. Adhesions are lysed until the course of the major pelvic blood vessels and the ureter can be traced and, if necessary, dissected. The ovarian blood supply is coagulated with bipolar forceps, and the ovarian tissue is excised and submitted for histologic examination.

When the remnant is adherent to the bowel, adhesions are lysed, using hydrodissection and the CO_2 laser. Ovarian tissue embedded in the muscularis of the bowel is removed superficially, skinning the mucosa beneath it. The serosa and muscularis layers are imbricated with one to three interrupted 4-0 polydioxanone sutures in one layer. All remnant ovarian tissue should be removed. When the lesion is embedded in the bowel or bladder muscularis or when the ureter is involved or possibly obstructed, partial removal of the organ and repair are necessary.

References

1. Yuzpe AA, Rioux JE. The value of laparoscopic ovarian biopsy. *J Reprod Med* 1975; 15:57.
2. Nezhat C, Nezhat F. Postoperative adhesion formation after ovarian cystectomy with and without ovarian reconstruction. American Fertility Society Annual Meeting, Orlando, FL, October 21, 1991. (Abstract)
3. Semm K, Course of endoscopic abdominal surgery, in Friedrich E, ed., *Operative Manual for Endoscopic Abdominal Surgery*. Chicago: Year Book, 1984.
4. Nezhat F, Nezhat C, Silfen SL. Videolaseroscopy for oophorectomy. *Am J Obstet Gynecol* 1991; 165:1323.
5. Silva PD, Juffel ME, Beguin EA. Open laparoscopy simplifies instrumentation required for laparoscopic oophorectomy and salpingo-oophorectomy. *Obstet Gynecol* 1991; 77:482.
6. Russell JB. Laparoscopic oophorectomy. *Curr Opin Obstet Gynecol* 1995; 7:295.
7. Nezhat C, Nezhat F, Silfen SL. Laparoscopic hysterectomy and bilateral salpingo-oophorectomy using multifire GIA surgical stapler. *J Gynecol Surg* 1990; 6:287.
8. Daniell JF, Jurtz BR, Lee JY. Laparoscopic oophorectomy: Comparative study of ligatures, bipolar coagulation and automatic stapling devices. *Obstet Gynecol* 1992; 80:325.
9. Nezhat C, Nezhat F, Winer W. Salpingectomy via laparoscopy: A new surgical approach. *J Laparosc Surg* 1991; 1:91.
10. Nezhat C, Nezhat F. Operative laparoscopy for the management of ovarian remnant syndrome. *Fertil Steril* 1992; 57:1003.
11. Sigel B, Dunn MR. The mechanism of blood vessel closure by high frequency electrocoagulation. *Surg Gynecol Obstet* 1965; 121(4):823.
12. Nezhat C, Nezhat F. Laparoscopic electrosurgical oophorectomy: Risk of using "blanching" as the end point [letter to the editor]. *Am J Obstet Gynecol* 1992; 167:1151.
13. Semm K. *Operative Manual for Endoscopic Abdominal Surgery*. Chicago: Year Book, 1984.
14. Campo S, Garcia N. Laparoscopic gonadectomy in two patients with gonadal dysgenesis. *J Am Assoc Gynecol Laparosc* 1998; 5:305.
15. Kriplani A, Abbi M, Ammini AC, et al. Laparoscopic gonadectomy in male pseudohermaphrodites. *Eur J Obstet Gynecol Reprod Biol* 1998; 81:37.
16. Ulrich U, Keckstein J, Buck G. Removal of gonads in Y-chromosome-bearing gonadal dysgenesis and in androgen insensitivity syndrome by laparoscopic surgery. *Surg Endosc* 1996; 10:422.
17. Droesch K, Dorexch J, Chumas J, et al. Laparoscopic gonadectomy for gonadal dysgenesis. *Fertil Steril* 1990; 53:360.
18. Seifer DB. Laparoscopic adnexectomy in a prepubertal Turner mosaic female with isodicentric Y. *Human Reprod* 1991; 6:566.
19. Nezhat C, Nezhat F. Safe laser excision or vaporization of peritoneal endometriosis. *Fertil Steril* 1989; 52:1:149.
20. Nezhat C, Nezhat F, Welander CE, et al. Four ovarian cancers diagnosed during laparoscopic management of 1,011 adnexal masses. *Am J Obstet Gynecol* 1992; 167:790.
21. Nezhat F, Brill AI, Nezhat CH, et al. Adhesion formation after endoscopic posterior colpotomy. *J Reprod Med* 1993; 38:534.
22. Stein IF, Leventhal ML. Amenorrhea associated with bilateral polycystic ovaries. *Am J Obstet Gynecol* 1935; 29:181.
23. Gjonnaess H. Polycystic ovarian syndrome treated by ovarian electrocautery through the laparoscope. *Fertil Steril* 1984; 41:20.
24. Judd HL, Rigg LA, Anderson DC, et al. The effects of ovarian wedge resection on circulating gonadotropin and ovarian steroid levels in patients with polycystic ovarian syndrome. *J Clin Endocrinol* Metab 1976; 43:347.
25. Kojima E. Ovarian wedge resection with contact Nd:YAG laser irradiation used laparoscopically. *J Reprod Med* 1989; 34:444.
26. Campo S, Garcia N, Caruso A, et al: Effect of celioscopy ovarian resection in patients with polycystic ovaries. *Gynecol Obstet Invest* 1983; 15:213.
27. Aakvaag A. Hormonal response to electrocautery of the ovary in patients with polycystic ovarian disease. *Br J Obstet Gynaecol* 1985; 92:1258.
28. Casper RF, Greenblatt EM. Laparoscopic ovarian cautery for induction of ovulation in women with polycystic ovary disease. *Semin Reprod Endocrinol* 1990; 8:209.
29. Kovacs G, Buckler H, Bangah M, et al. Treatment of anovulation due to polycystic ovarian syndrome by laparoscopic ovarian electrocautery. *Br J Obstet Gynaecol* 1991; 98:30.
30. Keckstein G, Rossmanith W, Spatzier K, et al. The effect of laparoscopic treatment of poly-

cystic ovarian disease by CO_2 laser or ND-YAG laser. *Surg Endosc* 1990; 4:103.
31. Daniell JF, Miller W. Polycystic ovaries treated by laparoscopic laser vaporization. *Fertil Steril* 1989; 51(2):232.
32. Sumioki H, Utsunomyiya T, Matsuoka K, et al. The effect of laparoscopic multiple punch resection of the ovary on the hypothalamo-pituitary axis in polycystic ovary syndrome. *Fertil Steril* 1988; 50:567.
33. Adashi EY, Rock JA, Guzick D, et al. Fertility following bilateral ovarian wedge resection: a critical analysis of 90 consective cases of the polycystic ovary syndrome. *Fertil Steril* 1981; 36:320.
34. Campo S. Ovulatory cycles, pregnancy outcome and complications after surgical treatment of polycystic ovary syndrome. *Obstet Gynecol Surv* 1998; 53:297.
35. Saravelos H, Li TC. Post-operative adhesions after laparoscopic electrosurgical treatment for polycystic ovarian syndrome with the application of Interceed to one ovary: A prospective randomized controlled study. *Hum Reprod* 1996; 11:992.
36. Oelsner G, Bider D, Goldenberg M, et al. Long-term follow-up of the twisted ischemic adnexa managed by detorsion. *Fertil Steril* 1993; 60:976.
37. Shalev E, Bustan M, Yarom I, Peleg D. Recovery of ovarian function after laparoscopic detorsion. *Hum Reprod* 1995; 10:2965.
38. Steyaert H, Meynol F, Valla JS. Torsion of the adnexa in children: The value of laparoscopy. *Pediatr Surg Int* 1998; 13:384.
39. Way S. Ovarian cystectomy of twisted cysts. *Lancet* 1946; 2:47.
40. Taskin O, Birincioglu M, Aydin A, et al. The effects of twisted ischaemic adnexa managed by detorsion on ovarian viability and histology: An ischaemia-reperfusion rodent model. *Hum Reprod* 1998; 13:2823.
41. Mage G, Canis M, Manhes H, et al. Laparoscopic management of adnexal torsion. *J Reprod Med* 1989; 34:520.
42. Wagaman R, Williams RS. Conservative therapy for adnexal torsion. *J Reprod Med* 1990; 35:833.
43. Ben-Rafael Z, Bider D, Mashiach S. Laparoscopic unwinding of twisted ischemic hemorrhagic adnexum after in vitro fertilization. *Fertil Steril* 1990; 53:569.
44. Petit PD, Lee RA. Ovarian remnant syndrome: Diagnostic dilemma and surgical challenge. *Obstet Gynecol* 1988; 71:580.
45. Siddall-Allum J, Rae T, Rogers V, et al. Chronic pelvic pain caused by residual ovaries and ovarian remnants. *Br J Obstet Gynaecol* 1994; 101:979.
46. Orford VP, Kuhn RJ. Management of ovarian remnant syndrome. *Aust N Z J Obstet Gynaecol* 1996; 36:468.
47. Minke T, DePond W, Winkelmann T, Blythe J. Ovarian remnant syndrome: Study in laboratory rats. *Am J Obstet Gynecol* 1994; 171:1440.
48. Price FV, Edwards R, Buschsbaum HJ. Ovarian remnant syndrome: Difficulties in diagnosis and management. *Obstet Gynecol Surv* 1990; 45:151.
49. Fleischer AC, Tait D, Mayo J, et al. Sonographic features of ovarian remnants. *J Ultrasound Med* 1998; 17:551.
50. Siddall-Allum J, Rae T, Rogers V, et al. Chronic pelvic pain caused by residual ovaries and ovarian remnants. *Br J Obstet Gynaecol* 1994; 101:979.
51. Kaminski PF, Sorosky JI, Mandell MJ, et al. Clomiphene citrate stimulation as an adjunct in locating ovarian tissue in ovarian remnant syndrome. *Obstet Gynecol* 1990; 76:924.
52. Nezhat F, Nezhat C, Nezhat CH, et al. Use of laparoscopic ultrasonography to detect ovarian remnants. *Am J Obstet Gynecol* 1996; 174:641.
53. Nezhat C, Nezhat F, Silfen SL. Videolaseroscopy: The CO_2 laser for advanced operative laparoscopy. *Obstet Gynecol Clin North Am* 1991; 18:3:585.
54. Lafferty HW, Angioli R, Rudolph J, Penalver MA. Ovarian remnant syndrome: Experience at Jackson Memorial Hospital, University of Miami, 1985 through 1993. *Am J Obstet Gynecol* 1996; 174:641.
55. Kamprath S, Possover M, Schneider A. Description of a laparoscopic technique for treating patients with ovarian remnant syndrome. *Fertil Steril* 1997; 68:663.
56. Goldzeiher JW, Green JA. The polycystic ovary: Clinical and histological features. *J Clin Endocrinol Metab* 1962; 22:325.
57. Buttram VC, Vaquero C. Post-ovarian wedge resection adhesive disease. *Fertil Steril* 1975; 26:874.
58. Lunde O. Polycystic ovarian syndrome: A retrospective study of the therapeutic effect of ovarian wedge resection after unsuccessful treatment with clomiphene citrate. *Ann Chir Gynaecol* 1982; 71:330.
59. Hjortrup A, Kehlet H, Lockwood K, et al. Long term clinical effects of ovarian wedge

resection in polycystic ovarian syndrome. *Acta Obstet Gynecol Scand* 1983; 62:55.

60. Ronnberg L, Ylostalo P, Ruokonen A. Hormonal parameters and conception rate during 5 different types of treatment of polycystic ovarian syndrome. *Int J Gynaecol Obstet* 1985; 23:177.
61. Stein IF. Wedge resection of the ovaries: The Stein Leventhal syndrome, in Greenblatt RB, ed., *Ovulation.* Philadelphia: Lippincott, 1966.
62. Weinstein D, Polishuk WZ. The role of wedge resection of the ovary as a cause for mechanical sterility. *Surg Gynecol Obstet* 1975; 141:417.
63. Toaff R, Toaff ME, Peyser MR. Infertility following wedge resection of the ovaries. *Am J Obstet Gynecol* 1976; 124:92.
64. Portuondo JA, Melchor JC, Neyro JL, et al. Periovarian adhesions following ovarian wedge resection or laparoscopic biopsy. *Endoscopy* 1984; 16:143.
65. Greenblatt R, Casper RF. Endocrine changes after laparoscopic ovarian cautery in polycystic ovary syndrome. *Am J Obstet Gynecol* 1987; 156:279.
66. Armar NA, McGarrigle HHG, Honour J, et al. Laparoscopic ovarian diathermy in the management of ovulatory infertility in women with polycystic ovaries: Endocrine changes and clinical outcome. *Fertil Steril* 1990; 53:45.
67. Gjonnaess H. Ovarian electrocautery in the treatment of women with polycystic ovary syndrome (PCOS): Factors affecting the results. *Acta Obstet Gynecol Scand* 1994; 73:407.
68. Campo S, Felli A, Lamanna MA, et al. Endocrine changes and clinical outcome after laparoscopic ovarian resection in women with polycystic ovaries. *Hum Reprod* 1993; 8:359.
69. Armar NA, Lachelin GC. Laparoscopic ovarian diathermy: An effective treatment for anti-oestrogen resistant anovulatory infertility in women with the polycystic ovary syndrome. *Br J Obstet Gynaecol* 1993; 100:161.
70. Gurgan T, Urman B, Aksu T, et al. The effect of short-interval laparoscopic lysis of adhesions on pregnancy rates following Nd-YAG laser photocoagulation of polycystic ovaries. *Obstet Gynecol* 1992; 80:45.
71. Naether OG, Baukloh V, Fischer R, Kowalczyk T. Long-term follow-up in 206 infertility patients with polycystic ovarian syndrome after laparoscopic electrocautery of the ovarian surface. *Hum Reprod* 1994; 9:2342.
72. Gurgan T, Kisnisci H, Yarali H, et al. Evaluation of adhesion formation after laparoscopic treatment of polycystic ovarian disease. *Fertil Steril* 1991; 56:1176.
73. Dabirashrafi H, Mohamad K, Behjantia Y, et al. Adhesion formation after ovarian electrocauterization on patients with polycystic ovarian syndrome. *Fertil Steril* 1991; 55:1200.
74. Naether OG, Fischer R. Adhesion formation after laparoscopic electrocoagulation of the ovarian surface in polycystic ovary patients. *Fertil Steril* 1993; 60:95.
75. Naether OG, Fischer R, Weise HC, et al. Laparoscopic electrocoagulation of the ovarian surface in infertile patients with polycystic ovarian disease. *Fertil Steril* 1993; 60.
76. Keckstein G, Rossmanith W, Spatzier K, et al. The effect of laparoscopic treatment of polycystic ovarian disease by CO_2-laser or Nd:YAG laser. *Surg Endosc* 1990; 4:103.

12

Laparoscopic Treatment of Endometriosis

Endometriosis is a progressive, often debilitating disease that affects 10 to 15% of women during their reproductive years[1,2] and accounts for 25% of laparotomies carried out by gynecologists. Among gynecologic disorders, endometriosis is surpassed in frequency only by leiomyomas.[3]

Patients who have endometriosis present with different clinical complaints at various stages of the disease. Treatment depends on age of the patient, extent of the disease, severity of the symptoms, and desire for fertility. Intervention usually is indicated for pain, infertility, or impaired function of the bladder, ureter, or intestine. Medical and surgical forms of management are available.

Historical Perspectives

Rokitansky described pelvic endometriosis of the fallopian tubes, ovaries, and uterus in 1860.[4] Before 1960, therapy often required hysterectomy and bilateral salpingo-oophorectomy.[5] Conservative operations to relieve pain and preserve fertility have been modified significantly since the introduction of such therapy. After recognition of the negative impact of surgical trauma and postoperative adhesions on success rates, microsurgical techniques were developed and applied with improved results.[6] Nevertheless, recurrences were not eliminated.[7] Both laparotomy and operative laparoscopy are effective for the treatment of endometriosis in that they reduce the incidence of implants, relieve dysmenorrhea and pelvic pain, and improve fertility potential.[8–12] Unlike radical operations, conservative procedures frequently are not curative.[13,14]

Surgical Approach

The goals of conservative operative procedures are to remove all implants, resect adhesions, relieve pain, reduce the risk of recurrence and postoperative adhesions, and restore the involved organs to a normal anatomic and physiologic condition. For infertile patients, restoration of the normal tubo-ovarian relationship is essential to enhance fertility. These goals may be achieved by using various surgical instruments (scalpel, scissors, lasers, or electrodes) and a variety of techniques (laparoscopy, laparotomy, combined endoscopy and minilaparotomy).

Since 1980, surgical instruments and techniques with varying degrees of efficacy have been introduced, including lasers, video cameras, monitors, electric generators, hydrodissection, microelectrodes, microsurgery, and operative laparoscopy.[15] There are definite advantages to using a high-powered CO_2 laser (especially the Ultrapulse 5000 L) as a long knife through the operative channel of the laparoscope. Because this laser does not penetrate water, it can be used with hydrodissection[16] to selectively treat sensitive areas in the bowel, bladder, ureters, and blood vessels. The recognized advantages of operative laparoscopy include faster patient recovery and reduced cost.[17] In addition, as gynecologists become more proficient, pregnancy rates after operative laparoscopy should improve and surpass the results after laparotomy.

Laparoscopy and Laparotomy

The results of endoscopy and laparotomy are judged by many factors.[18] Three studies compared postoperative adhesion formation and re-formation after a standardized laser injury and laser adhesiolysis by both surgical approaches.[19–21] Laparoscopy caused fewer postoperative adhesions compared with laparotomy. After microsurgical salpingoplasty or adhesiolysis by laparotomy, adhesion recurrence rates were 40 to 72% and new adhesions occurred in more than 50% of patients.[22–26] However, when comparable operations are carried out laparoscopically, recurrence of postoperative adhesions appears to be less common,[27] and new adhesions were either absent or less than 20%.[28] Lundorff and colleagues[25] evaluated the formation of adhesions after laparoscopy and laparotomy in patients treated for tubal pregnancy. Those authors stratified 105 women with tubal pregnancy by age and risk factors and prospectively randomized them to treatment by laparoscopy or laparotomy. Second-look laparoscopy revealed more adhesions in the laparotomy group.[25]

Data from animal[19–21] and clinical studies[22–26] suggest that laparoscopic operations are more effective for adhesiolysis, cause fewer new adhesions than does laparotomy, and reduce impairment of tubo-ovarian function.[25] The efficacy of laparotomy or laparoscopy has not been evaluated for restoring fertility or reducing pelvic pain. However, it has been reported that pain relief and pregnancy rates after operative laparoscopy are comparable to or better than those after laparotomy[7–12,17,18,25,29–32] for endometriosis (mild to severe), hydrosalpinges, and ectopic pregnancy.

Gomel[33] described the therapeutic efficacy of laparoscopic adhesiolysis in 1975. In a follow-up publication, he stated that "in trained hands, laparoscopic salpingo-ovariolysis is a low-risk procedure associated with a surprisingly good success rate." In his series of 92 patients with moderate to severe adnexal adhesive disease, the intrauterine pregnancy rate was 62.5%.[34] Subsequent studies confirmed that the results of laparoscopy were better than those obtained by laparotomy, especially in the case of severe endometriosis.[11,12,18,29–32] Even extensive endometriosis can be treated more effectively at laparoscopy and with better results than at laparotomy.[9,10]

Fayez and Collazo[30] noted pregnancy rates of 58% after laparoscopy and 36% after laparotomy. Chong and colleagues[35] assessed the relative efficacy of CO_2 laser surgery by laparoscopy and laparotomy in treating infertile patients with severe endometriosis; the mean revised American Fertility Society (rAFS) scores were 59 (laparoscopy) and 58 (laparotomy) with similar pregnancy rates. In two studies, CO_2 laser laparoscopy was compared with laparotomy as a treatment for all stages of endometriosis associated with infertility.[11,12] Operative laparoscopy was found to be safe and effective for all stages of endometriosis. Only if the results with laparoscopy are equal to or better than those with laparotomy should the endoscopic approach be considered.[9,16,35] The reduced hospital cost and recovery period obtained with the laparoscopic approach cannot compensate for failure to achieve the optimal treatment.

The outcome of laparoscopy was compared with that of laparotomy in conservative surgical treatment for severe endometriosis.[36] A nonrandomized group of 216 patients underwent conservative surgical treatment for severe endometriosis by either laparoscopy ($n = 67$) or laparotomy ($n = 149$). The results from laparoscopy and laparotomy were equal for the treatment of infertility and chronic pelvic pain associated with severe endometriosis. However, a trend toward a higher pregnancy rate and less dyspareunia was observed after operations done for severe endometriosis by laparotomy compared with laparoscopy.

Laser laparoscopy was compared with traditional laparoscopy or laparotomy in the treatment of 309 infertile women with moderate or severe endometriosis.[37] These patients were treated with one of four options: operative laparoscopy with the CO_2 laser vaporization or resection, operative laparoscopy with electrocoagulation and sharp dissection, laparotomy with electrocoagulation and sharp dissection, and medical treatment with danazol. Pregnancy rates in the laparoscopy group were equal to or higher than those in the laparotomy group for both the entire population and the endometriosis-only subset. When the CO_2 laser was used as an adjuvant option, the rates were better, especially in patients with advanced disease and with endometriosis as the only infertility factor.

Radical Operations

Hysterectomy and bilateral salpingo-oophorectomy are indicated for patients with severe symptoms who have not responded to medical or conservative surgical treatment and are not interested in pregnancy. Fibrosis obliterates tissue planes and sometimes causes a suspicion of malignancy because of extensive involvement of the intestinal and urinary tracts. In advanced disease, the ovaries may be encased and densely adherent to the pelvic side wall. Ovarian dissection entails the risk of injury to the ureter, major blood vessels, and bowel. A retroperitoneal approach can isolate the ureter throughout its course to ensure complete removal of ovarian tissue and prevent ovarian remnant syndrome.[38] Bilateral oophorectomy must be done to eliminate the estrogen that sustains and stimulates the ectopic endometrium.[39] Although conserving one ovary has resulted in reasonable cure rates,[14,40,41] failure rates of 13% and 40% at 3 and 5 years, respectively, have been reported after laparotomy when ovarian function is preserved.[42] Consequently, in patients who do not desire fertility and whose complaints justify definitive treatment, concomitant removal of both ovaries is recommended as the best chance for relief, particularly if endometriosis is severe.

Hormone Replacement

After hysterectomy and bilateral salpingo-oophorectomy, patients often require hormone replacement therapy to relieve menopausal symptoms. Administering the minimal effective dose of estrogen is associated with only a small risk of recurrence.[43–45] In a retrospective study of 85 women with endometriosis, Henderson and coworkers[44] reported a recurrence rate of 1.1% in women receiving estrogen replacement. In contrast, 25% of women with comparable disease and residual ovarian tissue required additional operations.

Hormone replacement therapy should begin postoperatively. Patients with residual disease may benefit from receiving progestin for 3 to 6 months, followed by combined estrogen and progestin for an additional 9 months. A single intramuscular injection of 100 mg medroxyprogesterone acetate (Depo-Provera) administered on the second postoperative day can suppress hot flashes for up to 12 weeks and, with the hypoestrogenemia that follows castration, cause regression of residual implants.[46] Similar effects may be achieved with oral medroxyprogesterone acetate (20 to 30 mg/day) for 3 to 6 months postoperatively.[47] Subsequently, combined estrogen and progestin may be administered for up to 12 months postoperatively.[45,48] These patients are treated with conjugated estrogen (0.625 mg) or estradiol (Estrace) (1.0 mg daily) and medroxyprogesterone acetate (2.5 mg or 5.0 mg daily) to minimize the risk of recurrence and prevent menopausal symptoms. Estrogen-progestin therapy is continued for the first postoperative year to induce further regression of residual disease. Women who are treated with estrogen only are protected against bone loss and cardiovascular disease and have a lower risk of recurrence of endometriosis. The use of estradiol pellets (25 to 50 mg) and testosterone (75 mg) administered subcutaneously every 4 to 6 months has been reported with good results.[49]

Chetkowski and colleagues[50] suggested that there are varying degrees of responsiveness of the various organs to blood estradiol levels. Although the precise serum concentration of estrogen required to prevent the growth of endometriosis has not been ascertained, it seems that the serum concentration of estradiol required to induce growth and proliferation of endometriosis is significantly higher (greater than 50 pg/mL) than that required to stabilize bone mineral density (20 to 50 pg/mL), and prevent osteoporosis.[43,50] Transdermal estrogen may be substituted (50 mg semiweekly) if circulating levels of estradiol are kept between 40 and 70 pg/mL to maximize the therapeutic effects and minimize the risk of symptom recurrence.[45]

Conservative Operations

Women who desire pregnancy and whose disease is responsible for their symptoms of pain or infertility should have conservative operations. Although seldom curative, such procedures improve the likelihood of pregnancy and offer at least temporary pain relief. Approximately 25% of patients undergoing conservative operations will require a subsequent operation because of recurrence of endometriosis or progression of residual (microscopic) disease.[51] The rate of repeat interventions is related directly to the extent of disease and the ability to conceive postoperatively. Among those who achieve pregnancy after the initial operation, only 10% require another operation.[42,51] Conservative methods are cytoreductive, and recurrence of symptoms most likely is caused by the progression of existing microscopic disease that was not seen during the initial operation.[52–54]

An extensive meta-analysis of published studies showed that either no treatment or surgery is superior to medical treatment for the management of minimal and mild endometriosis associated with infertility.[55] A randomized, controlled Canadian trial studied 341 infertile women to ascertain whether laparoscopic operations enhanced fecundity in infertile women with minimal or mild endometriosis.[56] The women were assigned randomly during diagnostic laparoscopy to undergo either resection or ablation of visible endometriosis or diagnostic laparoscopy only. Among the 172 women who had resection or ablation of endometriosis, 29 percent became pregnant 36 weeks after the laparoscopy and had pregnancies that continued for 20 weeks or longer, compared with 17.2% of the 169 women in the diagnostic laparoscopy group. Laparoscopic resection or ablation of minimal and mild endometriosis significantly improved fecundity in infertile women. Another prospective study assessed the efficacy of CO_2 laser laparoscopy in treating 176 infertile women with minimal to mild endometriosis according to the American Society of Reproductive Medicine (ASRM) classification in terms of pregnancy rates.[57] The patients were treated with one of four methods: 49 underwent operative laparoscopy with newly developed CO_2 laser vaporization or resection, 45 were treated by operative laparoscopy with simple monopolar electrocoagulation, 43 who had undergone only diagnostic laparoscopy did not receive any treatment, and 39 received danazol 800 mg/day for 3 months after diagnostic laparoscopy. Advanced laparoscopic operations with a laser were more efficient than were other modalities in treating infertile women with minimal to mild endometriosis in terms of pregnancy rates. Tulandi and al-Took[58] found no difference in the pregnancy rates of 101 infertile women with mild endometriosis treated laparoscopically either by excision or by electrocoagulation.

Appearances of Endometriosis

Complete removal of endometriotic implants is difficult because of their variability in appearance and visibility. Powder burn lesions represent foci of inactive disease containing stroma and glands embedded in hemosiderin deposits.[59] These lesions are more common in older women and may not cause pain or infertility.[60] When implants involve the uterosacral ligaments, they are palpable as tender nodularities and can cause dysmenorrhea and dyspareunia. Atypical and nonpigmented lesions, which are seen as clear vesicles, pink vascular patterns, white scarred lesions, red lesions, yellow-brown patches, and peritoneal windows, represent active endometriosis and secrete prostaglandin in the peritoneal fluid.[61]

The depth of endometrial implants may be related to the level of disease activity and symptoms (Figure 12-1, A and B). Cornillie and coworkers[62] reported that cellular activity of endometriosis was greater for both superficial and deep implants (58% and 68%, respectively) than for intermediate implants (25%). They postulated that early lesions result from proliferation of retrograde menstrual tissue and present as superficial implants. These lesions progress to an intermediate depth, where they either become inactive or progress and infiltrate deeper layers, usually more than 5 mm. Implants continue their biologic activity and proliferate, being stimulated by circulating steroid hormones because they are no longer dependent on the steroids in the peritoneal fluid.[61,63]

Microscopic endometriosis can be overlooked during surgical exploration but is identified by light and electron microscopy in normal-appearing peritoneum. This finding has been noted in patients with visible endometriosis in other areas of the pelvis[52,53] and patients with unexplained infertility in whom no endometriosis was seen at laparoscopy.[54,64] Microscopic presentation may preclude total resection, but two techniques can enhance visual detection. Near-contact laparoscopy magnifies the peritoneal area. In a series of 20 women with pelvic endometriosis, biopsy specimens were taken from peritoneum that appeared normal. The histologic studies of this tissue revealed only one case of microscopic endometriosis, and an additional two cases were suspicious for endometriosis.[53] The second technique for improved detection of microscopic endometriosis is "painting" the peritoneum and broad ligament with blood or serosanguinous fluid to render atypical lesions more evident.[65] Retroperitoneal hydrodissection of the anterior cul-de-sac, posterior broad ligaments, and pelvic side wall sometimes facilitates the identification of lesions (Figure 12-2, A and B).

The peritoneum must be examined from different angles and at different degrees of illumination to see vesicles or whitish lesions. The peritoneal folds must be stretched and searched for small, atypical lesions. Although the resolution of cameras has improved, it is still not comparable to that of direct vision through the laparoscope. Reinspection of the peritoneal cavity for endometrial implants should be accomplished by direct vision to ensure identification of all foci.

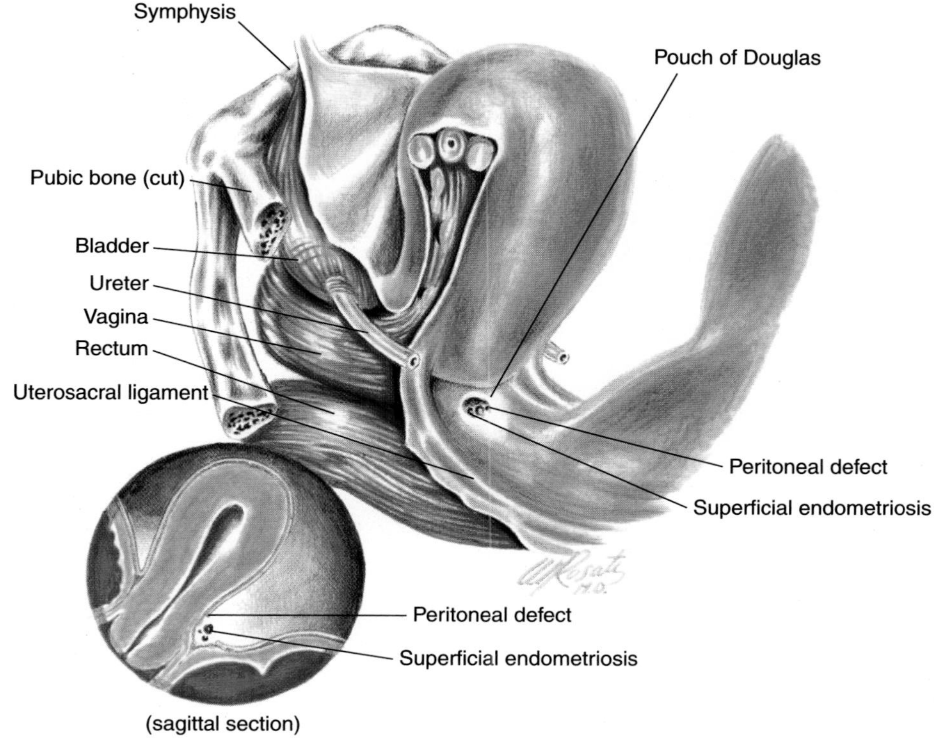

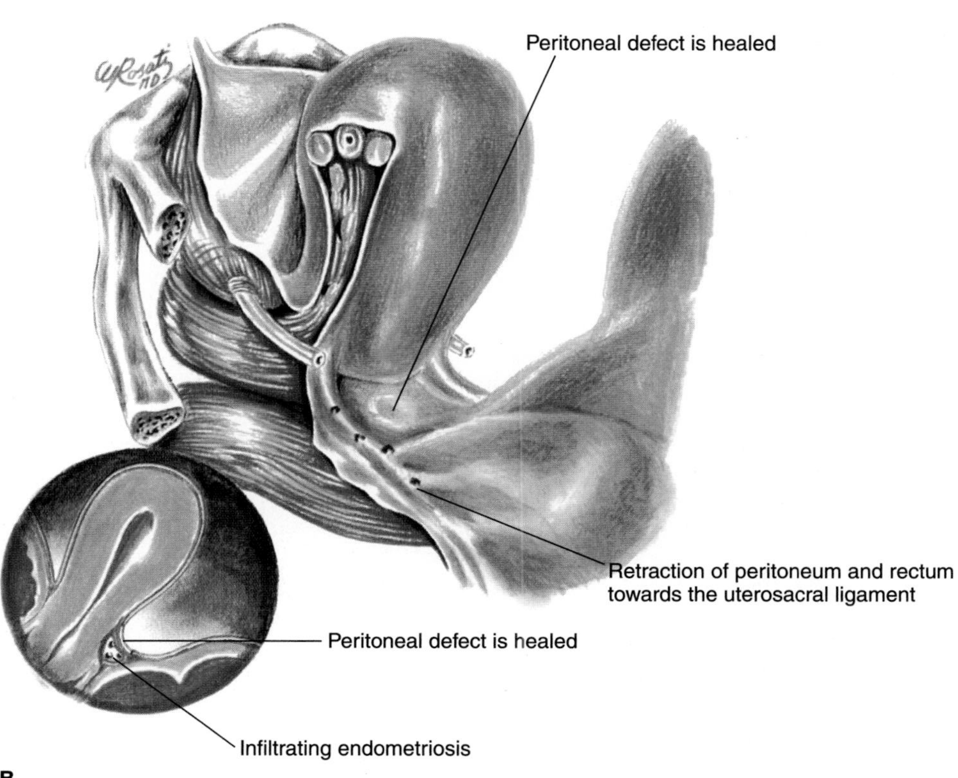

Figure 12-1. **A.** A peritoneal defect in the pouch of Douglas has an endometrial implant at its base. The inset reveals a healed peritoneal defect with infiltrating endometrosis beneath it. **B.** Sagittal view of endometrial implants involving the uterosacral ligament. Inset shows infiltrating endometriosis beneath the peritoneum.

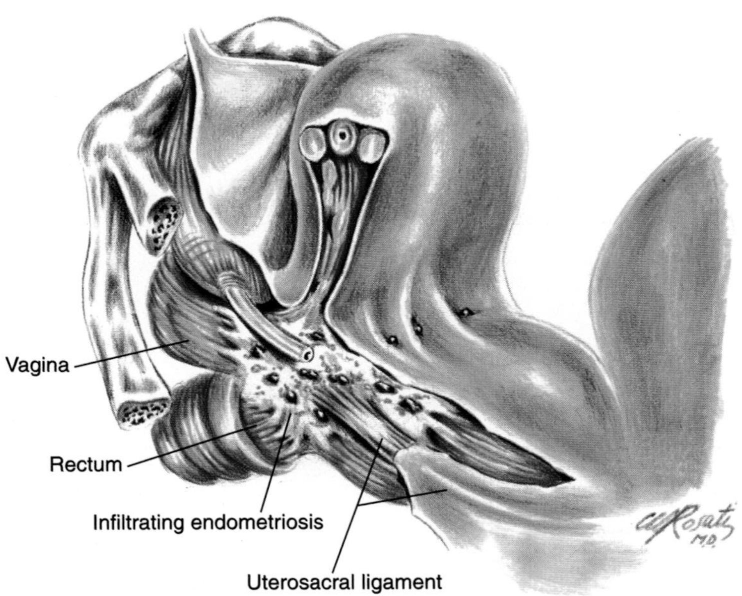

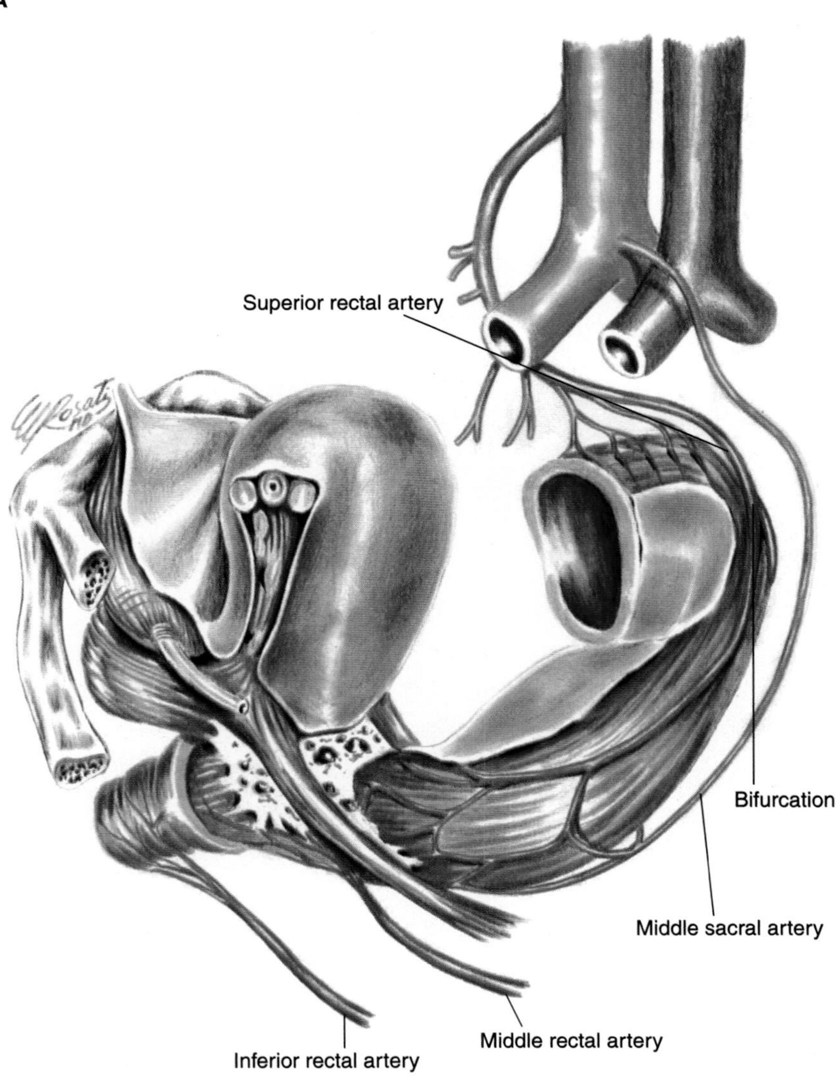

Figure 12-2. **A.** Anatomic representation of the pelvic structures involved with implants of endometriosis. **B.** The ureters are at risk because of infiltrating endometriosis.

Normal-appearing ovaries can contain endometriosis under an apparently normal cortex. By inserting a needle deep in the stroma and aspirating the ovary, Candiani and coworkers[66] identified small endometriomas in 48% of otherwise normal-appearing or slightly enlarged ovaries. They suggested that preoperative ultrasonographic evaluation is useful to screen for small subcortical ovarian cysts, which should be explored surgically with needle aspiration. The diagnosis of endometriosis is missed in at least 7% of patients and understaged in as many as 50%.[53] A careful examination of the pelvis is essential to diagnose and stage endometriosis and to be aware of its various appearances, including its presence as microscopic implants on visually normal peritoneal surfaces or as small, deep endometriomas within slightly enlarged but otherwise normal ovaries.

Using patient-assisted laparoscopy Demco[67] studied the relationship of lesions of endometriosis to pelvic pain. He found that pain from endometriosis has little relationship to the location or color of lesions. However, red and vascular lesions were the most painful, followed by clear and white scar lesions. Least painful were black lesions. Pain extended beyond lesions to normal-looking peritoneum for up to 27 mm but was not consistent with respect to the type of lesion.

Treatment of Endometrial Implants

Diagnostic Laparoscopy

Initially, the surgeon explores the pelvic cavity to assess the extent of disease and identify abnormalities or distortions of the pelvic organs. Photographs and video recordings have been very useful for documenting the surgeon's findings. In a recent opinion statement, however, the American College of Obstetricians and Gynecologists' Committee on Professional Liability advised against physicians recording laparoscopic procedures because of a growing fear among clinicians that procedural tapes can be edited, enhanced, or otherwise manipulated for the purposes of winning liability suits against doctors.[68a] The committee further cautioned that if a recording is made, the health care facility should keep the original tape and provide an exact copy to the patient. The location and boundaries of the bladder, ureter, colon, rectum, pelvic gutters, uterosacral ligaments, and major blood vessels are noted. The upper abdominal organs, abdominal walls, liver, and diaphragm should be evaluated for endometriosis or any other condition that may contribute to the patient's symptoms. The omentum and the small bowel are evaluated for disease and to ensure that they were not injured during insertion of the Veress needle or trocar. A rectovaginal examination is accomplished to evaluate deep and retroperitoneal endometriosis found in the lower pelvis at the rectovaginal septum, uterosacral ligament, lower colon, and pararectal area. Deep retroperitoneal endometriosis is rare without a connection to the surface peritoneum.

In 15% of patients with endometriosis, the appendix is involved and should be examined.[68] An implant that has penetrated retroperitoneally several centimeters is called an "iceberg" lesion. It can be detected laparoscopically by palpating areas of the pelvis and bowel with the suction-irrigator probe. With the forceps or probe, endometriotic implants are examined to gauge size, depth, and proximity to normal pelvic structures. The diagnostic laparoscopy is extended to an operative procedure if the patient has been advised of this possibility.

Operative Laparoscopy

The operative procedure begins by lysing adhesions between the bowel and the pelvic organs to expose the pelvic cavity adequately. The ovaries are dissected from the cul-de-sac or pelvic side wall, and the tubes are freed from adhesions and chromopertubated. Endometrial implants and endometriomas are resected or vaporized, and if the patient has significant central pelvic pain, uterosacral nerve ablation or presacral nerve resection is done.

Lysis of bowel adhesions

Bowel adhesions vary in thickness, vascularity, and cohesiveness. Some adhesions are stretched without tearing the tissue, excised with a laser Harmonic scalpel or electrosurgery at the points of attachment to the pelvic organs, and removed. Dense adhesions are excised with scissors or any other cutting instrument The CO_2 laser has more controlled penetration than do electrosurgery and fiber lasers. The structures requiring separation are pulled apart with forceps, and a cleavage plane is formed. Hydrodissection is useful to identify and develop the dissection plane, which is ablated or excised, using a laser or dissecting scissors or any other cutting instrument.

Peritoneal implants

In treating peritoneal endometriosis, the implants should be destroyed in the most effective and least traumatic manner to minimize postoperative adhesions. Although different modalities have been used, hydrodissection and a high-power superpulse or ultrapulse CO_2 laser are the best choices for treatment.[69] This laser does not penetrate water, and a fluid backstop (hydrodissection) allows the surgeon to work on selected tissue with a greater safety margin than would otherwise be available (Figure 12-3). A small opening is made in the retroperitoneum with the laser or scissors, and lactated Ringer's solution is injected beneath the lesion to provide a protective cushion of fluid between the lesion to be excised and the underlying ureter or blood vessels. The fluid under the implant absorbs the CO_2 laser energy, buffering the underlying tissue. For retroperitoneal disease, the lesion is picked up with grasping forceps, pulled medially, and removed, using sharp or blunt dissection.

Superficial peritoneal endometriosis is vaporized with the laser, coagulated with monopolar or bipolar current, or excised. Implants less than 2 mm are coagulated, vaporized, or excised. When lesions exceed 3 mm, vaporization or excision is needed. For lesions greater than 5 mm, deep vaporization or excisional techniques are used. Superficial implants on the pelvic side wall are ablated with the CO_2 laser (3500 to 5500 W/cm^2). Low-power densities cause greater damage and

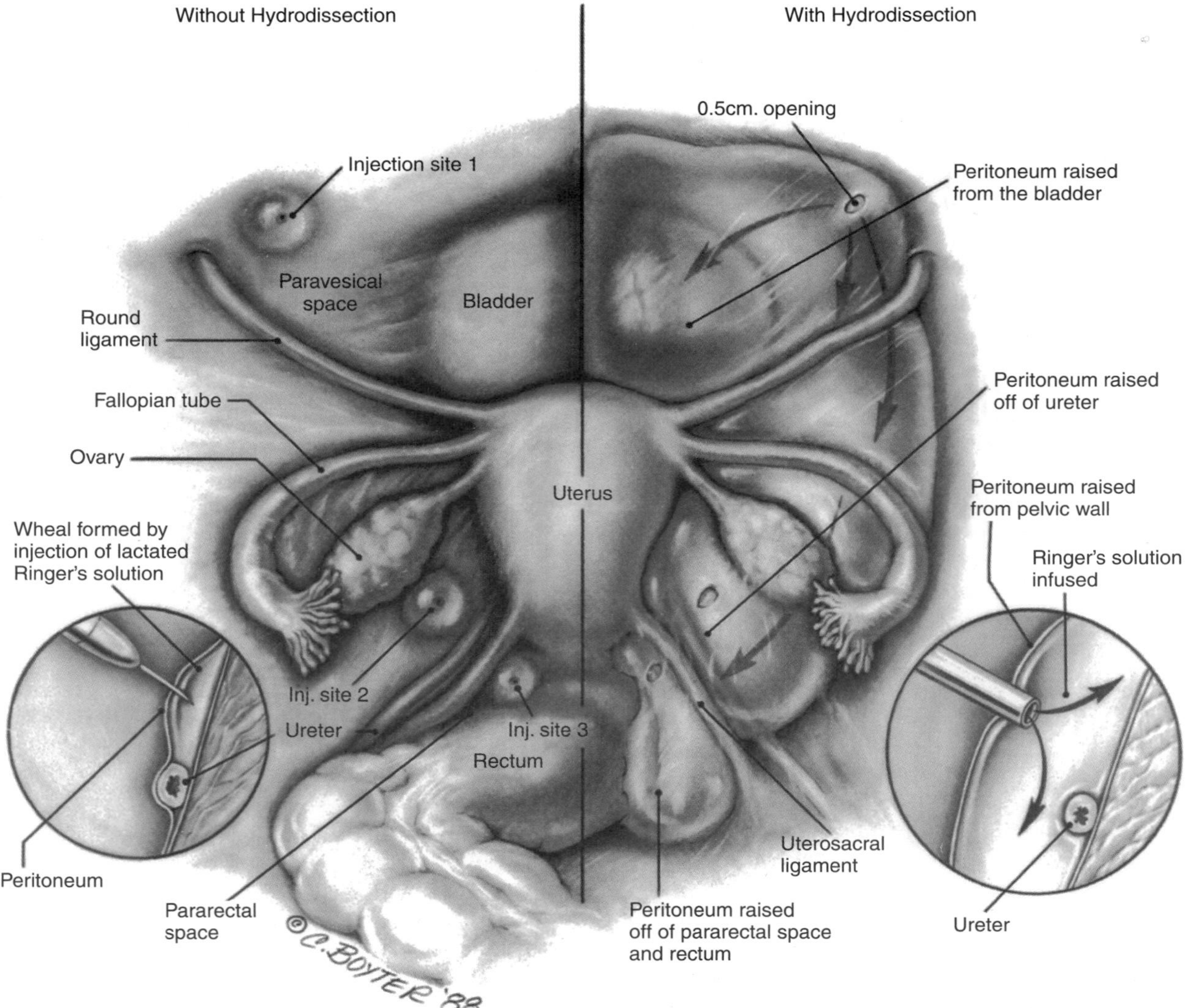

Figure 12-3. Hydrodissection protects retroperitoneal structures such as the bladder, ureter, and blood vessels from the CO_2 laser. Insets show creation of retroperitoneal space.

more charring. High-power densities penetrate too deeply and injure underlying normal structures or cause unnecessary bleeding. Firing in a continuous mode will ablate the lesion from the surface to its base, where the peritoneal fat should appear as unpigmented and soft rather than fibrotic like endometriosis or scars. To suction the laser plume and irrigate the lesion base, the suction-irrigator is placed next to or behind the lesion, removing char and identifying any vascular structure within the operative field. If carbon is allowed to accumulate, the field is obscured. In either situation, carbon can be mistaken for endometriosis. Therefore, if vaporization is chosen, it is important to copiously irrigate and remove the charred areas to confirm complete removal of the lesion and avoid confusing endometriosis with a carbon deposit. When used in the superpulse/ultrapulse mode, this laser achieves more rapid vaporization and decreased carbonization.

Resection of ovarian endometriosis

The ovaries are a common site for endometriosis. Ovarian endometriosis causes adhesions between the ovarian surface and the broad ligament. In 1921, Sampson[70] noted that the histologic findings varied in different portions of the same cyst. Some implants also developed from spilling of the contents of endometriomas after rupture, resulting in the invasion of functional cysts by these surface implants. Large endometriomas could develop because of secondary involvement of follicular or luteal cysts by surface implants. Ovarian implants are similar to endometriosis in extraovarian sites and are limited in size by fibrosis and scarring. Endometriomas might originate from metaplasia of the celomic epithelium that lines the cystic epithelial inclusions that frequently are found in the ovaries.[71,72] Sampson believed that there was local spread of endometriosis by salpingeal reflux.

The accepted histologic criterion for the diagnosis of endometriosis is the presence of endometrial glands and stroma.[73] Chernobilsky and Morris[74] described a variety of epithelial characteristics found in ovarian endometriosis. Nissole-Pochet and associates[75] studied 113 instances of ovarian endometriosis before and after hormone therapy. Those authors could identify typical endometrial glandular epithelium and stroma. In 18%, only the endometrial epithelium lined the cyst. Areas with ciliated cells representing oviduct-like epithelium were observed in 47%. In the others, flattened endometrial epithelium and typical glandular and stromal structures were seen. Martin and Berry[76] examined 41 "chocolate" cysts and found that 61% were endometriomas, 27% were corpora lutea, and in 12% no lining was found. Vercellini and coworkers[77] confirmed 97.7% of visually diagnosed endometriomas by using at least two of the following microscopic patterns to diagnose them: (1) the presence of endometrial epithelium, (2) endometrial glands or gland-like structures, (3) endometrial stroma and hemosiderin-laden macrophages.

Endometrial implants or endometriomas less than 2 cm in diameter are coagulated, laser ablated, or excised, using scissors, biopsy forceps, lasers, or electrodes (Figure 12-4). For successful eradication, all visible lesions and scars must be removed from the ovarian surface. Entrapment of oocytes within the luteinized ovarian follicle, as reported in experimental animal models, must be avoided.[78] Draining the endometrioma or partially resecting its wall is inadequate because the endometrial tissue lining the cyst can remain functional and can cause the symptoms to recur.[79] However, photocoagulation of the cyst wall has been equally therapeutic and occasionally less difficult.[30,80,81] Brosens and Puttemansi[80] recommended cystoscopy and biopsy of the cyst wall before ablating the cyst. When a double optic laparoscope, which involves the passage of a smaller operative endoscope through the channel of the main laparoscope, is used, the ovarian cyst is punctured and drained, the fluid is sent for cytology, and the lining is inspected visually. Any suspicious area is biopsied, and the specimen is sent for frozen section. Once it has been ascertained that the cyst is not malignant, its wall is ablated to a depth of 3 to 4 mm, using a laser or an electrocoagulator introduced through the operative channel of the second laparoscope. This procedure is analogous to endometrial ablation and seems to be successful, with no recurrence on follow-up ultrasound or second-look laparoscopy.

Type I endometriomas are 1 to 2 cm in size and contain dark fluid (Figure 12-5). They develop from surface endometrial implants and are difficult to excise. Microscopically, endometrial tissue is seen in all of them. While small, these endometriomas are difficult to remove intact because of associated fibrosis and adhesions. They can be biopsied, drained, and vaporized by using a laser or electrosurgery or removed in pieces.

Type IIA endometriomas are hemorrhagic cysts and grossly look like endometriomas. The cyst wall is separated easily from the ovarian tissue. Endometrial implants are superficial and adjacent to a hemorrhagic cyst, which is either follicular or

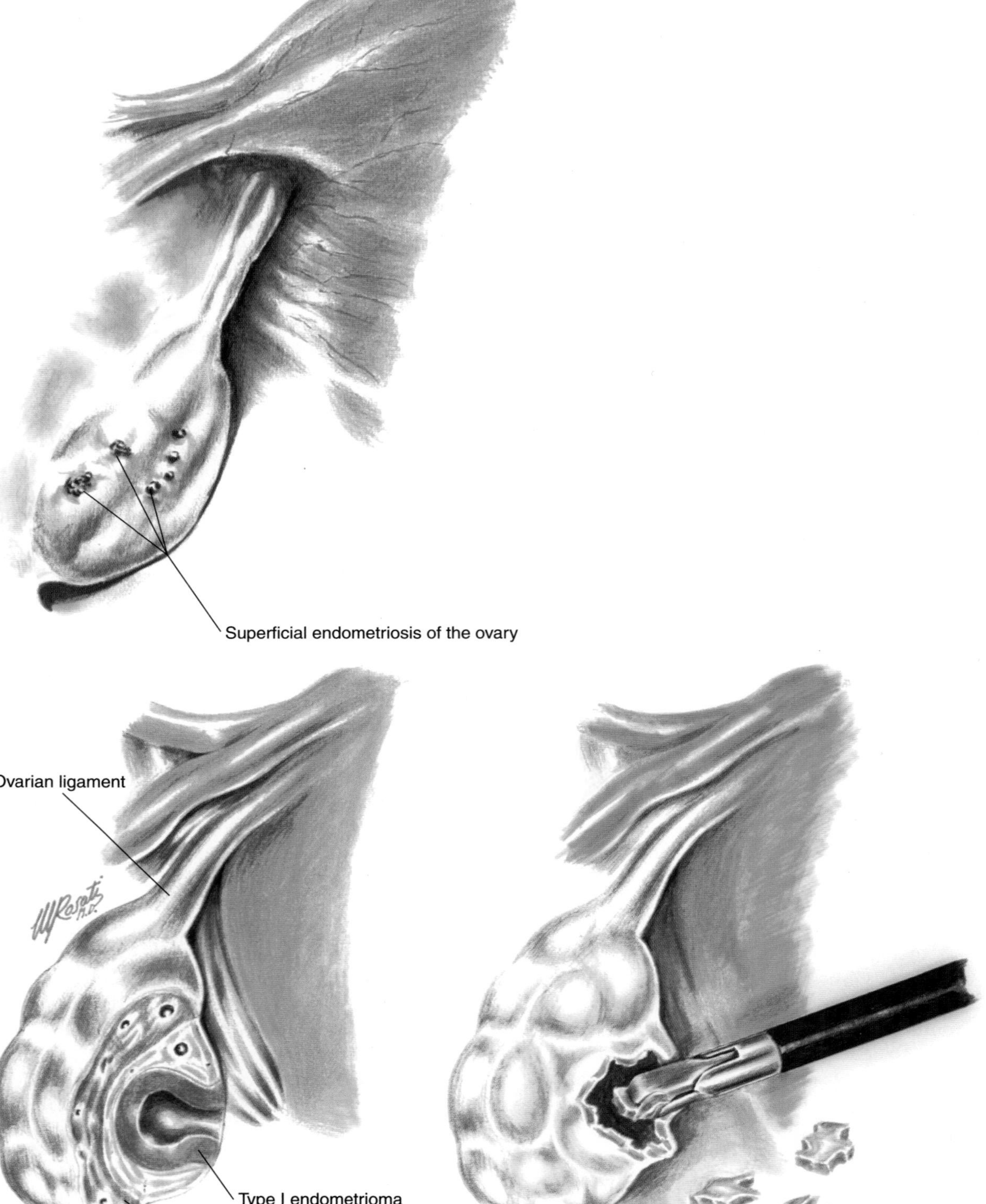

Figure 12-4. Superficial implants are seen on this ovary.

Figure 12-5. **A.** Type I endometriomas are small, contain dark fluid, and develop from surface implants. **B.** They are difficult to remove intact because of associated adhesions and fibrosis.

luteal in origin; microscopically, no endometrial lining is seen.

In type IIA lesions, the periovarian adhesions are lysed, the ovarian cortex is evaluated, and the cyst is aspirated. Superficial ovarian implants adjacent to the cyst are vaporized or excised. The cyst is opened, its wall is examined, and a biopsy specimen is taken for frozen section. If it has a yellowish appearance, removal is easy (Figure 12-6). Postoperatively, either danazol 800 mg/day or a gonadotropin-releasing hormone (GnRH) analog is used for 6 to 8 weeks.

In type IIB lesions, the cyst lining is separated easily from the ovarian capsule and stroma except near the endometrial implant. In type IIC lesions, surface endometrial implants penetrate deeply into the cyst wall, making excision difficult. Histologic findings of endometriosis are seen in the cyst wall in these two subtypes. The basis for differentiating between these two subtypes is the progressive difficulty in removing the cyst wall.

Type IIB and type IIC endometriomas are large and are associated with periovarian adhesions that attach them to the pelvic side wall and the back of the uterus. When suction and irrigation are alternated, the contents are removed. The inside of the cyst is examined, and the portion of ovarian cortex involved with endometriosis is removed. Using the grasping forceps and the suction-irrigator probe, the cyst wall is grasped and separated from the ovarian stroma by traction and countertraction.[82] Small blood vessels from the ovarian bed and bleeding from the ovarian hilum are controlled with bipolar electrocoagulation.

In type IIC lesions, it is difficult to develop a cleavage plane between the cyst wall and the ovarian stroma. The portion of the ovary attached to the cyst wall is removed until a clear boundary is found so that the entire cyst can be extirpated. The remainder of the procedure is similar to that which was described above. The edges of the ovarian defect are brought together with a low-power laser or electrosurgery. Low-power, continuous laser or bipolar coagulation applied to the inside wall of the redundant ovarian capsule causes it to invert. Excessive coagulation of the adjacent ovarian stroma must be avoided. If sutures are needed, they are placed inside the capsule, and 4-0 polyglycolic material is used. Fewer sutures result in fewer adhesions.[83]

The least invasive and technically simplest approach to endometriomas involves laparoscopic fenestration and removal of "chocolate" fluid without cystectomy or ablation of the cyst wall. However, fenestration and irrigation are ineffective, as evidenced by a 50% recurrence rate. Fayez and

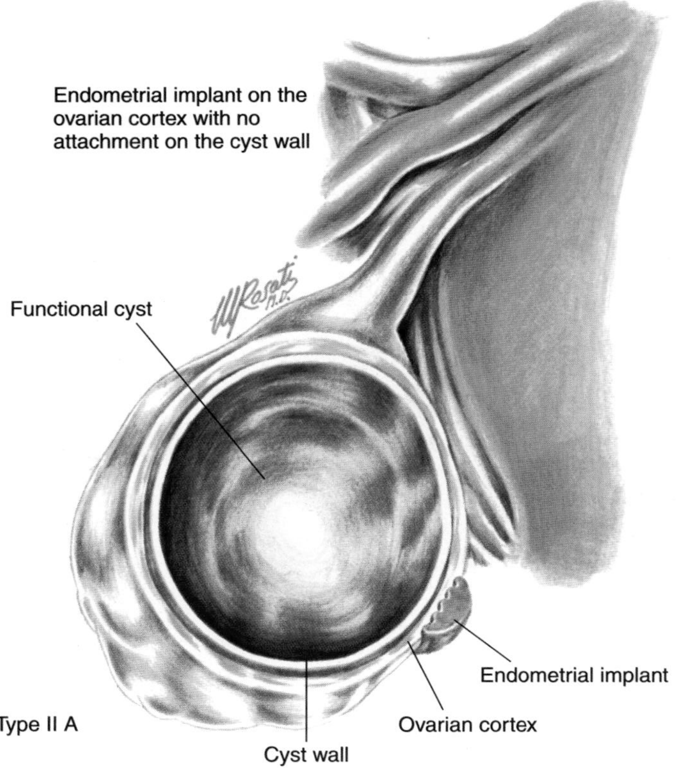

Figure 12-6. A functional cyst with a small endometrial implant.

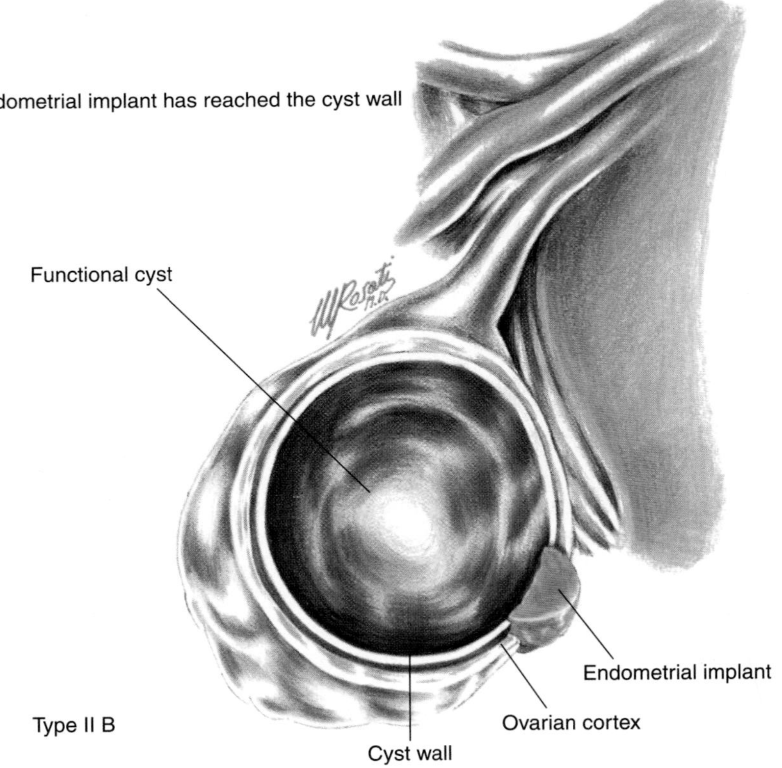

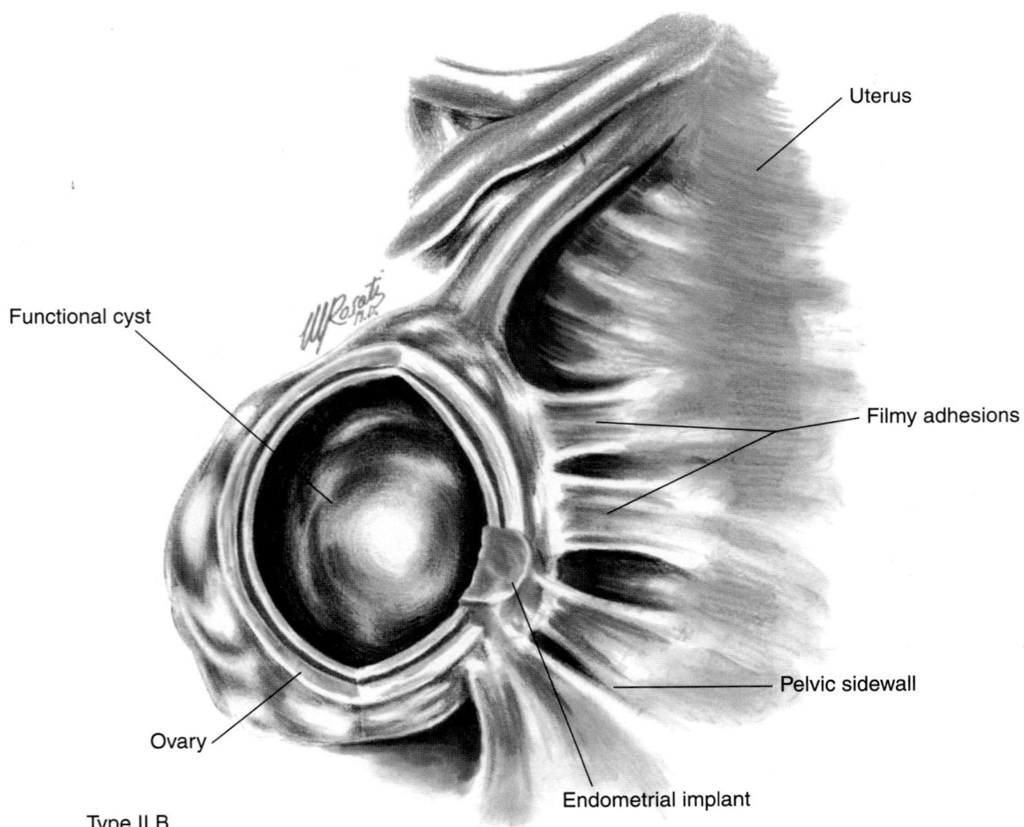

Figure 12-7. **A.** A type IIB endometrioma with features of a functional cyst involved deeply with histologic findings of endometriosis in the cyst wall. The cyst wall is separated easily from the ovarian capsule and stroma except adjacent to the areas of endometriosis. **B.** In this type IIB lesion, the endometrial implant has reached the cyst wall.

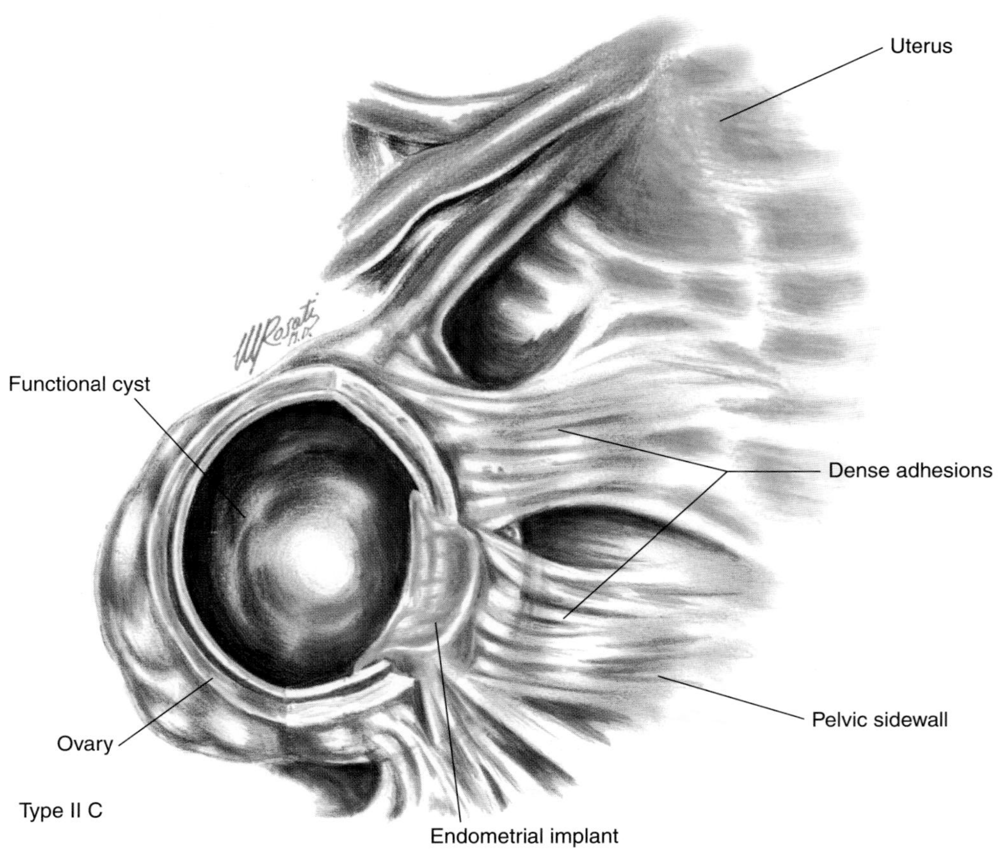

Figure 12-7. (*Continued*) **C.** Extensive periovarian adhesions are present, and there is more extensive involvement of the cyst wall with endometrial implants. When suction and irrigation are alternated, the inside of the cyst can be explored.

Vogel[84] made a wide opening in the cyst wall to drain its contents. They claimed that their technique created fewer periadnexal adhesions (27%). Vercellini and associates[77] showed that aspiration of the cyst and irrigation of the endometriomas were ineffective. In 33 women, most endometriomas recurred, although many patients took GnRH analogs postoperatively. Hasson[85] noted recurrences in eight of nine endometriomas treated by fenestration alone.

For endometriomas over 2 cm in diameter, the cyst is punctured with the 5-mm trocar and aspirated with the suction-irrigator probe. Using high-pressure irrigation at 500 to 800 mm Hg, the cyst is irrigated, causing it to expand, and is aspirated several times.[86] This procedure allows examination of the cyst wall. After the repeated expansion and shrinkage with irrigation and suction, the cyst wall should separate from the surrounding ovarian stroma (Figure 12-7, A through C). If it does not, 5 to 20 mL of lactated Ringer's solution is injected between the stroma and the cyst wall. The cyst wall is removed by grasping its base with laparoscopic forceps and peeling it from the ovarian stroma (Figure 12-8). If this is not successful, the wall is separated from the ovarian cortex with forceps at the puncture site. A cleavage plane is created by pulling the two forceps apart and cutting between the structures. The laser or electrosurgery minimizes bleeding because the blood vessels supplying the endometrioma are usually small enough to be cut and coagulated simultaneously. Another method involves hydrodissection of the plane between the cyst wall and the ovarian stroma.[16,32] These techniques can be applied successfully to completely remove the cyst wall, which should be sent for histologic evaluation to rule out malignancy. If the entire cyst cannot be separated from the ovary, the adherent sections are ablated or coagulated.[79,80,81,86] When the entire

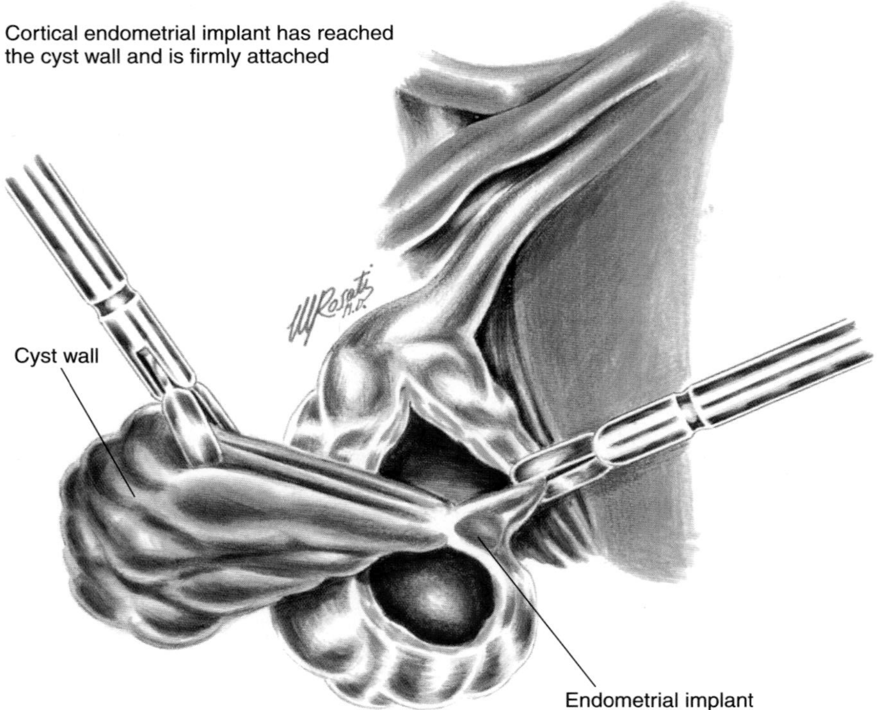

Figure 12-8. A. The lining is separated easily from the ovarian capsule and stroma except adjacent to the areas of endometriosis. B.. The cyst wall has been removed, and a piece of the ovarian cortex with the endometrial implant has been excised. Using the grasping forceps and the suction-irrigator probe, the cyst wall is separated from the ovarian cortex by traction and countertraction.

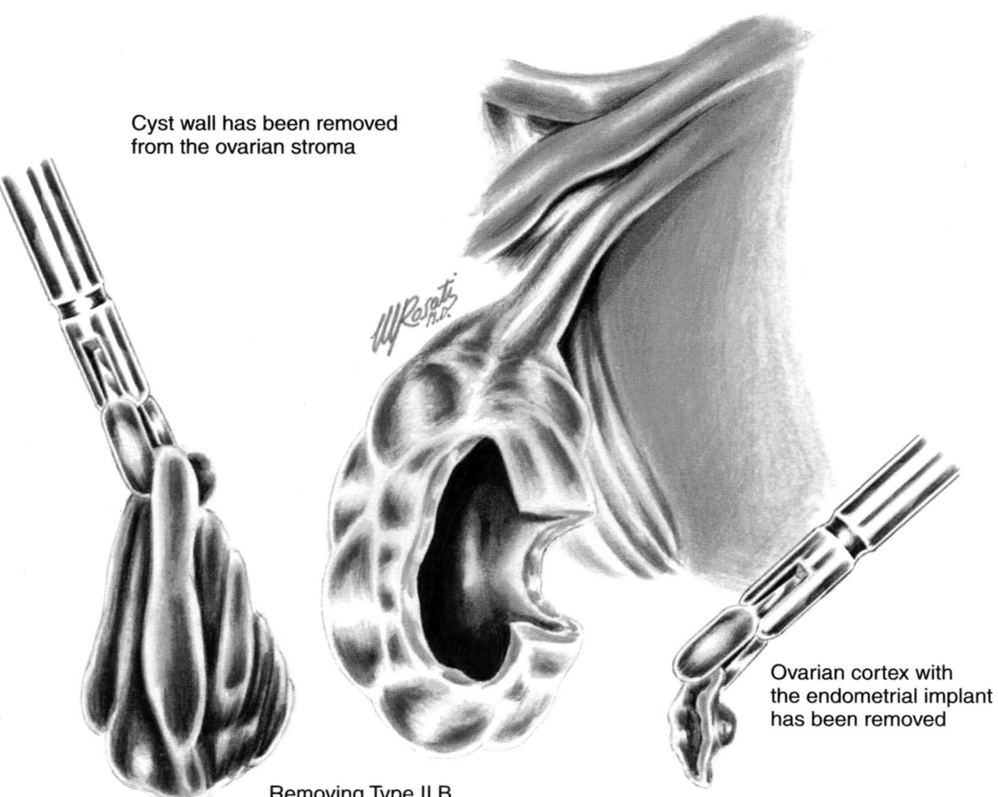

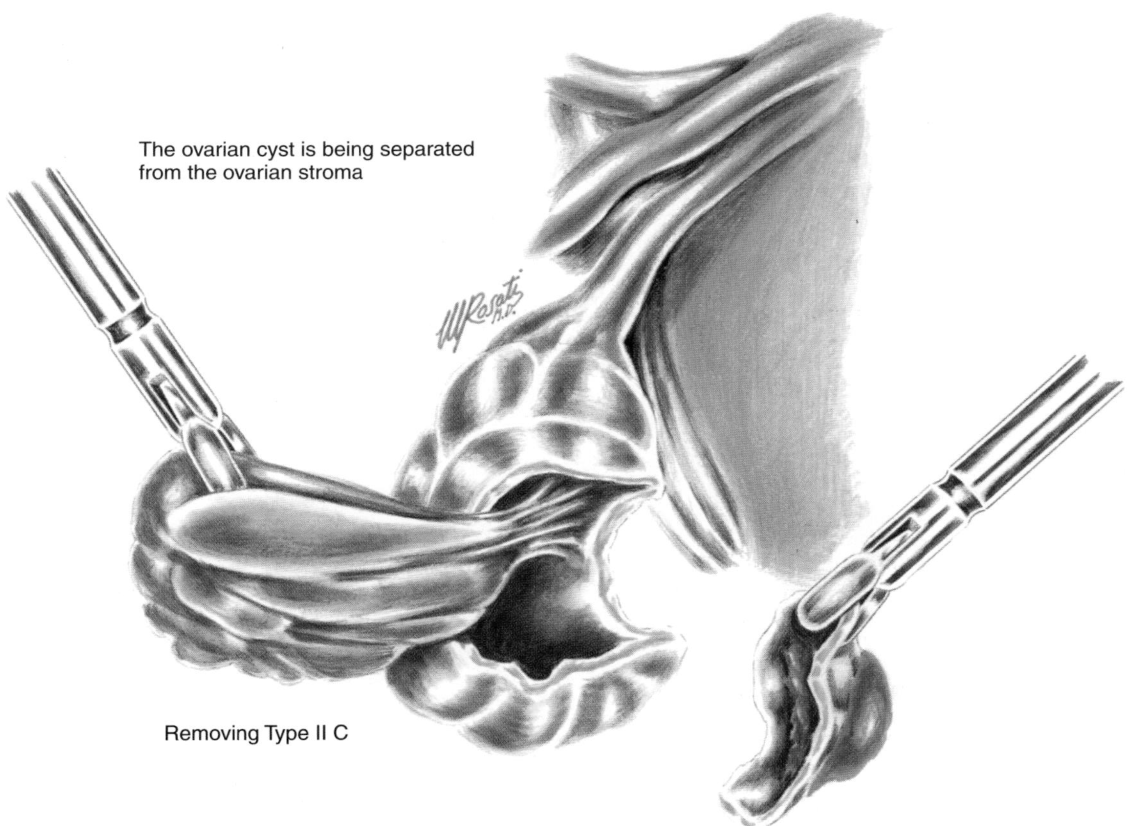

Figure 12-8. (*Continued*) **C.** Surface implants penetrate the cyst wall deeply, making excision difficult. The degree of invasion of the cyst wall forms the basis for differentiating these subgroups.

cyst wall is ablated, representative biopsy specimens are taken for histologic diagnosis. These endometriomas tend to rupture during separation because of their adherence to other pelvic structures. Since it is difficult to develop a plane between the cyst wall and the ovarian stroma, the portion of the ovary attached to the cyst wall is removed until an area is located to produce a line of cleavage.

Cyst wall closure is not necessary, according to animal experiments[87] and clinical experience.[88] For large defects that result from resecting endometriomas larger than 5 cm, the edges of the ovarian cortex are approximated with a single suture placed within the ovarian stroma. The knot is tied inside the ovary so that no part of the suture penetrates the ovarian cortex or is exposed to the ovarian surface to minimize adhesion formation. Fibrin sealant has been described to atraumatically approximate the edges of large ovarian defects (Figure 12-9).[89]

Rare patients present with localized symptoms and severe involvement of the ovary with disease and adhesions while the opposite ovary is normal, requiring unilateral salpingo-oophorectomy. When the diseased ovary is removed, the risk of disease recurrence is minimized, and the fertility potential is improved by limiting ovulation to the healthy side. In a prospective trial, Beretta and coauthors[90] randomly allocated 64 patients with

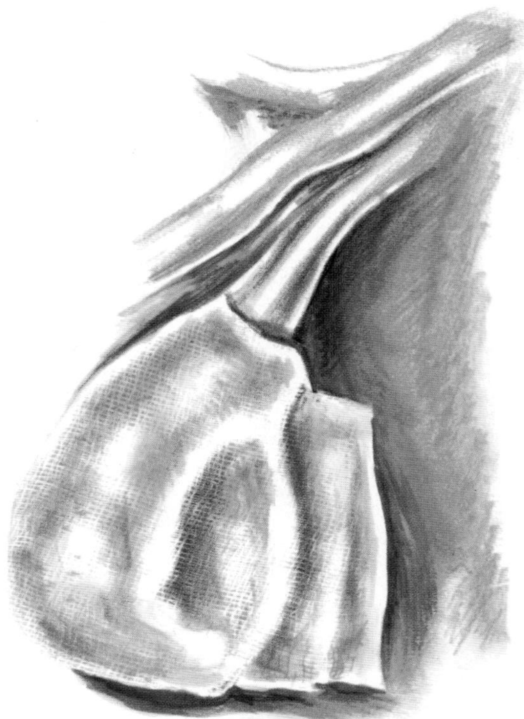

Figure 12-9. The resected ovary and adjacent side wall of the pelvis are wrapped with Interceed.

advanced stages of endometriosis to undergo either cystectomy of the endometrioma or drainage of the endometrioma and bipolar coagulation of the inner lining. The 24-month cumulative recurrence rates of dysmenorrhea, deep dyspareunia, and nonmenstrual pelvic pain were lower in the patients who underwent cystectomy than in those who did not (dysmenorrhea: 15.8% compared to 52.9%; deep dyspareunia: 20% compared to 75%; nonmenstrual pelvic pain: 10% compared to 52.9%). The median interval between the operation and the recurrence of moderate to severe pelvic pain was longer after cystectomy: 19 months compared with 5 months. The 24-month cumulative pregnancy rate was higher after cystectomy: 66.7% compared with 23.5%. For the treatment of ovarian endometriomas, a better outcome with a similar rate of complications is achieved with laparoscopic cystectomy than with drainage and coagulation.

The efficacy of laparoscopy done by applying the stripping technique was compared retrospectively to that of microsurgery by laparotomy in 132 women under 40 years of age with ovarian endometriotic cysts at least 3 cm in diameter, stage III and IV endometriosis, rAFS classification.[91] The recurrence rate of ovarian cysts, symptomatic improvement, and the reproductive outcome were found to be comparable for the two groups. However, as was expected, laparoscopy resulted in less postoperative febrile morbidity and a significantly shorter duration of hospitalization. The long-term results of laparoscopic fenestration and coagulation of ovarian endometriomas were investigated in a case-control study and compared with the results of ovarian cystectomy done by either laparotomy or laparoscopy.[92] The study enrolled 156 premenopausal women with ovarian endometriomas at least 3 cm in diameter, stage III and IV endometriosis, rAFS classification. The mean time to first pregnancy was shorter in the 80 patients who underwent laparoscopic ovarian fenestration and coagulation (1.4 years) than it was in the 23 patients who underwent laparoscopic ovarian cystectomy (2.2 years) or the 53 patients who underwent ovarian cystectomy by laparotomy and a microsurgical technique (2.4 years). The difference in the recurrence rate and between the cumulative clinical pregnancy rates in the three groups was not statistically significant after 36 months of follow-up. The investigators concluded that laparoscopic ovarian fenestration and coagulation of endometriomas led to faster conception than did ovarian cystectomy by laparotomy. Furthermore, laparoscopic ovarian fenestration and coagulation of endometriomas were associated with cumulative clinical pregnancy rates and recurrence rates over 36 months that were similar to those associated with ovarian cystectomy.

Genitourinary endometriosis

Ureteral involvement has been reported in 1 to 11% of women diagnosed with endometriosis.[93] Endometriosis of the urinary tract tends to be superficial but can be invasive and cause complete ureteral obstruction. Decreased bladder capacity and stability unresponsive to conventional therapy can result. Goldstein and Brodman[94] reported one case of bladder endometriosis that they monitored cystometrically for 4 years. They found that decreased bladder capacity and bladder instability that were not responsive to conventional parasympatholytic therapy were corrected after surgical destruction of superficial bladder endometriosis. When bladder symptoms recurred 2 years later, a course of danazol again reversed bladder instability. Clinicians should consider endometriosis in cases of refractory and unexplained urinary complaints. If urinary tract endometriosis is suspected, an intravenous pyelogram, ultrasound of the kidneys, and a routine blood and urine workup are indicated. In selected cases of recurrent hematuria, cystoscopy is suggested.

Superficial implants over the ureter are treated with a variation of hydrodissection. Approximately 20 to 30 mL of lactated Ringer's solution is injected subperitoneally on the lateral pelvic wall; this elevates the peritoneum and backs it with a bed of fluid. The CO_2 laser may be used to create a 0.5-cm opening on this elevation. The opening in the peritoneum is made anteriorly and laterally, close to the corresponding round ligament. The hydrodissection probe is inserted into the opening, and approximately 100 mL of lactated Ringer's solution is injected under 300 mm Hg pressure into the retroperitoneal space along the course of the ureter. The fluid surrounds the ureter, moves it posteriorly, and allows superficial laser dissection or vaporization of the area.

After a water bed is created, a superpulse or ultrapulse CO_2 laser or any other cutting device (20 to 80 W) may be used to vaporize or excise the lesion with a circumference of 1 to 2 cm. When the lesions are large or excision is preferred, a circular line with a 1- to 2-cm margin is made around the lesion. The peritoneum is held with an atraumatic grasping forceps and peeled away with the help of a cutting instrument and the suction-irrigator probe. If the endometrial implant is embedded and has formed scarring down to the subperitoneal connective tissue, hydrodissection allows water to tunnel beneath the lesion, often separating scar tissue. Then the lesion can be treated safely. After vaporization or excision of these lesions, the area is irrigated and washed to remove all charcoal and verify that the nonpenetrating endometriosis (to the lumen of ureter bladder) has been treated properly. In over 500 consecutive procedures (275 bladder and 250 ureter), there were no major complications involving vesical or ureteral injury.[15] Two patients were unable to void immediately postoperatively. An indwelling catheter was placed and removed the day after surgery, and then those women were able to void. Four patients with bladder endometriosis experienced minimal hematuria that resolved several hours postoperatively. After hydrodissection of the broad ligaments and the pelvic side wall, about 5% of the patients developed swelling of the external genitalia, most likely from the penetration of water through the inguinal canal to the labia major. This swelling resolved in most patients within 1 to 2 hours without sequelae.

The surgical management of 28 women who had deeply infiltrating urinary tract endometriosis has been described.[95] All procedures were accomplished laparoscopically: Seven involved the bladder, and 21 the ureter. Patients who had vesical endometriosis underwent partial cystectomy and primary repair. Partial ureteral obstruction was found in 17 women; 10 underwent ureterolysis and excision of endometriosis, and 7 had partial wall resection. Four patients with ureteral involvement had complete obstruction. Three underwent partial resection and ureteroureterostomy, and one had ureteroneocystostomy. Severe infiltrative endometriosis of the bladder and the ureter can present without specific symptoms and can cause silent compromise of renal function.

Laparoscopic closure of intentional or unintentional bladder lacerations during operative laparoscopy was done in 19 women with one layer, using interrupted absorbable polyglycolic suture or polydioxanone suture followed by 7 to 14 days of transurethral drainage.[96] Complications were limited to one vesicovaginal fistula that required reoperation. After 6 to 48 months of follow-up, all these patients had a good outcome. A new laparoscopic technique for the treatment of infiltrative ureteral endometriosis, a laparoscopic vesicopsoas hitch, was described. In this 36-year-old woman with infiltrative endometriosis of the ureter after partial ureteral resection, it was noted that a tension-free anastomosis to the bladder was not possible. Thus, a laparoscopic vesicopsoas hitch was done.[97]

Ureteral obstruction

The incidence of ureteral obstruction by endometriosis is low, and conventional therapy previously consisted of laparotomy and resection of the obstructed segment of the ureter. Laparoscopic ureteroureterostomy was accomplished in 1990 by Nezhat and colleagues[98] on a 36-year-old woman with long-term ureteral obstruction caused by endometriosis. The condition had been diagnosed previously at laparoscopy. The patient refused conventional laparotomy and had a nephrostomy tube for 4 years. At laparoscopy, a 3- to 4-cm fibrotic nodule over the left ureter was seen approximately 4 cm above the bladder, distorting the course of the ureter (Figure 12-10). This corresponded to the level of obstruction seen on radioimaging techniques. Under direct laparoscopic observation, an attempt to place a retrograde catheter was unsuccessful, and so the nodule was excised. The left retroperitoneal space was entered at the pelvic brim. After all associated endometriosis, fibrosis, or adhesions were treated, the ureter was dissected (Figure 12-11). The nodule involved the

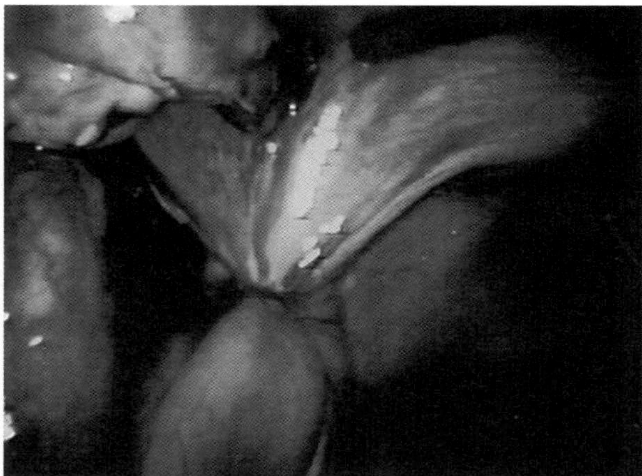

Figure 12-10. At laparoscopy, a 3-to 4-cm nodule was found over the left ureter about 4 cm above the bladder, distorting the course of the ureter.

entire thickness of the ureter; a partial resection was done (Figure 12-12).

Under cystoscopic guidance, a 7 French ureteral catheter was passed through the ureterovesical junction, at which level the ureter was excised. Indigo carmine was injected into the patient's intravenous line to ensure patency of the proximal ureter. The distal ureter was transected over the stent, and the obstructed portion was removed. The ureteral stent was introduced into the proximal ureter and advanced into the renal pelvis (Figure 12-13). Finally, the edges of the ureter were reapproximated with sutures. To accomplish anastomosis, four interrupted 4-0 polydioxanone sutures (PDS) were placed at 6, 12, 9, and 3 O'-clock to approximate the proximal and distal ureteral ostia (Figure 12-14). The patient went home the next day. The postoperative course was

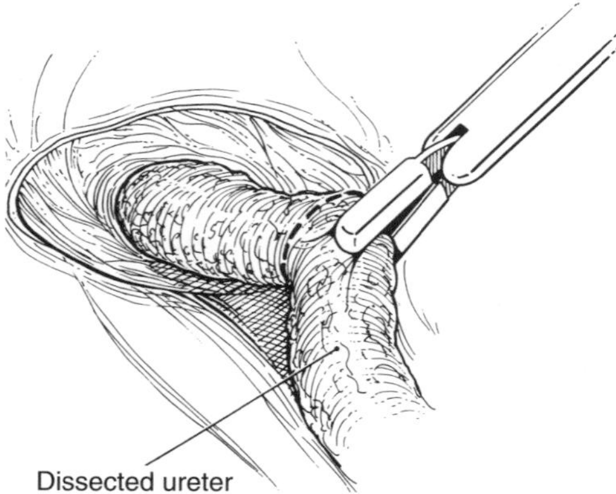

Figure 12-11. After all associated endometriosis, fibrosis, or adhesions were treated, the ureter was dissected with the CO_2 laser.

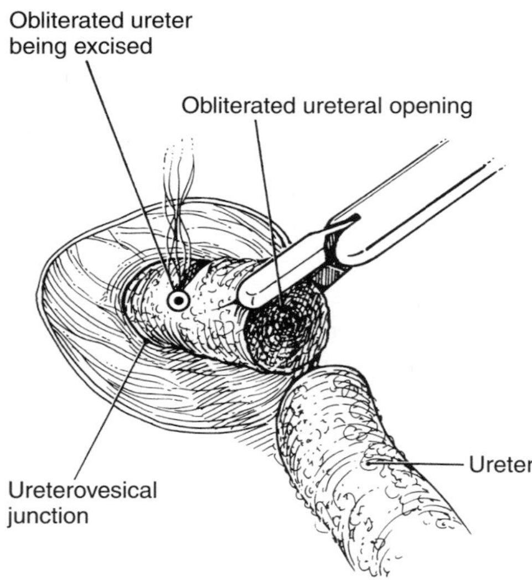

Figure 12-12. During dissection, it was discovered that the nodule involved the entire thickness of the ureter; a partial resection was done.

uncomplicated. An intravenous pyelogram (IVP) confirmed ureteral patency and renal function (Figure 12-15). Estimated blood loss was less than 100 mL, and the procedure lasted 117 minutes. The pathology report confirmed severe endometriosis and fibrosis of the resected ureter.

Since that time, 12 more patients with severe ureteral endometriosis have been treated in whom endometriosis and fibrosis caused partial or complete ureteral obstruction. All these patients had a known history of endometriosis and underwent different surgical and medical treatments. In four women, the ureteral endometriosis was removed completely without entering the ureteral lumen. In three women, the obstructed ureter required a complete segmental resection. One right and one left ureteroureterostomy and one anastomosis of the left ureter to the bladder (ureteroneocystostomy) were achieved, using four through-and-through interrupted 4.0 PDS to approximate the edges over the ureteral catheter. In five women, the ureter was involved partially. The severe retroperitoneal and ureteral endometriosis was excised or vaporized cautiously with the CO_2 laser until ureterotomy occurred.

In three women, the ureterotomy was very small and was detected by intravenous injection of indigo carmine. A ureteral stent was left in place, and no suture was required. In two patients, the ureterotomy was repaired using 4-0 PDS to overlap the laceration after stent placement. Histologic examination of the resected specimen revealed fibrosis, endometriosis, or both in all the women.

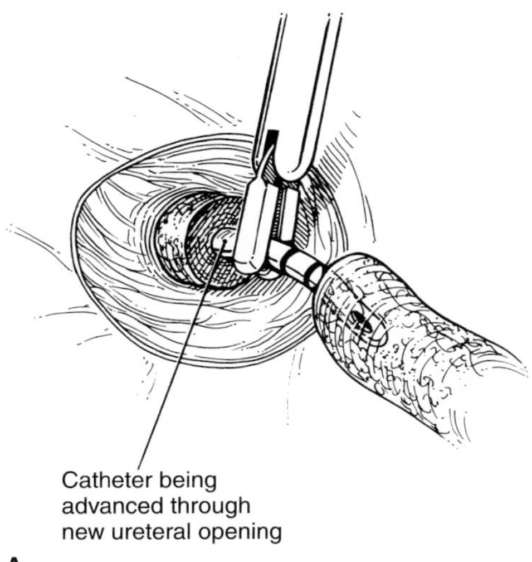

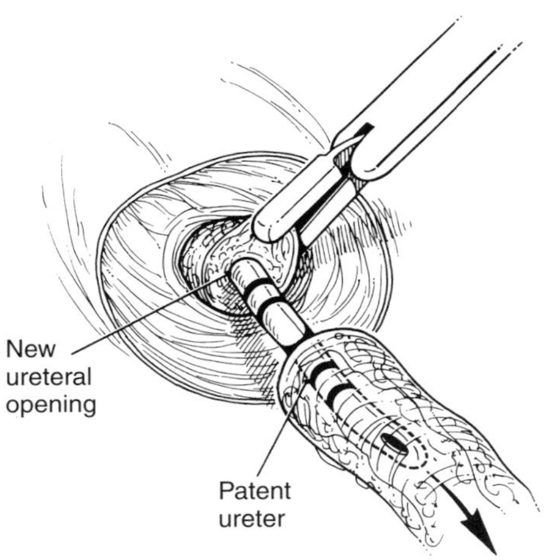

Figure 12-13. The ureteral stent was introduced into the proximal ureter and advanced into the renal pelvis.

A rare case of endometriosis with focal severely atypical hyperplasia was found in the specimen of a 46-year-old woman. She had undergone total abdominal hysterectomy and bilateral salpingo-oophorectomy followed by hormone replacement therapy at another institution. All the patients had an uneventful intra- and postoperative course and reported symptomatic relief of their symptoms. Imaging techniques revealed patent ureters with a functioning kidney in all these patients except one, a 24-year-old woman who had been diagnosed several months earlier with pelvic endometriosis that was treated partially at initial laparoscopy, followed by GnRH analog therapy postoperatively. During a second laparoscopy, she had severe left uterosacral, left pelvic side wall, and left ureteral endometriosis that had caused complete ureteral

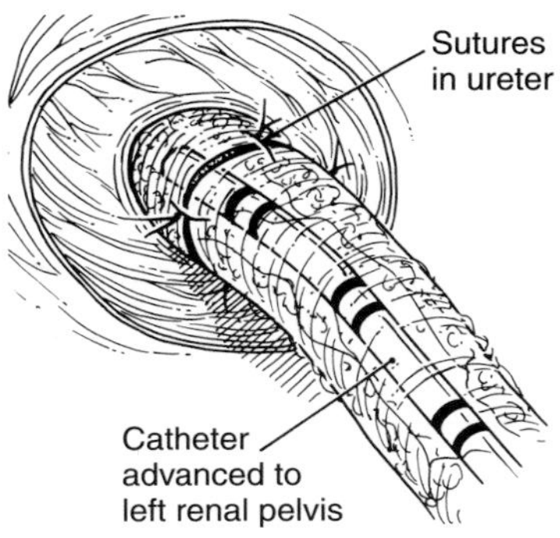

Figure 12-14. To do an anastomosis, four interrupted 4-0 polydioxanone sutures were placed at 6, 12, 9, and 3 o'clock to approximate the proximal and distal ureteral edges.

obstruction. Segmental resection and ureteroureterostomy were accomplished. Intraoperative intravenous injection of indigo carmine did not reveal any leakage from the ureter and raised the question of a nonfunctioning kidney. Postoperative follow-up and imaging revealed a 10 to 20% functioning kidney. However, the ureter was patent. In such cases, a ureteral stent is left in the ureter. This stent remains in place for approximately 2 months postoperatively. The patient's follow-up should include IVP, ultrasound, or excretion scans.

Vesical endometriosis

The bladder wall is one of the sites least frequently involved with endometriosis.[94] If the lesions are superficial, hydrodissection and vaporization, or

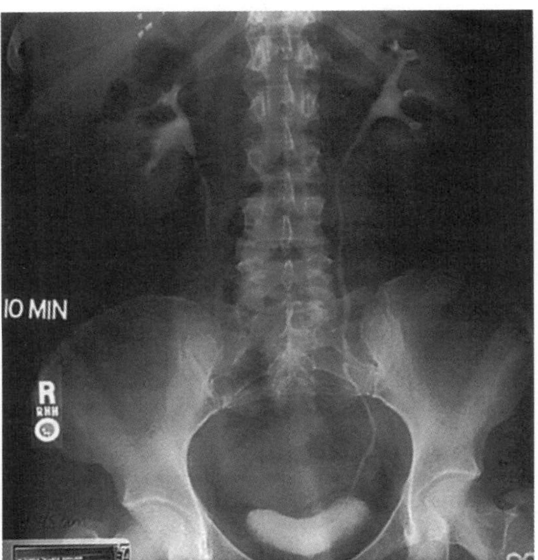

Figure 12-15. An IVP confirmed bilateral patency and renal function.

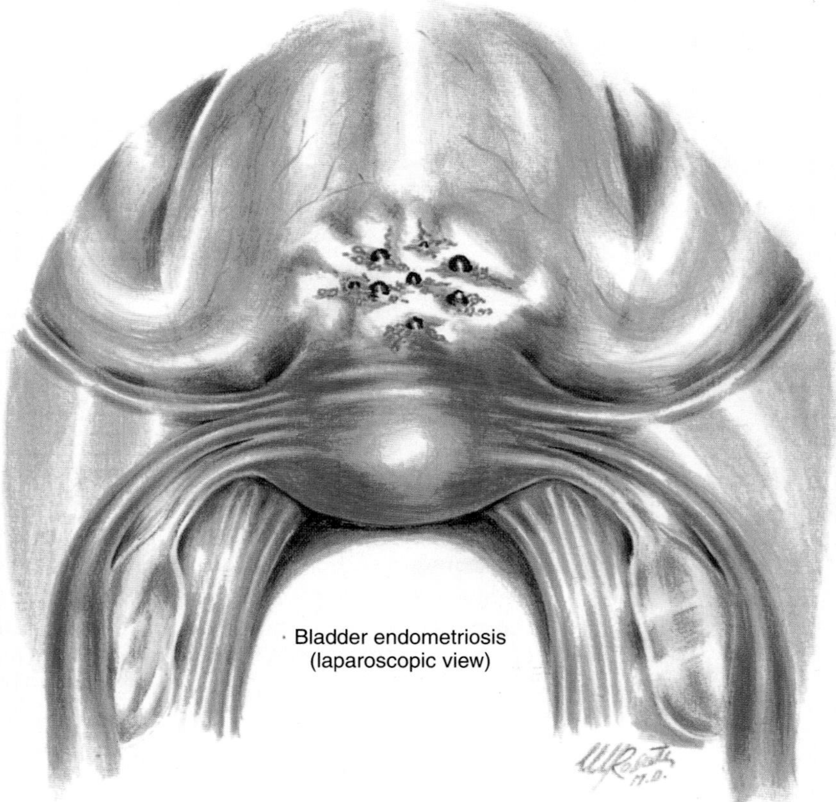

A

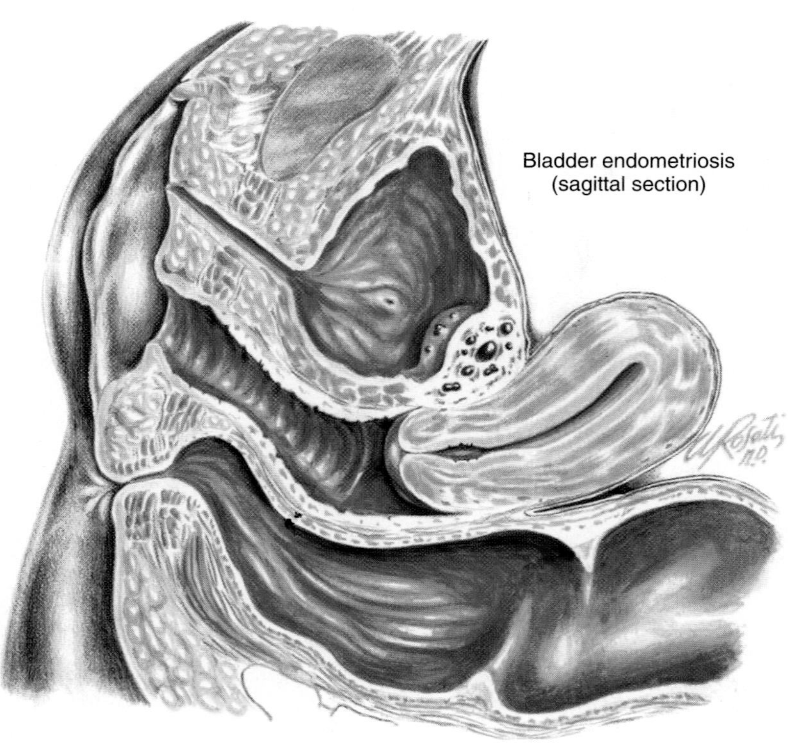

B

Figure 12-16. **A.** Endometriosis involves the anterior lower uterine segment and the bladder. The extent of vesical involvement cannot be ascertained from this view. **B.** The sagittal sections show that the muscularis and mucosal surface of the bladder are involved.

excision may be adequate for removal (Figure 12-16, A and B). Using hydrodissection, the areolar tissue between the serosa and muscularis beneath the implants is dissected. The lesion is circumcised, and fluid is injected into the resulting defect. The lesion is grasped with forceps and dissected. Frequent irrigation is necessary to remove char, ascertain the depth of vaporization or excision, and ensure that the lesion does not involve the muscularis and the mucosa.

Endometriosis extending to the muscularis but without mucosal involvement can be treated laparoscopically, and any residual or deeper lesions may be treated successfully with postoperative hormone therapy. When endometriosis involves full bladder wall thickness, the lesion is excised and the bladder is reconstructed.[99] Four cases of full-thickness bladder endometriosis were treated by excision and a one-layer reconstruction. The exposure seemed to be better than that at laparotomy. Simultaneous cystoscopy is performed, and bilateral ureteral catheters are inserted. The bladder dome is held near the midline with the grasping forceps, and the endometriotic nodule is excised 5 mm beyond the lesion (Figure 12-17). An incision is made. The specimen is removed from the abdominal cavity with a long grasping forceps through the operative channel of the laparoscope. CO_2 gas distends the bladder cavity, allowing excellent observation of its interior (Figure 12-18). After the ureters have been identified and the bladder mucosa have been examined again, the bladder is closed with several interrupted or continuous 4-0 polydioxanone through-and-through sutures, using extracorporeal or intracorporeal knotting (Figure 12-19). Cystoscopy is done to identify possible leaks. The duration of laparoscopic segmental cystectomy is approximately 35 minutes. Patients are discharged the following day and instructed to take trimethoprim-sulfamethoxazole for 2 weeks. The Foley catheter is removed 5 to 14 days later, depending on the

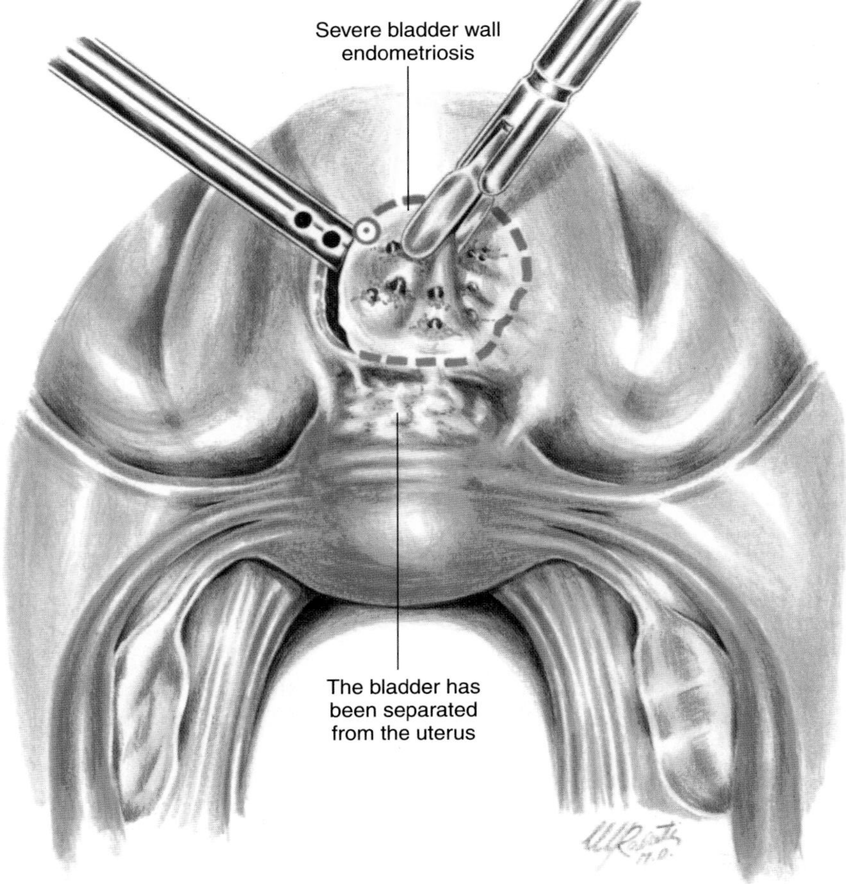

Figure 12-17. Endometriosis involving the bladder is being excised with the CO_2 laser after the bladder has been separated from the uterus. The lesion involves the full thickness of the bladder. Bilateral ureteral catheters were inserted during simultaneous cystoscopy. The endometrial implants were excised 5 mm beyond the lesion.

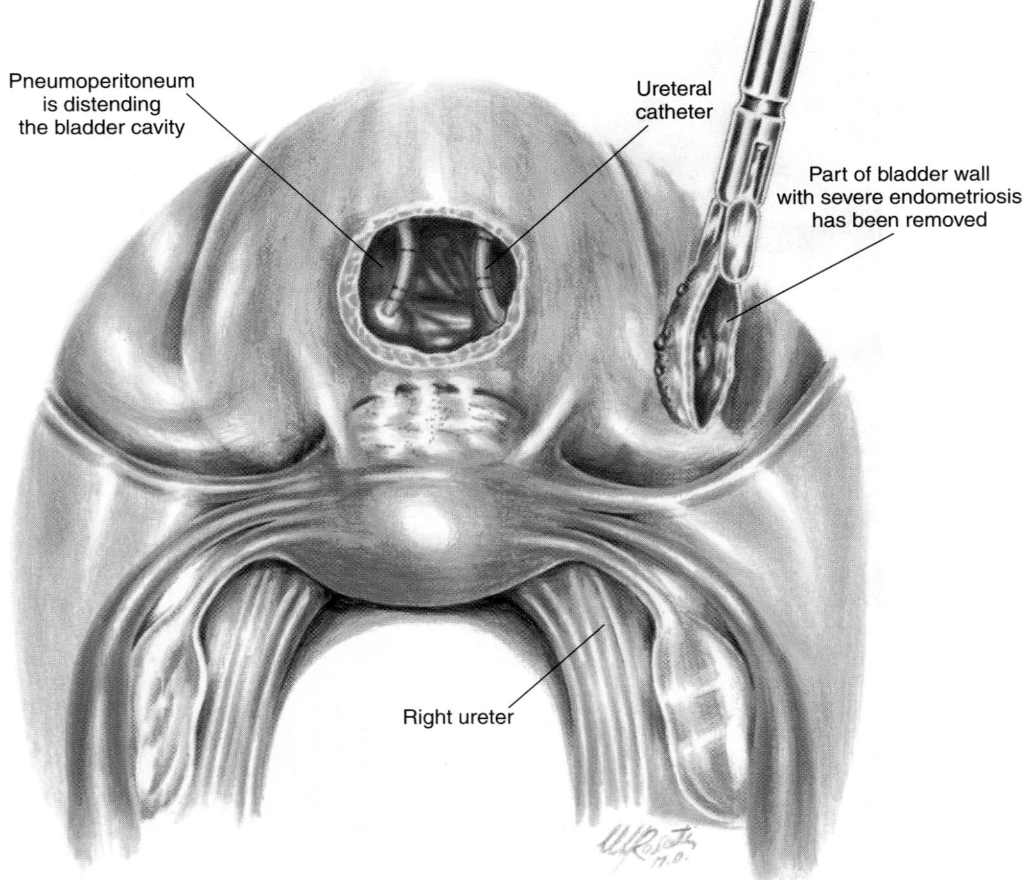

Figure 12-18. The lesion is be removed with a grasping forceps through a 10-mm trocar sleeve.

size of the lesion and condition of the tissue, and cystograms are done. Blood loss is minimal. In this group of four patients, the pathology report confirmed severe endometriosis and fibrosis of the resected bladder wall. No intraoperative or postoperative complications were noted. Ten to 13 months postoperatively, the women were doing well, with no menouria.

Gastrointestinal involvement

Gastrointestinal endometriosis was described in 1909 by Sampson[100] during the histologic examination of resected sigmoid colon that had been diagnosed intraoperatively as a carcinoma. The gastrointestinal tract is believed to be involved in 3 to 37% of women with endometriosis.[101,102] However, in a specialized practice, the number of patients with bowel involvement can be as high as 50% if patients with serosal and subserosal lesions are included. Endometrial implants may be found between the small intestine and the anal canal. The clinical presentation varies from an incidental finding at celiotomy to bowel obstruction.[103]

Severe endometriosis commonly involves the uterosacral ligaments, rectovaginal septum, and rectosigmoid colon with partial or complete posterior cul-de-sac obliteration. Patients can present with lower abdominal pain, back pain, dysmenorrhea, dyspareunia, diarrhea, constipation, tenesmus, and occasionally rectal bleeding.[101] Symptoms usually occur cyclically at or about the time of menstruation.

Intestinal endometriosis should be suspected in women of childbearing age who present with gastrointestinal symptoms and a history of endometriosis. Proctoscopy and colonoscopy are suggestive, but the lesions usually are not identified before laparoscopy. Although microscopic examination of the bowel mucosa may reveal endometrial glands, colonoscopic biopsy is usually not diagnostic.[104] In patients with severe symptoms,

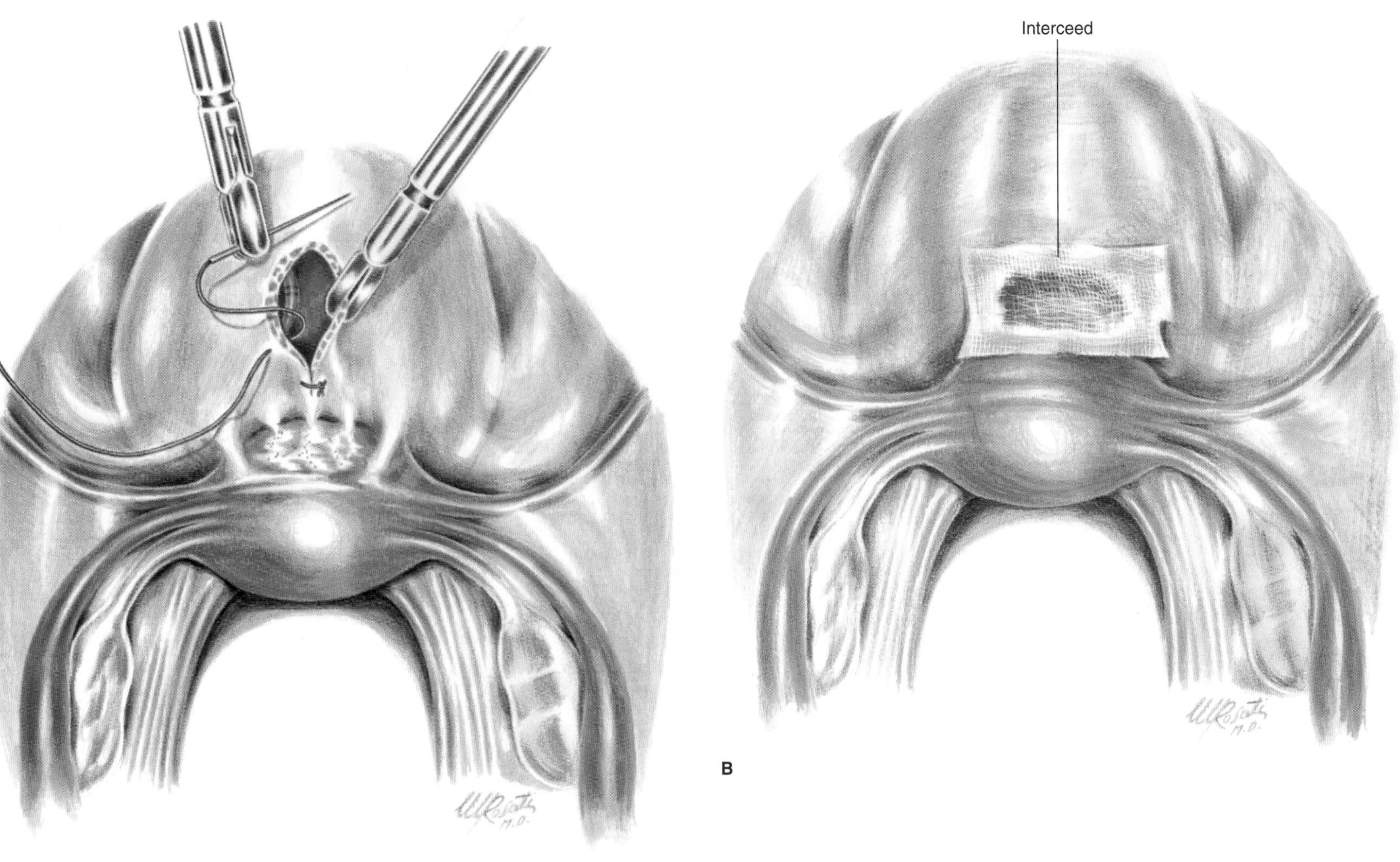

Figure 12-19. **A.** After the ureteral orifices and the ureteral catheters have been identified, the bladder is closed with several interrupted polydioxanone through-and-through sutures, using extracorporeal and intracorporeal knot tying. Cystoscopy in done to identify any leaks. **B.** The suture line is covered with Interceed.

medical therapy rarely yields satisfactory long-term results. Surgical intervention is necessary to dissect and resect infiltrating bowel endometriosis. These patients generally undergo videolaparoscopy after previous surgical or hormonal management fails to relieve their discomfort. Large bowel resection for obstructing endometriosis of the sigmoid colon was reported in 1909 by Mackenrodt.[105] Colonic resection has been shown to be safe with low morbidity, providing satisfactory pain relief and favorable pregnancy rates.[106]

Intestinal endometriosis involves the rectum and sigmoid colon in 76% of cases, the appendix in 18%, and the cecum in 5%. Operative laparoscopy is done to treat endometrial implants on the intestinal wall, appendix, and rectovaginal space.

Appendiceal endometriosis

Appendiceal lesions may be noted only by palpation, and so incidental appendectomy is recommended for patients with severe endometriosis.

Bowel resection

In patients who have severe disease of the bowel wall, resection may be necessary. Laparoscopically assisted anterior rectal wall resection and anastomosis were described in 1991 to treat symptomatic, infiltrative rectosigmoid endometriosis.[107,108] Preoperative mechanical and antibiotic bowel preparation is necessary. Three 5-mm suprapubic trocars are placed, one each in the midline and right and left lower quadrants for the insertion of grasping forceps, Endoloop suture applicators, a suction-irrigator probe, and a bipolar electrocoagulator.

The technique includes laparoscopic mobilization of the lower colon, transanal or transvaginal prolapse, resection, and anastomosis.[109-112] When the lesion involves only the anterior rectal wall near the anal verge, the rectovaginal septum is delineated by simultaneous vaginal and rectal examinations effected by an assistant. The rectum is mobilized along the rectovaginal septum anteriorly to within 2 cm of the anus. Mobilization continues along the left and right pararectal spaces by electrodesiccating and dividing branches of the hemorrhoidal artery and partially posteriorly. When the rectum is mobilized sufficiently, the tumor is prolapsed vaginally or anally and the nodule is excised. Two staple applications may be required to traverse the width of the involved mucosa. The rectum is returned to the pelvis under direct observation, and closure is confirmed by insufflating the rectum while the cul-de-sac is filled with lactated Ringer's solution.

In patients with circumferential lesions, the entire rectum is mobilized, the lateral rectal pedicles are electrocoagulated, and the presacral space is entered to the level of the levator ani muscles to allow mobilization of the bowel. The branches of the inferior mesenteric vessels of the bowel segment to be resected are coagulated and cut. The rectum is transected proximal to the lesion, and the proximal limb is either prolapsed vaginally or into the distal limb, using Babcock clamps (Figure 12-20). A 2-0 purse-string suture is inserted to the end of the proximal bowel to secure the opposing anvil of a no. 29 or 33 ILA stapler (Ethicon) (Figure 12-21). The anvil is replaced transanally or transvaginally into the pelvis along with the proximal bowel.

The rectal stump, containing the endometrial lesion, is prolapsed through the anal canal or vagina and transected proximal to the lesion, using

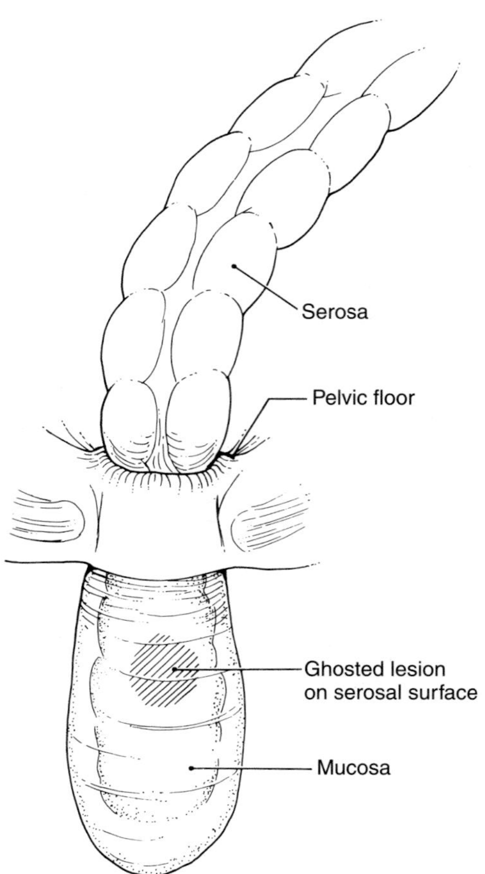

Figure 12-20. In patients with circumferential lesions, the rectum is transected distal to the lesion and the proximal limb is prolapsed into the distal bulb.

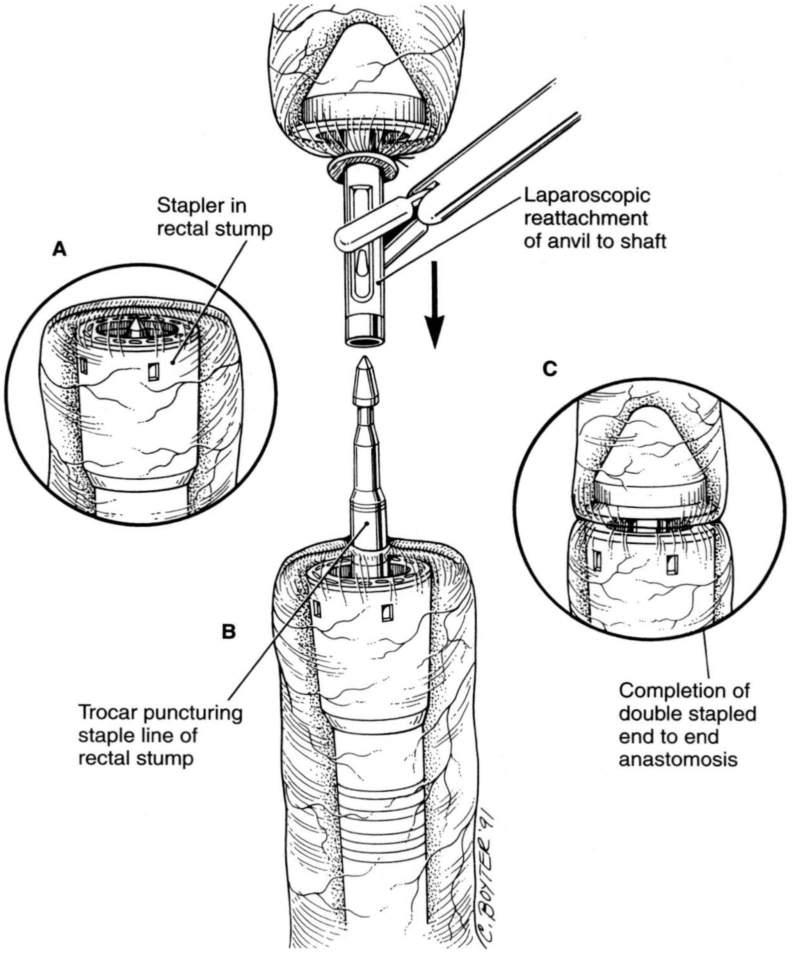

Figure 12-21. **A.** The ILS stapler is placed into the rectum. **B.** The anvil trocar within the proximal bowel is inserted into the stapling device, using the laparoscope. **C.** The device is fired, creating an end-to-end anastomosis.

an RL60 linear stapler [Ethicon] (Figure 12-22). The resected segment is sent for pathologic diagnosis. The rectal stump is replaced through the anal canal or vagina into the pelvis. The ILS stapler is placed into the rectum, and the anvil in the proximal limb of the bowel is inserted into the stapling device by using the laparoscope. The device is fired, creating an end-to-end anastomosis. A proctoscope is used to examine the anastomosis for structural integrity and bleeding. The pelvis is filled with lactated Ringer's solution and observed with the laparoscope as the rectum is insufflated with air to check for leakage. Air leaks can be corrected with 2-0 polyglactin sutures placed transanally. This technique is identical to resection at laparotomy.[113]

Another method utilizes a 60-mm Endostapler (Ethicon) to resect the bowel intraabdominally. The Endostapler is fired distal to the lesion. The proximal limb of the colon is delivered from the abdomen and exteriorized through a small (2–4 cm) incision. The lesion is amputated, and the anvil of the stapler is inserted in the lumen after the placement of a purse-string suture. At this stage, anastomosis is completed with the stapler gun.

Another method to treat severe disease of the anterior wall of the colon eliminates stapling devices.[114] The extent of the lesion is evaluated visually and by palpation, using the tip of the suction-irrigator probe. If the lesion is low enough, an assistant can identify it by doing a rectal examination. A sigmoidoscope is used to further delineate the lesion and guide the surgeon. After the ureters are identified to avoid inadvertent injury, the lower colon is mobilized in all aspects except posteriorly. Depending on the location of the lesion, the right or left pararectal area is entered, and the colon is separated from the adjacent organs. Full-thickness shaving excision, if necessary, is carried out, beginning above the area of visible disease. After the normal tissue is identified, the lesion is

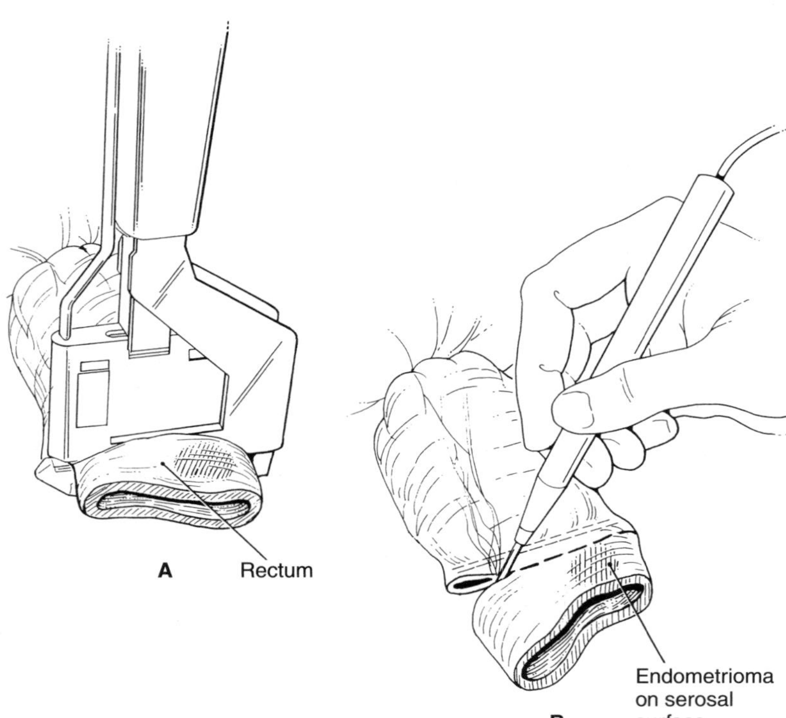

Figure 12-22. The rectal stump, containing the endometrial lesion, is prolapsed through the anal canal. **A.** The RL60 linear stapler is applied. **B.** Using a sharper electrosurgical knife (Ethicon), the rectal stump is transected proximal to the lesion.

held at its proximal end with grasping forceps. An incision is made through the bowel serosa and muscularis, and the lumen is entered. The lesion is excised entirely from the anterior rectal wall. After complete excision of the lesion, the pelvic cavity is irrigated and suctioned. Debris is extracted through the operative channel of the laparoscope by using a long grasping forceps or from the anus by using polyp forceps and submitted for pathology. The bowel is repaired transversely in one layer. Two traction sutures are applied to each side of the defect, transforming it to a transverse opening (Figure 12-23, A through D). The stay sutures are brought out through the right and left lower quadrant trocar sleeves. The sleeves are removed and then replaced in the peritoneal cavity next to the stay sutures, and the sutures are secured outside the abdomen. The bowel is repaired by placing several interrupted through-and-through sutures in 0.4- to 0.6-cm increments until it is completely anastomosed (Figure 12-24). Polyglactin or polydioxanone sutures with a straight needle (Ethicon) and extracorporeal knot tying are used. At the end of the procedure, sigmoidoscopy is done to ensure that the closure is watertight and that there is no bowel stricture. As an alternative, at times it is possible to excise the nodule and staple it; the defect closes simultaneously by articulated vascular staplers.

Cul-de-sac restoration

Cul-de-sac obliteration, which is common among patients with severe endometriosis and pain, suggests rectovaginal involvement with deep endometriosis and dense adhesions and significant distortion of the regional anatomy involving the bowel, vaginal apex, posterior cervix, ureter, and major blood vessels (Figure 12-25). Transrectal ultrasonography is sensitive and specific for diagnosing the presence of rectovaginal endometriosis.[115] In one study, infiltration of the rectal and vaginal walls was identified correctly in all the patients in whom it was present, but rectal infiltration in three women was not confirmed by the surgeon and the pathologic specimen. Rectal endoscopic ultrasonography was shown by other researchers to provide a reliable indication of the presence of deep bowel infiltration in patients with retroperitoneal endometriotic lesions.[116] The preoperative use of endoscopic ultrasonography as a diagnostic instrument may facilitate preparing a patient for laparoscopic surgery.

Cul-de-sac restoration should not be attempted by an inexperienced laparoscopist or a gynecologist unfamiliar with bowel and urinary tract operations. Most of these situations involve the rectum and the rectovaginal spectrum and do not require bowel resection. To aid in identifying anatomic

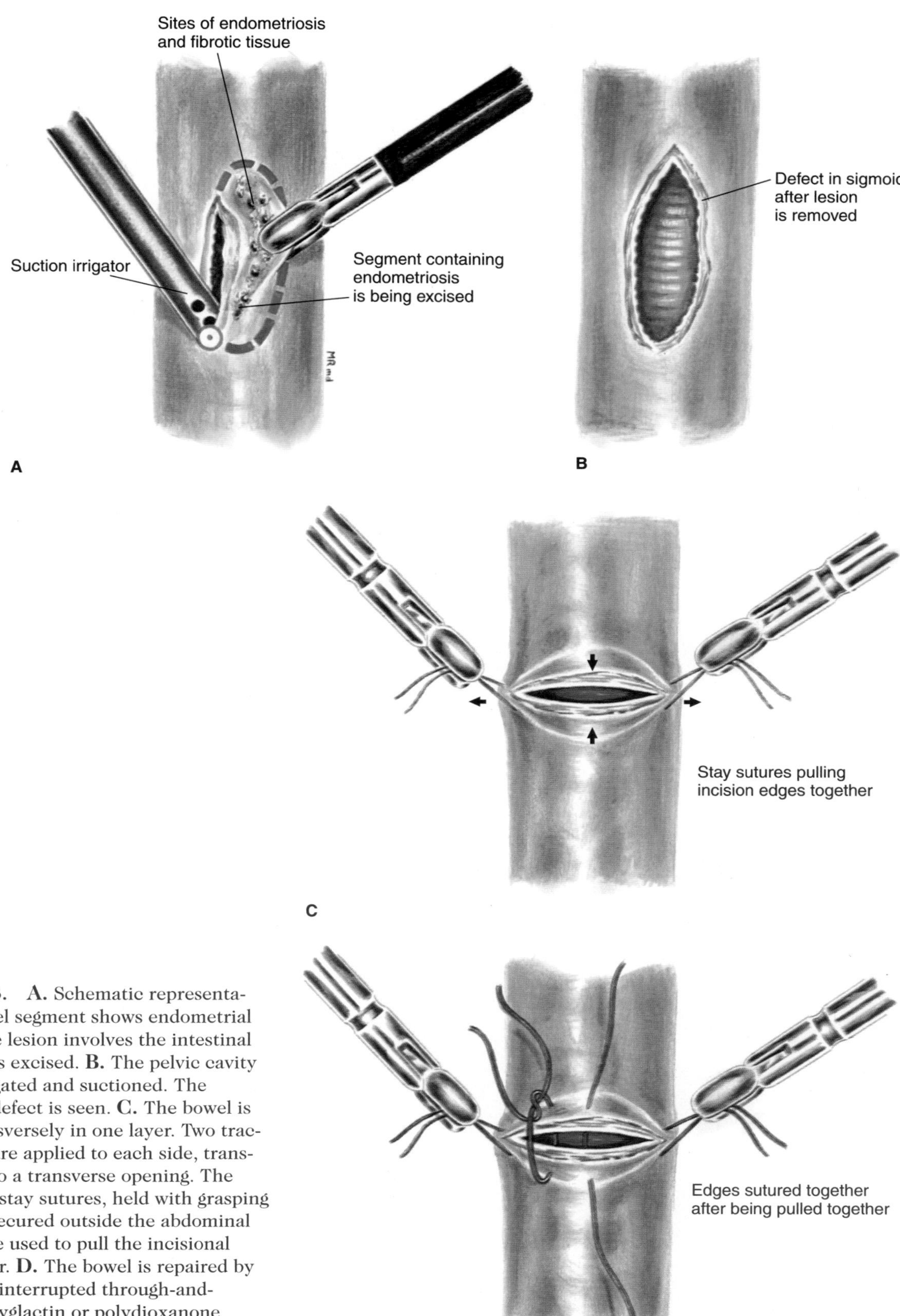

Figure 12-23. **A.** Schematic representation of a bowel segment shows endometrial implants. The lesion involves the intestinal mucosa and is excised. **B.** The pelvic cavity has been irrigated and suctioned. The longitudinal defect is seen. **C.** The bowel is repaired transversely in one layer. Two traction sutures are applied to each side, transforming it into a transverse opening. The right and left stay sutures, held with grasping forceps, are secured outside the abdominal cavity and are used to pull the incisional edges together. **D.** The bowel is repaired by using several interrupted through-and-through 0 polyglactin or polydioxanone sutures on a straight needle. Extracorporeal knot tying is used.

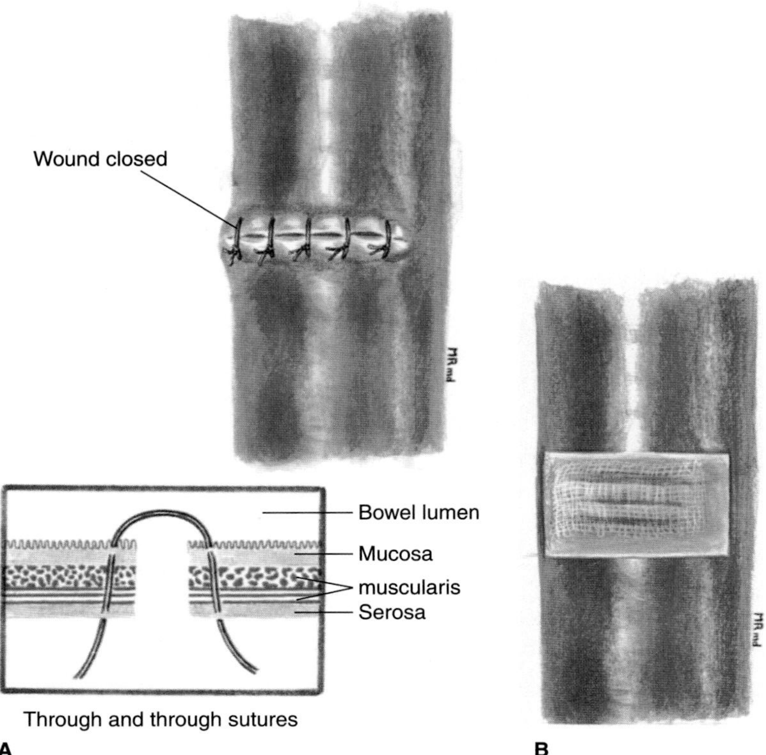

Figure 12-24. **A.** The wound has been closed. At the end of the operation, sigmoidoscopy is done to ensure that the closure is watertight and that there is no bowel stricture. The inset shows the through-and-through suture technique to close the defect. **B.** Interceed has been applied to cover the suture line.

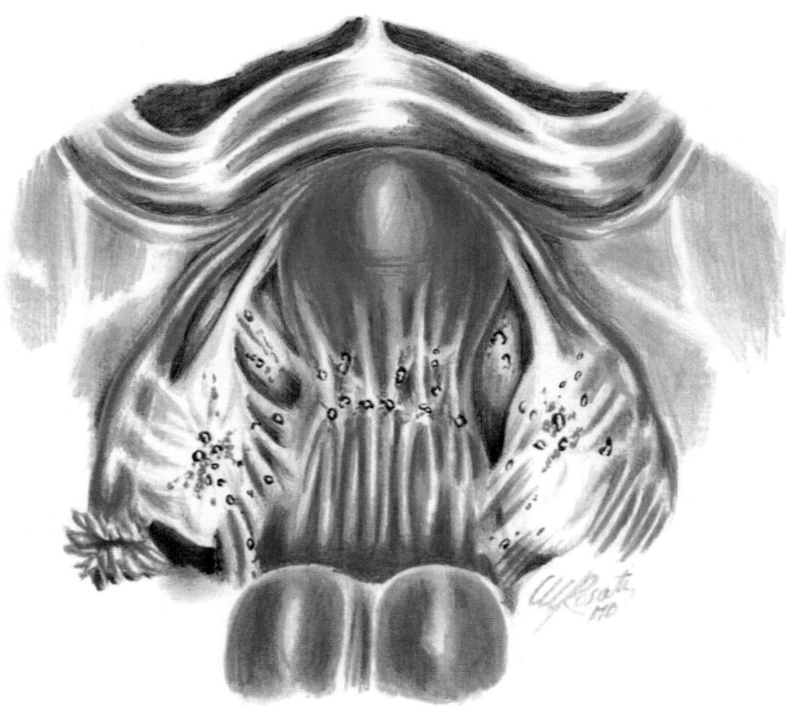

Figure 12-25. **A.** Diffuse endometriosis involves the posterior cul-de-sac and both ovaries associated with dense periadnexal adhesions.

Figure 12-25. (*Continued*) **B.** Sagittal view reveals obliteration of the posterior fornix with cul-de-sac nodularity and dense adhesions between the rectum and uterus. **C.** Dissection and resection of these nodularities require an assistant to palpate them to assure their removal. The inset shows endometrial implants on the posterior vaginal wall.

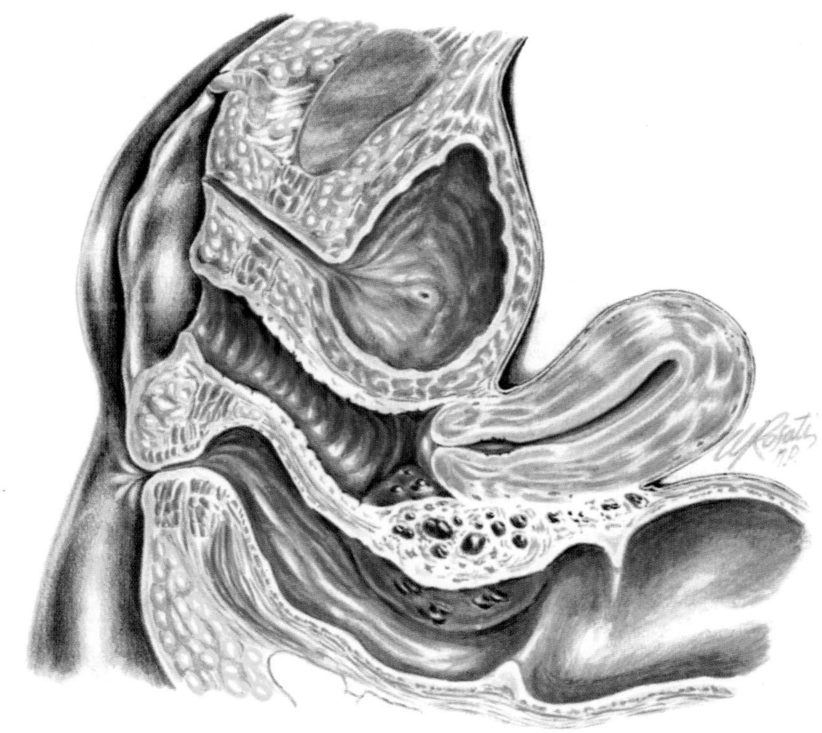

B

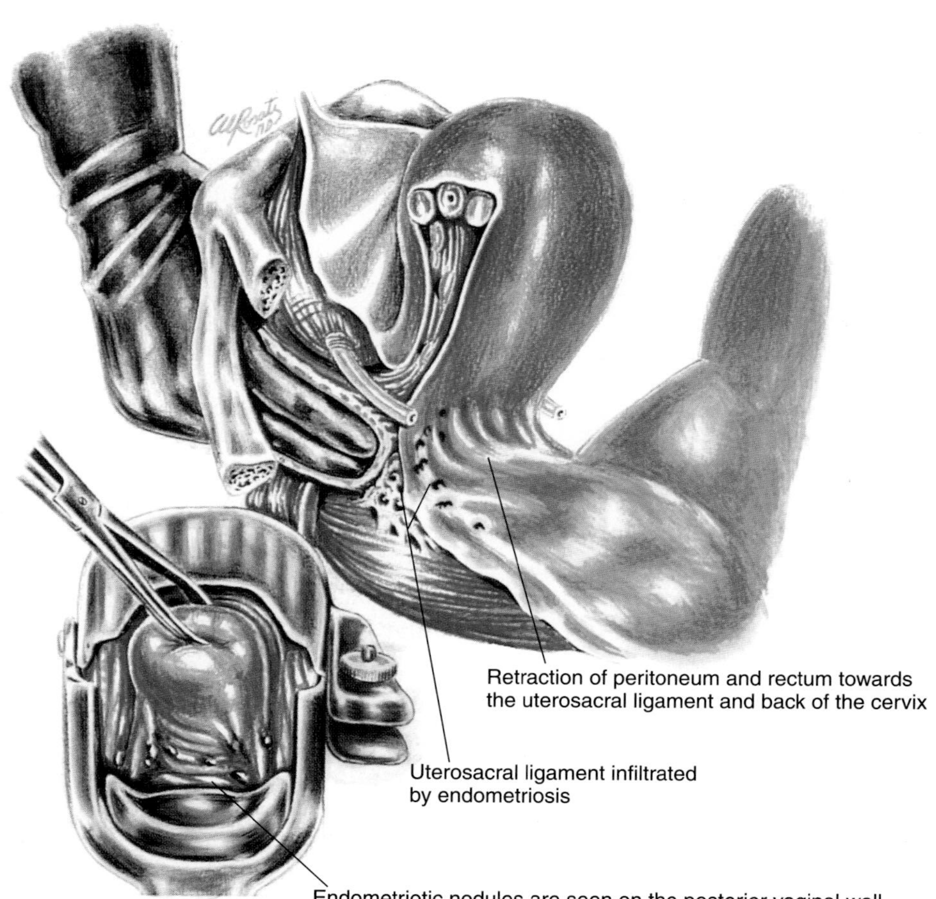

C

landmarks and tissue planes, an assistant stands between the patient's legs and does a rectovaginal examination with one hand while holding the uterus up with a rigid uterine elevator. An uninvolved area of peritoneum is identified and injected with 5 to 8 mL of diluted vasopressin (10 U in 100 mL of lactated Ringer's solution) with an 18-gauge laparoscopic needle. Using the CO_2 laser, scissors, electrosurgical knife, needle, or harmonic scalpel the peritoneal adhesions are cut. With the high-power CO_2 laser and hydrodissection, the rectum attached to the uterosacral ligaments and the back of the cervix is separated. If rectal involvement is more extensive, a sigmoidoscope can be used to guide the surgeon and rule out bowel perforation. After complete separation of the rectum, lesions on the rectum or rectovaginal septum are removed or vaporized (Figure 12-26). The cul-de-sac is filled with irrigation fluid and is observed through the laparoscope while air is introduced into the rectum through the sigmoidoscope. Air bubbles observed in the cul-de-sac fluid indicate perforation. As the assistant guides the gynecologist by doing a rectovaginal examination, the rectum is freed from the back of the cervix. Generalized oozing or bleeding is controlled with an injection of 3 to 5 mL vasopressin solution (1 ampule in 100 mL of lactated Ringer's solution), laser, or bipolar electrocoagulator. Bleeding from the stalk vessels caused by dissection or vaporization of the fibrotic uterosacral ligaments and pararectal area is controlled with a bipolar electrocoagulator, clips or sutures.

The ureters are usually lateral to the uterosacral ligaments. If the dissection is extended lateral to the uterosacral ligaments, the ipsilateral ureter should be identified by opening the overlying peritoneum and tracing it to the area of the lesion. The ureter, uterine arteries, and uterine veins are exposed. Bipolar forceps or hemoclips must be available and fully functional to control unexpected bleeding.

For patients who have posterior cul-de-sac nodularity and infiltration of endometriosis toward the vagina, dissection and resection of the nodularity continue as an assistant palpates the nodule to ensure its removal.[117–119] Endometriosis rarely penetrates the mucosa of the colon but commonly involves the serosa, subserosa, and muscularis. When significant portions of both muscularis layers have been excised or vaporized and the mucosa is reached, the bowel wall is reinforced by interrupted 4-0 PDS. The procedure requires maximal coordination between the assistant and the surgeon.

When the rectovaginal space is dissected and hemostasis is accomplished, the pelvis is filled with lactated Ringer's solution to observe the cul-de-sac and the area of dissection under water. This magnifies and clarifies the dissected tissue to help identify residual disease, verify the intact anatomy of the ureters and bowel, and coagulate small bleeders. The raw surfaces of the rectum or cul-de-sac are not reperitonealized because several studies have demonstrated that reperitonealization is not necessary and promotes adhesion formation.[75,76,101,102]

This procedure was accomplished in 185 women age 25 to 41 years. Eighty patients had complete posterior cul-de-sac obliteration. All were managed successfully by laparoscopy and discharged within 24 hours except for nine patients with bowel perforation and one with a partial bowel resection, who were discharged after 2 to 4 days. The procedures lasted from 55 to 245 minutes. Among 185 patients, 174 were available for follow-up after 1 to 5 years. Moderate to complete pain relief was observed in 162 of 174 patients (93%). Thirteen (8%) required two procedures, and four required three procedures. Twelve (7%) had persistent or worse pain postoperatively.[120]

In a series of 356 women who underwent laparoscopic treatment of bowel endometriosis with different techniques, 2 patients required intraoperative laparotomy early in the authors' experience. The first patient underwent laparotomy for repair of enterotomy after treatment of infiltrative rectal endometriosis. The other patient required laparotomy for anastomosis after an unsuccessful attempt to place a purse-string suture around the patulous rectal ampulla. Significant postoperative complications occurred in 1.7% of these patients. Two women developed leaks and pelvic infections. One required a temporary laparoscopic colostomy with subsequent takedown and repair, and one was managed with prolonged drainage. One woman had a bowel stricture requiring resection and anastomosis by laparotomy. One developed a pelvic abscess and subsequently underwent laparoscopic right salpingo-oophorectomy. One patient had an immediate rectal prolapse that was reduced without surgical management. Her original bowel symptoms persisted, and she finally had a colectomy.

Minor complications included skin ecchymosis, temporary urinary retention, temporary diarrhea or constipation, and dyschezia. Donnez and coworkers[117] described a series of 500 women who underwent a laparoscopic procedure with exci-

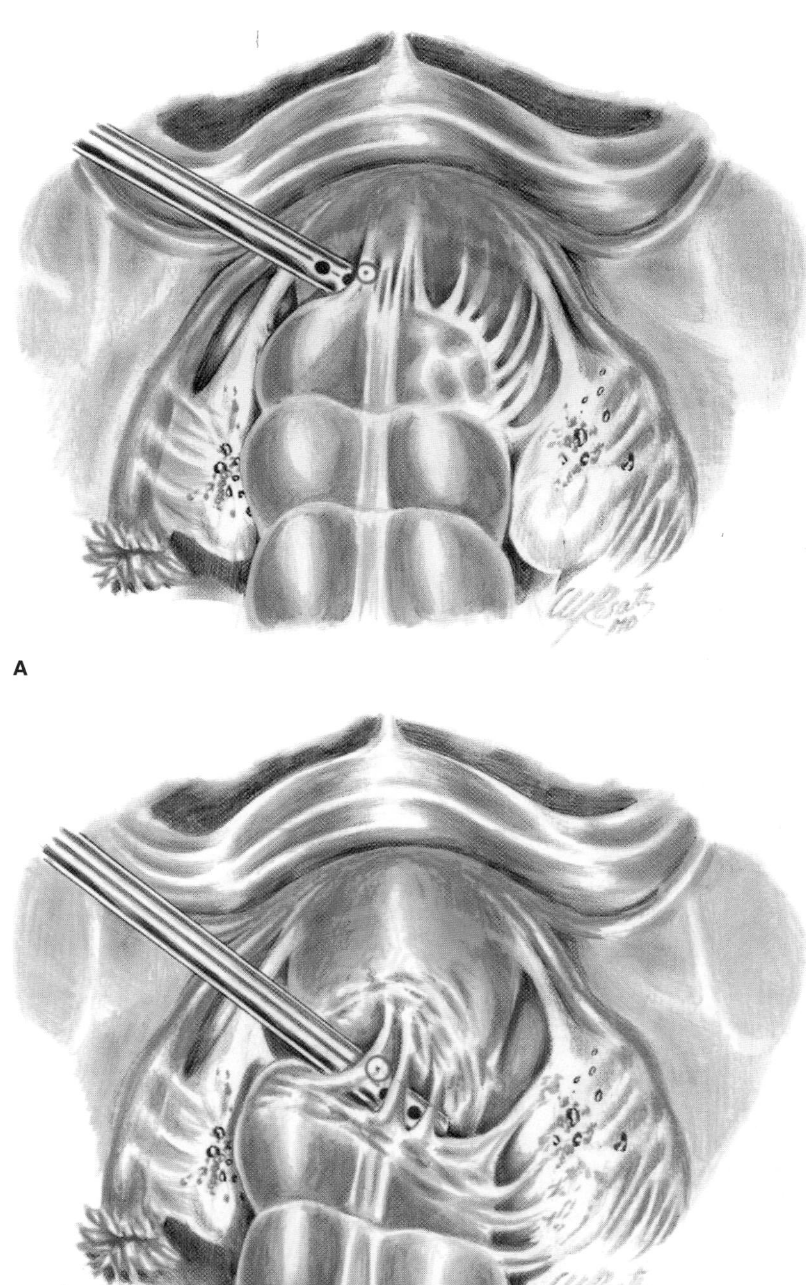

Figure 12-26. **A.** Adherent sigmoid is removed from the posterior aspect of the uterus. The probe serves as a backstop for the laser, for irrigation, and to put the adhesions on stretch. **B.** The dissection continues.

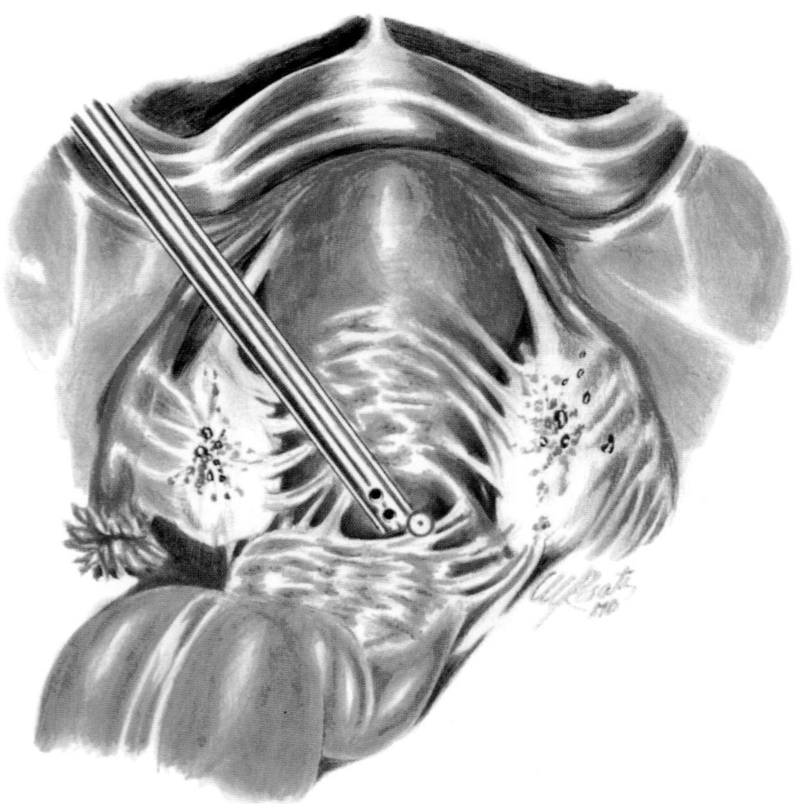

C

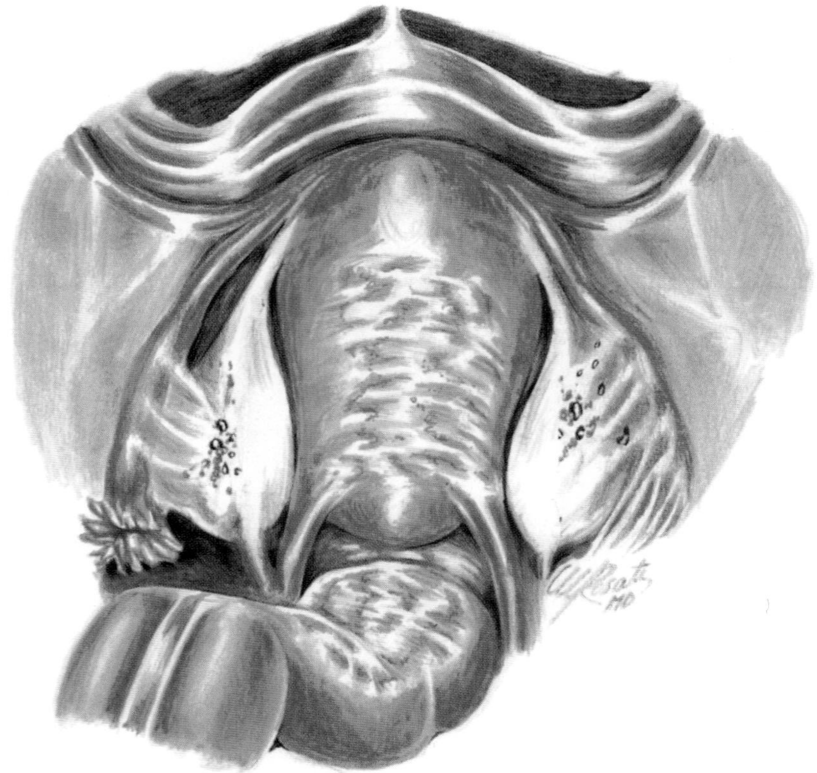

D

Figure 12-26. (*Continued*) **C.** Adhesiolysis proceeds until the back of the cervix and the uterosacral ligaments come into view. **D.** The rectosigmoid colon is mobilized, and most of the adhesions have been removed.

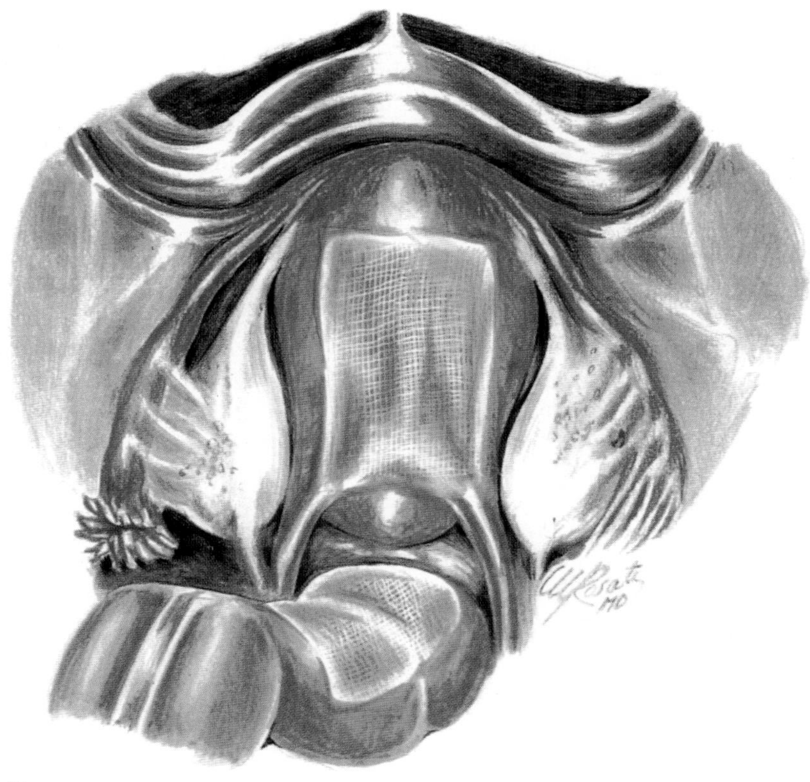

E

Figure 12-26. (*Continued*) **E.** Interceed has been placed over the raw surfaces.

sion of deep fibrotic endometriotic nodules of the rectovaginal septum for pelvic pain or infertility. Excision of the endometriotic nodules resulted in considerable pain relief. Histologically, the rectovaginal nodule was similar to an adenomyoma, as it was a circumscribed nodular aggregate of smooth muscle and endometrial glands and stroma. The variations in estrogen receptor and progesterone receptor content suggested a regulatory mechanism different from that of eutopic endometrium. On the basis of these observations, the authors suggested that nodules of the rectovaginal septum should be considered an entity distinct from peritoneal and ovarian endometriosis and originating from the müllerian rests present in the rectovaginal septum.[121]

Diaphragmatic endometriosis

The diaphragm rarely is a reported site of endometriosis.[122] Women should be asked about pleuritic, shoulder, or upper abdominal pain occurring with menses because they do not make the connection between these distant anatomic landmarks. The laparoscope is excellent for diagnosing and possibly treating endometriosis on the diaphragm that is difficult to reach by laparotomy.[123]

Before diaphragmatic endometriosis is treated by laparotomy or laparoscopy, other options are discussed with the patient because an operation at this location can injure the diaphragm, phrenic nerve, lungs, or heart.

For women interested in preserving their reproductive organs, medical treatment should be administered. If the patient does not want to preserve her reproductive organs, bilateral oophorectomy may relieve her symptoms and further intervention may not be necessary. However, if she does want to preserve her fertility potential and symptoms are not responsive to medical therapy, surgical intervention can be attempted after all possible complications have been discussed.

Most implants are superficial and cause no discomfort. Symptomatic diaphragmatic lesions were found in 8 of 4875 patients at our center. Most women prefer bilateral salpingo-oophorectomy, and so it rarely is necessary to treat these implants surgically. Others benefit from medical therapy, and the chance of recurrence on the diaphragm is low.

Endoscopic treatment begins by introducing a 10-mm laparoscope at the umbilical port and placing three additional trocars in the upper quadrant (right or left, according to implant location), similar to the arrangement for laparoscopic cholecystectomy. Two grasping forceps are used to push the liver from the operative field and allow better exposure of the diaphragm. Lesions are removed with hydrodissection and vaporization or excision. If a diaphragmatic defect is formed, it is repaired with 4-0 PDS or staples.

After the procedure, the patient should be evaluated by a cardiopulmonary consultant. The pharynx, larynx, and trachea are examined with a rigid bronchoscope. A flexible scope is introduced to examine the distal trachea and proximal main bronchi. Symptomatic diaphragmatic endometriosis implants were treated in eight women at our center. In three patients, the lesions were directly over the phrenic nerve or the diaphragmatic vasculature. The lesions were excised in three, and vaporization was accomplished in three others. In one patient, the lesion was treated by combined laser and ultrasound [Cavitational Ultrasonographic Surgical Aspirator (CUSA), Valley Lab, Boulder, CO]. In the remaining patient, only a bilateral salpingo-oophorectomy was done. No intraoperative or postoperative complications were noted. Six patients were without pain 6 to 36 months later. In one woman, the pain returned after 1 year, and another experienced no significant pain relief. Both responded to hormone suppressive therapy.

Experience with 24 women with endometriosis of the diaphragm was summarized.[124] Operative findings in 17 patients included two to five spots of endometriosis on the diaphragm measuring < 1 cm. Some women had numerous lesions scattered across the diaphragm. Lesions were bilateral in 8 patients, limited to the right hemidiaphragm in 14 patients, and limited to the left hemidiaphragm in 2 patients. In seven patients, six endometriosis lesions were directly in the line of the left ventricle and three lesions were adjacent to the phrenic nerve. Endometriosis was infiltrating into the muscular layer of the diaphragm in seven patients. The symptoms in all seven symptomatic patients decreased significantly after treatment, with a minimal follow-up period of 12 months. No postoperative complications occurred.

Restoration of Tubo-Ovarian Anatomy

Once all lesions are resected or ablated and the adnexa are freed of adhesions, the anatomic relation between the ovary and ipsilateral tube is evaluated and any distortion caused by adhesions is corrected. The mesosalpinx often adheres to the ovarian cortex along the ampullary segment of the tube. These adhesions cover a significant part of the surface of the ovarian cortex and can interfere with the ovulatory process at oocyte release. Moreover, the fimbriae frequently are agglutinated, inhibiting their ability to capture the oocyte. Adhesiolysis along the ovarian surface and mesosalpinx can be accomplished, the ovary and tube are grasped with atraumatic forceps and pulled apart, and the plane between them is dissected with a laser, electrode, or scissors. However, fimbrial adhesions should be resected with laparoscopic microscissors only under water or with an ultrapulse CO_2 laser with high millijoules. Adhesiolysis effected under water offers a clearer view of the anatomy than is provided with the pneumoperitoneum alone. The pelvis is filled with lactated Ringer's solution to allow the fimbriae to float freely in the clear fluid away from each other and from the filmy adhesions. The lighter fimbriae float higher and separate from the normal tissue. As they float away from the fimbrial folds, adhesions are grasped with a fine forceps and atraumatically divided with microscissors without bleeding or injury to the normal tissues.

Relief of Pain

Besides infertility, the most common complaint of patients with endometriosis is pain, usually in the pelvis, frequently worse at menses and occasionally during coital activity. The classic symptom triad of infertility, dysmenorrhea, and dyspareunia, although not diagnostic of endometriosis, strongly suggests the disease. Focal or localized pain associated with endometriosis usually responds to removal or destruction of endometriosis and associated adhesions. However, in some women, the pain is disproportionate to the extent of the disease or does not improve after resection of endometriosis and adhesions. For intractable or diffuse pain, interruption of pelvic nerves by uterosacral resection or presacral neurectomy is advised.[125–127]

Sutton and coworkers[128] were able to assess in a prospective, randomized, double-blind controlled clinical study the efficacy of laser laparoscopic operations in the treatment of pain associated with minimal, mild, and moderate endometriosis. At the time of laparoscopy, they randomized 63 patients with pain (dysmenorrhea, pelvic pain, or dyspareunia) and minimal to moderate endometriosis to laser ablation of endometriotic deposits and laparoscopic uterine nerve ablation or expectant management. The study was unique, since both the women and nurse who assessed them postoperatively were unaware of the treatment. The study showed that laser laparoscopy results in significant pain relief compared with expectant management 6 months postoperatively. Among the patients treated by laser laparoscopy, 62.5% reported improvement or resolution of symptoms, compared with 22.6% in the expectant group. Results were poorest for those with minimal disease, and if patients with mild and moderate disease only are included, 73.7% of the patients achieved pain relief. There were no operative or laser complications in this series. A long-term follow-up of this study revealed that symptom relief continued at 1 year in 90% of those who initially responded.[129] All symptomatic controls had a second-look procedure, which showed disease progression in 7 (29%), disease regression in 7 (29%), and 10 (42%) with static disease. The benefits of laser laparoscopy for painful pelvic endometriosis continue in the majority of patients at 1 year. In most untreated patients, painful endometriosis progresses or remains static, but it may spontaneously improve in others.

Minimizing Recurrences

The surgical treatment of endometriosis involves destroying endometrial implants (coagulation, vaporization, resection) and associated adhesions, and restoring normal anatomy. The anatomic, physiologic, and genetic factors that predispose each patient to developing endometriosis are not altered by the treatment. Therefore, recurrence is unavoidable unless endometrial proliferation, menstruation, or the predominantly estrogenic environment of the patient is altered. For those who desire pregnancy, an early success will be therapeutic since the 9-month gestational period, besides precluding menstrual flow, results in a predominantly progestational medium that reduces endometrial proliferation and the extent of disease. Patients who do not desire pregnancy have an increased risk of earlier recurrence and may benefit from preventive measures targeted at decreasing known risk factors, such as short length of menstrual cycles, lack of exercise, menorrhagia, and outflow obstruction. Müllerian anomalies that predispose a patient to outflow obstruction should be corrected.[130] Postoperatively, exercise and hormone therapy (progestational agents or low-dose oral contraceptives) are suggested. For the first 9 months postoperatively, medroxyprogesterone (Provera) 30 mg daily is ordered to induce amenorrhea in more than 75% of patients and regression of residual disease.[131] Continuous oral contraceptive pills may be prescribed for certain patients. In using the Provera regimen, a change to low-dose oral contraceptives can cause hypomenorrhea and can be therapeutic. If symptoms recur, medroxyprogesterone acetate therapy or a GnRH analog can control pain. Second-look laparoscopy may be necessary to treat recurrent or persistent endometriosis. Supracervical hysterectomy is not advisable for patients with severe endometriosis because persistent pelvic pain subsequently requires the removal of the cervical stump.

Future Development

New developments in fiberoptic endoscopes with diameters less than 1 mm have enabled a gynecologist to diagnose and stage the disease in an office setting under local anesthesia, possibly at earlier stages. Further development of laser surgery and photodynamic therapy may make therapeutic microendoscopy possible in an office setting.[132] Manyak and colleagues[132] conducted experiments evaluating photodynamic therapy for endometriosis using rabbit endometrial implants. After the intravenous injection of dihydroporphyrin ether (DHE), the rabbits were treated with a low-energy argon laser, which is absorbed mainly by the endometrial implants but not the surrounding normal tissues. The selective absorption of the laser energy by the DHE enables the low-power laser energy to destroy only the endometriotic lesions containing DHE, sparing the normal tissue. Since DHE is absorbed by both gross and microscopic disease, a more thorough resection of endometriosis is possible with photodynamic therapy, which is less invasive and safer. The ability to diagnose and treat disease at earlier stages and in an office setting may prevent the progression and invasion of endometriosis, reducing its adverse impact on health, quality of life, and fertility potential. Operative microlaparoscopy can be safe in the office under local anesthesia with conscious sedation for the diagnosis and treatment of chronic pelvic pain.[134] The diagnostic accuracy achieved for endometriosis with 2-mm microlaparoscopy is comparable to that achieved with standard 10-mm laparoscopy.[135] However, one study found discordant findings for mild or minimal endometriosis.[136]

Microlaparoscopy allows conscious pain mapping, fulguration of endometriotic lesions, adhesiolysis, and laparoscopic uterosacral nerve ablation.[137]

Pelvic pain mapping during laparoscopy under conscious sedation can provide useful information about visceral and somatic sources of chronic pelvic pain. A diagnostic superior hypogastric plexus block under direct laparoscopic observation is possible. The pelvis is mapped to ascertain whether painful areas are supplied by hypogastric plexuses. The results of mapping allow a more informed selection of patients for presacral neurectomy.[137]

After intravenous and oral delivery of 5-amino-levulinic acid and protoporphyrin IX in experimentally induced endometriosis in a rat, fluorescence was greater in the implants than the fluorescence detected in adjacent normal peritoneum.[138]

References

1. Hasson HM. Incidence of endometriosis in diagnostic laparoscopy. *J Reprod Med* 1976; 16:135.
2. Schmidt LC. Endometriosis: A reappraisal of pathogenesis and treatment. *Fertil Steril* 1985; 44:157.
3. Williams TJ, Pratt JHL. Endometriosis in a 1000 consecutive celiotomies: Incidence and management. *Am J Obstet Gynecol* 1977; 129:245.
4. Rokitansky C. Ueber Uterusdrusen-Neubildung in uterus and ovarial sarcomen. *Z Gesellschaft Aertz Wein* 1860; 16:755.
5. Williams TJ. Endometriosis, in Thompson JD, Rock JA, eds., *Te Linde's Gynecology*, 7th ed. Philadelphia: Lippincott, 1992.
6. Gomel V, McComb P. Microsurgery in gynecology, in Silver JS, ed., *Microsurgery*. Baltimore: Williams & Wilkins, 1979.
7. Cook AS, Rock JA. The role of laparoscopy in the treatment of endometriosis. *Fertil Steril* 1991; 4:663.
8. Martin DC. CO_2 laser laparoscopy for the treatment of endometriosis associated with infertility. *J Reprod Med* 1985; 30:409.
9. Nezhat C, Crowgey S, Nezhat F. Surgical treatment of endometriosis via laser laparoscopy. *Fertil Steril* 1986; 45:778.
10. Nezhat C, Crowgey S, Nezhat F. Videolaseroscopy for the treatment of endometriosis associated with infertility. *Fertil Steril* 1989; 51:123.
11. Adamson DG, Subak LL, Pasta DJ, et al. Comparison of CO_2 laser laparoscopy with laparotomy for the treatment of endometriomata. *Fertil Steril* 1992; 57:965.
12. Adamson DG, Hurd SJ, Pasta DJ, et al. Laparoscopic endometriosis treatment: Is it better? *Fertil Steril* 1993; 59:35.
13. Ranney BR. Endometriosis III: Complete operations. *Am J Obstet Gynecol* 1971; 109:1137.
14. Wilson EA. Surgical therapy for endometriosis. *Clin Obstet Gynecol* 1988; 31:857.
15. Nezhat C, Nezhat F, Nezhat CH. Operative laparoscopy (minimally invasive surgery): State of the art. *J Gynecol Surg* 1992; 8:111.
16. Nezhat C, Nezhat FR. Safe laser endoscopic excision or vaporization of peritoneal endometriosis. *Fertil Steril* 1989; 52:149.
17. Luciano AA, Lowney J, Jacobs SL. Endoscopic treatment of endometriosis-associated infertility: Therapeutic, economic and social benefits. *J Reprod Med* 1992; 37:573.
18. Olive DL, Martin DC. Treatment of endometriosis associated infertility with CO_2 laser laparoscopy: The use of 1- and 2-parameter exponential models. *Fertil Steril* 1987; 48:18.
19. Filmar S, Gomel V, McComb P. Operative laparoscopy versus open abdominal surgery: A comparative study on postoperative adhesion formation in the rat model. *Fertil Steril* 1987; 48:486.
20. Luciano AA, Maier DB, Nulsen ZC, et al. A comparative study of postoperative adhesion formation following laser surgery by laparoscopy versus laparotomy in the rabbit model. *Obstet Gynecol* 1989; 74:220.
21. Maier DB, Klock A, Nulsen J, et al. Laser laparoscopy vs laparotomy in lysis of dense and incidental pelvic adhesions. *J Reprod Med* 1992; 37:965.
22. Diamond MP, Daniell SF, Feste J, et al. Adhesion reformation and de novo formation after reproductive pelvic surgery. *Fertil Steril* 1987; 47:864.
23. Luciano AA, Moufauino-Oliva M. Comparison of postoperative adhesion formation—laparoscopy versus laparotomy. *Infert Reprod Med Clin North Am* 1994; 5:437.
24. Marana R, Luciano AA, Morendino VE, et al. Reproductive outcome after ovarian surgery:

Microsurgery versus CO_2 laser. *J Gynecol Surg* 1991; 7:159.
25. Lundorff P, Hahlin M, Kallfelt B, et al. Adhesion formation after laparoscopic surgery in ectopic pregnancy: A randomized trial versus laparotomy. *Fertil Steril* 1991; 55:91.
26. Trimbos-Kemper TCM, Trimbos JB, van Hall EV. Adhesion formation after tubal surgery: Results of the 8 day laparoscopy in 188 patients. *Fertil Steril* 1985; 43:395.
27. Nezhat C, Nezhat F, Metzger DA, et al. Adhesion reformation after reproductive surgery by videolaseroscopy. *Fertil Steril* 1990; 53:1008.
28. Operative Laparoscopy Study Group: Postoperative adhesion development after operative laparoscopy evaluation at early second look procedures. *Fertil Steril* 1991; 55:700.
29. Donnez J. Carbon dioxide laser laparoscopy in infertile women with endometriosis and women with adnexal adhesions. *Fertil Steril* 1987; 48:190.
30. Fayez JA, Collazo LM. Comparison between laparotomy and operative laparoscopy in the treatment of moderate and severe endometriosis. *Int J Fertil* 1990; 35:272.
31. Nezhat C, Silfen SL, Nezhat F, et al. Surgery for endometriosis. *Curr Opin Obstet Gynecol* 1991; 3:385.
32. Nezhat C, Winer W, Cooper J, et al. Endoscopic infertility surgery. *J Reprod Med* 1989; 34:127.
33. Gomel V. Laparoscopic tubal surgery in infertility. *Obstet Gynecol* 1975; 46:4752.
34. Gomel V. Salpingo-ovariolysis by laparoscopy in infertility. *Fertil Steril* 1983; 40:607.
35. Chong AP, Luciano AA, O'Shaughnessy AM. Laser laparoscopy versus laparotomy in the treatment of infertility patients with severe endometriosis. *J Gynecol Surg* 1990; 6:179.
36. Crosignani PG, Vercellini P, Biffignandi F, et al. Laparoscopy versus laparotomy in conservative surgical treatment for severe endometriosis. *Fertil Steril* 1996; 66:706.
37. Soong YK, Chang FH, Chou HH, et al. Life table analysis of pregnancy rates in women with moderate or severe endometriosis comparing danazol therapy after carbon dioxide laser laparoscopy plus electrocoagulation or laparotomy plus electrocoagulation versus danazol therapy only. *J Am Assoc Gynecol Laparosc* 1997; 4:225.
38. Nezhat C, Nezhat F. Operative laparoscopy for the management of ovarian remnant syndrome. *Fertil Steril* 1992; 57:1003.
39. Nezhat F, Nezhat C, Silfen SL. Videolaseroscopy for oophorectomy. *Am J Obstet Gynecol* 1991; 165:1323.
40. Betts WJ, Buttram CVJ. A plan for managing endometriosis. *Contemp Ob/Gyn* 1980; 15:121.
41. Ranney BR. Endometriosis: Conservative operations. *Am J Obstet Gynecol* 1970; 107:743.
42. Wheeler JH, Malinak LR. Recurrent endometriosis: Incidence, management, and prognosis. *Am J Obstet Gynecol* 1983; 146:247.
43. Barbieri RL. Hormonal therapy of endometriosis. *Infertil Reprod Med North Am* 1992; 3:187.
44. Henderson AF, Studd JW, Watson N. A retrospective study of estrogen replacement therapy following hysterectomy for the treatment of endometriosis, in Shaw RW, ed., *Advances in Reproductive Endocrinology*, vol. 1: *Endometriosis*. Carnforth, Lancs, Parthenon, 1989.
45. Luciano AA. Hormone replacement therapy in post menopausal women. *Infert Reprod Med Clin North Am* 1992; 3:109.
46. Luciano AA, Manzi D. Treatment options for endometriosis—surgical therapies. *Infert Reprod Med Clin North Am* 1992; 3:657.
47. Luciano AA, Turksoy RN, Carleo J. Evaluation of oral medroxyprogesterone acetate in the treatment of endometriosis. *Obstet Gynecol* 1988; 72:323.
48. Luciano AA, Roy M, De Souza MJ, et al. Evaluation of low dose estrogen and progestin therapy in postmenopausal women. *J Reprod Med* 1993; 38:207.
49. Greenblatt RB, Nezhat C, Natrajan PK. Update on the male and female climacteric. *J Am Geriatr Soc* 1979; 27:481.
50. Chetkowski RJ, Meldrum DR, Steingold KA, et al. Biological effects of transdermal estradiol. *J Clin Endocrinol Metab* 1986; 314:1615.
51. Schenken SR, Malinak RL. Reoperation after initial treatment of endometriosis with conservative surgery. *Am J Obstet Gynecol* 1978; 131:416.
52. Murphy AA, Green WR, Bobbie D, et al. Unsuspected endometriosis documented by scanning electron microscopy in visually normal peritoneum. *Fertil Steril* 1986; 46:522.
53. Nezhat F, Allan JC, Nezhat C, et al. Nonvisualized endometriosis at laparoscopy. *Int J Fertil* 1991; 36:340.

54. Vasquez G, Cornille F, Brosens IA. Peritoneal endometriosis: Scanning electron microscopy and histology of minimal pelvic endometriotic lesions. *Fertil Steril* 1984; 42:696.
55. Adamson GD, Pasta DJ. Surgical treatment of endometriosis-associated infertility: Meta-analysis compared with survival analysis. *Am J Obstet Gynecol* 1994; 171:1488.
56. Marcoux S, Maheux R, Berube S. Canadian Collaborative Group on Endometriosis: Laparoscopic surgery in infertile women with minimal or mild endometriosis. *N Engl J Med* 1997; 337:217.
57. Chang FH, Chou HH, Soong YK, et al. Efficacy of isotopic $13CO_2$ laser laparoscopic evaporation in the treatment of infertile patients with minimal and mild endometriosis: A life table cumulative pregnancy rates study. *J Am Assoc Gynecol Laparosc* 1997; 4:219.
58. Tulandi T, al-Took S. Reproductive outcome after treatment of mild endometriosis with laparoscopic excision and electrocoagulation. *Fertil Steril* 1998; 69:229.
59. Martin DC, Hubert GD, Vander-Zwaag R, et al. Laparoscopic appearances of pelvic endometriosis. *Fertil Steril* 1989; 51:63.
60. Redwine DB. Age-related evolution in color appearance of endometriosis. *Fertil Steril* 1987; 48:1062.
61. Vernon MW, Beard JS, Graves K, et al. Classification of endometriotic implants by morphologic appearance and capacity to synthesize prostaglandin. *Fertil Steril* 1990; 53:984.
62. Cornillie FJ, Ooosterlynck D, Lauweryns JM, et al. Deeply infiltrating pelvic endometriosis: Histology and clinical significance. *Fertil Steril* 1990; 53:978.
63. Crain LJ, Luciano AA. Peritoneal fluid evaluation in infertility. *Obstet Gynecol* 1983; 61:1591.
64. Nisolle M, Paindavene B, Boudon A, et al. Histologic study of peritoneal endometriosis in infertile women. *Fertil Steril* 1990; 53:984.
65. Redwine DB. Peritoneal blood painting: An aid in the diagnosis of endometriosis. *Am J Obstet Gynecol* 1989; 161:865.
66. Candiani GB, Vercelli P, Fedele L. Laparoscopic ovarian puncture to correct staging of endometriosis. *Fertil Steril* 1990; 53:984.
67. Demco L. Mapping the source and character of pain due to endometriosis by patient-assisted laparoscopy. *J Am Assoc Gynecol Laparosc* 1998; 5:241.
68. Prystowsky JB, Stryker SJ. Ujiki GT, et al. Gastrointestinal endometriosis: Incidence and indications for resection. *Arch Surg* 1988; 7:855.
68a. Goldman EL. ACOG advises against videotaping of deliveries. *OB/GYN News* 1999; 28. (Newsletter)
69. Nezhat CH, Nezhat F, Roemisch M, et al. Laparoscopic trachelectomy for persistent pelvic pain and endometriosis after supracervical hysterectomy. *Fertil Steril* 1996; 66:925.
70. Sampson JA. Perforating hemorrhagic (chocolate) cysts of the ovary. *Arch Surg* 1921; 3:245.
71. Blaustein A, Kantius M, Kaganowicz A, et al. Inclusions in ovaries of females aged 1–30 years. *Int J Gynecol Pathol* 1982; 1:145.
72. Kerner H, Gaton E, Czernobilsky B. Unusual ovarian, tubal and pelvic mesothelial inclusions in patients with endometriosis. *Histopathology* 1981; 5:277.
73. Sternberg SS, ed. *Histology for pathologists*. Philadelphia: Lippincott/Williams & Wilkins, *Publishers.* 1992.
74. Chernobilsky B, Morris WJ. A histologic study of ovarian endometriosis with emphasis on hyperplastic and atypical changes. *Obstet Gynecol* 1979; 53:318.
75. Nissole-Pochet M, Casanas-Roux F, Donnez J. Histologic study of ovarian endometriosis after hormonal therapy. *Fertil Steril* 1988; 49:423.
76. Martin DC, Berry JD. Histology of chocolate cysts. *J Gynecol Surg* 1990; 6:43.
77. Vercellini P, Vendola N, Bocciolone L, et al. Reliability of the visual diagnosis of ovarian endometriosis. *Fertil Steril* 1991; 56:1198.
78. Luciano AA, Marana R, Krakta S, et al. Ovarian function after incision of the ovary by scalpel, CO_2 laser and microelectrode. *Fertil Steril* 1991; 56:349.
79. Hasson HM. Laparoscopic management of ovarian cysts. *J Reprod Med* 1990; 25:863.
80. Brosens I, Puttemansi P. Double optic laparoscopy. *Ballieres Clin Obstet Gynecol* 1989; 3:595.
81. Keye WR, Hansen LW, Astin M, et al. Argon laser therapy of endometriosis: A review of 92 consecutive patients. *Fertil Steril* 1987; 47:208.
82. Nezhat F, Nezhat C, Allan CJ, et al. A clinical and histologic classification of en-

dometriomas: Implications for a mechanism of pathogenesis. *J Reprod Med* 1992; 37:771.

83. Nezhat C, Nezhat F. Postoperative adhesion formation after ovarian cystectomy with and without ovarian reconstruction. Presented at the 75th Annual Meeting of the American Fertility Society, Orlando, FL, October 19–24, 1991.
84. Fayez JA, Vogel MF. Comparison of different treatment methods of endometriomas by laparoscopy. *Obstet Gynecol* 1991; 78:660.
85. Hasson HM. Laparoscopic management of ovarian cysts. *J Reprod Med* 1990; 25:863.
86. Nezhat F, Nezhat C, Allan CJ, et al. A clinical and histologic classification of endometriomas: Implications for a mechanism of pathogenesis. *J Reprod Med* 1992; 37:771.
87. Marana R, Luciano AA, Muzii L, et al. Reproductive outcome after ovarian surgery. Suturing versus nonsuturing of the ovarian cortex. *J Gynecol Surg* 1991; 7:155.
88. Nezhat C, Nezhat F. Postoperative adhesion formation after ovarian cystectomy with and without ovarian reconstruction. Abstract O-012, 47th annual meeting of the American Fertility Association, Orlando, FL, October 21-24, 1991.
89. Donnez J, Nisolle M. Laparoscopic management of large ovarian endometrial cyst: Use of fibrin sealant. *Surgery* 1991; 7:163.
90. Beretta P, Franchi M, Ghezzi F, et al. Randomized clinical trial of two laparoscopic treatments of endometriomas: Cystectomy versus drainage and coagulation. *Fertil Steril* 1998; 70:1176.
91. Catalano GF, Marana R, Caruana P, et al. Laparoscopy versus microsurgery by laparotomy for excision of ovarian cysts in patients with moderate or severe endometriosis. *J Am Assoc Gynecol Laparosc* 1996; 3:267.
92. Hemmings R, Bissonnette F, Bouzayen R. Results of laparoscopic treatments of ovarian endometriomas: Laparoscopic ovarian fenestration and coagulation. *Fertil Steril* 1998; 70:527.
93. Stanley EK, Utz DC, Dockerty MB. Clinically significant endometriosis of the urinary tract. *Surg Gynecol Obstet* 1965; 120:491.
94. Goldstein MS, Brodman ML. Cystometric evaluation of vesical endometriosis before and after hormonal or surgical treatment. *Mt Sinai J Med* 1990; 57:109.
95. Nezhat C, Nezhat F, Nezhat CH, et al. Urinary tract endometriosis treated by laparoscopy. *Fertil Steril* 1996; 66:920.
96. Nezhat CH, Seidman DS, Nezhat F, et al. Laparoscopic management of intentional and unintentional cystotomy. *J Urol* 1996; 156:1400.
97. Nezhat CH, Nezhat FR, Freiha F, Nezhat CR. Laparoscopic vesicopsoas hitch for infiltrative ureteral endometriosis. *Fertil Steril* 1999; 71:376.
98. Nezhat C, Nezhat F, Green B. Laparoscopic treatment of obstructed ureter due to endometriosis by resection and ureteroureterostomy: A case report. *J Urol* 1992; 148:659.
99. Nezhat C, Nezhat F. Laparoscopic segmental bladder resection for endometriosis: A report of two cases. *Obstet Gynecol* 1993; 81:882.
100. Sampson JA. Intestinal adenomas of endometrial type. *Arch Surg* 1922; 5:217.
101. Jenkinson EL. Brown WH. Endometriosis: A study of 117 cases with special reference to constricting lesions of the rectum and signoid colon. *JAMA* 1943; 122:349.
102. Samper ER, Sagle GW, Hand AM. Colonic endometriosis, its clinical spectrum. *South Med J* 1984; 77:912.
103. Ponka JL, Brush BE, Hodgkinson CP. Colorectal endometriosis. *Dis Colon Rectum* 1973; 16:490.
104. Meyers WC, Kelvin FM, Jones RS. Diagnosis and surgical treatment of colonic endometriosis. *Arch Surg* 1979; 114:169.
105. Mackenrodt R. Uber entzundliche heterage Epithelwucherungen in weiblichen Genitalgebiete und uber eine bir in die Wurzel des Mescolon ausgedehnte benigne Wucherung des Darmepithels. *Virchows Arch Pathol Anat* 1909; 195:487.
106. Coronado C, Franklin RR, Lotze EC, et al. Surgical treatment of symptomatic colorectal endometriosis. *Fertil Steril* 1990; 3:411.
107. Nezhat C, Pennington E, Nezhat F, Silfen SL. Laparoscopically assisted anterior rectal wall resection and reanastomosis for deeply infiltrating endometriosis. *Surg Laparosc Endosc* 1991; 1:106.
108. Nezhat C, Nezhat F, Pennington E. Laparoscopic proctectomy for infiltrating endometriosis of the rectum. *Fertil Steril* 1992; 57:1129.
109. Nezhat F, Nezhat C, Pennington E, Ambroze W. Laparoscopic segmental resection for in-

filtrating endometriosis of the rectosigmoid colon: A preliminary report. *Surg Laparosc Endosc* 1992; 2:212.

110. Sharpe DR, Redwine DB: Laparoscopic Segmented resection of the Sigmoid and the recto Sigmoid colon for endometriosis. *Surgical Laparoscopy Endoscopy* 1992; 2:120
111. Redwine DB, Koning M, Sharpe DR. Laparoscipically assisted transvaginal Segmental resection of the rectosigmoid colon for Endometriosis. *Fertil Steril,* 1996; 65:193.
112. Jerby, BL, Kessler H, Falcon S. Milsom J.W. Laparoscopic Management of Colorectal Endometriosis. *Surg Endosc* 1999; 13:1125.
113. Nezhat C, Nezhat F, Pennington E, et al. Laparoscopic disk excision and primary repair of the anterior rectal wall for the treatment of full-thickness bowel endometriosis. *Surg Endosc* 1994; 8:682.
114. Nezhat C, Nezhat F, Ambroze W, Pennington E. Laparoscopic repair of small bowel, colon, and rectal endometriosis: A report of twenty-six cases. *Surg Endosc* 1993; 7:88.
115. Fedele L, Bianchi S, Portuese A, et al. Transrectal ultrasonography in the assessment of rectovaginal endometriosis. *Obstet Gynecol* 1998; 91:444.
116. Chapron C, Dumontier I, Dousset B, et al. Results and role of rectal endoscopic ultrasonography for patients with deep pelvic endometriosis. *Hum Reprod* 1998; 13:2266.
117. Donnez J, Nisolle M, Gillerot S, et al. Rectovaginal septum adenomyotic nodules: A series of 500 cases. *Br J Obstet Gynaecol* 1997; 104:1014.
118. Martin DC. Laparoscopic and vaginal colpotomy for the excision of infiltrating cul-de-sac endometriosis. *J Reprod Med* 1988; 33:806.
119. Redwine DB. Laparoscopic en bloc resection for treatment of the obliterated cul-de-sac in endometriosis. *J Reprod Med* 1992; 37:695
120. Nezhat C, Nezhat F, Pennington E. Laparoscopic treatment of lower colorectal and infiltrative rectovaginal septum endometriosis by the technique of video-laseroscopy. *Br J Obstet Gynaecol* 1992; 99:664.
121. Donnez J, Nisolle M, Smoes P, et al. Peritoneal endometriosis and "endometriotic" nodules of the rectovaginal septum are two different entities. *Fertil Steril* 1996; 66:362.
122. Shiraishi T. Catamenial pneumothorax: Report of a case and review of the Japanese and non-Japanese literature. *Thorac Cardiovasc Surg* 1991; 39:304.
123. Nezhat F, Nezhat C, Levy JS. Laparoscopic treatment of symptomatic diaphragmatic endometriosis: A case report. *Fertil Steril* 1992; 58:614.
124. Nezhat C, Seidman DS, Nezhat F, Nezhat C. Laparoscopic surgical management of diaphragmatic endometriosis. *Fertil Steril* 1998; 69:1048.
125. Black WT. Use of presacral sympathectomy in the treatment of dysmenorrhea: A second look after twenty-five years. *Am J Obstet Gynecol* 1964; 89:16.
126. Lee RB, Stone K, Magelssen D, et al. Presacral neurectomy for chronic pelvic pain. *Obstet Gynecol* 1986; 68:517.
127. Tjaden B, Schlaff WD, Kimball A, et al. The efficacy of presacral neurectomy for the relief of midline dysmenorrhea. *Obstet Gynecol* 1990; 76:89.
128. Sutton CJ, Ewen SP, Whitelaw N, Haines P. Prospective, randomized, double-blind, controlled trial of laser laparoscopy in the treatment of pelvic pain associated with minimal, mild, and moderate endometriosis. *Fertil Steril* 1994; 62:696.
129. Sutton CJ, Pooley AS, Ewen SP, Haines P. Follow-up report on a randomized controlled trial of laser laparoscopy in the treatment of pelvic pain associated with minimal to moderate endometriosis. *Fertil Steril* 1997; 68:1070.
130. Olive DL, Henderson DY. Endometriosis and müllerian anomalies. *Obstet Gynecol* 1987; 69:412.
131. Moghissi KS, Boyce CR. Management of endometriosis with oral medroxyprogesterone acetate. *Obstet Gynecol* 1976; 47:265.
132. Henzi MR, Corson SL, Moghissi K, et al. Photodynamic therapy of rabbit endometrial implants: A model treatment of endometriosis. *Fertil Steril* 1989; 52:140.
133. Manyak MJ, Nelson LM, Solomon D, et al. Photodynamic therapy of rabbit endometrial implants: A model treatment of endometriosis. *Fertil Steril* 1989; 52:140.
134. Almeida OD Jr, Val-Gallas JM. Office microlaparoscopy under local anesthesia in the diagnosis and treatment of chronic pelvic pain. *J Am Assoc Gynecol Laparosc* 1998; 5:407.
135. Faber BM, Coddington CC 3d. Microlaparoscopy: A comparative study of diagnostic accuracy. *Fertil Steril* 1997; 67:952.
136. Evans SF, Petrucco OM. Microlaparoscopy for suspected pelvic pathology—a compari-

son of 2mm versus 10mm laparoscope. *Aust N Z J Obstet Gynaecol* 1998; 38:215.

137. Steege JF. Superior hypogastric block during microlaparoscopic pain mapping. *J Am Assoc Gynecol Laparosc* 1998; 5:265.

138. Yang JZ, Van Dijk-Smith JP, Van Vugt DA, et al. Fluorescence and photosensitization of experimental endometriosis in the rat after systemic 5-aminolevulinic acid administration: A potential new approach to the diagnosis and treatment of endometriosis. *Am J Obstet Gynecol* 1996; 174:154.

13

Management of the Ectopic Pregnancy

A tubal pregnancy entails certain death of the gestation, a threat to the woman's life, and a subsequent successful pregnancy in less than 50% of patients. Until 1970, more than 80% of ectopic pregnancies were recognized after rupture. With the excellent resolution afforded by transvaginal sonography (TVS), the high sensitivity of radioimmunoassay of the beta subunit of human chorionic gonadotropin (hCG), and the increased vigilance of clinicians, more than 80% of ectopic pregnancies now are detected before rupture.

Incidence

Although earlier diagnosis has resulted in decreased maternal mortality and morbidity, hospitalizations for this condition increased from 17,800 in 1970 to 88,400 in 1989, representing a nearly fivefold rise.[1,2] Ranging in frequency from 1 in 250 to 1 in 87 live births, tubal pregnancy has emerged as a leading cause of maternal death, accounting for 10% of all maternal mortalities.[3] In 1986, the Centers for Disease Control reported 36 maternal deaths attributable to tubal pregnancy, accounting for 13.2% of all maternal deaths in the United States.

From 1970 through 1989, more than 1 million ectopic pregnancies were estimated to have occurred among women in the United States.[4] The general trend was for the numbers and rates of ectopic pregnancy to increase over that 20-year period. The rate has increased by almost fourfold, from 4.5 to 16.0 ectopic pregnancies per 1000 reported pregnancies. Although ectopic pregnancies accounted for less than 2% of all reported pregnancies during that period, complications of this condition were associated with approximately 13% of all pregnancy-related deaths.[4] However, during that period, the risk of death associated with ectopic pregnancy decreased 90%. The case fatality rate declined from 35.5 deaths per 10,000 ectopic pregnancies in 1970 to 3.8 in 1989.

The risk of ectopic pregnancy is higher in nonwhite women (all races including African-American, Asian, and American Indian women; relative risk is 1.6). Among inner-city African-American women, cigarette smoking is an independent, dose-related risk factor for ectopic pregnancy.[5] The hazard is correlated with age. It increases three to four times in women between ages 35 and 44 compared with those 15 to 24.[6] The "epidemic" of tubal pregnancies in the 1970s and 1980s has been associated with the "baby boom" cohort (1945 to 1954), who were in their fertile period.[7]

About 61% of these women conceive subsequently, but only 38% of them deliver a living infant. The others either have a spontaneous abortion or suffer repeated extrauterine gestation.[8,9] About 95% of such pregnancies occur in the ampulla, where fertilization takes place, but they can develop elsewhere in the tube, cervix, ovary, or abdominal cavity (Figure 13-1). A higher risk of ovarian implantation exists in women who conceive while using intrauterine contraceptive devices.[10] A woman with an intrauterine device (IUD) in place who conceives is more likely to have an extrauterine pregnancy (EUP) than is a woman who conceives while using other contraceptive methods. Although an IUD is more effective in preventing an intrauterine pregnancy (IUP) than an EUP, women are not at increased risk of

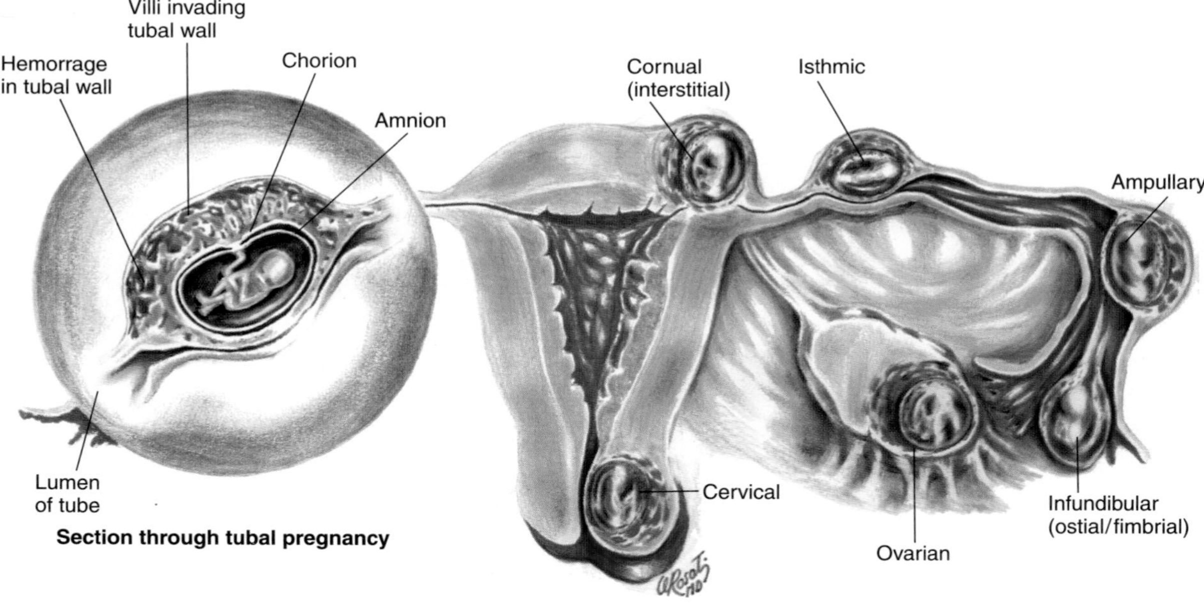

Figure 13-1. The sites of implantation of ectopic pregnancies, along with a section through an advanced tubal pregnancy.

developing an EUP compared with the general population solely because they are wearing an IUD.

The increase in tubal pregnancy also is attributed to a greater incidence of sexually transmitted diseases, previous tubal operations (either reconstruction or sterilization), delayed childbearing, and more successful clinical detection. Major risk factors for this life-threatening condition are listed in Table 13-1. Any condition that prevents or retards migration of the fertilized ovum to the uterine cavity predisposes a woman to an EUP.

TABLE 13-1. Major Factors and Associated Relative Risks for Tubal Pregnancy

Risk Factors	Relative Risk, %
Current use of intrauterine devices	11.9
Use of clomiphene citrate	10.0
Prior tubal surgery	5.6
Pelvic inflammatory disease	4.0
Infertility	2.9
Induced abortion	2.5
Adhesions	2.4
Abdominal surgery	2.3
T-shaped uterus	2.0
Myomas	1.7
Progestin-only oral contraceptives	1.6

Source: Marchbanks et al.[10]

Diagnosis

Symptoms

The usual pregnancy symptoms, including nausea, vomiting, breast fullness, fatigue, and interruption of the normal menstrual pattern, also occur with tubal pregnancies. Other symptoms more typical of EUP include lower abdominal pain of varying intensity and abnormal uterine bleeding ranging from amenorrhea to spotting or heavy bleeding. The presence of shoulder pain suggests possible rupture, with intraperitoneal blood flowing toward the diaphragm causing phrenic nerve irritation.

Physical Findings

Fever of more than 101°F is unusual. About one-third of patients with ruptured tubal pregnancies experience syncope because of hypotension caused by hypovolemia. Signs of ectopic pregnancy, including lower abdominal tenderness with or without rebound, are more severe on the affected side. There may be tenderness with cervical motion. The uterus usually is enlarged and soft. An adnexal mass is present in 50% of these patients (Table 13-2).

Patients with abdominal peritoneal signs or definite cervical motion tenderness constitute a

TABLE 13-2. Symptoms and Signs Suggesting Tubal Pregnancy

1. Nausea, breast fullness, fatigue, interruption of menses
2. Lower abdominal pain, heavy cramping, shoulder pain
3. Uterine bleeding, spotting
4. Pelvic tenderness, enlarged soft uterus
5. Adnexal mass, tenderness
6. Positive pregnancy test
7. Serum levels of hCG <6000 mIU/mL at 6 weeks
8. Less than 66% increase in hCG titers in 48 hours
9. Positive culdocentesis (83%)
10. Absence of gestational sac in the uterus by TVS
11. Gestational sac outside the uterus by TVS

high-risk group, while patients with only midline menstrual-like cramping constitute a low-risk group.[11] Abdominal pain, rebound tenderness on abdominal examination, fluid in the pouch of Douglas at transvaginal ultrasound examination, and a low serum hemoglobin level are independent predictors of tubal rupture.[12] Another study discovered no constellation of physical examination findings that could confirm or exclude the diagnosis reliably.[13] Rebound tenderness and muscular rigidity were associated with a high likelihood of an EUP, while findings on speculum inspection and vaginal examination contributed little to confirm the diagnosis. Information provided by physical examination for the diagnosis is limited compared with that obtained from TVS and serum hCG measurements. A pelvic digital examination for patients with a suspected EUP is of limited value.[14]

Laboratory Studies

The presence of a pregnancy can be discovered as early as 10 days after ovulation with sensitive serum assays for the beta subunit of hCG. Isolated values of hCG can aid in the diagnosis only when used in combination with other diagnostic tests. It is the pattern of the rise and fall that is meaningful. Doubling of the hCG levels every 48 hours in the fifth gestational week is an indication of a normally growing IUP. However, using this criterion, 15% of normal IUPs could fall in the EUP category and 13% of EUPs would be missed. Besides having lower titers and slower increases in serum concentrations of hCG compared with normal pregnancies, ectopic pregnancies have slower declines in the hCG titers than do spontaneous abortions.

Kadar and colleagues [15] noted that the absence of an intrauterine gestational sac on abdominal ultrasound and serum beta hCG levels of 6000 to 6500 mIU/mL suggest an EUP. The presence of an apparent intrauterine gestational sac with levels below 6500 mIU/mL implies an EUP or a missed or spontaneous abortion. More accurate diagnostic studies are obtained with high-frequency vaginal transducers that can discover a normal gestational sac in 98% of women after the fifth week of pregnancy, when the hCG levels are between 1000 mIU/mL and 1500 mIU/mL, the so-called discriminatory zone.[16] In one study, the sensitivity of TVS for the prediction of EUP was 87% and the specificity was 94%.[17] The positive and negative predictive values were 92.5% and 90%, respectively. When a level of 1500 IU/L is associated with an ectopic mass or fluid in the pouch of Douglas or in patients without these clinical findings, a level of at least 2000 IU/L suggests an EUP.[18]

A single progesterone assay is predictive of an abnormal pregnancy but not specific for an extrauterine one. A value of 25 ng/mL or more suggests a normal IUP. Serum progesterone values of 15 ng/mL or less imply an abnormal pregnancy, ectopic pregnancy, or threatened abortion. A meta-analysis incorporating 26 studies evaluating one serum progesterone measurement for the diagnosis of EUP showed a good discriminative capacity for the diagnosis of pregnancy failure and that of a viable IUP. However, one measurement could not discriminate between an EUP and an IUP.[19]

Culdocentesis revealing nonclotting blood is found in more than 50% of unruptured tubal pregnancies.[20] When it is used in combination with a positive pregnancy test, positive results suggest the presence of an EUP.

Treatment

Once the diagnosis is made, treatment choices include laparotomy, laparoscopy, chemotherapy, and expectant management. Hemodynamic instability previously was considered an indication for immediate laparotomy. The availability of optimal anesthesia and advanced cardiovascular monitoring and the ability to convert rapidly to laparotomy if required enable the safe performance of operative laparoscopy in most women with hypovolemic shock.[21] The superior exposure with laparoscopy provides the possibility of a rapid diagnosis and control of the bleeding, making laparoscopy a good choice.

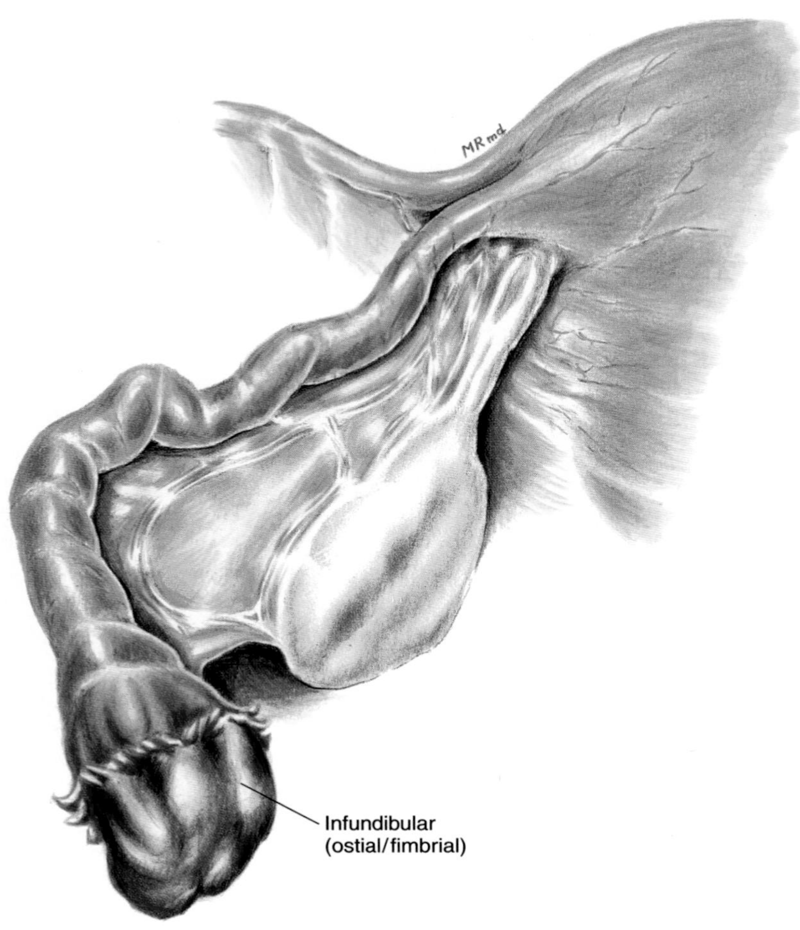

Figure 13-2. This infundibular pregnancy is about to be extruded. At laparoscopy, such conditions can be managed by grasping the tissue and completing the process. Bleeding usually is minimal.

Since 1970, a conservative approach to unruptured EUP has been advocated to preserve tubal function (Table 13-3). Several types of tubal operations have been done successfully.[22] These operations include linear salpingostomy, "milking" the pregnancy from the distal ampulla (Figure 13-2), and partial salpingectomy followed by anastomosis. Postoperative viable births or repeat EUPs are similar after salpingectomy with or without ipsilateral oophorectomy and salpingostomy.[23] In 321 tubal pregnancies treated conservatively by laparoscopy, it was reported that 15 (4.8 %) required subsequent laparotomy or a second laparoscopic procedure as hCG levels failed to return to normal.[24]

The preferred operative approach is by laparoscopy.[25] This technique yields pregnancy rates comparable to those reported after laparotomy.[23–28] This laparoscopic procedure was proved in prospective randomized trials to be superior to laparotomy.[29] Vermesh and associates[25] prospectively randomized patients with unruptured EUP to either laparoscopy or laparotomy. Those authors analyzed postoperative morbidity, length of hospital stay, duration of convalescence, hospital cost, postoperative tubal patency by hysterosalpingography, and pregnancy rates. The two procedures were similarly safe and effective, but the laparoscopic approach was more cost-effective and required a shorter recovery period. The laparoscopic approach results in improved fertility rates because of reduced formation of postoperative adhesions.[30]

Animal[31] and clinical[32] studies confirmed the impression that laparoscopic procedures were associated with reductions of new adhesions and re-formation of preexisting adhesions. Tubal healing and the extent of pelvic adhesions were assessed at repeat laparoscopy within 15 weeks of the initial operation.[33] Although tubal patency did

TABLE 13-3. Comparative Results of Conservative Operations for Tubal Pregnancy by Laparotomy and Laparoscopy

Authors	No. Cases	Percent Intrauterine Pregnancy	Percent Tubal Pregnancy
Laparotomy			
Vermesh et al[20*]	30	42	16
DeCherney and Kase[23]	49	40	12
Stromme[26]	45	71	15
Timonen and Nieminen[27]	240	38	16
Total	364	47.75	14.75
Laparoscopy			
DeCherney and Diamond[22]	79	62	16
Pouly et al[24]	118	64	22
Vermesh et al[25*]	30	50	6
Total	227	58.67	14.67

*Controlled and prospectively randomized to laparotomy and laparoscopy.

not differ between the two groups, patients who were treated by laparotomy developed more adhesions. Brumsted and coworkers[34] reported a shorter convalescence of 8.7 ± 7.8 days in the laparoscopy group compared with 25.7 ± 16.2 days among the laparotomy patients ($p < 0.01$) and reduced postoperative analgesia requirements in the laparoscopy patients of 0.84 ± 2.3 doses compared with 4.64 ± 2.9 doses ($p < 0.01$) in the laparotomy group.

With adequate experience in operative endoscopy and with proper instruments, most patients with ectopic pregnancies can be treated successfully by laparoscopy regardless of the gestation's size or location, the number of gestations, or the presence of tubal rupture.[35] At the initial exploratory procedure, both fallopian tubes are examined to avoid missing multiple ectopic pregnancies. Because of delayed childbearing and the expanded use of assisted reproductive technology, multiple EUPs may become more prevalent. After a nonstimulated menstrual cycle, three separate gestational sacs were identified in one woman at initial operative laparoscopy, one in the right tube and two in the left tube.[36]

In the management of a tubal gestation, the gynecologist must consider the patient's desire for further childbearing. The patient is informed of the possibility of laparotomy with salpingectomy or more extirpative procedures because of uncontrollable bleeding or unexpected findings. If neither tube is salvageable, the uterus and at least one ovary is preserved to retain the possibility of in vitro fertilization.[37]

Laparoscopic Techniques

The location, size, and nature of the tubal pregnancy are established. Ruptured tubal pregnancies are treated successfully endoscopically if the bleeding has ceased or is stopped adequately. Once bleeding is controlled, the products of conception and blood clots are removed. A 10-mm suction instrument cleanses the abdominal cavity quickly. Forced irrigation with lactated Ringer's solution dislodges clots and trophoblastic tissue from the serosa of the peritoneal organs with minimal trauma to those structures.

Salpingotomy

For unruptured tubal pregnancies, the tube is identified and mobilized. To reduce bleeding, a 5- to 7-mL diluted solution containing 20 units of vasopressin (Pitressin) in 100 mL of normal saline is injected with a 20-gauge spinal or laparoscopic needle in the mesosalpinx just below the EUP and over the antimesenteric surface of the tubal segment containing the gestational products (Figure 13-3A). The needle must not be within a blood vessel because intravascular injection of vasopressin solution can cause acute arterial hypertension, bradycardia, and death.[32]

Using a laser, microelectrode, or scissors, a linear incision is made on the antimesenteric surface extending 1 to 2 cm over the thinnest portion of the tube containing the pregnancy. The pregnancy usually protrudes through the incision and slowly slips out of the tube; it is removed by using

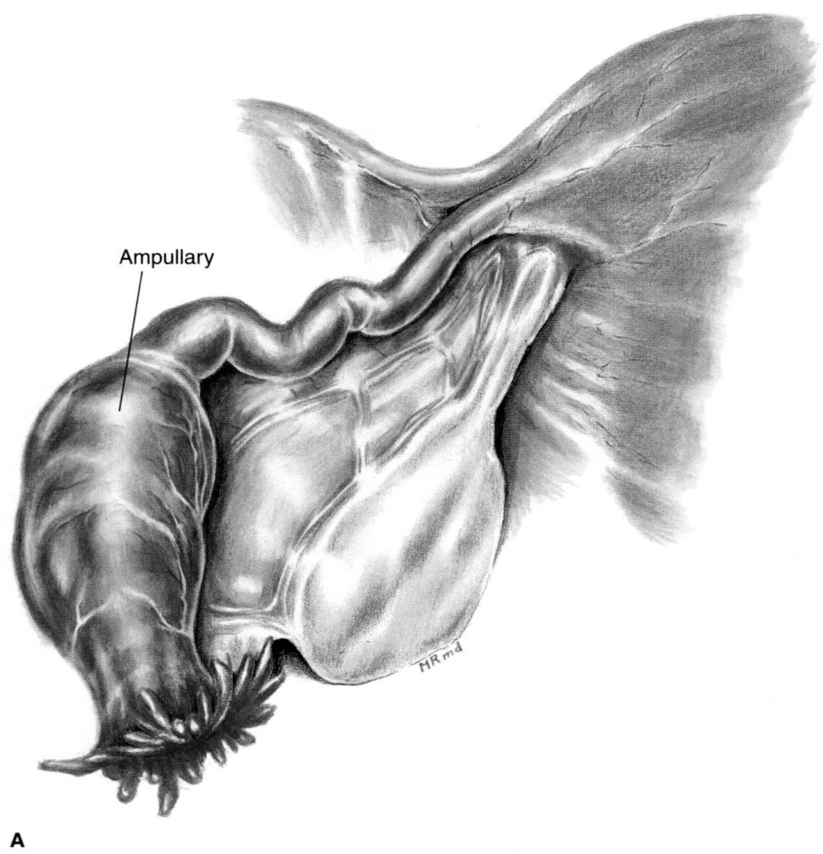

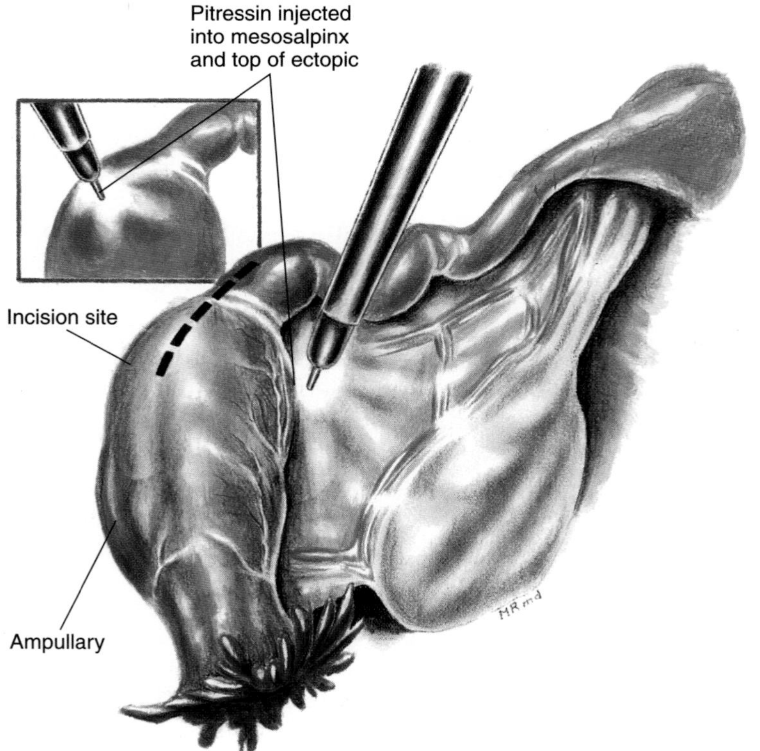

Figure 13-3. **A.** An unruptured ampullary pregnancy. **B.** Injection is done into the top of the tube (inset) and into the mesosalpinx—with 5 to 7 mL of diluted Pitressin.

hydrodissection or laparoscopic forceps (Figure 13-3B). Forceful irrigation in the tube's opening can dislodge the gestation from its implantation. As the pregnancy is pulled out or extrudes from the tube, some products of conception can adhere to the implantation site by a ligamentous structure containing blood vessels (Figure 13-4). Using the electrocoagulator, this structure is coagulated before the tissue is removed. Oozing from the tube is common but usually ceases spontaneously. Occasionally, coagulation is necessary with a defocused laser beam or an electrocoagulator. Depending on the size, the products of conception are removed through a 5- or 10-mm trocar sleeve.

Tubal resection

Resection of the tubal segment that contains the gestation is preferable to salpingotomy for an isthmic pregnancy or a ruptured tube or if hemostasis is difficult to obtain. Segmental resection is done with bipolar electrosurgery, fiber lasers (potassium titanyl phosphate, argon, or neodymium-yttrium aluminum garnet), CO_2 laser, sutures, or stapling devices.

Bloodless segmental resection is achieved by grasping the proximal and distal boundaries of the tubal segment containing the gestation with a Kleppinger forceps and coagulating them from the antimesenteric surface to the mesosalpinx. The segment is cut with laparoscopic scissors or a laser, with little risk of bleeding. The mesosalpinx under the pregnancy is coagulated, with particular attention given to the arcuate anastomosing branches of the ovarian and uterine vessels.[38] After coagulation, the mesosalpinx is cut (Figure 13-5 and 13-6).

Salpingectomy

Guidelines for choosing salpingectomy include the presence of uncontrolled bleeding, tubal destruction by the EUP, and a recurrent pregnancy in the same tube. Preoperative counseling should have included the desire of the patient for future childbearing.

This operation is done by progressively coagulating and cutting the mesosalpinx, beginning with the proximal isthmic portion and progressing to the fimbriated end of the tube. It is separated from the uterus by using bipolar coagulation and scissors or a laser (Figure 13-7). A multifire stapling device for salpingectomy requires a 12-mm trocar and is expensive. Alternatively, one or two Endoloops (Ethicon) can be applied around the salpinx and then cut. The isolated segment containing the EUP is removed intact or in sectioned parts through the 10-mm trocar sleeve. Products of conception can be placed in a bag (Endopouch, Ethicon, Inc.) and

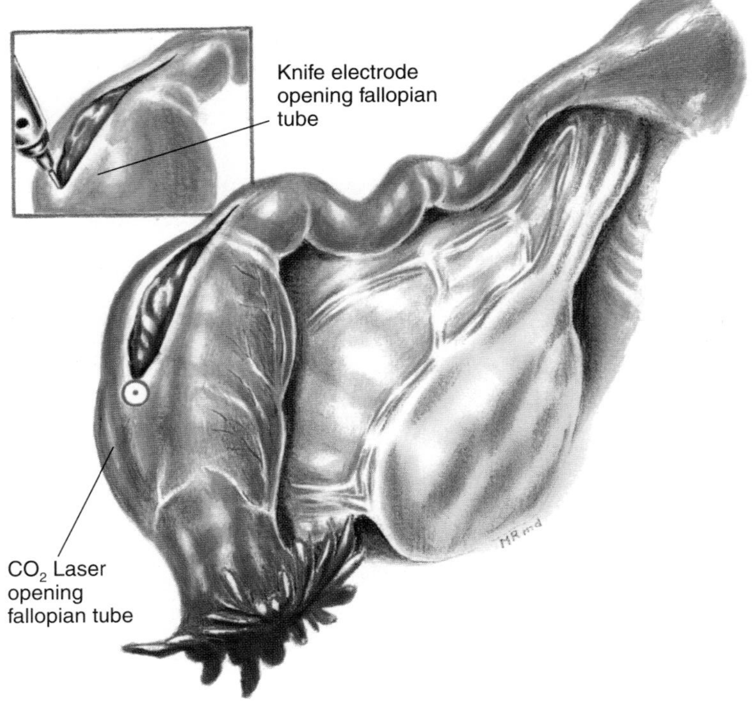

Figure 13-4. **A.** The pregnancy is revealed by either a CO_2 laser or knife electrode (inset) after a tubal incision is made.

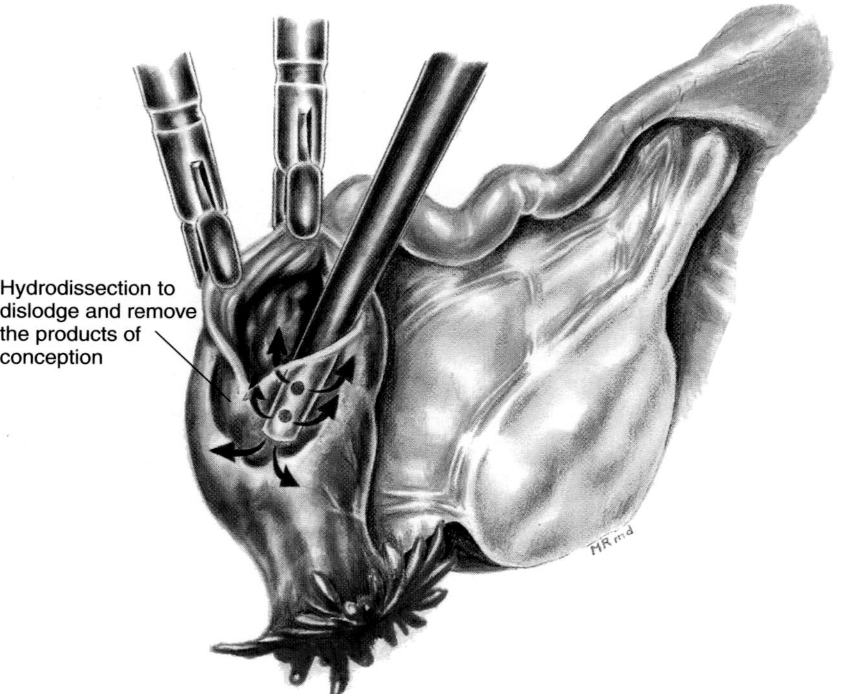

Figure 13-4. (*Continued*) B. Products of conception are being separated from the tube.

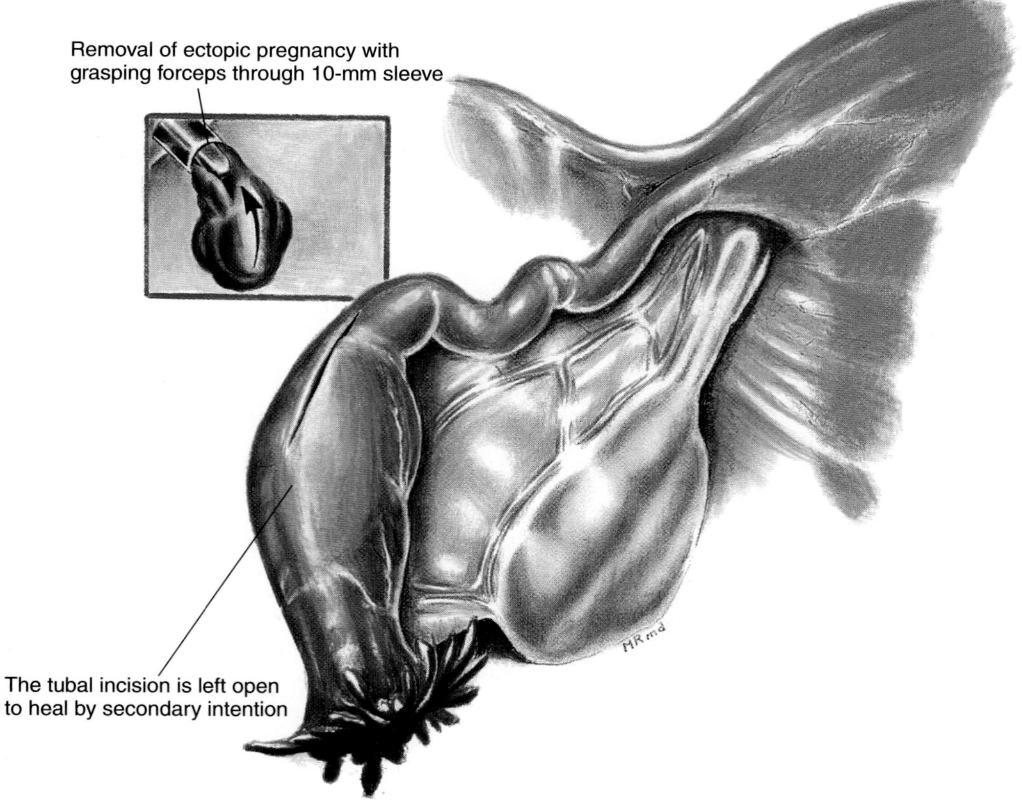

C. Depending on the size of the ectopic pregnancy, the products of conception can be removed through a 5- or 10-mm trocar sleeve (*inset*). The tubal incision is not sutured and usually heals spontaneously.

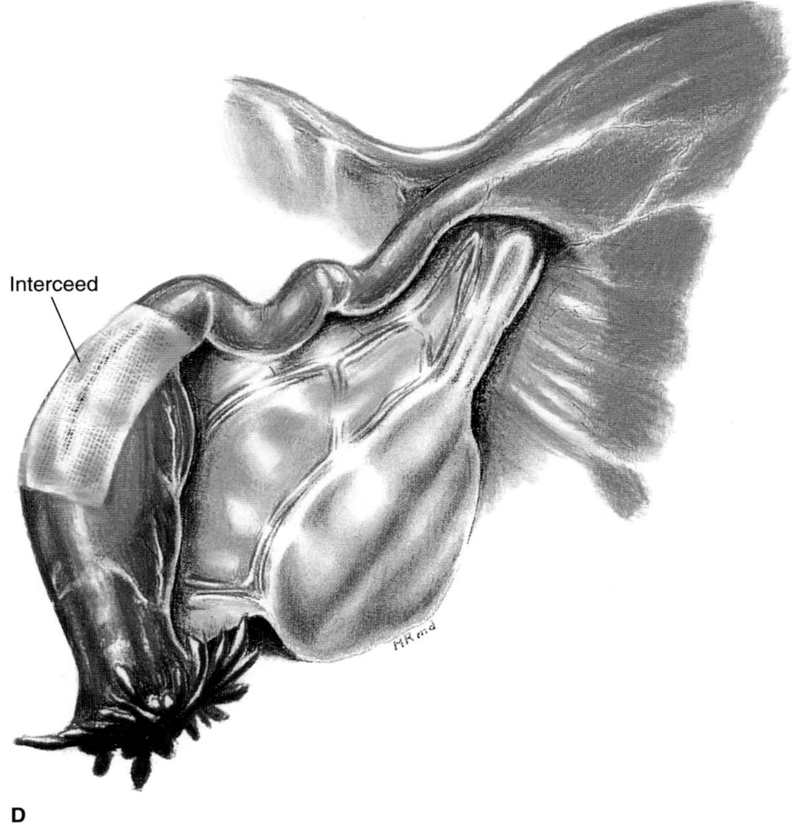

Figure 13-4. (*Continued*) **D.** In some instances, the incision can be covered with Interceed.

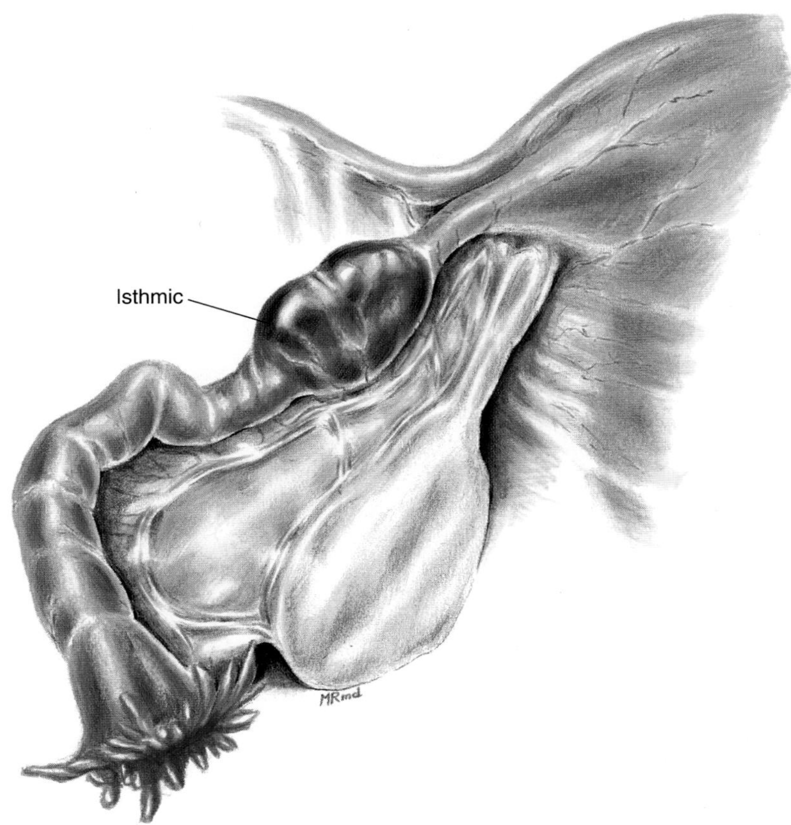

Figure 13-5. **A.** An isthmic pregnancy is illustrated.

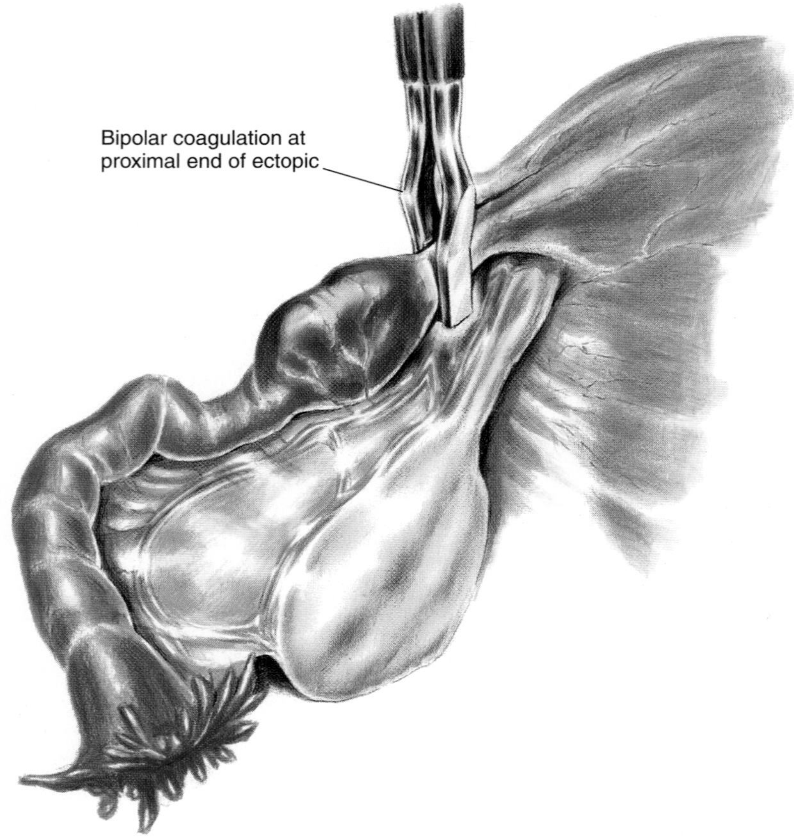

Figure 13-5. (***Continued***) **B.** The bipolar forceps coagulates proximal ishthmic segment.

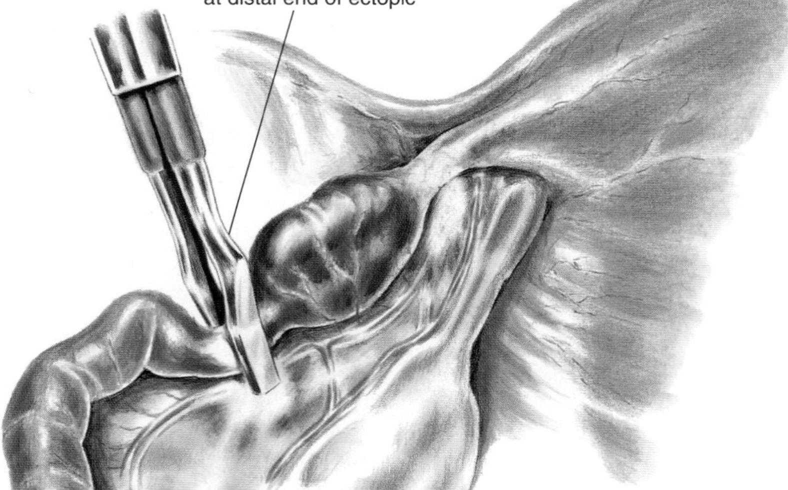

C. Electrocoagulation of the tube distal to the ectopic.

Figure 13-6. A. Either a scissors or a CO_2 laser is employed to transect the areas.

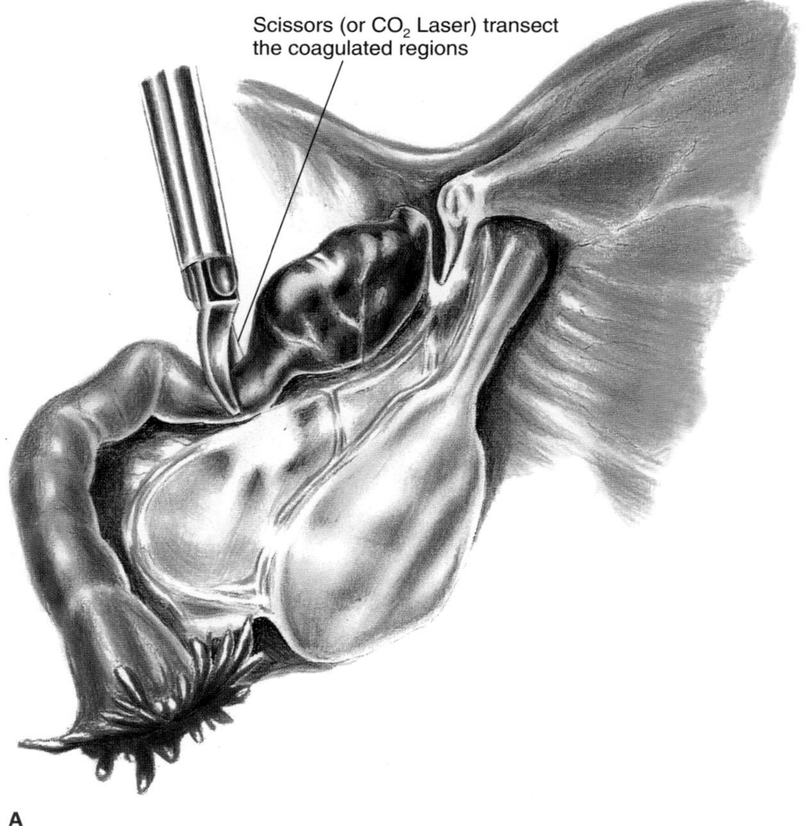

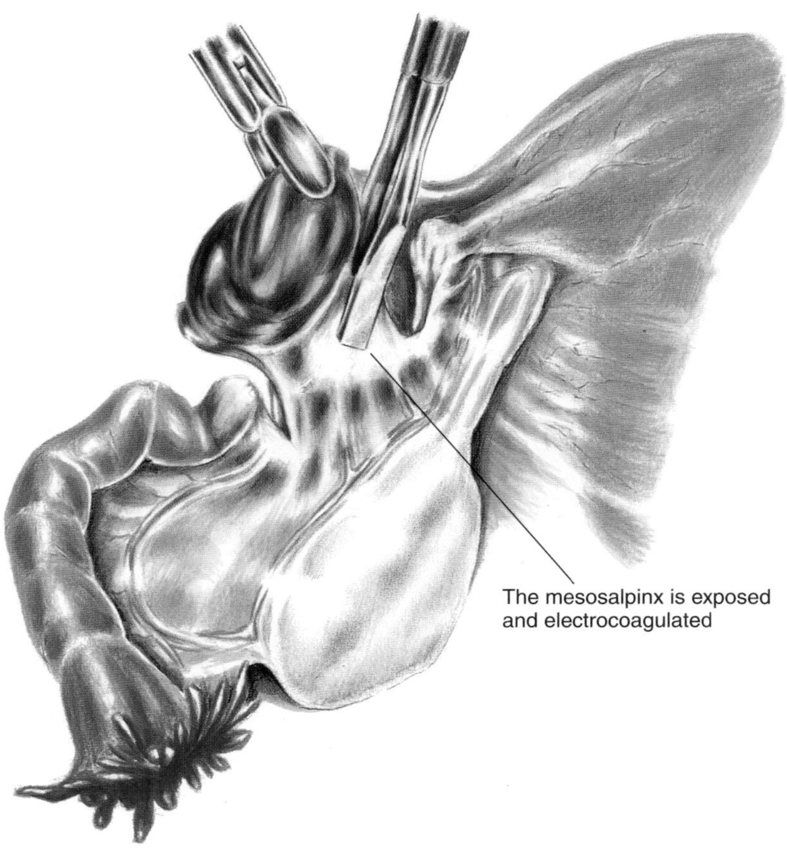

B. The adjacent mesosalpinx is coagulated.

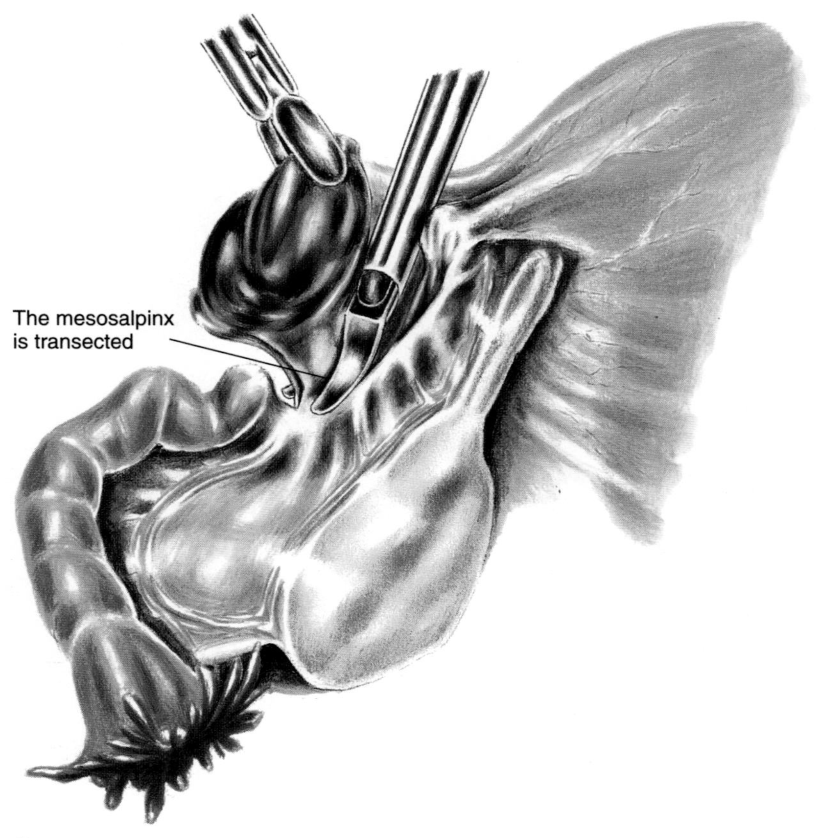

Figure 13-6. (*Continued*) **C.** The isthmic ectopic pregnancy is removed.

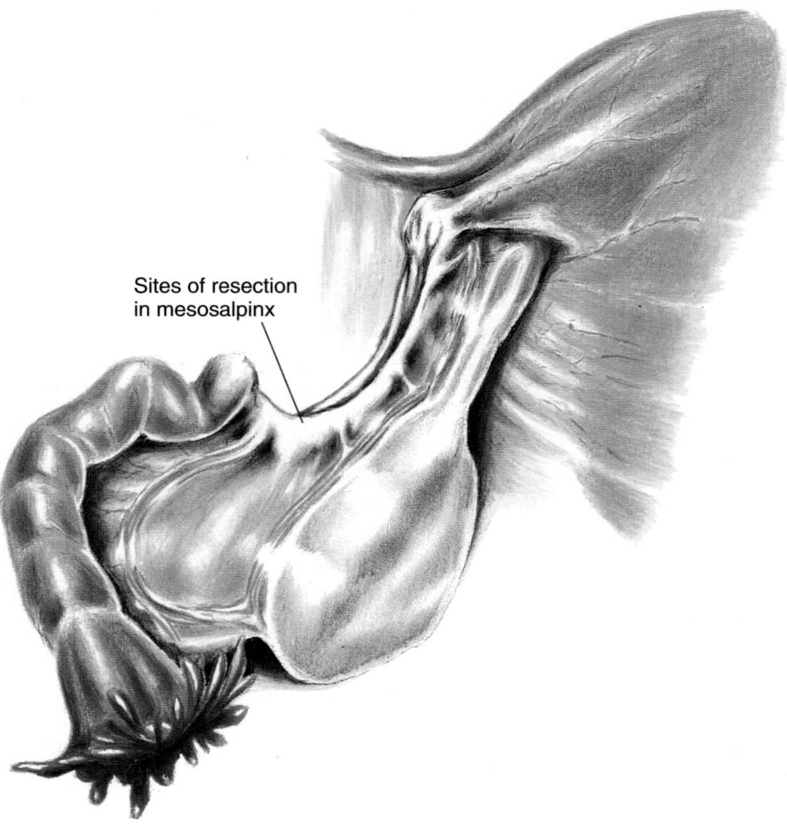

D. The resected segments and mesosalpinx are seen.

Figure 13-6. (*Continued*) **E.** Interceed is placed over the coagulated surfaces.

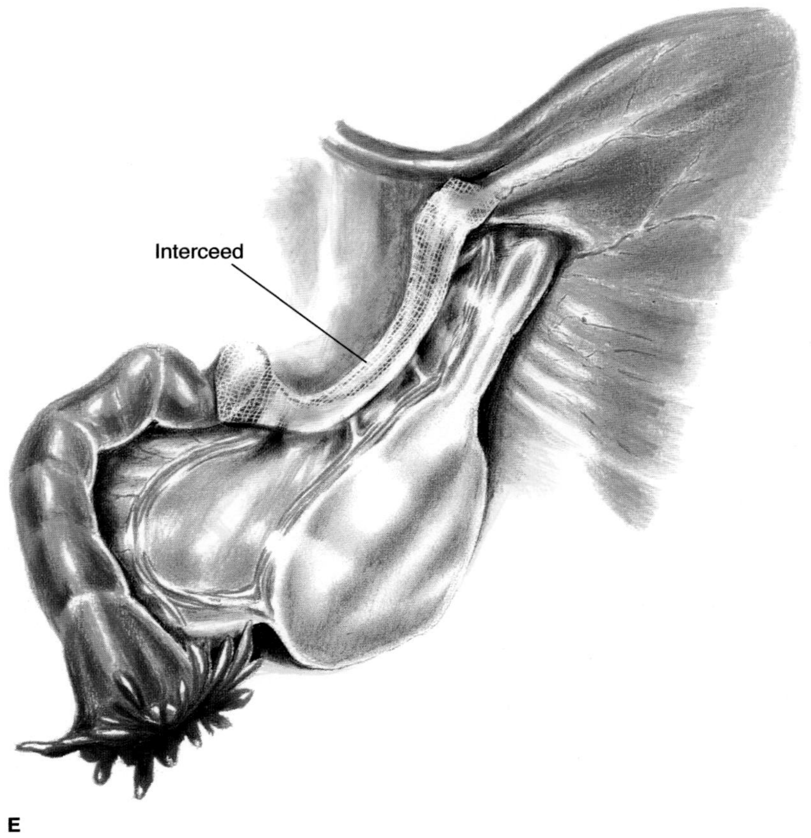

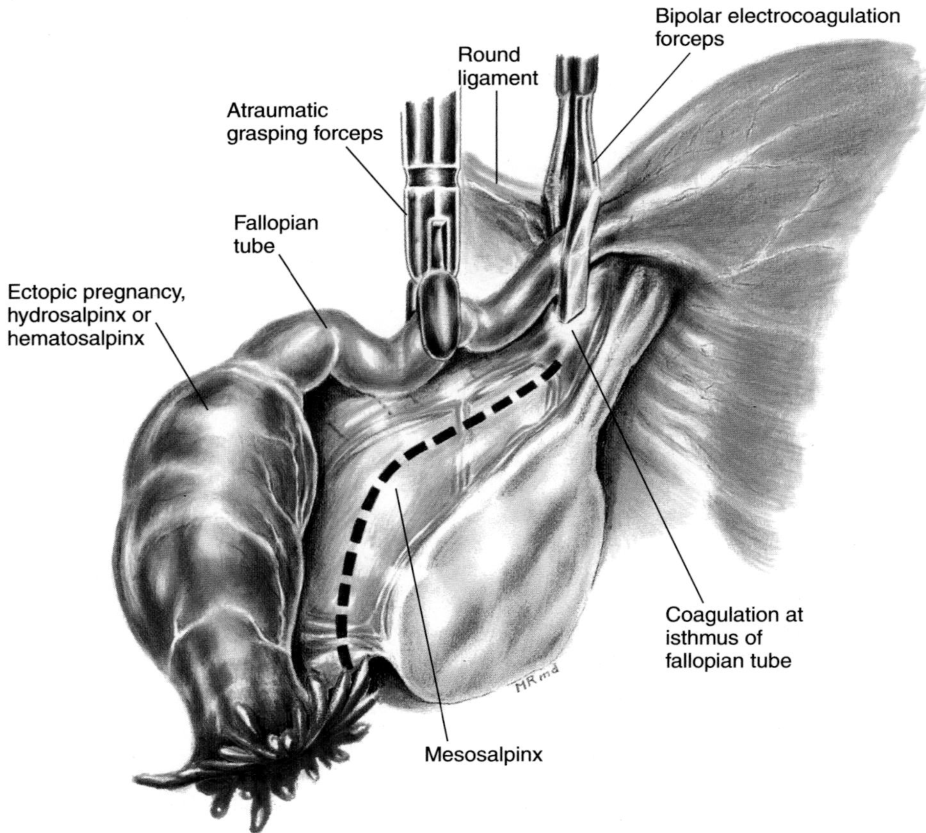

Figure 13-7. **A.** Total salpingectomy is done by progressively coagulating and cutting the mesosalpinx, beginning with the isthmic segment.

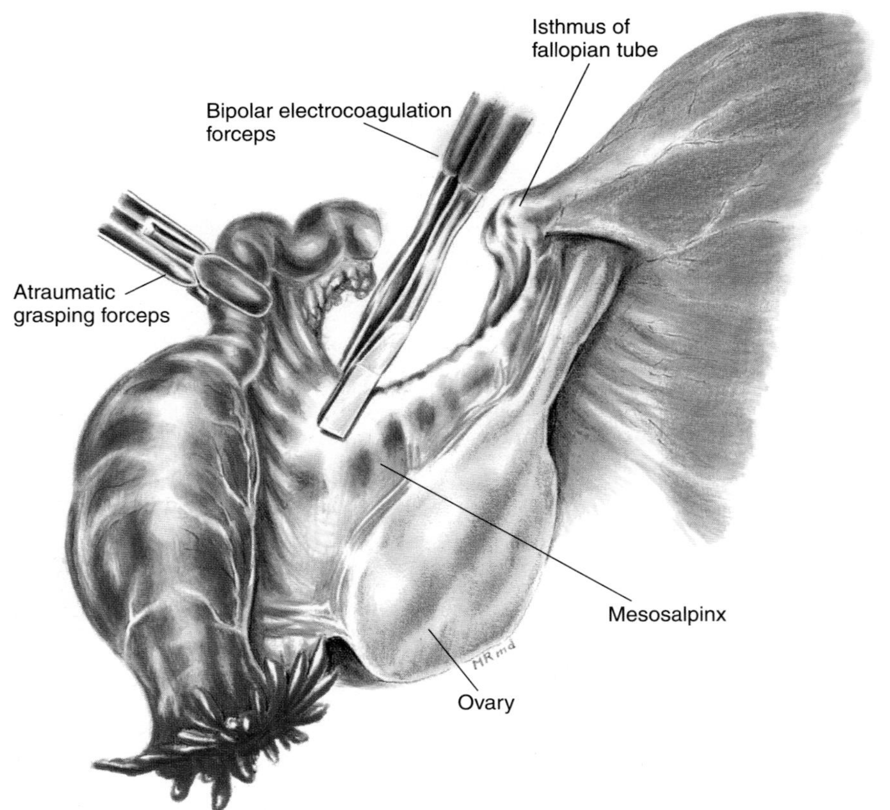

Figure 13-7. (*Continued*) **B.** The mesosalpinx is coagulated with bipolar forceps.

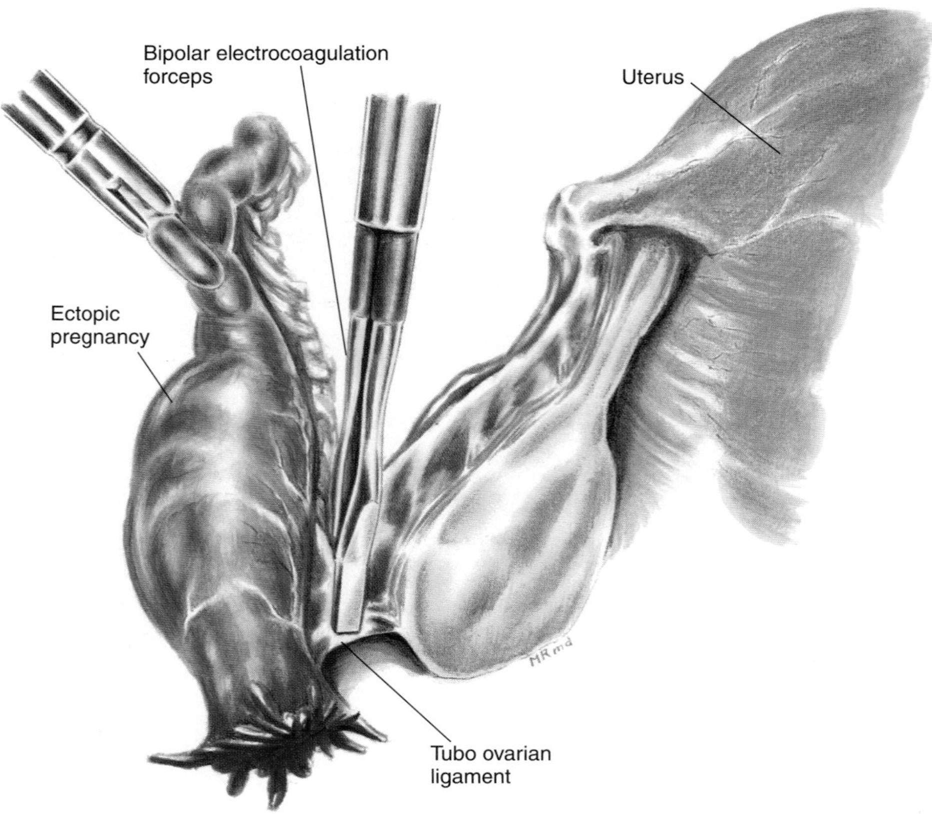

C. The procedure is continued.

Figure 13-7. (*Continued*)
D. The tube is separated from the uterus by using bipolar coagulation and scissors or the laser (*inset*). The isolated tubal segment is removed intact or in sections through the 10-mm sleeve.

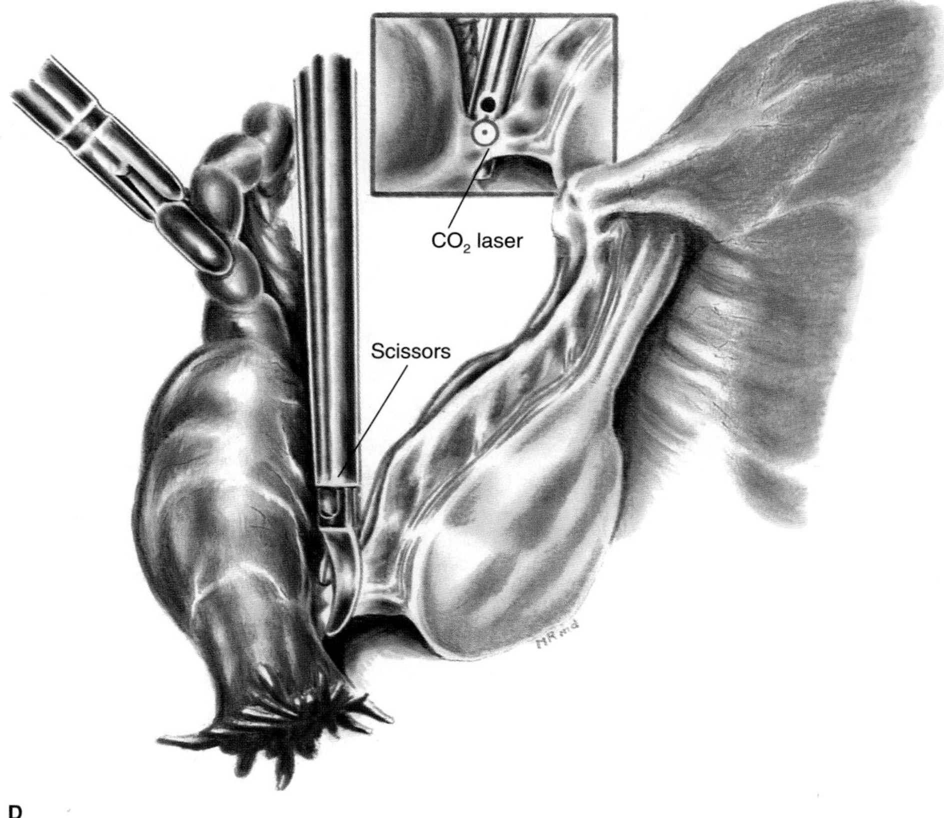

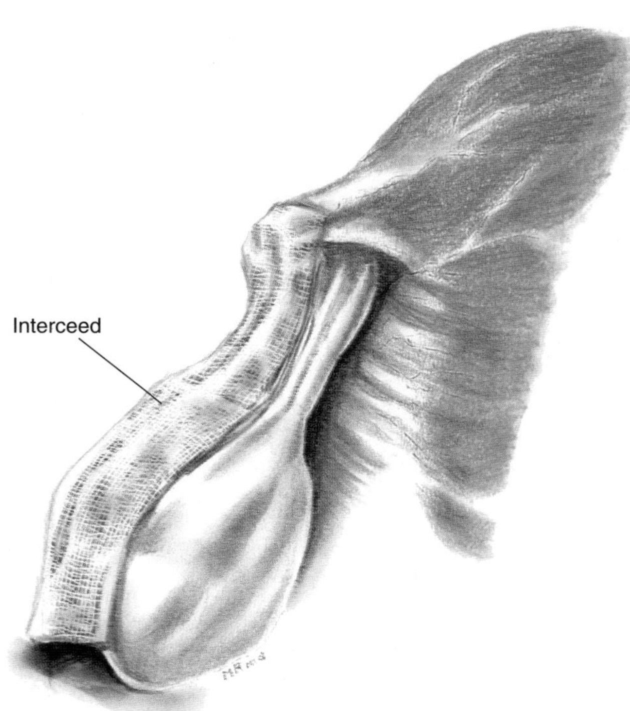

E. Interceed can be placed over the resected area to prevent postoperative adnexal adhesions.

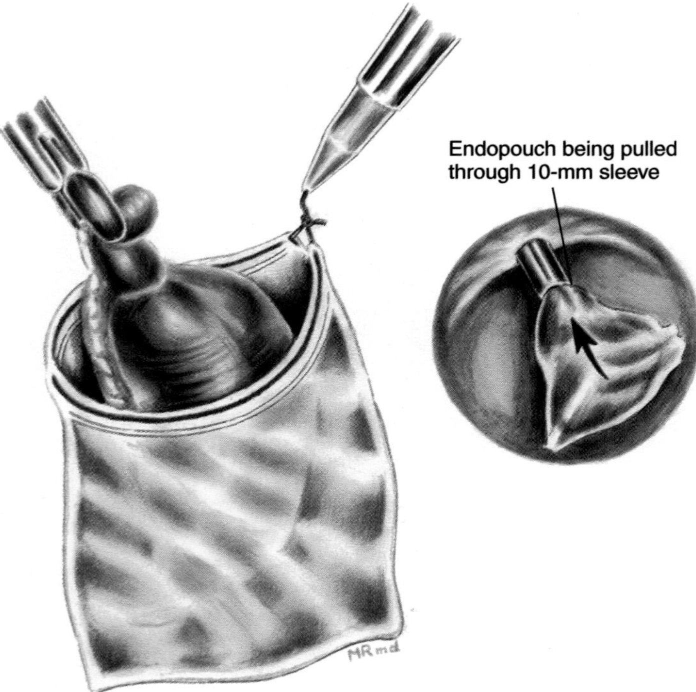

Figure 13-8. The resected tube containing the pregnancy is placed in an Endopouch. The inset shows removal through a 10-mm trocar sleeve.

removed (Figure 13-8). Adhesions and other pathologic processes such as endometriosis are treated during removal of the EUP without prolonging the operation. Occasionally, a patient is admitted overnight to be observed for postoperative bleeding and to receive emotional support from the infertility team.

Follow-Up

In 1 week, the patient returns for a serum hCG to ascertain resolution of the ectopic gestation. The hCG level should be undetectable or very low. If it is above 20 mIU/mL, a repeat blood test is ordered 1 to 2 weeks later, when the hCG should be undetectable.[39] If the levels persist, other treatment options must be considered.

Interstitial Pregnancy

Interstitial (cornual) pregnancies occur rarely; the prevalence ranges from 1 in 2500 to 1 in 5000 live births. Since the morbidity and mortality are high, the correct diagnosis must be made and treatment must be begun promptly. This type of EUP is associated with an increased risk of traumatic rupture and hemorrhagic shock, with a mortality rate of 2 to 2.5%. Later diagnosis and the increased vascularity of this area account for these increased risks. Two to 4% of ectopic gestations are interstitial. The anatomy favors the growing gestation, accounting for the late onset of symptoms and occasional reports of term interstitial pregnancies. The traditional management for interstitial (cornual) pregnancy is salpingectomy with or without cornual resection and sometimes hysterectomy. In selected women, more conservative and less radical approaches are employed if the diagnosis is made early and the patient is stable. Other options include methotrexate (MTX) injections (local or systemic), potassium chloride injections (local), and prostaglandin administration. In a series of 15 patients, unruptured interstitial pregnancies were managed with local MTX administration of 1 mg/kg body weight under transvaginal ultrasound or laparoscopy.[40]

Interstitial pregnancy is suspected in women with an enlarged asymmetric uterus and an eccentrically placed gestational sac on sonography. Differential diagnoses include ovarian and abdominal pregnancy and a pregnancy in one horn of a bicornuate uterus. The diagnosis is confirmed by

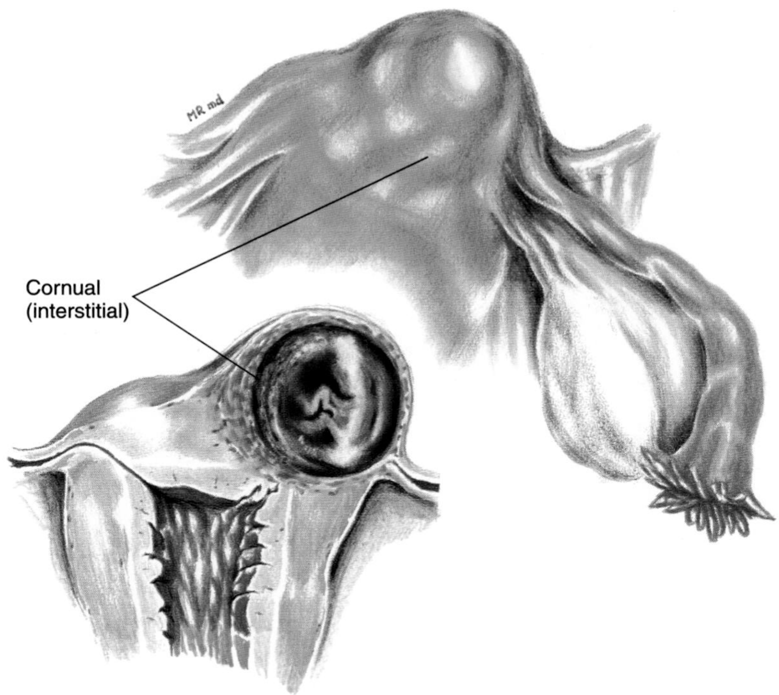

Figure 13-9. An interstitial pregnancy is recognized as a cornual bulge in the myometrium and serosal surface.

laparoscopy, and the treatment involves immediate laparotomy or a combined laparoscopic and hysteroscopic approach in certain patients.

At laparoscopy, the interstitial pregnancy is recognized as a cornual bulge stretching the myometrium and serosal surface (Figure 13-9). If the overlying myometrium is thick and intact, removal of the pregnancy by hysteroscopy is preferable. Early detection of an interstitial pregnancy can be managed by combining MTX and hysteroscopy.[41] A diagnostic laparoscopy is done to identify the location and accessibility of the gestation. If it is accessible by hysteroscopy, it is suctioned or resected using forceps, scissors, or electrosurgery under hysteroscopic control. For larger pregnancies, it is better and faster to do a gentle curettage of the dilated interstitial–cornual area under laparoscopic control. To verify complete removal of the products of conception, hysteroscopic observation of the curetted cornu and the interstitial area is done.

If the pregnancy has eroded through the cornual myometrium, it is prudent to do a laparotomy to remove the pregnancy. In some patients, a laparoscopic approach is considered after the patient is counseled concerning the possibility of a laparotomy.[42–44] The cornu is vascular, and profuse bleeding can occur quickly.

Nonsurgical Management

Other approaches to tubal pregnancy include expectant management and MTX. Since some tubal pregnancies end in tubal abortions or complete reabsorption, particular patients are monitored with repeated levels of hCG until tubal abortion or reabsorption occurs as suggested by falling hormonal levels.[45] With declining values and a starting hCG above 2000 mIU/mL, 93.3% failed on expectant management, whereas below 2000 mIU/mL, 60.0% succeeded.[46] This choice preserves tubal function and fertility, but tubal occlusion can result from retained products of conception.[47] Shalev and coworkers[46] found no difference in the resultant ipsilateral tubal patency or 1-year fertility rates of women succeeding or failing on expectant management. Rantala and coauthors[48] reported a pregnancy rate of 88% and a rate of repeat ectopic pregnancy of 4.2%. Patients who were treated expectantly had a good fertility outcome. Spontaneous regression of the EUP did not lead to increased tubal damage because of the risk for a repeat EUP.

The difficulty with such management lies in the selection of the proper patients. A patient with low or falling titers must understand the risks involved and have the ability to comply with instructions concerning follow-up.

MTX has been recommended for women with a cornual pregnancy or an incomplete resolution of surgically treated ectopic gestation and for residual trophoblastic tissue. Patients who are poor risks because of induced ovarian hyperstimulation syndrome and those suspected of having extensive intraperitoneal abdominal adhesions can be treated medically if they are hemodynamically stable. Single- and multiple-dose treatment plans have been used. In one study, patients were treated with MTX 1 mg/kg intravenously and leucovorin 0.1 mg/kg intramuscularly every other day for 4 days. These patients were admitted to the hospital and monitored during therapy with serum levels of aspartate aminotransferase, lactate dehydrogenase, hCG, and progesterone and with complete blood counts and platelet counts.[49]

A single intramuscular injection of MTX (50 mg/m^2) without citrovorum rescue was used in 29 of 30 consecutive patients with unruptured ectopic pregnancies. Six patients experienced an increase in abdominal pain, and two were hospitalized for overnight observation.[50] This single-dose plan administered on an outpatient basis decreases the expense and lessens the side effects associated with the treatment of EUPs 3 to 5 cm or less in diameter.

Injection of MTX into the gestational sac under ultrasound guidance or at laparoscopy is feasible, and 17 of 24 patients were treated successfully with this technique.[51] Seven of those patients required additional systemic injections, and one patient experienced tubal rupture 3 days after the initial injection. The tubal injection consisted of 10 to 20 mL of adrenaline 1:80,000 dilution injected into the mesosalpinx with a 22-gauge needle, followed by 100 mg MTX injected into the tubal gestation. Leucovorin 15 mg was given orally 30 hours after the administration of MTX. Subsequent systemic MTX injections were given intramuscularly, 50 mg every 2 to 4 days, according to the level of serum hCG. The relative efficacies of MTX and prostaglandin sulprostone (Nalador, Schering Laboratory, Lys-Lez-Lannoy, France) have been compared.[52] The medication was administered into the gestational sac and intramuscularly on days 3, 5 and 7 after the day of diagnosis in 21 patients with an unruptured tubal pregnancy. Both therapies were effective. However, 34% of patients underwent either laparotomy or laparoscopy for a ruptured tubal pregnancy or a persistent rise in hCG levels despite the treatment.

Yao and Tulandi[53] summarized 13 studies that included 523 women treated with a single administration of MTX. The treatment succeeded in 74.4% of these women, with a range of 56.0% to 95.0%. The administration of repeat doses of MTX in 420 women achieved a success rate of 85.3%, with a range of 78.0% to 94.2%. Studies that examined the route of MTX administration reported that the success rate in 177 women treated with local injection of MTX under ultrasound was 81%, ranging between 70% and 95%, while treatment with MTX injection under ultrasound guidance succeeded in 79% of 191 women, ranging from 61% to 100%. These success rates were not significantly different from those reported after a single intra muscular injection, 98% in 172 women, ranging from 86% to 94%. Local injection under laparoscopic guidance offers no advantage over ultrasound guidance since the women must undergo a laparoscopy if the medical treatment fails. Local injection of MTX requires a sonographically visible EUP as well as technical skills and has less consistent success rates than does systemic MTX therapy.[54] Although local administration of MTX may be associated with a lower incidence of side effects, its administration is associated with more inconvenience to the patient and the medical staff.[55]

Medical treatment of EUP with MTX has become the standard of care in many areas of the United States. However, patients with an EUP treated with MTX may require an emergency operation for rupture.[56] Systemic MTX therapy had a more negative impact on patients' health-related quality of life than did laparoscopic salpingostomy.[57] This negative impact on patients' health-related quality of life of systemic MTX therapy should be taken into account in deciding on the appropriate therapy for a tubal pregnancy. Systemic MTX therapy would be preferred by most patients as part of a completely nonsurgical management strategy.[54]

Laparoscopy was as effective as laparotomy in the treatment of tubal pregnancy and reduced the cost considerably.[58,59] Among stable patients, laparoscopic excision of EUPs saved nearly 25% per case compared with laparotomy.[60] Hemodynamic instability increased the cost of management because of the longer length of stay and higher laboratory costs. The cost savings may be lost if patients undergoing laparotomy are discharged on or before postoperative day 2 or if laparoscopic treatment of the EUP is not associated with rapid postoperative discharge.[61]

Medical treatment with MTX is supposed to offer cost savings by minimizing hospitalization.[62,63] Follow-up of patients receiving MTX often is prolonged, necessitating additional blood tests, repeated sonographic evaluations, and loss of days from work. However, a financial analysis of EUP management at a large health plan revealed that total charges were similar for laparotomy and laparoscopy ($6720 and $6840), while outpatient MTX therapy cost less than did the two surgical procedures (average of $818 per case, $p < 0.001$).[64] Another economic analysis described the possible cost benefits of conservative tubal operations for EUP over salpingectomy.[65]

References

1. Rubin GL, Peterson HB, Dorfman SF, et al. Ectopic pregnancy in the United States: 1970 through 1978. *JAMA* 1983; 249:1725.
2. Ectopic pregnancy—Unite States, 1990–1992 *MMWR* 1995; 44:46.
3. Schneider J, Berger CJ, Cattell C. Maternal mortality due to ectopic pregnancy: A review of 102 deaths. *Obstet Gynecol* 1977; 49:557.
4. Goldner TE, Lawson HW, Xia Z, Atrash HK. Surveillance for ectopic pregnancy—United States, 1970–1989. *MMWR* 1993; 42:73.
5. Saraiya M, Berg CJ, Kendrick JS, et al. Cigarette smoking as a risk factor for ectopic pregnancy. *Am J Obstet Gynecol* 1998; 178 (3):493.
6. Ectopic pregnancy—United States, 1986. *MMWR* 1989; 38:481.
7. Makinen J, Rantala M, Vanha-Kamppa O. A link between the epidemic of ectopic pregnancy and the "baby-boom" cohort. *Am J Epidemiol* 1998; 148:369.
8. Schoen JA, Nowak RJ. Repeat ectopic pregnancy: A 16-year clinical survey. *Obstet Gynecol* 1975; 45:542.
9. Sandvei R, Bergsio P, Ulstein M, et al. Repeat ectopic pregnancy—a twenty-year hospital survey. *Acta Obstet Gynecol Scand* 1987; 66:607.
10. Marchbanks PA, Annegers JF, Coulam CB, et al. Risk factors for ectopic pregnancy: A population based study. *JAMA* 1988; 259:1823.
11. Buckley RG, King KJ, Disney JD, et al. Derivation of a clinical prediction model for the emergency department diagnosis of ectopic pregnancy. *Acad Emerg Med* 1998; 5:951.
12. Mol BW, Hajenius PJ, Engelsbel S, et al. Can noninvasive diagnostic tools predict tubal rupture or active bleeding in patients with tubal pregnancy? *Fertil Steril* 1999; 71:167.
13. Dart RG, Kaplan B, Varaklis K. Predictive value of history and physical examination in patients with suspected ectopic pregnancy. *Ann Emerg Med* 1999; 33:283.
14. Mol BW, Hajenius PJ, Engelsbel S, et al. Should patients who are suspected of having an ectopic pregnancy undergo physical examination? *Fertil Steril* 1999; 71:155.
15. Kadar N, DeVore G, Romero R. Discriminatory hCG zone: Its use in the sonographic evaluation for ectopic pregnancy. *Obstet Gynecol* 1981; 58:156.
16. Goldstein SR, Snyder JR, Watson C, et al. Very early pregnancy detection with endovaginal ultrasound. *Obstet Gynecol* 1988; 72:200.
17. Shalev E, Yarom I, Bustan M, et al. Transvaginal sonography as the ultimate diagnostic tool for the management of ectopic pregnancy: Experience with 840 cases. *Fertil Steril* 1998; 69:62.
18. Mol BW, Hajenius PJ, Engelsbel S, et al. Serum human chorionic gonadotropin measurement in the diagnosis of ectopic pregnancy when transvaginal sonography is inconclusive. *Fertil Steril* 1998; 70:972.
19. Mol BW, Lijmer JG, Ankum WM, et al. The accuracy of single serum progesterone measurement in the diagnosis of ectopic pregnancy: A meta-analysis. *Hum Reprod* 1998; 13:3220.
20. Vermesh M, Graczykowski JW, Sauer MV. Reevaluation of the role of culdocentesis in the management of ectopic pregnancy. *Am J Obstet Gynecol* 1990; 162:411.
21. Soriano D, Yefet Y, Oelsner G, et al. Operative laparoscopy for management of ectopic pregnancy in patients with hypovolemic shock. *J Am Assoc Gynecol Laparosc* 1997; 4:363.
22. DeCherney AH, Diamond MP. Laparoscopic salpingostomy for ectopic pregnancy. *Obstet Gynecol* 1987; 70:948.
23. DeCherney AH, Kase N. The conservative surgical management of unruptured ectopic pregnancy. *Obstet Gynecol* 1979; 54:451.
24. Pouly JL, Mahnes H, Mage G, et al. Conservative laparoscopic treatment of 321 ectopic pregnancies. *Fertil Steril* 1986; 46:1093.
25. Vermesh M, Silva PD, Rosen GF, et al. Management of unruptured ectopic gestation by linear salpingostomy: A prospective, randomized clinical trial of laparoscopy versus laparotomy. *Obstet Gynecol* 1989; 73:400.
26. Stromme WB. Conservative surgery for ectopic pregnancy: A 20-year review. *Obstet Gynecol* 1973; 41:215.
27. Timonen S, Nieminen U. Tubal pregnancy: Choice of operative method of treatment. *Acta Obstet Gynecol Scand* 1967; 46:327.

28. Lundorff P, Thornburn J, Lindblom B. Fertility outcome after conservative surgical treatment of ectopic pregnancy evaluated in a randomized trial. *Fertil Steril* 1992; 57:998.
29. Nagele F, Molnar BG, O'Connor H, Magos AL. Randomized studies in endoscopic surgery—where is the proof? *Curr Opin Obstet Gynecol* 1996; 8:281.
30. Bruhat MA, Manhes H, Mage G, et al. Treatment of ectopic pregnancy by means of laparoscopy. *Fertil Steril* 1980; 33:411.
31. Luciano AA, Maier DB, Koch EI, et al. A comparative study of postoperative adhesions following laser surgery by laparoscopy versus laparotomy in the rabbit model. *Obstet Gynecol* 1989; 74:220.
32. Nezhat C, Metzger MD, Nezhat F, et al. Adhesion reformation after reproductive surgery by videolaseroscopy. *Fertil Steril* 1990; 53:1008.
33. Lundorff P, Hahlin M, Kallfelt B, et al. Adhesion formation after laparoscopic surgery in tubal pregnancy: A randomized trial versus laparotomy. *Fertil Steril* 1991; 55:911.
34. Brumsted J, Kessler C, Gibson C, et al. A comparison of laparoscopy and laparotomy for the treatment of ectopic pregnancy. *Obstet Gynecol* 1988; 71:889.
35. Nezhat C, Nezhat F. Conservative management of ectopic gestation (letter to the editor). *Fertil Steril* 1990; 53:382.
36. Frishman GN, Steinhoff MM, Luciano AA. Triplet tubal pregnancy treated by outpatient laparoscopic salpingostomy. *Fertil Steril* 1990; 54:934.
37. Luciano AA. Ectopic pregnancy, in Quilling EJ, Zuspan FP, eds., *Current Therapy in Obstetrics and Gynecology*. Philadelphia: Saunders, 1990.
38. Nezhat F, Winer W, Nezhat C. Salpingectomy via laparoscopy: A new surgical approach. *J Laparoendosc Surg* 1991; 1:91.
39. Jafri SZH, Loginsky JS, Bouffard JA, et al. Sonographic detection of interstitial pregnancy. *J Clin Ultrasound* 1987; 15:253.
40. Benifla JL, Fernandez H, Sebban E, et al. Alternative to surgery of treatment of unruptured interstitial pregnancy: 15 cases of medical treatment. *Eur J Obstet Gynecol Reprod Biol* 1996; 70:151.
41. Groutz A, Wolf Y, Caspi B, et al. Successful treatment of advanced interstitial pregnancy with methotrexate and hysteroscopy: A case report. *J Reprod Med* 1998; 43:719.
42. Laury D. Laparoscopic treatment of an interstitial pregnancy. *J Am Assoc Gynecol Laparosc* 1995; 2:219.
43. Ostrzenski A. A new laparoscopic technique for interstitial pregnancy resection: A case report. *J Reprod Med* 1997; 42:363.
44. Grobman WA, Milad MP. Conservative laparoscopic management of a large cornual ectopic pregnancy. *Hum Reprod* 1998; 13:2002.
45. Kamreava MM, Taymor Ml, Berger MJ, et al. Disappearance of human chorionic gonadotropin following removal of ectopic pregnancy. *Obstet Gynecol* 1983; 62:486.
46. Shalev E, Peleg D, Tsabari A, et al. Spontaneous resolution of ectopic tubal pregnancy: Natural history. *Fertil Steril* 1995; 63:15.
47. Tulandi T, Ferenczy A, Berger E. Tubal occlusion as a result of retained ectopic pregnancy: A case report. *Am J Obstet Gynecol* 1988; 158:1116.
48. Rantala M, Makinen J. Tubal patency and fertility outcome after expectant management of ectopic pregnancy. *Fertil Steril* 1997; 68:1043.
49. Fernandez H, Rainhorn JD, Papiernik E. Spontaneous resolution of ectopic pregnancy. *Obstet Gynecol* 1988; 71 (2):171.
50. Stovall TG, Ling FW, Gray LA. Single doses of methotrexate for treatment of ectopic pregnancy. *Obstet Gynecol* 1991; 77:754.
51. Kooi S, Kock H CLV. Treatment of tubal pregnancy by local injection of methotrexate after adrenaline injection into the mesosalpinx: A report of 25 patients. *Fertil Steril* 1990; 54:580.
52. Fernandez H, Baton C, Lelaidier C, et al. Conservative management of ectopic pregnancy: Prospective randomized clinical trial of methotrexate versus prostaglandin sulprostone by combined transvaginal and systemic administration. *Fertil Steril* 1991; 55:746.
53. Yao M, Tulandi T. Current status of surgical and nonsurgical management of ectopic pregnancy. *Fertil Steril* 1997; 67:421.
54. Namnoum AB. Medical management of ectopic pregnancy. *Clin Obstet Gynecol* 1998; 41:382.
55. Parker J, Bisits A, Proietto AM. A systematic review of single-dose intramuscular methotrexate for the treatment of ectopic pregnancy. *Aust N Z J Obstet Gynaecol* 1998; 38:145.
56. Heard K, Kendall J, Abbott J. Rupture of ectopic pregnancy after medical therapy with methotrexate: A case series. *J Emerg Med* 1998; 16:857.

57. Nieuwkerk PT, Hajenius PJ, Ankum WM, et al. Systemic methotrexate therapy versus laparoscopic salpingostomy in patients with tubal pregnancy: I. Impact on patients' health-related quality of life. *Fertil Steril* 1998; 70:511.
58. Gray DT, Thornburn J, Lundorff P, et al. A cost-effectiveness study of a randomised trial of laparoscopy versus laparotomy for ectopic pregnancy. *Lancet* 1995; 345:1139.
59. Mol BW, Hajenius PJ, Engelsbel S, et al. An economic evaluation of laparoscopy and open surgery in the treatment of tubal pregnancy. *Acta Obstet Gynecol Scand* 1997; 76:596.
60. Foulk RA, Steiger RM. Operative management of ectopic pregnancy: A cost analysis. *Am J Obstet Gynecol* 1996; 175:90.
61. Learman LA, Grimes DA. Rapid hospital discharge following laparoscopy for ectopic pregnancy: A promise unfulfilled? *West J Med* 1997; 167:145.
62. Creinin MD, Washington AE. Cost of ectopic pregnancy management: Surgery versus methotrexate. *Fertil Steril* 1993; 60:963.
63. Yao M, Tulandi T, Kaplow M, Smith AP. A comparison of methotrexate versus laparoscopic surgery for the treatment of ectopic pregnancy: A cost analysis. *Hum Reprod* 1996; 11:2762.
64. Hidlebaugh D, O'Mara P. Clinical and financial analyses of ectopic pregnancy management at a large health plan. *J Am Assoc Gynecol Laparosc* 1997; 4:207.
65. Mol BW, Hajenius PJ, Engelsbel S, et al. Is conservative surgery for tubal pregnancy preferable to salpingectomy? An economic analysis. *Br J Obstet Gynaecol* 1997; 104:834.

14

Operations on the Fallopian Tube

Tubal abnormalities produce infertility in 20% of women who have difficulty conceiving. Pelvic inflammatory disease (PID), previous pelvic operations, a ruptured appendix, and endometriosis are the principal causes. The prevalence of some of these conditions has increased since 1980.[1]

Pelvic Inflammatory Disease

PID results from sexually transmitted diseases caused by infection with chlamydia or gonococcus, an intrauterine device (IUD), or postpartum endometritis. Sequelae cause infertility, tubal pregnancy, chronic pelvic pain, and recurrent upper genital tract infection. The extent of tubal damage and pelvic adhesions depends on the severity of the infection, the number of PID episodes, and the etiology. Peritonitis is associated with a 17% risk of infertility compared with 3% for a mild infection. With each successive episode, the risk of infertility increases. The risk of ectopic pregnancy is 6 to 10 times higher in women who have had PID. Chronic pelvic pain occurs in 15 to 18% of patients after PID because of adhesions. About 25% of these patients will have at least one recurrent infection.[2] Additional criteria that support a diagnosis of PID include oral temperature above 101°F (38.3°C), abnormal cervical or vaginal discharge, elevated erythrocyte sedimentation rate and C-reactive protein, and laboratory documentation of cervical infection with *Neisseria gonorrhoeae* or *Chlamydia trachomatis*.

The definitive criteria for diagnosing PID are histopathologic evidence of endometritis on an endometrial biopsy specimen, transvaginal sonography or other imaging techniques showing thickened fluid-filled tubes with or without free pelvic fluid or a tubo-ovarian complex, and laparoscopic abnormalities consistent with PID.

The Use of Laparoscopy for Diagnosis

The clinical diagnosis of PID is difficult because of the wide variation in symptoms and signs. Many women report subtle, nonspecific symptoms such as dyspareunia, postcoital spotting, and abnormal uterine bleeding. In these situations, a bimanual examination could reveal cervical motion or adnexal tenderness. Even in the presence of "classic" symptoms and signs such as lower abdominal pain, cervical motion and adnexal tenderness, elevated white cell count, fever, and a mass on ultrasound, other diseases are part of a differential diagnosis (Table 14-1). Several studies suggest that the diagnosis is correct in only 65% of patients.[3–5] Laparoscopy is used to make precise identification so that appropriate therapy can be instituted. Its routine use to diagnose acute salpingitis is widespread in Europe.[6]

Treatment

The objectives are to cure the initial infection and prevent sequelae. Initial treatment of a mild infection involves outpatient therapy with broad-spectrum antibiotics that are effective against both penicillin-resistant gonococcus and chlamydia (Table 14-2). Empirical treatment of PID should be started in women who are at risk if lower abdominal tenderness, adnexal tenderness, and cervical motion tenderness are present.[7]

TABLE 14-1. Differential Diagnosis of Pelvic Inflammatory Disease

Appendicitis
Endometriosis
Ruptured ovarian cyst
Torsion of adnexa
Gastroenteritis
Urinary tract infection

Treatment can be initiated before a bacteriologic diagnosis of *C. trachomatis* or *N. gonorrhoeae* infection. Such confirmation necessitates treating the sexual partners.

Droegemueller[8] recommended hospitalizing women suspected of having mild PID so that intravenous antibiotics can be administered. The criteria for admission are listed in Table 14-3.

Tubo-ovarian abscess (TOA) is a severe sequela and occurs in almost one-third of patients hospitalized with PID. Symptomatic or subclinical infections can progress rapidly into a TOA,[9] which can rupture and cause peritonitis. A TOA can be drained laparoscopically with the aid of accessory instruments, reducing the risk of serious morbidity associated with rupture.

TABLE 14-2. Oral Treatment for Pelvic Inflammatory Disease

Outpatient
Regimen A
Ofloxacin 400 mg orally twice a day for 14 days
Metronidazole 500 mg orally twice a day for 14 days
Regimen B
Ceftriaxone 250 mg IM once or
Cefoxitin 2 g IM plus probenecid 1 g orally in a single dose concurrently once or
Other parenteral third-generation cephalosporines (e.g., ceftizoxime or cefotaxime) plus
Doxycycline 100 mg orally twice a day for 14 days (include this regimen with one of the above regimens)
Inpatient (Parenteral)
Regimen A
Cefotetan 2 g IV every 12 hours or cefoxitin 2 g IV every 6 hours plus
Doxycycline 100 mg IV or orally every 12 hours
Regimen B
Clindamycin 900 mg IV every 8 hours plus gentamicin loading dose IV or IM (2 mg/kg body weight), followed by a maintenance dose (1.5 mg/kg) every 8 hours; single daily dosing may be substituted

Source: Centers for Disease Control and Prevention.[7]

TABLE 14-3. Criteria for Hospitalization

Surgical emergencies such as appendicitis cannot be excluded. The patient
Is pregnant
Does not respond clinically to oral antimicrobial therapy
Is unable to follow or tolerate an outpatient oral regimen
Has severe illness, nausea and vomiting, or high fever
Has a tubo-ovarian abscess
Is immunodeficient (i.e., has HIV infection with low CD4 counts, is taking immunosuppressive therapy, or has another disease)

Source: Centers for Disease Control and Prevention.[7]

The accepted treatment for a TOA has been total abdominal hysterectomy with bilateral salpingo-oophorectomy regardless of the patient's age because the risk from a rupture is avoided and the chance for a cure is excellent.

Laparoscopic procedures for treating pelvic abscesses have been described by several authors.[6,9,10] Two 5-mm trocars are inserted in the lower quadrants, and a suction-irrigator probe and grasping forceps are inserted through the trocars. The pelvis, upper abdomen, and pelvic viscera are examined for free or loculated purulent material, and the course of both ureters is identified. Collections are dispersed gently with the suction-irrigator, and purulent fluid is aspirated. Cultures are taken from the inflammatory exudate. If necessary, the suction-irrigator is used to bluntly mobilize the omentum, small bowel, rectosigmoid, and tubo-ovarian adhesions (Figure 14-1). After the abscess cavity is localized, it is drained, and the suction-irrigator separates the bowel and omentum completely from the reproductive organs. TOAs are separated by using a combination of blunt lysis and hydrodissection. Adhesions caused by acute PID are soft and can be disrupted by gentle blunt dissection and hydrodissection. Hydrodissection is done by placing the tip of the suction-irrigator between the tissues. The pressure of the fluid spray and the gentle force of the instrument create a plane for dissection (Figure 14-2). The 5-mm graspers provide traction and countertraction, improving observation of the affected area. After the abscess is mobilized, it is drained (Figure 14-3). Its walls are removed in sections by using the 5-mm

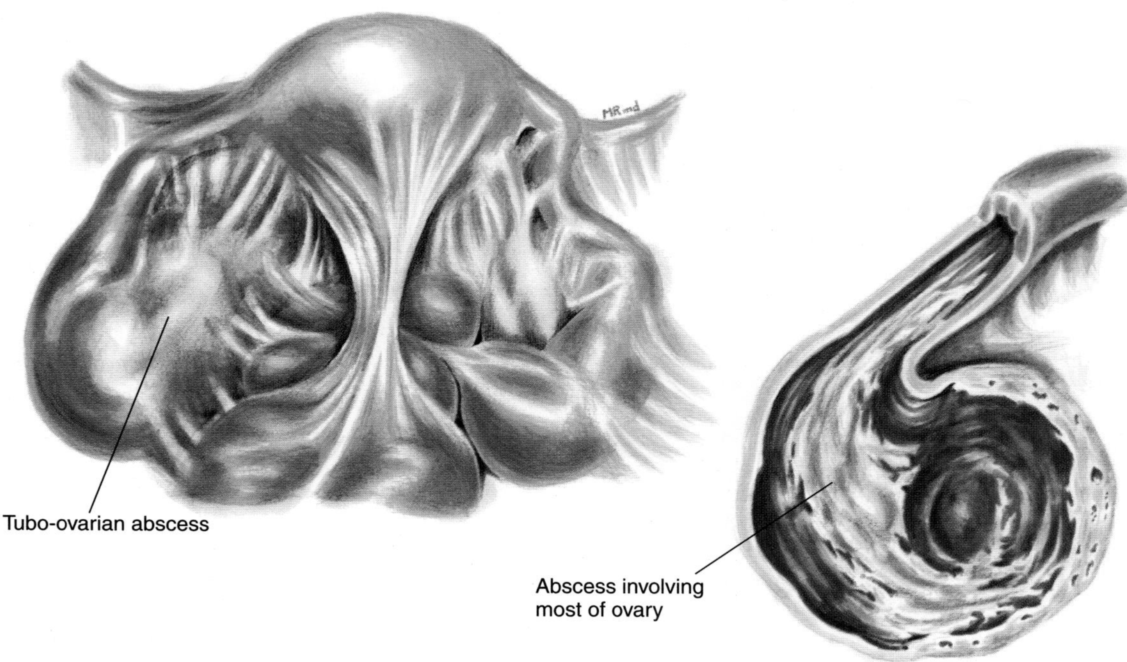

Figure 14-1. The abscess is localized and is prepared for drainage. The cut surface of the tubo-ovarian abscess is shown.

graspers (Figure 14-4). Though technically arduous, meticulous dissection of the abscess from the surrounding structures is important for success.

The infection can involve the site of ovulation. Once the ovary is mobilized, rents or holes in it are irrigated copiously. Sutures are not required to repair the ovary. Graspers are inserted into the tubal ostium to spread it and free agglutinated fimbriae. Chromopertubation is not suggested because edema in the interstitial tissue of the tube occludes the lumen. At the end of the procedure, the peritoneal cavity is irrigated with lactated Ringer's solution until the effluent is clear (Figure 14-5). The upper abdomen is irrigated also, and the remainder of the irrigation fluid is aspirated with the patient in a reverse Trendelenburg

Figure 14-2. Hydrodissection and gentle blunt dissection lessen the potential for intestinal injury.

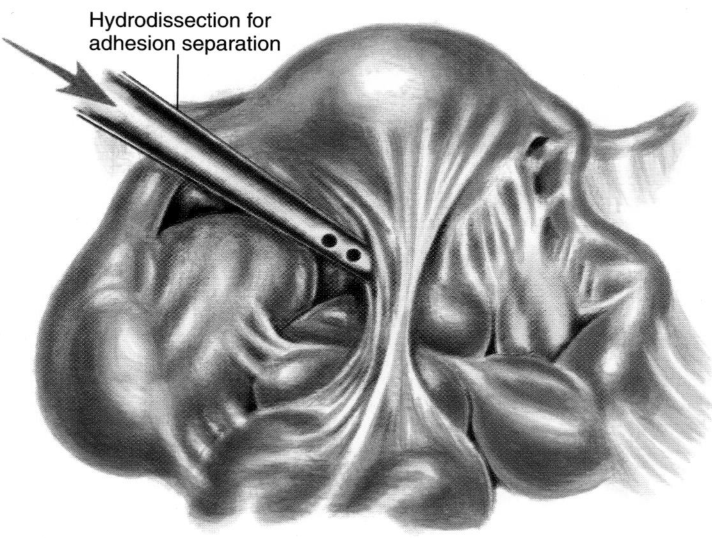

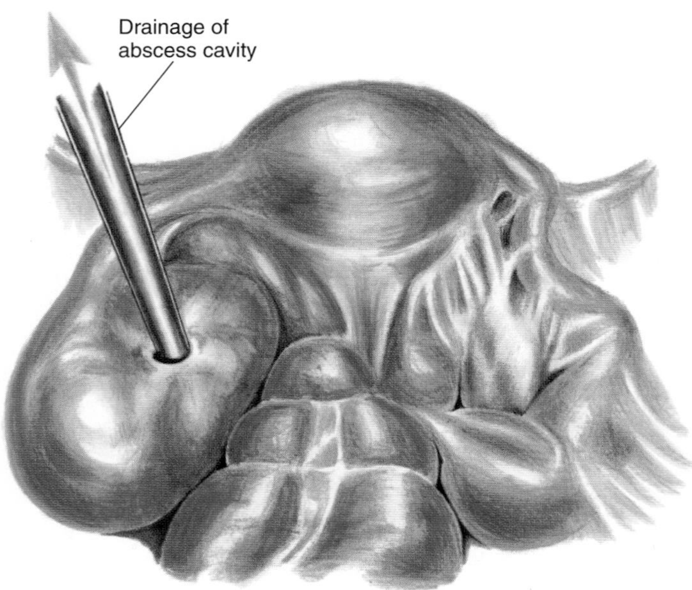

Figure 14-3. The abscess cavity is drained and irrigated.

position. Between 300 and 400 mL of irrigation fluid is left in the pelvis to separate these organs during the early healing phase. Hydrodissection and gentle blunt dissection decrease the potential for intestinal injury; the laser and electrosurgery should be used sparingly.

Henry-Suchet and associates[6] presented data on 50 patients with TOA and noted clinical improvement in 90% within 5 days of combined treatment consisting of laparoscopic abscess drainage and antibiotics. Eight patients required laparotomy for removal of some or all reproductive organs later. Second-look laparoscopy revealed bilateral adhesions with tubal obstruction in only 16% of these patients. Similar results were found in other studies.[10,11] Mecke and colleagues[11] described their results in 66 patients with pelvic abscesses. Twenty-five required laparotomy, but the others underwent operative laparoscopy. The choice was based on a patient's age, clinical presentation, and operative findings. Abscesses involving both adnexa and adnexal masses in older

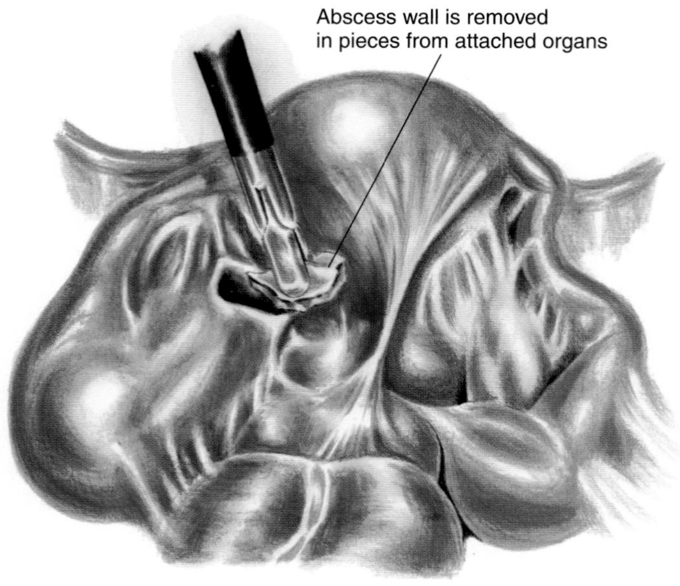

Figure 14-4. Sections of the abscess cavity removed in pieces, using a 5-mm grasper.

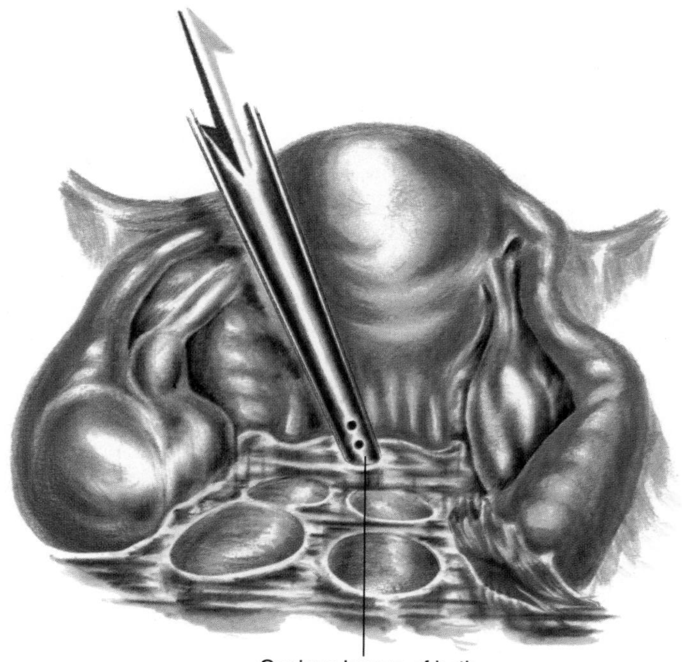

Figure 14-5. The pelvis is irrigated.

women were removed at laparotomy. In women over age 40, fertility is less a consideration and TOAs are associated more often with ovarian cancer and systemic illness such as diabetes rather than with sexually transmitted diseases.[12]

In contrast to the adhesions associated with an acute abscess, chronic TOAs have dense walls. The bowel often adheres to pelvic organs and is dissected with difficulty; the adnexa appear as a dense mass, making it difficult to distinguish between the pyosalpinx and the ovary. Adhesiolysis technically is difficult and is associated with a high risk of complications.[11]

Raiga and coauthors[13] studied 39 patients who were treated for adnexal abscesses. Those authors showed that laparoscopic surgery is a safe and efficient technique for treating this condition. No immediate repeat operation was necessary within the first 2 months after the initial laparoscopic procedure. At a second-look laparoscopy, an adhesiolysis was required in all the patients. A salpingostomy was done in 17 women, and 6 others were referred for in vitro fertilization–embryo transfer (IVF-ET). Subsequently, 12 of 19 patients who did not use any contraception became pregnant. While laparoscopy remains the technique of choice in the initial management of adnexal abscesses, the anatomic results observed at second-look laparoscopy suggest that a second-look procedure may be essential for patients who desire future pregnancy.

A laparoscopic study of acute PID conducted in Nairobi, Kenya, among patients with acute salpingitis showed that the likelihood of TOA was related to HIV-1 infection and advanced immunosuppression.[14]

Tubal Reconstruction

Distal tubal obstruction has been treated by laparotomy and microsurgical techniques with pregnancy rates of 20 to 30% 2 years postoperatively.[15] Fimbrioplasty and lysis of peritubal and periovarian adhesions result in the best outcome.[16] For some women with severe tubal damage, IVF offers a better chance of conception (72.3%) than does tuboplasty (27.3%).[17] Laparoscopy for tubal infertility is a significant factor in reducing medical costs and the duration of recuperation, although the technique has not increased pregnancy rates.[18]

Pregnancy after the repair of damaged fallopian tubes depends on many factors, the most important of which are the type of tubal occlusion and the severity of the periadnexal adhesions. Adhesions can be filmy, dense, and vascular and involve the tubes and ovaries. Other pelvic diseases, such as endometriosis and myomas, also affect the outcome. The principles of laparoscopic tuboplasty are listed in Table 14-4.

TABLE 14-4. Principles of Tubal Reconstruction

Magnification
Meticulous hemostasis
Prevention of tissue desiccation
Complete excision of pathologic tissue
Prevention of tissue ischemia/thermal damage
Avoidance or minimized use of sutures
Gentle/atraumatic handling of tissues
Adhesion-preventing regimens/devices

TABLE 14-5. Factors Associated with Increased Risk of Adhesions

Ischemia
Sutures
Peritoneal/omental grafts
Tissue drying
Blood clots
Infection
Tissue necrosis
Tissue abrasion

Techniques

Before refinements in laparoscopy were developed, most tubal operations were aided by an operating microscope or magnifying loupes. These instruments reduced tissue trauma and increased the detection of abnormalities. Magnification allowed the use of microsurgical instruments and fine, nonreactive sutures. It represented an improvement over macrosurgical techniques.

The combination of the laparoscope and the video monitor makes it possible to do tubal microsurgery with laparoscopic instruments. The serosa of the fallopian tube is delicate and easily traumatized, especially when graspers apply traction. Although laparoscopic Babcock clamps allow atraumatic manipulation of the tube, it is still possible to tear the mesosalpinx and lacerate vessels. It is preferable to use a manipulating probe, a closed grasper, or the suction-irrigator to position the tube and apply traction. The tubal serosa is held behind the fimbria on the antimesenteric aspect by using atraumatic grasping forceps. Fimbriae are very vascular and bleed with little cause. Bleeding is difficult to localize precisely, and frequent attempts to achieve hemostasis can damage tubes. Unless a large vessel is torn, most bleeding will stop spontaneously. An injection of 3 to 5 mL of dilute vasopressin (Pitressin) in the mesosalpinx can be used to decrease bleeding. The removal of clots is vital to prevent adhesions (Table 14-5).

Sutures

The use of sutures in the pelvis increases the risk of adhesions, but there are circumstances in which their judicious use can improve the operative outcome. During neosalpingostomy, if the defocused laser is unsuccessful in flaring back the tube or if the tubal mucosa is thick, a monofilament suture is recommended [4-0 polydiaxanone sutures (PDS) or a similar type].

Prophylactic Antibiotics

Surgical trauma can predispose a patient who has some latent salpingitis to a recurrence. Therefore, prophylactic antibiotics are recommended for any woman having reconstructive tubal surgery.

Distal Tubal Occlusion

A hydrosalpinx results from distal tubal occlusion and is characterized by a dilated tube filled with clear fluid. It is a consequence of infectious salpingitis and is associated with intrinsic tubal disease. Extrinsic diseases result from a ruptured appendix, adhesions from previous pelvic operations, or endometriosis and do not affect the tubal mucosa. Boer-Meisel and coworkers[19] and Schlaff and colleagues[20] found that the best pregnancy rates correlated with a normal endosalpinx and the absence of adhesions. The presence of numerous fixed adhesions and thick tubal walls are contraindications to attempting salpingoneostomy. Several scoring systems have been proposed to predict the probability of conception (Table 14-6).[21,22] Any patient who has had a tuboplasty is at increased risk for an ectopic pregnancy.

Several reports have shown the advantages of microsurgery compared with gross tuboplastic operations. No randomized studies have correlated the relative efficacy of tuboplasty by laparotomy, microsurgery, and laparoscopy (Table 14-7).[16,20–58] Pregnancy rates after laparoscopic tuboplasty are comparable to those after microsurgery (Table 14-8).[15,19–22,35,37–46,59–71] Results of CO_2 laser surgery and electrosurgery are similar (Table 14-9).[22,46]

TABLE 14-6. Classifications of Tubal Obstructions

Rock et al[21]

Mild (80% pregnancy rate)
- Absent or small hydrosalpinx <15 mm in diameter
- Inverted fimbria easily recognized when patency is achieved
- No significant peritubal or periovarian adhesions
- Preoperative hysterogram reveals a rugal pattern

Moderate (31% pregnancy rate)
- Hydrosalpinx 15 to 30 mm in diameter
- Fragments of fimbria not readily identified
- Periovarian and/or peritubular adhesions without fixation, minimal cul-de-sac adhesions

Severe (16% pregnancy rate)
- Large hydrosalpinx >30 mm in diameter
- No frimbia
- Dense pelvic or adnexal adhesions with fixation of the ovary and tube to the broad ligament, pelvic side wall, omentum, and/or bowel
- Obliteration of the cul-de-sac
- Frozen pelvis (adhesion formation so dense that limits of organs are difficult to define)

Boer-Meisel et al[19]

Four questions	Four answers	Factor score
1. Is the tube wall thin?	Yes	1
	No	2
2. Is the gross condition of the endosalpinx normal?	Yes	1
	No	2 or 3
3. Are there not many adhesions?	Yes	1 or 2
	No	3
4. Are the adhesions not fixed?	Yes	1 or 2
	No	3

Four yes answers—good prognosis (77% conception rate); three yes answers—intermediate prognosis (21% conception rate); two yes answers—poor prognosis (3% conception rate)

Mage et al[22]

Factors	Scoring
Tubal patency	Partial occulusion—2; total occlusion—5
Tubal mucosa (HSG)	Normal folds—0; decreased folds—5; no folds or honeycomb—10
Tubal wall (direct exam)	Normal—0; thin—5; thick or rigid—10

Grade I, 2–5 (58.8% pregnancy rate); grade II, 7–10 (36.6% pregnancy rate); grade III, 12–15 (9.5% pregnancy rate); grade IV, 12–15 (0% pregnancy rate)

Neosalpingostomy

After the laparoscope is inserted and two to three suprapubic trocars are placed, the suction-irrigator and grasping forceps are introduced. Adhesions surrounding the tubes and ovaries are lysed with the CO_2 laser (30 to 80 W) or any other cutting method. Once the adnexa are freely mobile, the distal portion of the tube is manipulated into position with the grasper and the uterine fundus is used as a shelf. Fluid distention of the tube with chromopertubation allows identification of the avascular central point that is the thinnest portion of the tube (Figure 14-6). A cruciate incision using the CO_2 laser or scissors creates several flaps (Figure 14-7). The edges are flared back by using

TABLE 14-7. Macrosurgery and Microsurgery for Tubal Occlusion

	n	Pregnancies, %	Ectopic, %
Macrosurgery			
Fayez and Suliman[16]	128	35	N/A
Rock et al[21]	87	28	20
Palmer[23]	51	35	22
Mulligan[24]	66	30	30
Garcia[25]	25	28	N/A
Crane and Woodruff[26]	34	26	22
O'Brien et al[27]	83	29	8
Young et al[28]	114	32	16
Grant[29]	217	22	10
Lamb and Moscovitz[30]	48	15	42
Umezaki et al[31]	52	23	17
Comninos[32]	30	43	15
Siegler and Kontopoulos[33]	26	35	55
Spadoni[34]	7	43	N/A
DeCherney and Kase[35]	9	22	N/A
Wallach et al[36]	24	20	N/A
Total	1001	28	
Microsurgery			
Fayez and Suliman[16]	73	50	N/A
Schlaff et al[20]	95	27	26
Mage et al[22]	76	35	25
Siegler and Kontopoulos[33]	32	47	26
DeCherney and Kase[35]	72	42	13
Swolin[37]	33	46	40
Marik[38]	52	23	N/A
Salat-Baroux et al[39]	42	33	7
Betz et al[40]	27	26	42
Gomel[41]	72	29	N/A
Frantzen and Schlosser[42]	85	14	N/A
Hulka[43]	61	9	N/A
Verhoeven et al[44]	115	29	9
Bellina[45]	56	48	4
Tulandi et al[46]	68	28	26
Russell et al[47]	72	58	14
Donnez and Casanas-Roux[48]	83	38	19
Kitchin et al[49]	103	38	35
Daniell et al[50]	48	21	10
Carey and Brown[51]	87	24	13
Jacobs et al[52]	161	32	18
Williams and Griffin[53]	69	42	41
Audibert et al[54]	211	40	24
Canis et al[55]	76	30	N/A
Chong[56]	34	32	18
Total	1903	34	

*Ectopic rate represents the proportion of total pregnancies that are extrauterine.

N/A—not available.

the defocused laser (10 W). The defocused laser causes the serosa and superficial underlying tissue to shrink, thus everting the edges of the tube without a suture.

Neosalpingostomy can be created by opening the distended tubal end and grasping the endosalpinx with an atraumatic grasping forceps, pulling it out and back over the tube like a sleeve.[72] The defocused laser is used to evert the edges further. If the tube is thick and does not flare back well with the laser, the edges are sutured to the tubal serosa by using 4-0 PDS (Ethicon) (Figure 14-8).

TABLE 14-8. Laparotomy and Laparoscopy for Tubal Occlusion

	n	Pregnancies, %	Ectopic, %	Follow-up, years
Laparotomy				
Boer-Meisel et al[19]	108	46	38	N/A
Schlaff et al[20]	95	27	26	N/A
Rock et al[21]	87	28	6	>4
Mage et al[22]	68	37	9	1.5
DeCherney and Kase[35]	54	44	17	2
Swolin[37]	33	63	24	>8
Tulandi et al[46]	45	24	2	1
Audibert et al[54]	211	40	24	2
Canis et al[55]	76	30	N/A	N/A
Gomel[57]	41	29	12	>1
Jansen[58]	91	18	?	>10
Kelly and Roberts[59]	28	11	4	1
Tulandi and Vilos[60]	67	26	4	2
Total	1011	33		
Laparoscopy				
Audibert et al[54]	55	20	15	2
Canis et al[55]	87	33	6	N/A
Gomel[57]	9	44	0	1
Mettler et al[61]	38	26	?	>1
Fayez[62]	19	10	10	2
Daniell and Herbert[63]	21	24	5	0.5–1.5
Dubuisson et al[64]	65	33	18	N/A
McComb and Paleologou[65]	22	22	N/A	>1
Nezhat et al[66]	42	35	15	
Total	370	30		
Since 1994				
Prapas et al[67]	32	31	6	>2
Filippini et al[68]	104	32	4	>1
Lavergne et al[69]	46	39	4	>1.5
Kasia et al[70]	194	27	4	>2
Audebert et al[71]	35	74	22	>2
Total	411	40		

Tubal patency is confirmed by injecting diluted indigo carmine through the uterine cannula. The presence of fimbrial adhesions is assessed on a close-up view as the dye is injected.

Oh[73] did a comparative study in 82 women to ascertain the best method of laparoscopic neosalpingostomy with respect to postoperative tubal patency and pregnancy. Clubbed fimbriae were incised with scissors and sutured after eversion in 26 patients (type 1 procedure); incised with an electrosurgical needle and everted by endocoagulator without suturing in 27 (type 2), with the original fimbrial shape being restored by traction with grasping forceps after a small hole was made with an electrosurgical needle; the fimbriae were sutured after eversion in 29 women (type 3). Tubal patency rates on hysterosalpingography 2 months after the three operations were 13 (50%) of 26 patients for type 1, 23 (85.1%) of 27 patients for type 2, and 28 (96.2%)

TABLE 14-9. CO_2 Laser and Electrosurgery by Laparoscopy for Treatment of Tubal Occlusion

	n	Pregnancies, %	Ectopic, %
Laser			
Mage et al[22]	38	42	18
Tulandi et al[46]	37	29	18
Electrosurgery			
Mage et al[22]	30	30	33
Tulandi et al[46]	30	23	14

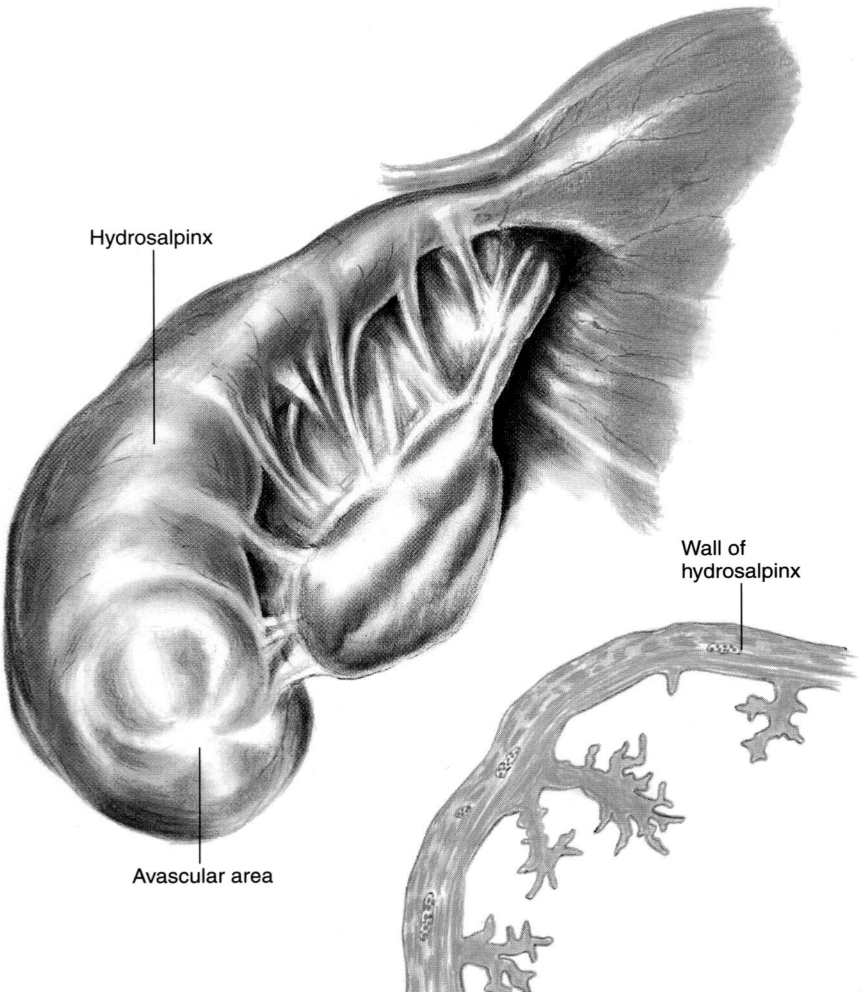

Figure 14-6. Chemopertubation is done, and an avascular central point of hydrosalpinx is identified. The section of tubal wall shows the endosalpinx with some luminal folds.

of 29 patients for type 3. Tubal patency for types 2 and 3 was significantly higher than it was for type 1 ($p < 0.01$). Conception rates within 3 years for the procedures were 5 (19.2%) of 26 women for type 1, 10 (37.2%) of 27 for type 2, and 14 (48.2%) of 29 for type 3. The conception rate for type 3 was significantly higher than that for type 1 ($p < 0.05$). The type 3 procedure was the most effective method, especially when done in patients with favorable prognostic factors.

Laparoscopic neosalpingostomies can be technically difficult and time-consuming and have suboptimal results in inexperienced hands. A laparoscopically assisted extracorporeal technique has been proposed,[10] followed by microsurgical neosalpingostomy. Operative time and cost can be reduced under such circumstances.

Fimbrioplasty

The goal of fimbrioplasty is to expose the fimbria to restore normal function. Tubal phimosis results from fimbrial agglutination and adhesions that bind the fimbriated end to the ovary or cover the distal end.

Chromopertubation distends the tube. If adhesions cover the ostia, they are incised with scissors and separated with the CO_2 laser, microscissors, a fiber laser, or a fine electrode tip. This is accomplished by first lysing any periadnexal adhesions so that the tube is freely mobile. The tube is immobilized by using the uterus as a shelf or by steadying its position with a blunt probe. To deagglutinate the fimbria, a closed 3-mm forceps is

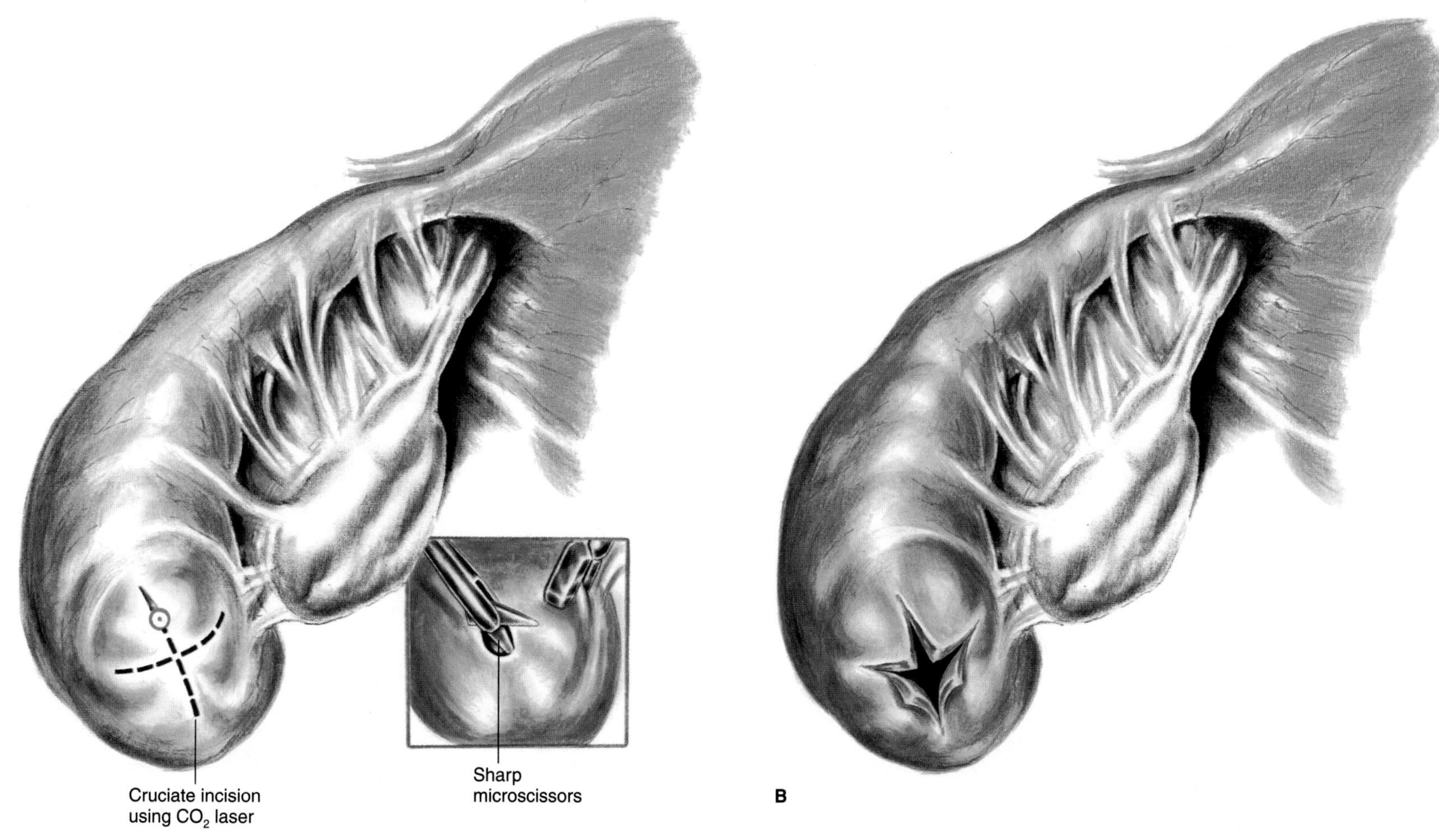

Figure 14-7. **A.** Cruciate incisions are made in distal end of the tube. Sharp microscissors (*inset*) or an ultrapulse CO_2 laser is used. **B.** Several flaps are created.

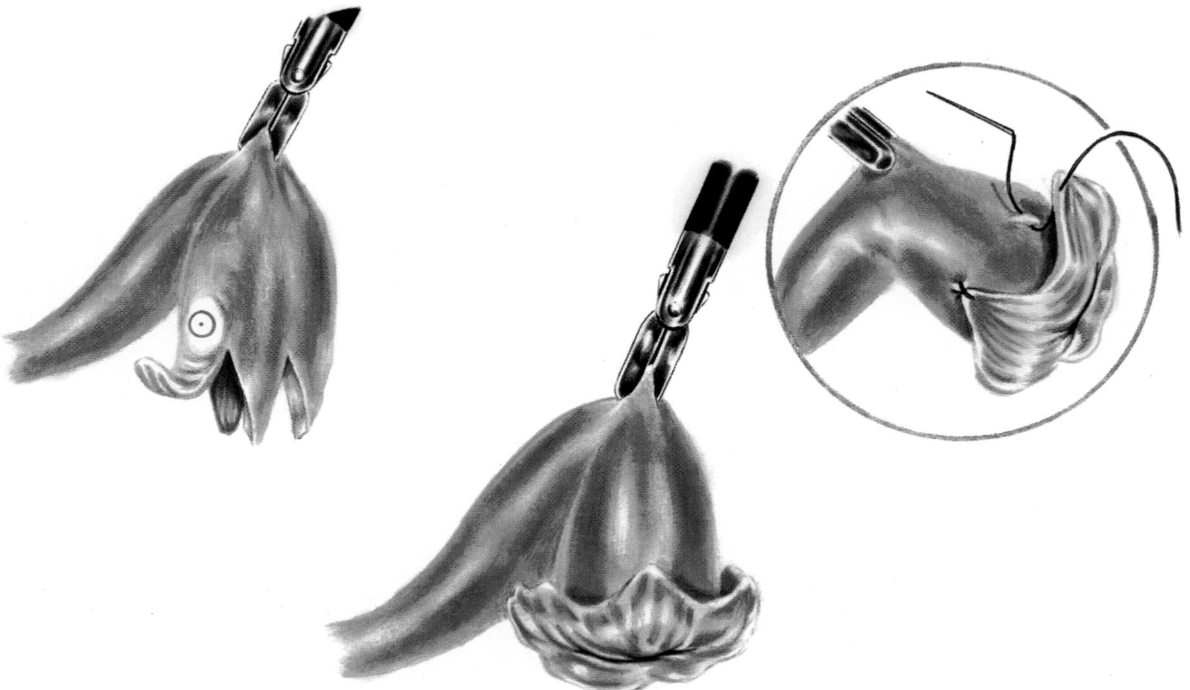

Figure 14-8. The ends of the tube are everted back, using the defocused laser beam or fine sutures (*inset*).

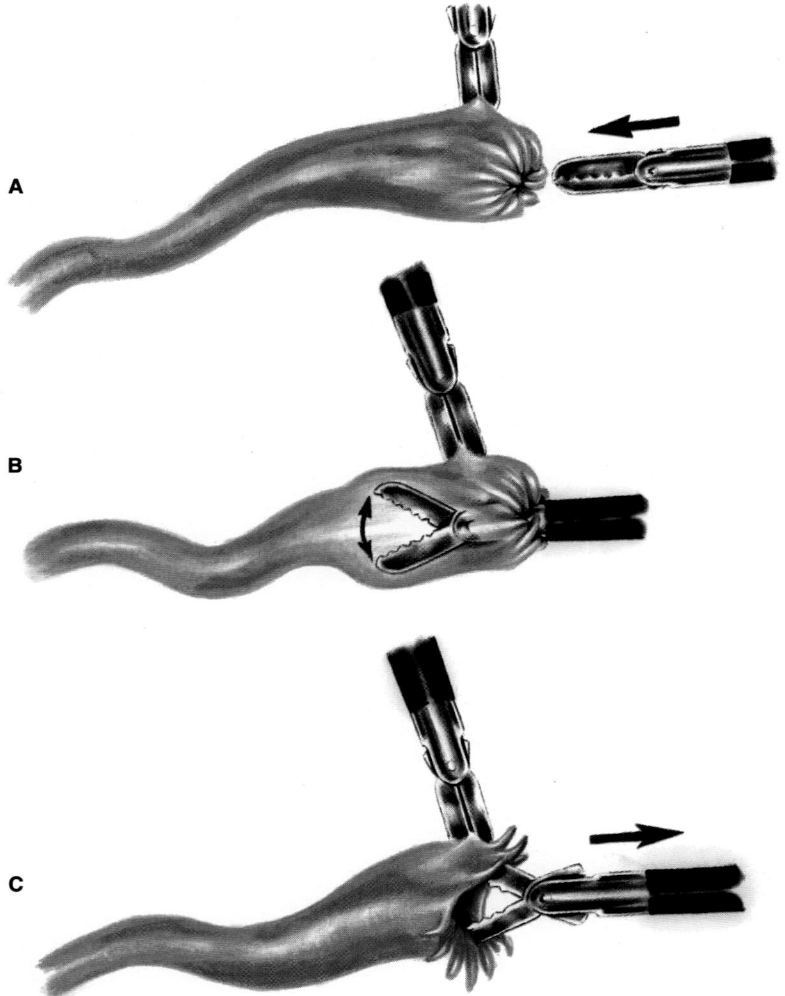

Figure 14-9. Fimbrial deagglutination. **A.** Introduction of grasping forceps. **B.** Forceps are opened. **C.** Withdrawing forceps.

inserted into the fallopian tube through the phimotic opening. The jaws of the forceps are opened within the tube; the open forceps are withdrawn. (Figure 14-9) This procedure is repeated until satisfactory deagglutination of the fimbria is obtained. Gentle manipulation decreases the chance of bleeding.[72] When the tube becomes patent, observation of the ostia is evident.

TABLE 14-10. Salpingoscopy Compared to Hysterosalpingography

	Salpingoscopy Normal, %	Salpingoscopy Abnormal, %
HSG normal (n = 61)	58	42
HSG abnormal (n = 52)	39	61

Source: Henry-Suchet et al.[75]

Salpingoscopy

The selection of patients who could benefit from tubal reconstructive operations is based mostly on the results from the preoperative hysterosalpingogram (HSG) and laparoscopic appearance of the tubes. Although mucosal folds can be seen on HSG, the correlation between radiologic studies and endoscopy in assessing the tubal mucosa is poor in many instances.

The severity and extent of intraluminal abnormalities assessed by transfimbrial salpingoscopy were correlated with the traditional criteria for evaluating distal tubal disease at laparoscopy in a prospective clinical trial in 55 infertile women who had suspected distal tubal disease or unexplained infertility.[74] Fallopian tubes with minimal disease suggested by laparoscopic examination had more abnormalities when viewed with the salpingoscope. Laparoscopic and salpingoscopic findings matched more closely in instances of severe distal disease. The prognosis for conception was poor in patients who had elevated mean salpingoscopic scores.

Henry-Suchet and coauthors[75] examined 231 tubes during tubal microsurgery and observed that lesions in the ampulla differed significantly from those predicted by HSG (Table 14-10). They found that if the tube had normal folds on HSG regardless of the presence of distal occlusion, there was agreement between the two diagnostic methods 55% of the time. Salpingoscopy revealed unsuspected synechiae and denuded areas in the endosalpinx in the other cases. When the tubal mucosa seemed abnormal on HSG, salpingoscopy revealed a normal mucosa 21% of the time. Salpingoscopy showed the condition of the tubal mucosa more accurately than did HSG. Cornier[76] used a flexible bronchoscope, and Brosens and coworkers[77] employed a specially designed rigid salpingoscope. Those authors reported similar discrepancies between HSG diagnosis and the salpingoscopic appearance of the tubal mucosa. Nezhat and coworkers[78] used a 3-mm 0-degree hysteroscope for salpingoscopy. Perhaps the findings should be used to decide upon the feasibility of a tuboplasty as opposed to IVF techniques.

Rigid salpingoscopy was evaluated during diagnostic laparoscopy for infertility in 158 patients.[79] Among 107 salpingoscopies in patients with endometriosis, 105 (98%) were normal. However, among patients with pelvic adhesions, only 42% were normal. Moreover, 9 of 50 abnormal salpingoscopies were found when no tubal factor was suspected during laparoscopy. A strong correlation was noted between the degree of intratubal damage and the extent of pelvic adhesions when the cause was previous PID but not when it was endometriosis. Since salpingoscopy can detect mucosal abnormalities, it can screen patients for assisted reproductive technology.[79]

Falloposcopy is a transvaginal microendoscopic technique that is used to explore the fallopian tube from the uterotubal ostium to the fimbria and may be used therapeutically to remove debris and cut filmy intraluminal adhesions. The images often are unable to describe the entire endosalpinx in detail. Nevertheless, on the basis of the greater accuracy of diagnosis with falloposcopy compared with hysterosalpingography and laparoscopy, it was suggested that falloposcopy should be incorporated into the initial screening of infertile patients.[80] The assessment of the ampullary conditions by falloposcopy agreed with the findings during salpingoscopy.[81]

A linear everting catheter can aid in safely guiding a falloposcope into the entire length of tube to observe the tubal lumen and also may be useful therapeutically for the recanalization of tubes. Falloposcopic tuboplasty was shown to be an effective and less invasive treatment of tubal infertility in selected patients.[82]

The feasibility of salpingoscopy as an office procedure using the transvaginal approach to the pelvic cavity has been demonstrated.[83] A transvaginal Veress needle puncture was used, and peritoneal distention was achieved with saline. The fimbriae were seen in all the patients. In combination with transvaginal hydrolaparoscopy and dye hydropertubation, the technique allows comprehensive screening of the tubo-ovarian structures in the early stages of an infertility investigation.[84]

Transvaginal hydrolaparoscopy is done under local anesthesia, using a small-diameter optic with the patient in the dorsal position. Cavity distention is achieved with normal saline. Transvaginal hydrolaparoscopy does not provide the familiar and panoramic view of the pelvis given by laparoscopy, but it does provide an accurate and atraumatic inspection of adnexal structures without manipulation. High patient acceptability may make this new procedure suitable as an early-stage investigation of infertility and as a repeat or second-look procedure. Although biopsy and adhesiolysis can be carried out, the precision and safety of transvaginal hydrolaparoscopy require additional evaluation.

Indications

Laparoscopic salpingoscopy permits detailed examination of the ampullary endosalpinx. It can

1. Detect unsuspected tubal lesions not previously identified on HSG
2. Discover the extent of mucosal damage in a woman who has PID
3. Evaluate the status of tubal mucosa in patients who have known tubal disease with or without a hydrosalpinx

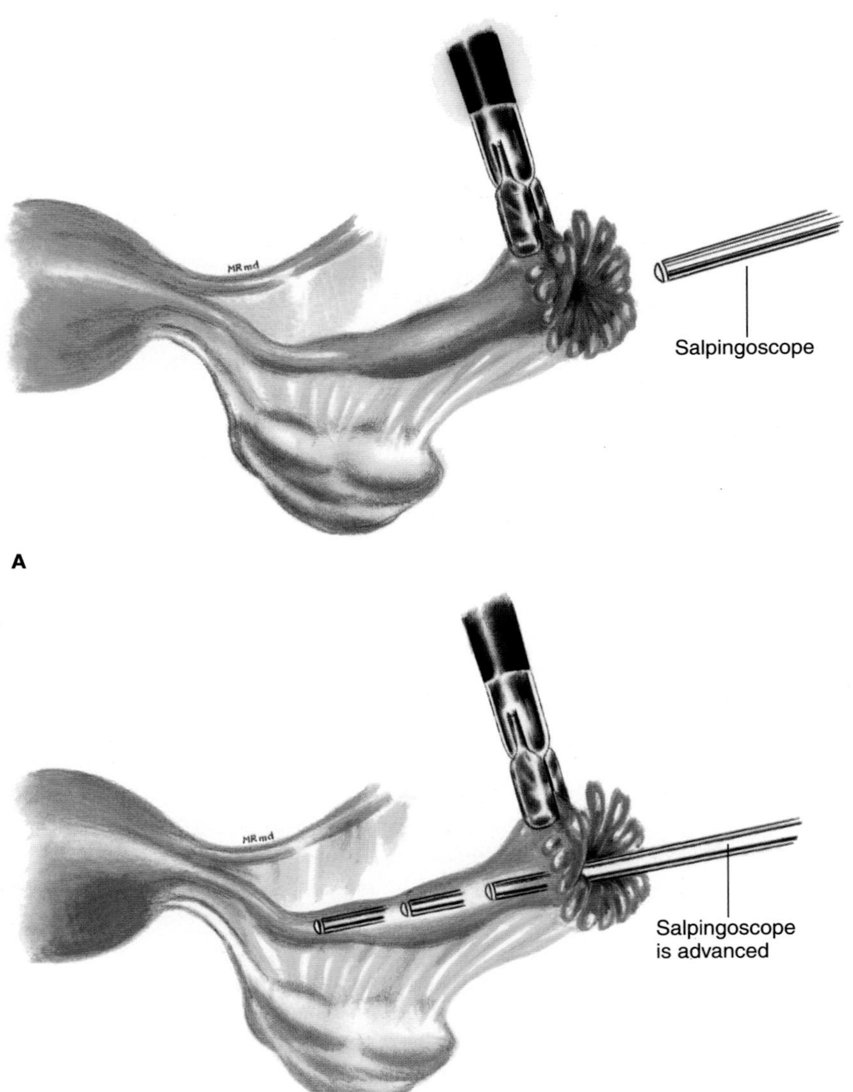

Figure 14-10. **A.** Manipulation of the tube with grasping forceps and placement of the salpingoscope. **B.** The salpingoscope is advanced under direct vision, and the tube is distended with saline.

4. Examine and decide upon treatment of the contralateral tube in a woman with an ectopic pregnancy
5. Observe tubes before a granulocyte immunofluorescence test (GIFT).

Technique

The laparoscope is inserted in the usual manner, and two suprapubic accessory trocars are added. The tube is manipulated with forceps applied to its antimesenteric serosal surface close to the fimbria. A 3-mm scope is inserted through the ipsilateral accessory trocar sleeve and placed in the tubal lumen (Figure 14-10). Saline is infused through the Cohen intrauterine cannula or a similar device. This infusion is essential because it creates space and makes the mucosal folds more visible. The end of the tube is occluded with an atraumatic grasper if distention is inadequate. The scope is advanced under direct vision into the infundibulum, where the major and minor folds are seen. In a normal tube, the folds are formed parallel to each other and freely move in the distending fluid. The lumen is followed into the ampulla by advancing the scope and maneuvering the bends. In the ampulla, there are four to six major folds, each

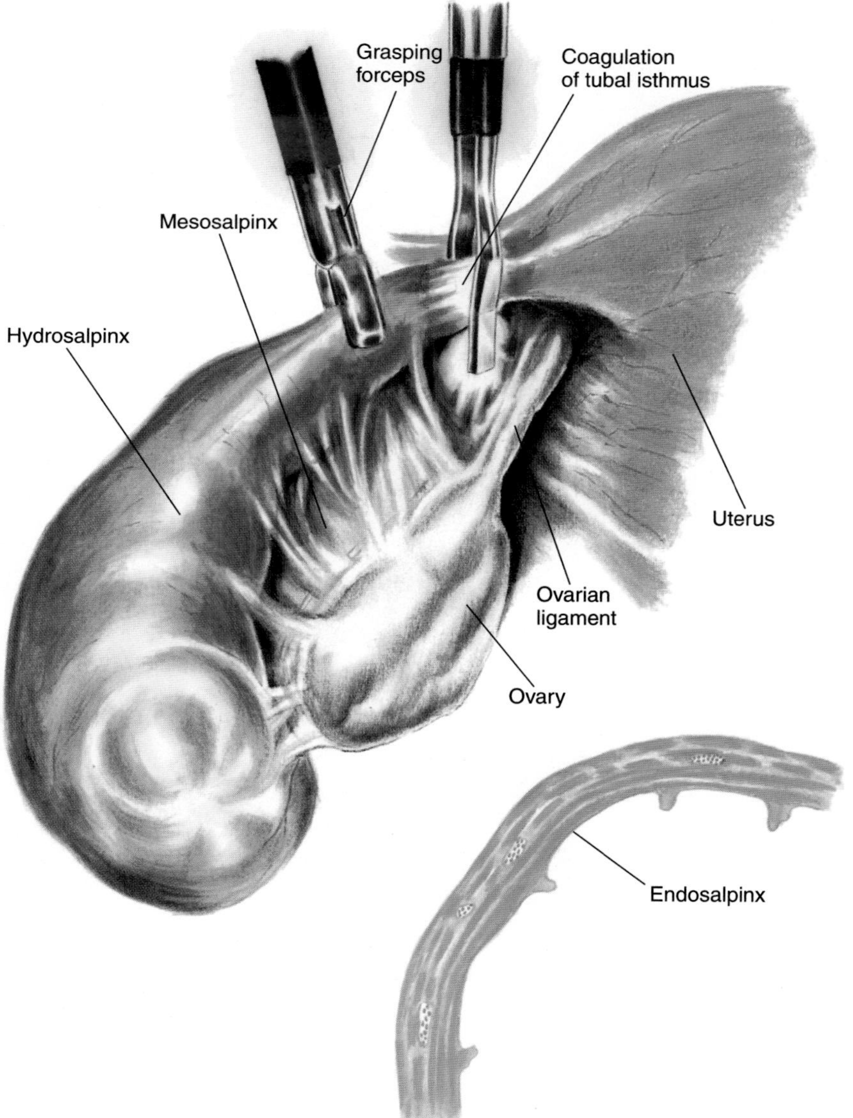

Figure 14-11. Salpingectomy is done with bipolar electrocoagulation for hemostasis. **A.** The isthmic portion of the tube is coagulated and cut close to the uterus.

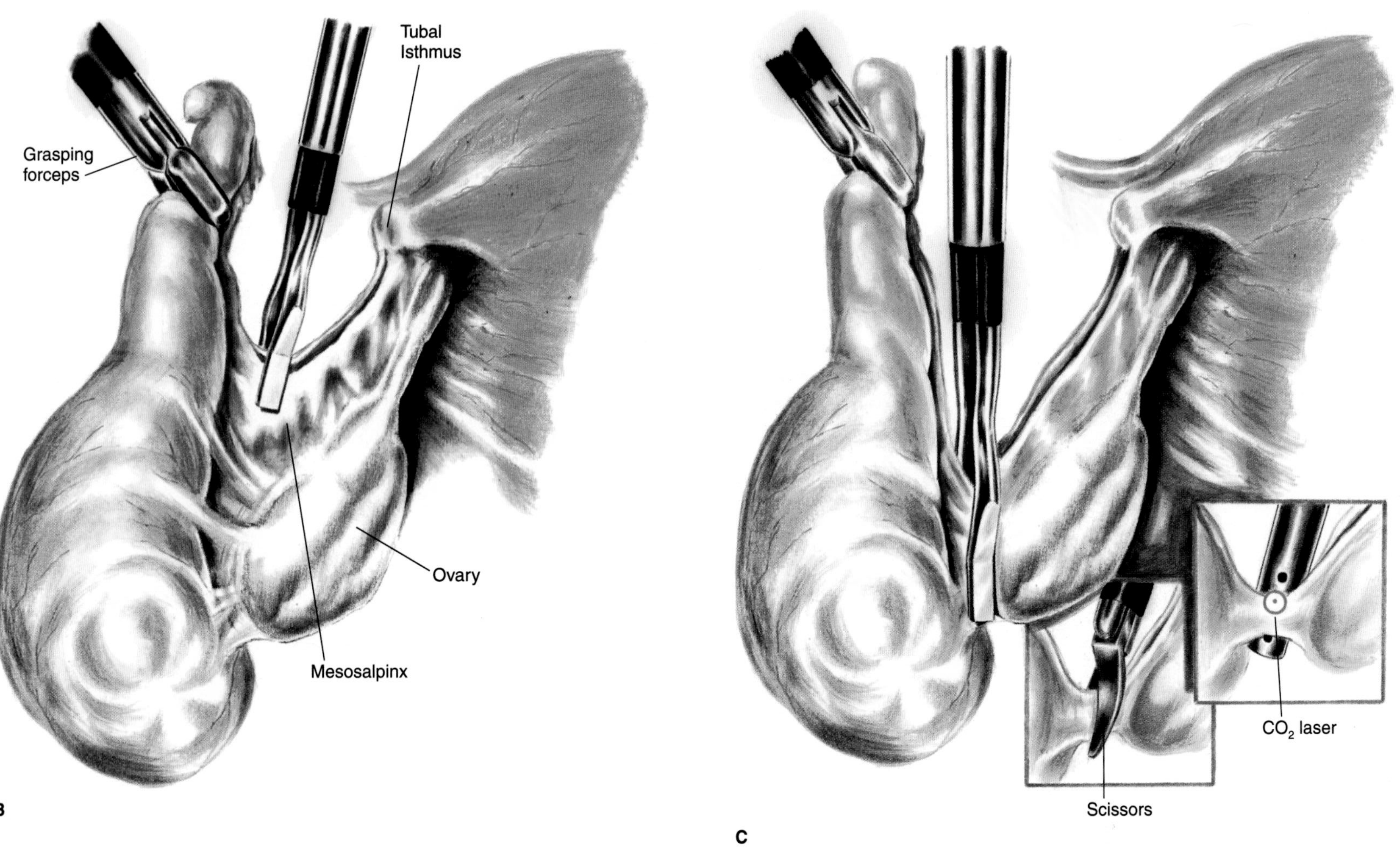

Figure 14-11. (*Continued*) **B.** while the tube is under traction, the mesosalpinx is coagulated and cut. **C.** Sharp scissors (*inset*) or the ultra pulse CO_2 laser is used for cutting.

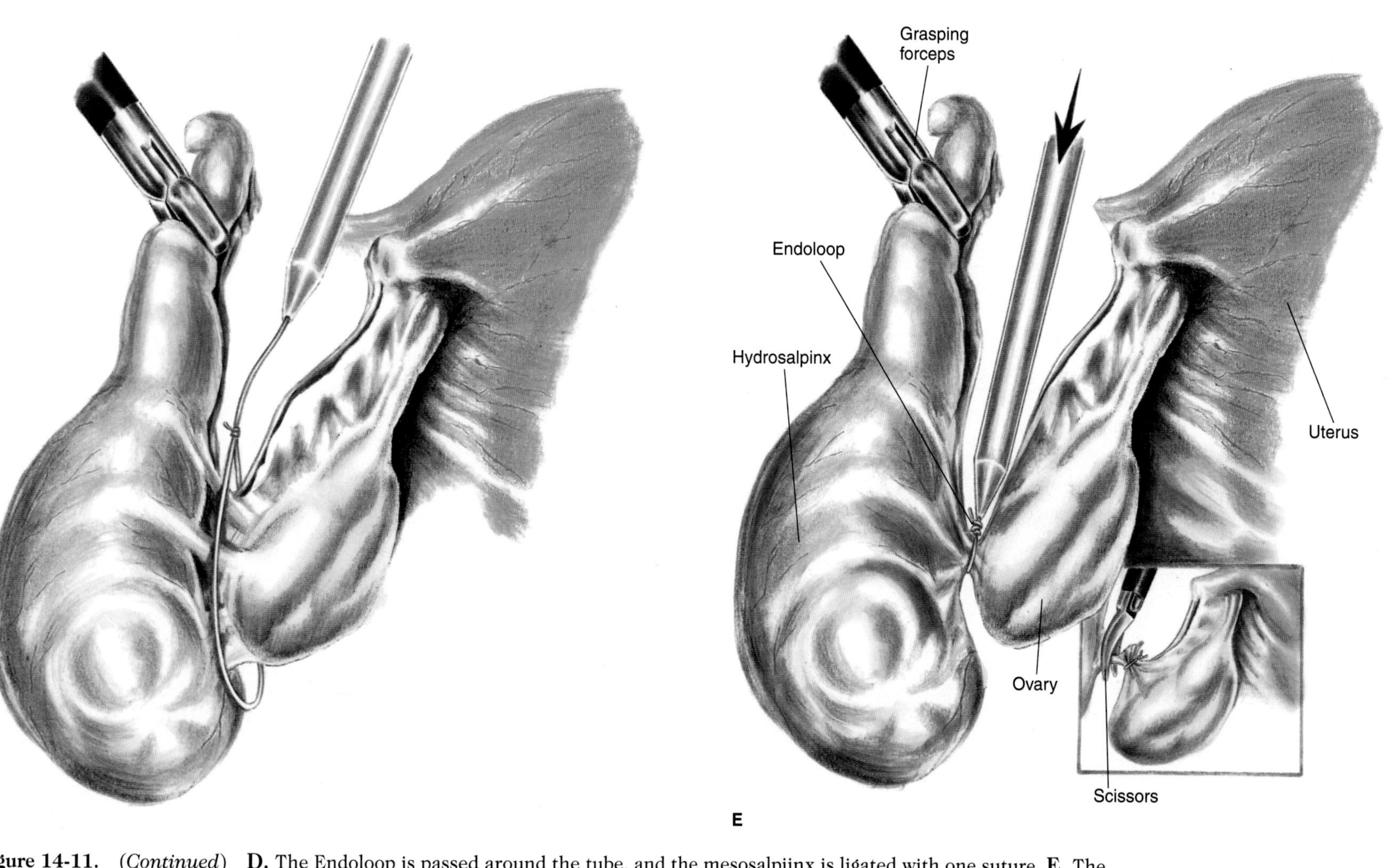

Figure 14-11. (*Continued*) **D.** The Endoloop is passed around the tube, and the mesosalpiinx is ligated with one suture. **E.** The mesosalpinx is cut above the tube. An adequate stump remains to prevent the ligature from slipping (*inset*).

about 4 mm in height, with accessory folds arising from them. Between the major folds, there are several minor folds approximately 1 mm high. When the junction of the ampulla and isthmus is reached, the major folds give way to three or four rounded folds that are 200 to 400 um high. With experience, it is usually possible to follow the lumen as far as the isthmic-ampullary junction.

Complications from this operation are rare; however, it is possible to damage the fimbriae with the forceps, causing minor bleeding or adhesions. The most serious complication—perforation of the tubal mucosa—can result if the scope is advanced without direct vision or with unnecessary force. Dechaud and coworkers[80] reported that their complication rate was 5.1% of pinpoint tubal perforations.

Occasionally, bleeding occurs at the fimbria, but it usually ceases spontaneously.

Salpingectomy

Salpingectomy is indicated for pathologic conditions such as ruptured ectopic pregnancy; more than two ectopic pregnancies in the same tube; severe tubal damage, particularly if the contralateral tube is normal; severe pelvic adhesions; pain caused by recurrent hydrosalpinx; and large hydrosalpinx or torsion with nonviability of the tube.

Salpingectomy has been recommended for patients with hydrosalpinx who will be undergoing IVF.[85,86] The hydrosalpinx had a negative effect on IVF because the hydrosalpingeal fluid was embryotoxic, leading to increased early pregnancy losses. Additionally, there was diminished endometrial receptivity. Three meta-analyses of multiple previous studies showed that hydrosalpinx present during IVF-ET has negative consequences on rates of pregnancy, implantation, live delivery, and early

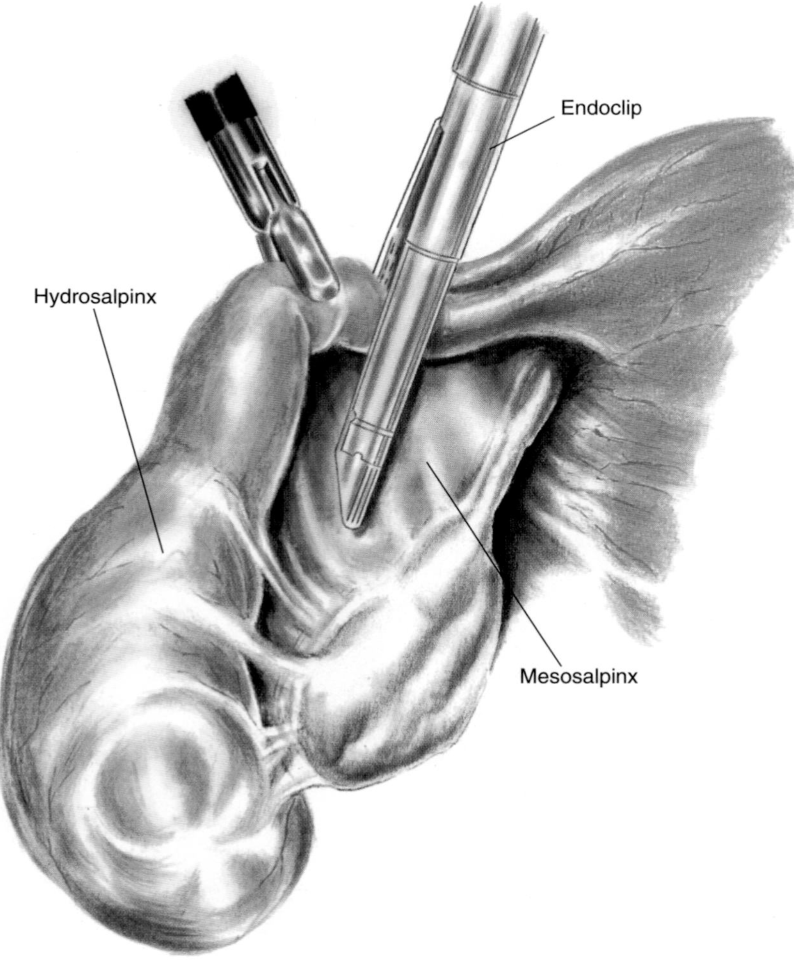

Figure 14-12. **A.** Salpingectomy is achieved with an automatic stapling device. The first application of the stapling device is to the proximal portion of the tube across the mesosalpinx. The tube is under traction.

Figure 14-12. (*Continued*) **B.** The second application completes the salpingectomy. *Inset*. A view of the mesosalpinx after the tube has been removed.

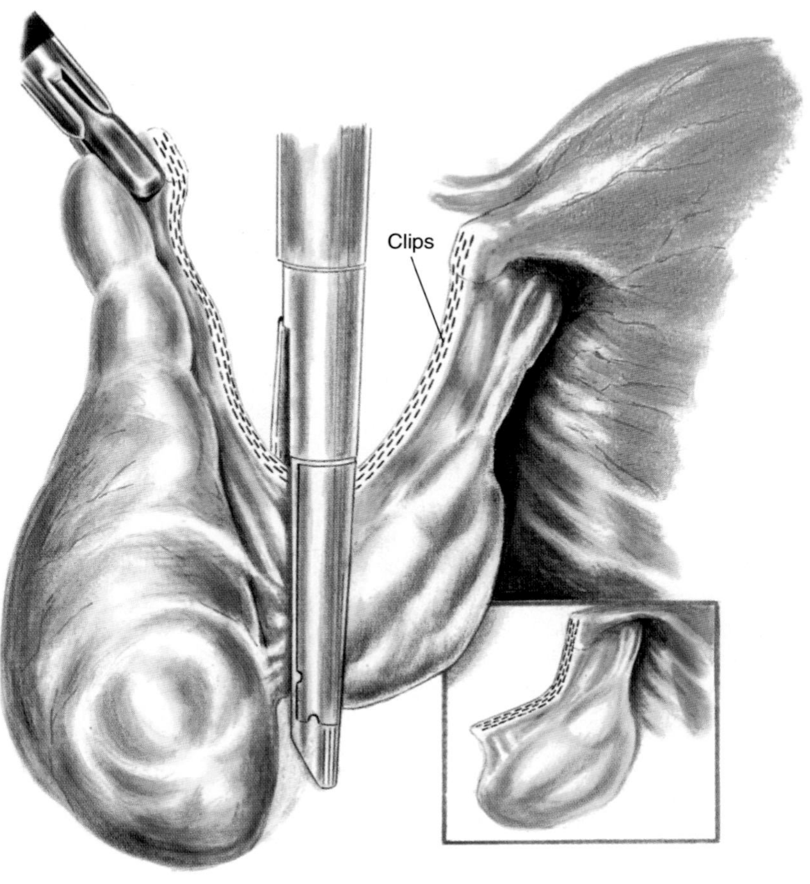

pregnancy loss.[86–88] However, prospective randomized trials have not been done to suggest that routine salpingectomy should be carried out on all patients with hydrosalpinx who are undergoing IVF.[89,90]

Salpingectomy is an easy procedure that requires instruments commonly used to do tubal electrocoagulation for sterilization.[91] The necessary instruments are a bipolar electrocoagulator, a grasping forceps, scissors, and a laparoscope. A CO_2 laser also can be used. The laparoscope and 5-mm suprapubic trocars are placed, through which the graspers and bipolar electrocoagulator are inserted. Peritubal adhesions are lysed, and the tube is grasped at the isthmic portion. The proximal portion of the isthmus is coagulated and cut, using either scissors or laser (Figure 14-11, A, B, and C). If scissors are used, the bipolar electrocoagulator must be removed and replaced with the scissors through the same secondary trocar, or a third accessory trocar can be placed. The laser is faster and more precise than the scissors. Cutting is done in layers so that there is less chance to overshoot the coagulated area and get into an area beyond the coagulated tissue. Once the tubal isthmus is transected, the mesosalpinx is coagulated alternately and cut at intervals of 1 to 2 cm in the direction of the tubo-ovarian ligament.

Alternatives to bipolar electrocoagulation of the mesosalpinx are the Endoloop sutures (Ethicon) and automated stapling device (Endo-path ELC 35, Ethicon). Before the Endoloop ligature is used, both the proximal portion of the tube and its distal attachment to the ovary (fimbria ovarica) are coagulated and cut. The Endoloop is passed around the tube, and the mesosalpinx is ligated with one Endoloop and removed. The mesosalpinx is cut above the ligature. An adequate stump is left to prevent the ligature from slipping (Figure 14-11, D and E). The stapling device is introduced through a 12-mm trocar incision. After adhesions are lysed and the tube is mobilized, it is pulled up and put under traction. The stapler is used from the proximal to be distal end to staple and cut the tube. One or two applications are sufficient for the entire tube (Figure 14-12). Once detached, the tube is removed from the pelvis through a suprapubic trocar sleeve or the operating channel of the laparoscope. Removal of a larger tube (a ruptured tubal pregnancy or hydrosalpinx) requires an Endopouch (Ethicon) or another method of removal. The pelvic cavity is irrigated. The intraabdominal pressure is decreased to reveal bleeding temporarily controlled by a pneumoperitoneum. This is especially important when one is using a stapling device.

Tubal Anastomosis

Successful tubal anastomosis depends on precise apposition of tissues to ensure and restore normal tubal patency. Fine suture material can reduce tissue reaction and excessive scar formation. Several obstacles limit tubal anastomosis at laparoscopy. There are no laparoscopic needle drivers available that can manipulate 8-0 sutures. It is difficult to tie fine sutures laparoscopically and precisely align the tissue. Sedbon and colleagues[92] reported five procedures done with fibrin glue with no subsequent pregnancies. Klink and associates[93] described a laser-welding technique to anastomose previously ligated rabbit uterine horns. The technique offered the theoretical advantages of reduced operating time, improved hemostasis, and precise microsurgery. It presented options for doing anastomosis with the laparoscope without microsuturing, but the results of laser welding were unsuccessful.

Lyon and coworkers[94] compared patency in the uterine horns of 12 rats that were randomized to undergo anastomosis by argon photocoagulation or microsuture. All the microsutured anastomoses were patent and contiguous, with no apparent fibrosis. In contrast, four of six laser subjects had complete occlusion and the other two had tubal stenosis. Although initially producing a satisfactory union, argon laser photocoagulation eventually proved traumatic and resulted in poor healing. Other studies showed that fallopian tube welding was accompanied by postoperative dehiscence.[95–97] Tulandi [98] did a randomized prospective study that compared microsurgical tubal anastomosis with anastomosis using fibrin glue. Postoperative adhesions and pregnancy rates did not differ between the two groups. Although this study was done by laparotomy, it may encourage the study of fibrin glue for laparoscopic tubal anastomosis.

Tubal anastomosis by welding tissue with a defocused CO_2 laser beam was attempted during laparotomy and with an endoscope in an animal experiment.[99] After sutureless anastomosis by laser welding, 50% of the laparotomy group and 40% of the laparoscopically operated group became pregnant. However, morphologic examination of oviducts showed dehiscence of the anastomosis in 20% of the welded tubes. Tubal anastomosis took three times longer laparoscopically than during laparotomy. Thus, the investigators suggested that laser welding as a sutureless alternative technique of tubal anastomosis should be viewed critically.

A comparison of rabbit oviduct anastomosis with autologous fibrin to 7-0 Vicryl, a conventional suture material used in tubal anastomosis, showed a significantly shortened time for the procedure and superior histopathologic union in the tissue adhesive group.[100] Patency rates, pregnancy rates, and the degree of adhesions were comparable in both groups.

Excising occluded portions of tubes with either the laser or the scalpel does not alter the outcome if the tubal segments are approximated by using microsurgical techniques (Figure 14-13, A through D).[97,101] The risk of adhesions is lower with laser preparation of the tubal segments before microsurgical anastomosis.[97,102] Improved hemostasis and precision and enhanced preservation of normal tissue were observed when the laser was used as an adjunct to microsurgical techniques. Scalpel preparation of the tubal ends has an advantage over the CO_2 laser for interstitial-isthmic anastomoses because the CO_2 laser cannot slice the interstitial segment of tube as well as the scalpel can.[101]

Silva and coauthors[103] described a combined laparoscopic minilaparotomy outpatient reversal of tubal sterilization with a conception rate of 71%. Outpatient microsurgical reversal of tubal sterilization combining laparoscopy and minilaparotomy is theoretically safe. The nonmicrosurgical aspects are similar to tubal sterilization by minilaparotomy, which has an excellent safety record on an outpatient basis.[104–106] The occluded portions are prepared laparoscopically by using the CO_2 laser or any other cutting modality, and the uterus or tubes are delivered into the operative field so that the tubal lumen can be approximated by microsurgical procedures. Patients selected for tubal reversal with this method should be less than 43 years old, be not more than 20% over ideal body weight, and have at least more than 2 cm of proximal fallopian tube. Original operative notes and pathology reports are reviewed to ascertain the type of sterilization procedure and the amount of tubal segment removed.

Patients are given one preoperative dose of prophylactic antibiotics. A single-tooth tenaculum with a Cohen cannula or Humi cannula is attached to the cervix to aid in uterine manipulation and allow retrograde dye studies. Laparoscopy is done to assess the length of distal tube present and lyse adhesions. The method described by Silva and coauthors[103] involves a 5- to 6-cm skin incision and uterine exteriorization with a Somers clamp. The adnexa is exteriorized by traction on the utero-ovarian ligaments. Significant adhesions are lysed laparoscopically to avoid blunt tearing of tissue. The uterus and adnexa are maintained in their exterior position by wedging gauze between the uterus and the incision. During resection of the occluded tubal portions and microsurgical anastomosis, constant irrigation of the exposed organs is used to prevent desiccation. Etidocaine 1% is injected into the peritoneal, fascial, and subcutaneous layers during closure of the abdominal wall to act as a long-acting anesthetic. Patients are monitored for 3 to 6 hours postoperatively before discharge or are admitted overnight. Most patients returned to work within 1 to 2 weeks. The data from the Silva study[107] show that sterilization reversal with the laparoscopic minilaparotomy approach compared with conventional laparotomy results in reduced cost and morbidity, and a shorter time to recuperation. It can be used for 75% of sterilization reversals. Most important, the pregnancy rate of 71% is comparable to previously published rates with microsurgical techniques.

A similar procedure has been done successfully in which the tubes are prepared laparoscopically by using sharp techniques, a CO_2 laser, or microelectrocoagulation. Hemostasis is obtained by using fine bipolar electrocoagulation. The ends of the tube are exteriorized through a minilaparotomy incision, and the lumens are approximated with an 8-0 or finer suture. Exteriorization is aided by using traction on the uterine manipulators to position the uterus properly. Patients are discharged the same day or the following morning.

With progress in laparoscopic microinstruments, refinement of three-dimensional video cameras, and further improvement of endoscopic surgical skills, it is likely that microsurgical tubal anastomosis will be possible entirely by laparoscopy. However, the success of the anastomosis must not be put at risk for the sake of doing the procedure laparoscopically.

Laparoscopic microsurgical tubal anastomosis was accomplished in 16 women by using a three-stitch technique with tubal cannulation.[107] Five pregnancies occurred. The surgical outcome depended on the patient's age, the method of tube interruption, and the length of the tube segments.

Outpatient laparoscopic procedures were completed in 14 women to reverse tubal sterilization, using titanium staples to approximate the oviducts.[108] The method involved excision of the tubal eschar, stenting of the severed remnants, and circumferential stapling of the muscularis and serosa. Approximation was possible in all these women. Within 6 months, there were six conceptions that resulted in one spontaneous abortion and five successful pregnancies. Among those not conceiving within 8 months, all had tubal patency on a follow-up HSG.

Yoon and colleagues[109] evaluated the fertility outcome after laparoscopic microsurgical tubal anastomosis in 44 patients who previously had undergone tubal sterilization. The overall pregnancy rate was 77.5%. The pregnancy success according to the method of previous tubal sterilization was 16 of 24 with the fallope-ring method, 14 of 15 in women whose tubes had been electrocoagulated, and 8 of 10 patients in whom the Pomeroy technique was used. Those authors[109] concluded that laparoscopic microsurgical tubal anastomosis could be an alternative procedure to laparotomy in patients who request the reversal of tubal sterilization.

Single-suture laparoscopic tubal anastomosis for tubal sterilization reversal was described by Dubuisson and Chapron.[110] After the tubal stumps were prepared and the edges of the mesosalpinx were brought together, laparoscopic anastomosis was achieved with one stitch placed at 12 o'clock on the antimesial edge of the tube. Those authors operated on 32 patients using this technique and carried out 48 tubal sterilization reversals. For the patients who underwent postoperative hysterosalpingography during the first or second month after the operation, the rate of patency was 87.5% (42 of 48 patients). The overall intrauterine pregnancy rate was 53.1%. Laparoscopic tubal sterilization reversal may be more feasible with this simplified technique. However, the surgeon should be experienced in both microsurgical tubal anastomosis by laparotomy and operative laparoscopic procedures.

New three-dimensional (3-D) technology may aid in the future performance of highly challenging procedures such as tubotubal anastomosis.[111] For microsurgical procedures of the adnexae, 3-D technology offers advantages compared with standard two-dimensional laparoscopy. In these operations,

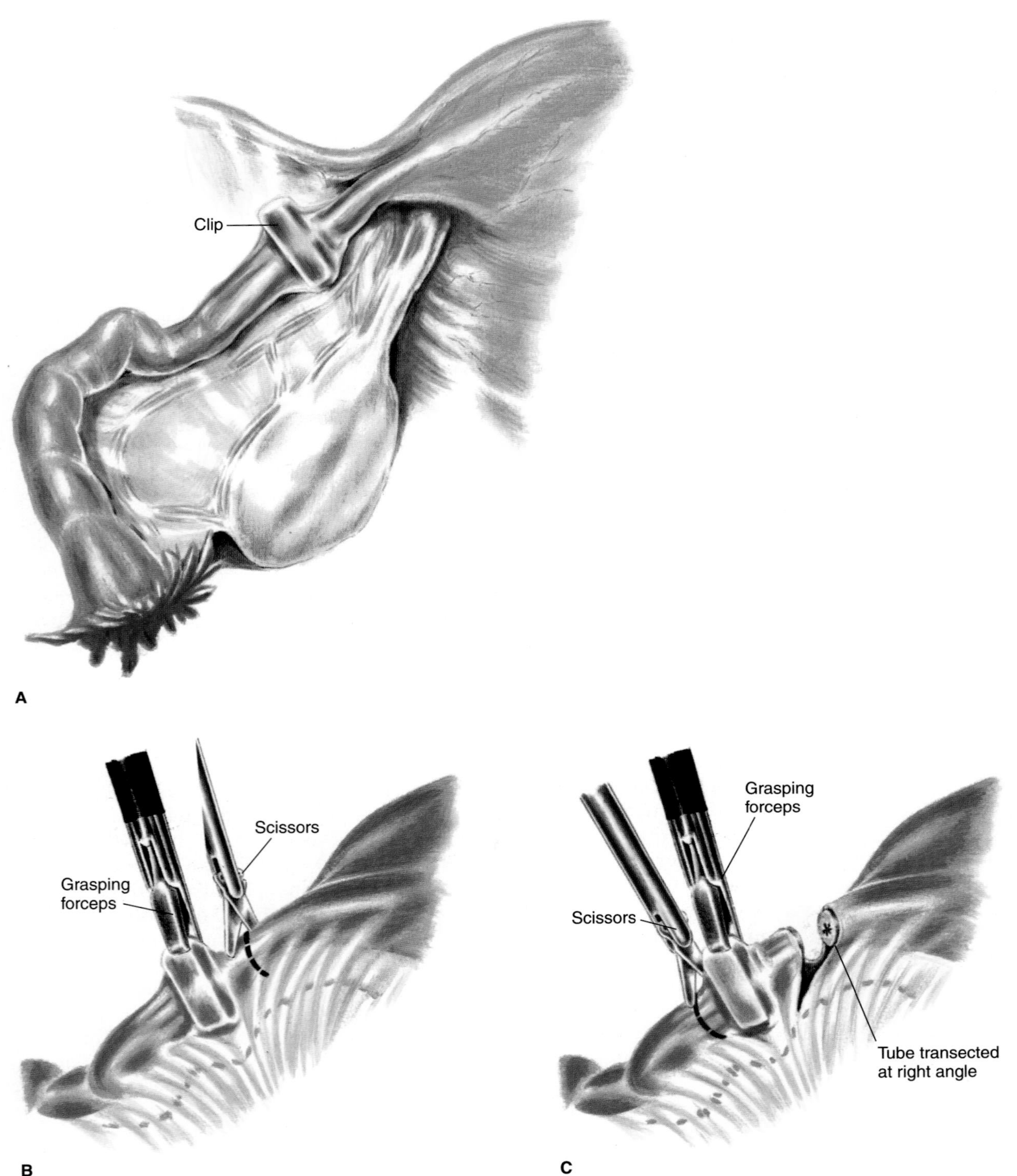

Figure 14-13. **A.** The tube was occluded previously with a clip. **B.** The clip is held by a grasper and the isthmic segment is cut. **C.** Another incision is made distal to the clipped segment.

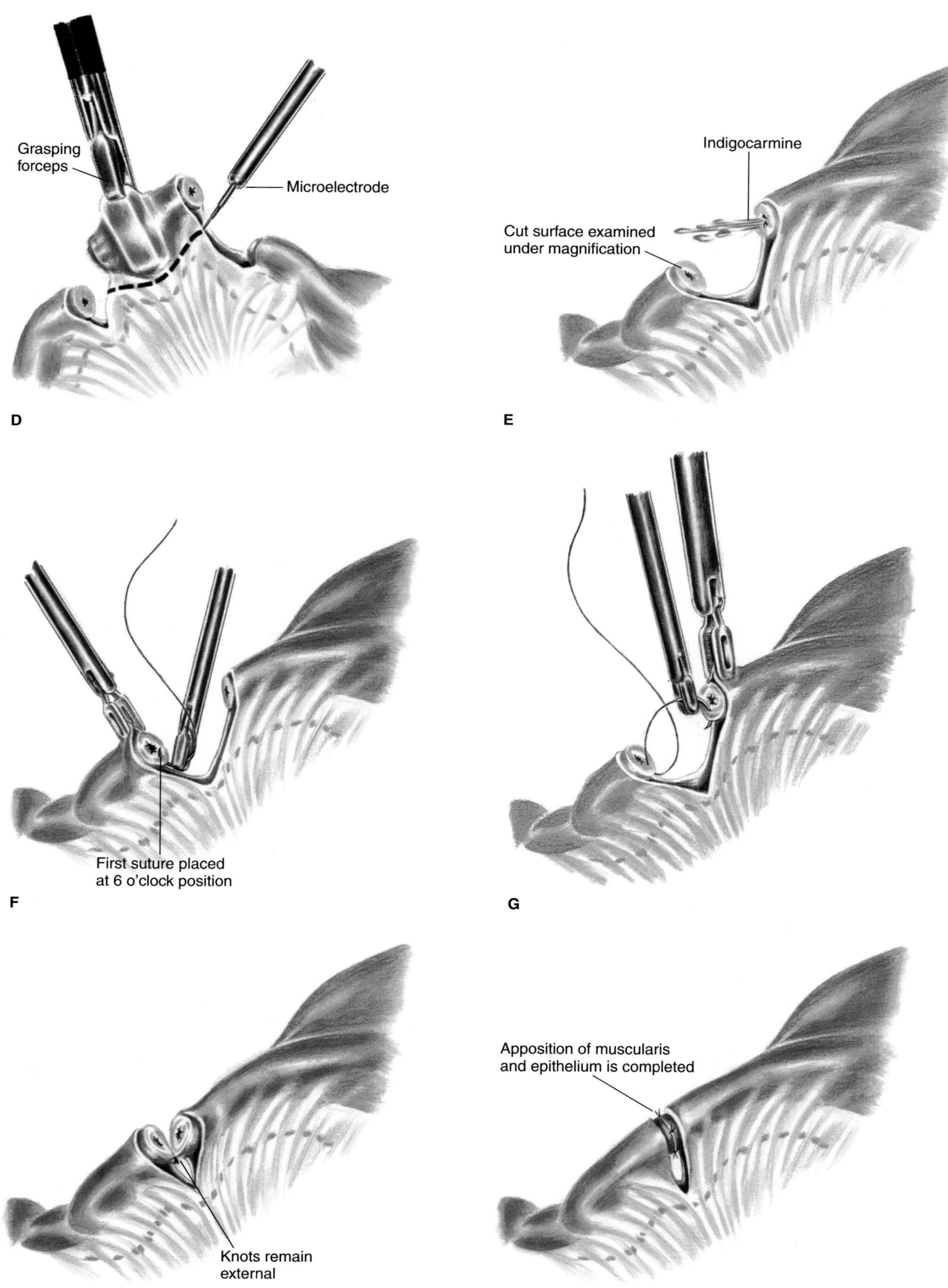

Figure 14-13. (*Continued*) **D.** The clipped segment is removed using a microelectrode. **E.** The patency of the proximal segment is tested with indigo carmine. **F.** The initial suture is placed in the 6 o'clock position. **G.** First the distal segment is sutured, and then the proximal one. **H.** The suture knots are tied to bring the edges together on the serosal surface. **I.** About four sutures are required.

the operating area is limited, and hence the disadvantages of the 3-D technology, such as limited depth of focus, are not important. The 3-D system allows improved observation of small structures and safe and exact handling.

Laparoscopic microsuturing may be difficult, since optical magnification and long instruments significantly increase tremors. Robotic assistance may facilitate laparoscopic tubal anastomosis by filtering tremor, reducing the surgeon's fatigue, and scaling the maneuvers.[112] Robotic technology has been used safely in creating laparoscopic microsurgical anastomoses in a live porcine model[113] and in a woman. Robotic technology has the potential to make laparoscopic microsuturing easier, increasing the acceptance of laparoscopic microsurgical tubal anastomosis.

References

1. Marana R, Muscatello P, Vanzetto M, et al. Laparoscopic salpingoscopy: Results, in Marana R, Brosens A, Mancuso S, eds., *Diagnostic and Operative Gynecological Endoscopy*. Tuttlingen, Germany, Braun Druck, 1991.
2. Centers for Disease Control: Pelvic inflammatory disease: Guidelines for prevention and management. *MMWR* 1991; 40:1.
3. Allen LA, Schoon MG. Laparoscopic diagnosis of acute pelvic inflammatory disease. *Br J Obstet Gynaecol* 1983; 90:966.
4. Jacobson L, Westrom L. Objective diagnosis of acute pelvic inflammatory disease. *Am J Obstet Gynecol* 1969; 105:1088.
5. Livengood CH, Hill BG, Addison WA. Pelvic inflammatory disease: Finding during inpatient treatment of clinically severe, laparoscopy-documented disease. *Am J Obstet Gynecol* 1992; 166:519.
6. Henry-Suchet J, Soler A. Loffredo V. Laparoscopic treatment of tubo-ovarian abscesses. *J Reprod Med* 1984; 8:579.
7. Centers for Disease Control and Prevention. 1998 Guidelines for Treatment of Sexually Transmitted Diseases. *MMWR* 1998; 1-111.
8. Droegemueller W. Pelvic inflammatory disease: Changing management concepts. *Drug Ther* 1984:67.
9. Walker CK, Landers DV. Pelvic abscesses: New trends in management. *Obstet Gynecol Surg* 1991; 46:615-624.
10. Anducci JE. Laparoscopy in the diagnosis and treatment of pelvic inflammatory disease with abscess formation. *Int Surg* 1981; 66:359.
11. Mecke H, Semm K, Freys I, et al. Pelvic abscesses: Pelviscopy or laparotomy. *Gynecol Obstet Invest* 1991; 31:231.
12. Vasilev SA, Roy S, Essin DJ. Pelvic abscesses in postmenopausal women. *Surg Gynecol Obstet* 1989; 169:243.
13. Raiga J, Canis M, Le Bouedec G, et al. Laparoscopic management of adnexal abscesses: Consequences for fertility. *Fertil Steril* 1996; 66:712.
14. Cohen CR, Sinei S, Reilly M, et al. Effect of human immunodeficiency virus type 1 infection upon acute salpingitis: A laparoscopic study. *J Infect Dis* 1998; 178:1352.
15. Bateman BG, Nunley WC, Kitchin JD. Surgical management of distal tubal obstruction—are we making progress? *Fertil Steril* 1987; 48:523.
16. Fayez JA, Suliman SO. Infertility surgery of the oviduct: Comparison between macrosurgery and microsurgery. *Fertil Steril* 1982; 37:73.
17. Holst N, Maltau JM, Forsdahl F, Hansen LJ. Handling of tubal infertility after introduction of in vitro fertilization: Changes and consequences. *Fertil Steril* 1991; 55:140.
18. Tulandi T: Reconstructive tubal surgery by laparoscopy. *Obstet Gynecol Surg* 1987; 42:193.
19. Boer-Meisel ME, teVelde ER, Haffeman JDF, et al. Predicting the pregnancy outcome in patients treated for hydrosalpinx: A prospective study. *Fertil Steril* 1986; 45:23.
20. Schlaff WD, Hassiakos DK, Damewood MD, et al. Neosalpingostomy for distal tubal obstruction: Prognostic factors and impact of surgical technique. *Fertil Steril* 1990; 54:984.
21. Rock JA, Katayma KF, Martin EJ, et al. Factors influencing the success of salpingostomy techniques for distal fimbrial obstruction. *Obstet Gynecol* 1978; 52:591.
22. Mage G, Pouly JL, DeJolinieres JB, et al. A preoperative classification to predict the intrauterine and ectopic pregnancy rates after distal tubal microsurgery. *Fertil Steril* 1986; 46:807.
23. Palmer R. Salpingostomy: A critical study of 396 personal cases operated upon without polyethylene tubing. *Proc R Soc Med* 1960; 53:357.
24. Mulligan WJ. Results of salpingostomy. *Int J Fertil* 1966; 11:424.
25. Garcia CR. Surgical reconstruction of the oviduct in the infertile patient, in *Progress in*

Infertility, 1st ed. Behrman SJ, Kistner RW, eds., Boston: Little, Brown, 1968.
26. Crane M, Woodruff JD. Factors influencing the success of tuboplastic procedures. *Fertil Steril* 1968; 19:810.
27. O'Brien JR, Arenet GH, Eduljee SY. Operative treatment of fallopian tube pathology in human fertility. *Am J Obstet Gynecol* 1969; 103:520.
28. Young DE, Egan JE, Barlow JJ, et al. Reconstructive surgery for infertility at the Boston Hospital for Women. *Am J Obstet Gynecol* 1970; 108:1092.
29. Grant A. Infertility surgery of the oviduct. *Fertil Steril* 1971; 22:496.
30. Lamb EJ, Moscovitz W. Tuboplasty for infertility. *Int J Fertil* 1972; 17:53.
31. Umezaki C, Katayama KP, Jones HW. Pregnancy rates after reconstructive surgery on the fallopian tubes. *Obstet Gynecol* 1974; 43:418.
32. Comninos AC. Salpingostomy: Results of two different methods of treatment. *Fertil Steril* 1977; 28:1211.
33. Siegler AM, Kontopoulos V. An analysis of macrosurgical and microsurgical techniques in the management of tuboperitoneal factor in infertility. *Fertil Steril* 1979; 32:377.
34. Spadoni LR. Tubal and peritubular surgery without magnification: An analysis. *Am J Obstet Gynecol* 1980; 137:198.
35. DeCherney AH, Kase N. A comparison of treatment for bilateral fimbrial occlusion. *Fertil Steril* 1981; 35:162.
36. Wallach EE, Manara LR, Eisenberg E. Experience with 143 cases of tubal surgery. *Fertil Steril* 1983; 39:609.
37. Swolin K. Electromicrosurgery and salpingostomy: Long-term results. *Am J Obstet Gynecol* 1974; 121:418.
38. Marik J: Microsurgical repair of hydrosalpinx, in Phyllips JM, ed., *Microsurgery in Infertility*. St. Louis: St. Louis Board of Publication, 1977.
39. Salat-Baroux J, Cornier E, Rotman J. Analyse de 65 salpingostomies microchirugicales. *J Gynecol Obstet Biol Reprod* 1979; 8:647.
40. Betz G, Engel T, Penney LL. Tuboplasty comparison of the methodology. *Fertil Steril* 1980; 34:534.
41. Gomel V. Clinical results of infertility microsurgery, in Crosignani PG, Rubin BL, eds., *Microsurgery in Female Infertility*. London: Academic Press, 1980.
42. Frantzen C, Schlosser HW. Microsurgery and postinfectious tubal infertility. *Fertil Steril* 1983; 38:397.
43. Hulka JF. Adnexal adhesions: A prognostic staging of fertility surgery results at Chapel Hill, North Carolina. *Am J Obstet Gynecol* 1982; 144:141.
44. Verhoeven HC, Berry H, Frantzen C, et al. Surgical treatment for distal tubal occlusion: A review of 167 cases. *J Reprod Med* 1983; 28:293.
45. Bellina JH. Microsurgery of the fallopian tube with the carbon dioxide laser: Analysis of 230 cases with a two-year follow-up. *Laser Surg Med* 1983; 3:255.
46. Tulandi T, Farag R, McInnes RA, et al. Reconstructive surgery of hydrosalpinx with and without the carbon dioxide laser. *Fertil Steril* 1984; 42:839.
47. Russell JB, DeCherney AH, Laufer N, et al. Neosalpingostomy: Comparison of 24 and 72 month follow-up time show increased pregnancy rate. *Fertil Steril* 1986; 45:296.
48. Donnez J, Casanas-Roux F. Prognostic factors of fimbrial microsurgery. *Fertil Steril* 1986; 46:200.
49. Kitchin JD, Nunley WC, Bateman BG. Surgical management of distal tubal occlusion. *Am J Obstet Gynecol* 1986; 155:524.
50. Daniell JF, Diamond MP, McLaughlin DS, et al. Clinical results of terminal salpingostomy with the use of the CO_2 laser: Report of the intraabdominal laser study group. *Fertil Steril* 1986; 45:175.
51. Carey M, Brown S. Infertility surgery for pelvic inflammatory disease: Success rates after salpingolysis and salpingostomy. *Am J Obstet Gynecol* 1987; 156:296.
52. Jacobs LA, Thie J, Patton PE, et al. Primary microsurgery for postinflammatory tubal infertility. *Fertil Steril* 1988; 50:855.
53. Williams KM, Griffin WT. Distal tuboplasty: Is it appropriate? *South Med J* 1988; 81:872.
54. Audibert F, Hedon B, Arnal F, et al. Therapeutic strategies in tubal infertility with distal pathology. *Hum Reprod* 1991; 6:1439.
55. Canis M, Mage G, Pouly JL, et al. Laparoscopic distal tuboplasty: Report of 87 cases and a 4 year experience. *Fertil Steril* 1991; 46:616.
56. Chong AP. Pregnancy outcome in neosalpingostomy by the Cuff vs Bruhat technique using the carbon dioxide laser. *J Gynecol Surg* 1991; 7:207.

57. Gomel V. Salpingostomy by laparoscopy. *J Reprod Med* 1977; 18:265.
58. Jansen RPS. Surgery-pregnancy time interval after salpingolysis, unilateral salpingostomy, and bilateral salpingostomy. *Fertil Steril* 1980; 34:222.
59. Kelly RW, Roberts DK. Experience with the carbon dioxide laser in gynecologic microsurgery. *Am J Obstet Gynecol* 1983; 145:585.
60. Tulandi T, Vilos GA. A comparison between laser surgery and electrosurgery for bilateral hydrosalpinx: A 2 year followup. *Fertil Steril* 1985; 44:846.
61. Mettler L, Giesel H, Semm K. Treatment of female infertility due to tubal obstruction by operative laparoscopy. *Fertil Steril* 1979; 32:384.
62. Fayez JA. An assessment of the role of operative laparoscopy in tuboplasty. *Fertil Steril* 1983; 39:476.
63. Daniell JF, Herbert CM. Laparoscopic salpingostomy utilizing the CO_2 laser. *Fertil Steril* 1984; 41:558.
64. Dubuisson JB, DeJolinieres JB, Aubriot FX, et al. Terminal tuboplasties by laparoscopy: 65 consecutive cases. *Fertil Steril* 1990; 54:401.
65. McComb PF, Paleologou A. The intussusception salpingostomy technique for the therapy of distal oviductal occlusion at laparoscopy. *Obstet Gynecol* 1991; 78:443.
66. Nezhat C, Nezhat F, Nezhat C. Operative laparoscopy (minimally invasive surgery): State of the art. *J Gynecol Surg* 1992; 8:111.
67. Prapas Y, Prapas N, Papanicolaou A, et al. Laparoscopic tubal surgery: A retrospective comparative study of open microsurgery versus laparoscopic surgery. *Acta Eur Fertil* 1995; 26:81.
68. Filippini F, Darai E, Benifla JL, et al. Distal tubal surgery: A critical review of 104 laparoscopic distal tuboplasties. *J Gynecol Obstet Biol Reprod* 1996; 25:471.
69. Lavergne N, Krimly A, Roge P, Erny R. Results and indications of laparoscopic distal tuboplasty. *Contracept Fertil Sex* 1996; 24:41.
70. Kasia JM, Raiga J, Doh AS, et al. Laparoscopic fimbrioplasty and neosalpingostomy: Experience of the Yaounde General Hospital, Cameroon (report of 194 cases). *Eur J Obstet Gynecol Reprod Biol* 1997; 73:71.
71. Audebert AJ, Pouly JL, Von Theobald P. Laparoscopic fimbrioplasty: An evaluation of 35 cases. *Hum Reprod* 1998; 13:1496.
72. Gomel V. *Microsurgery in Female Infertility*. Boston: Little, Brown, 1983.
73. Oh ST. Tubal patency and conception rates with three methods of laparoscopic terminal neosalpingostomy. *J Am Assoc Gynecol Laparosc* 1996; 3:519.
74. Surrey ES, Surrey MW. Correlation between salpingoscopic and laparoscopic staging in the assessment of the distal fallopian tube. *Fertil Steril* 1996; 65:267.
75. Henry-Suchet J, Loffredo V, Tesquier L, et al. Endoscopy of the tube (tuboscopy): Its prognostic value for tuboplasties. *Acta Eur Fertil* 1985; 16:139.
76. Cornier E. L'amullosalpingoscopie percoelioscopique. *J Gynecol Obstet Biol Reprod* 1985; 14:459.
77. Brosens IA, Broeckx W, Delattin P, et al. Salpingoscopy: A new preoperative diagnostic tool in tubal infertility. *Br J Obstet Gynaecol* 1987; 94:760.
78. Nezhat F, Winer WK, Nezhat C. Fimbrioscopy and salpingoscopy in patients with minimal to moderate pelvic endometriosis. *Obstet Gynecol* 1990; 75:15.
79. Heylen SM, Brosens IA, Puttemans PJ. Clinical value and cumulative pregnancy rates following rigid salpingoscopy during laparoscopy for infertility. *Hum Reprod* 1995; 10:2913.
80 Dechaud H, Daures JP, Hedon B. Prospective evaluation of falloposcopy. *Hum Reprod* 1998; 13:1815.
81. Scudamore IW, Dunphy BC, Bowman M, et al. Comparison of ampullary assessment by falloposcopy and salpingoscopy. *Hum Reprod* 1994; 9:1516.
82. Sueoka K, Asada H, Tsuchiya S, et al. Falloposcopic tuboplasty for bilateral tubal occlusion: A novel infertility treatment as an alternative for in-vitro fertilization? *Hum Reprod* 1998; 13:71.
83. Gordts S, Campo R, Rombauts L, Brosens I. Transvaginal salpingoscopy: An office procedure for infertility investigation. *Fertil Steril* 1998; 70:523.
84. Gordts S, Campo R, Rombauts L, Brosens I. Transvaginal hydrolaparoscopy as an outpatient procedure for infertility investigation. *Hum Reprod* 1998; 13:99.
85. Murray DL, Sagoskin AW, Widra EA, Levy MJ. The adverse effect of hydrosalpinges on in vitro fertilization pregnancy rates and the benefit of surgical correction. *Fertil Steril* 1998; 69:41.

86. Nackley AC, Muasher SJ. The significance of hydrosalpinx in in vitro fertilization. *Fertil Steril* 1998; 69:373.
87. Camus E, Poncelet C, Goffinet F, et al. Pregnancy rates after in-vitro fertilization in cases of tubal infertility with and without hydro-salpinx: A meta-analysis of published comparative studies. *Hum Reprod* 1999; 14:1243.
88. Zeyneloglu HB, Arici A, Olive DL. Adverse effects of hydrosalpinx on pregnancy rates after in vitro fertilization–embryo transfer. *Fertil Steril* 1998; 70:492.
89. Aboulghar MA, Mansour RT, Serour GI. Controversies in the modern management of hydrosalpinx. *Hum Reprod Update* 1998; 4:882.
90. Blazar AS, Hogan JW, Seifer DB, et al. The impact of hydrosalpinx on successful pregnancy in tubal factor infertility treated by in vitro fertilization. *Fertil Steril* 1997; 67:517.
91. Nezhat C, Nezhat F, Winer W. Salpingectomy via laparoscopy: A new surgical approach. *J Laparosc Surg* 1991; 1:91.
92. Sedbon E, Delajolinieres JB, Boudouris O, et al. Tubal desterilization through exclusive laparoscopy. *Hum Reprod* 1989; 4:158.
93. Klink F, Grosspietzsch R, von Klitzing L, et al. Animal in vivo studies and in vitro experiments with human tubes for end-to-end anastomotic operation by a CO_2 laser technique. *Fertil Steril* 1978; 30:100.
94. Lyon DR, Vontver LA, Patton DL, et al. A comparison between argon laser and microsuture anastomosis of the rat uterine horn. *Fertil Steril* 1987; 47:329.
95. Baggish MS, Chong AP. Carbon dioxide laser microsurgery of the uterine tube. *Obstet Gynecol* 1981; 58:111.
96. Fayez JA, McComb JS, Harper MA. Comparison of tubal surgery with the CO_2 laser and the unipolar microelectrode. *Fertil Steril* 1983; 40:476.
97. Choe JK, Dawood MY, Bardawil WA, et al. Clinical and histologic evaluation of laser reanastomosis of the uteri tube. *Fertil Steril* 1984; 41:755.
98. Tulandi T. Effects of fibrin sealant on tubal anastomosis and adhesion formation. *Fertil Steril* 1991; 56:136.
99. Wallwiener D, Meyer A, Bastert G. Carbon dioxide laser tissue welding: An alternative technique for tubal anastomosis? *J Clin Laser Med Surg* 1997; 15:163.
100. Rajaram S, Rusia U, Agarwal S, Agarwal N. Autologous fibrin adhesive in experimental tubal anastomosis. *Int J Fertil Menopausal Stud* 1996; 41:458.
101. Chong AP, Pepi M, Lashgari M. Pregnancy outcome in microsurgical anastomosis using cold knife versus CO_2 laser. *J Gynecol Surg* 1989; 5:99.
102. Choe JK, Dawood MY, Andrews AH: Conventional versus laser reanastomosis of rabbit ligated uterine horns. *Obstet Gynecol* 1983; 61:689.
103. Silva PD, Schapes AM, Meisch JK, et al. Outpatient microsurgical reversal of tubal sterilization by a combined approach of laparoscopy and minilaparotomy. *Fertil Steril* 1991; 55:696.
104. Penfield AF. Minilaparotomy for female sterilization. *Obstet Gynecol* 1979; 54:184.
105. Uchida HL. Uchida tubal sterilization. *Am J Obstet Gynecol* 1975; 121:153.
106. Osathanondh V. Suprapubic minilaparotomy, uterine elevation technique: Simple, inexpensive and outpatient procedure for interval female sterilization. *Contraception* 1974; 10:251.
107. Barjot PJ, Marie G, Von Theobald P. Laparoscopic tubal anastomosis and reversal of sterilization. *Hum Reprod* 1999; 14:1222.
108. Stadtmauer L, Sauer MV. Reversal of tubal sterilization using laparoscopically placed titanium staples: Preliminary experience. *Hum Reprod* 1997; 12:647.
109. Yoon TK, Sung HR, Cha SH, et al. Fertility outcome after laparoscopic microsurgical tubal anastomosis. *Fertil Steril* 1997; 67:18.
110. Dubuisson JB, Chapron C. Single suture laparoscopic tubal re-anastomosis. *Curr Opin Obstet Gynecol* 1998; 10:307.
111. Koster S, Volz J, Melchert F. Indications for 3-D laparoscopy in gynecology. *Geburtshilfe Frauenheilkd* 1996; 56:431.
112. Falcone T, Goldberg J, Garcia-Ruiz A, et al. Full robotic assistance for laparoscopic tubal anastomosis: A case report. *J Laparoendosc Adv Surg Tech* 1999; 9:107.
113. Margossian H, Garcia-Ruiz A, Falcone T, et al. Robotically assisted laparoscopic microsurgical uterine horn anastomosis. *Fertil Steril* 1998; 70:530.

15

Laparoscopic Operations on the Uterus

Benign diseases of the uterus are found commonly in gynecologic patients and account for most laparotomies and hysterectomies. Myomas are the most common uterine neoplasm, affecting approximately 20 to 25% of women of reproductive age.[1, 2] They can develop in any area where there are smooth muscle cells of müllerian origin, such as the fallopian tubes, the uterine corpus, and cervix. These growths arise from the benign transformation and proliferation of smooth muscle cells. Increased estrogen stimulation alone or acting synergistically with growth hormone or human placental lactogen is the major growth regulator. Progesterone appears to inhibit the growth of myomas but under certain circumstances promotes their growth.[3]

Myoma

The severity of the symptoms associated with uterine leiomyomas depends on their number, size, and location. These tumors can cause abnormal uterine bleeding, abdominal pressure, urinary frequency, and constipation. The tumors are seldom the only cause of infertility, but data from several studies show a link between myomas, fetal wastage, and premature delivery.[1] Indications for treatment are summarized in Table 15-1. Factors such as the size, number, and location of the tumors influence the choice of the operation.

Preoperative Evaluation

In women who complain of menorrhagia, the hematocrit is used to assess the degree of anemia. For anemic patients, preoperative gonadotropin-releasing hormone (GnRH) treatment may enable restoration of a normal hematocrit, decrease the size of the myoma,[4] and reduce the need for transfusion.[1] While some studies show a decrease in intraoperative blood loss after a course of GnRH therapy,[5] others do not.[6] GnRH therapy is associated with hypoestrogenic side effects[4] and possibly an increased risk of tumor recurrence.[4]

The presence of large broad ligament myoma shows the need for an intravenous pyelogram to search for ureteral obstruction. Periodic pelvic and ultrasound examinations help monitor the growth rate of asymptomatic myomas. Submucous tumors can be detected by pelvic ultrasound, a hysterogram, or hysteroscopy. Since small interstitial myomas palpated during laparotomy can be missed at laparoscopy, a vaginal ultrasound should be done preoperatively.[4, 5]

Depending on the tumor's size and location, preoperative autologous blood donation is suggested. Patients are counseled about the potential for intraoperative and postoperative bleeding and the possible need for a laparotomy.

Laparoscopic Myomectomy

Women who have large intramural fibroids should be managed laparoscopically only if they no longer wish to have children because meticulous repair is difficult. Nezhat and associates[7] reported on myomectomy in 137 women from whom 196 leiomyomas were removed. The fibroids ranged in size from 2 to 14 cm. The operations lasted from 50 to 160 minutes (mean, 116 minutes). Estimated blood loss was between 10 and 600 mL, and two women received transfusions because of intraoperative blood loss. The hospital stay

TABLE 15-1. Indications for Myomectomy

Menometrorrhagia and anemia
Pelvic pain and pressure
Enlarging leiomyoma and possibility of neoplasia
Associated fetal wastage or infertility
Gestational size more than 12 weeks and inability to evaluate the adnexa
Obstructed ureter

ranged from 7 to 48 hours, with a mean of 19.6 hours.

In 114 women undergoing laparoscopic myomectomy (LM) who desired future pregnancy,[8] the average number of myomas was 3.0 ± 2.9 and the mean size was 5.9 ± 3.0 cm. In 52.4% of the cases the deepest infiltrating myoma was intramural, in 42.9% subserosal, and in 4.7% pedunculated. Thirty-one pregnancies occurred in 29 women. Of the 26 that could be followed, 5 ended with vaginal delivery at term. Cesareans were done for 14 women: 9 at term, 1 at 26 weeks, and 4 at an unknown gestational age. Six women miscarried in the first trimester, and one had an ectopic pregnancy. No spontaneous uterine rupture was noted. Compared with women with ectopic pregnancies, miscarriages, and preterm deliveries, those who delivered at term were younger (33.1 ± 1.9 versus 36.6 ± 4.8 years., $p < 0.05$) and had fewer myomas at surgery (1.9 ± 2.0 versus 4.8 ± 3.0, $p < 0.05$). Those who had intramural myomas were most likely to develop complications during pregnancy. In another study,[9] 28 infertile patients with at least one uterine leiomyoma of > 5 cm in diameter underwent laparoscopic myomectomy. The average size of the myomas removed was 6 cm (range, 4 to 13.3 cm). The postoperative intrauterine pregnancy rate was 64.3% (n = 18), including one of two patients who underwent concomitant hysteroscopic myomectomy. Four patients had spontaneous abortions, and 14 delivered viable term neonates. Six patients had a vaginal delivery without complications, and eight had a cesarean delivery.

Technique

Essential instruments include a CO_2 laser, a unipolar electrode or a harmonic scalpel for cutting, a bipolar Kleppinger forceps, and clawed grasping forceps. In addition, dilute vasopressin (Pitressin)

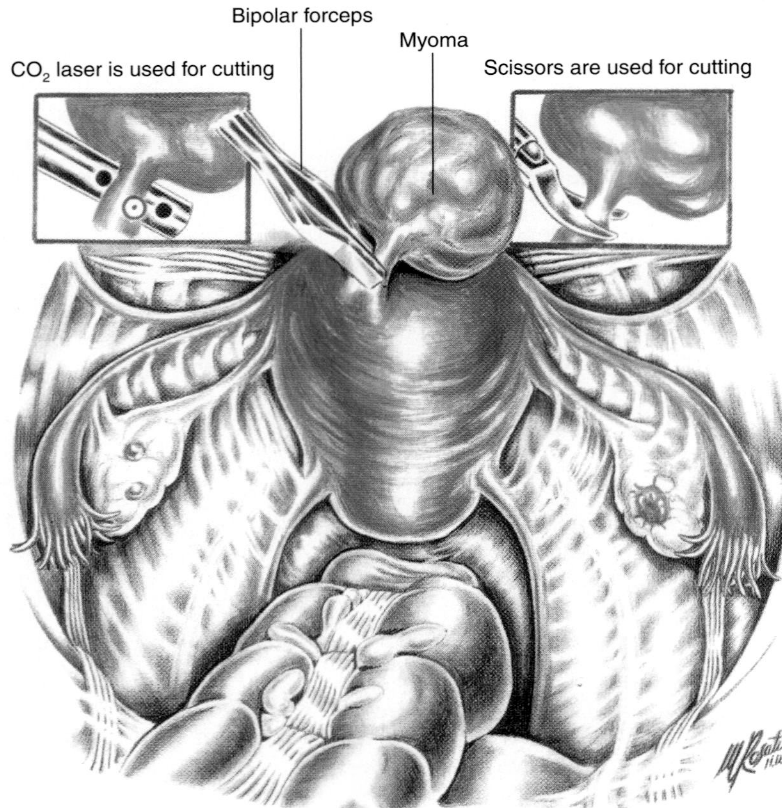

Figure 15-1. A pedunculated myoma is seen and its pedicle is electrocoagulated with a bipolar forceps. After this maneuver, the myoma can be cut with the CO_2 laser (*left inset*) or the electrosurgical scissors (*right inset*).

(1 IU in 100 mL lactated Ringer's solution) helps control uterine bleeding.

Dilute Pitressin (3 to 5 mL) is injected into the base of the stalk at the junction of the uterine fundus (Figure 15-1). Pedunculated leiomyomas are removed by coagulating and cutting the stalk. Bleeding areas are coagulated with bipolar forceps. For intramural myomas, the technique of myomectomy is different (Figure 15-2 A through E). Dilute vasopressin is injected in multiple sites between the myometrium and the fibroid capsule. An incision is made on the serosa overlying the leiomyoma, using the CO_2 laser (superpulse or ultrapulse mode), a monopolar electrode, a fiber laser or harmonic scapel. The incision is extended until it reaches the capsule. The myometrium retracts as the incision is made, exposing the tumor. Two grasping, toothed forceps hold the edges of the myometrium, and the suction-irrigator is used as a blunt probe to shell the leiomyoma from its capsule. A myoma screw is inserted into the tumor to apply traction while the suction-irrigator is used as a blunt dissector. Vessels are electrocoagulated before being cut. After complete removal of the myoma, the uterine defect is irrigated. Bleeding points are identified and controlled with electrocoagulation. The edges of the uterine defect are approximated by superficial suturing.

If the defect is deep or large, the myometrium and serosa are approximated by using a 4-0 polydioxanone or 1-0 polyglactin suture. While two layers of sutures can be applied, this maneuver may be difficult. The repair mainly involves the serosal and subserosal layers and can be accomplished in one layer. The sutures are applied in 1-cm increments, using extracorporeal or intracorporeal knot tying (Figure 15-3). After repair, the uterine surface is irrigated with warmed lactated Ringer's solution and Interceed (Ethicon, Somerville, NJ) is applied over the suture line

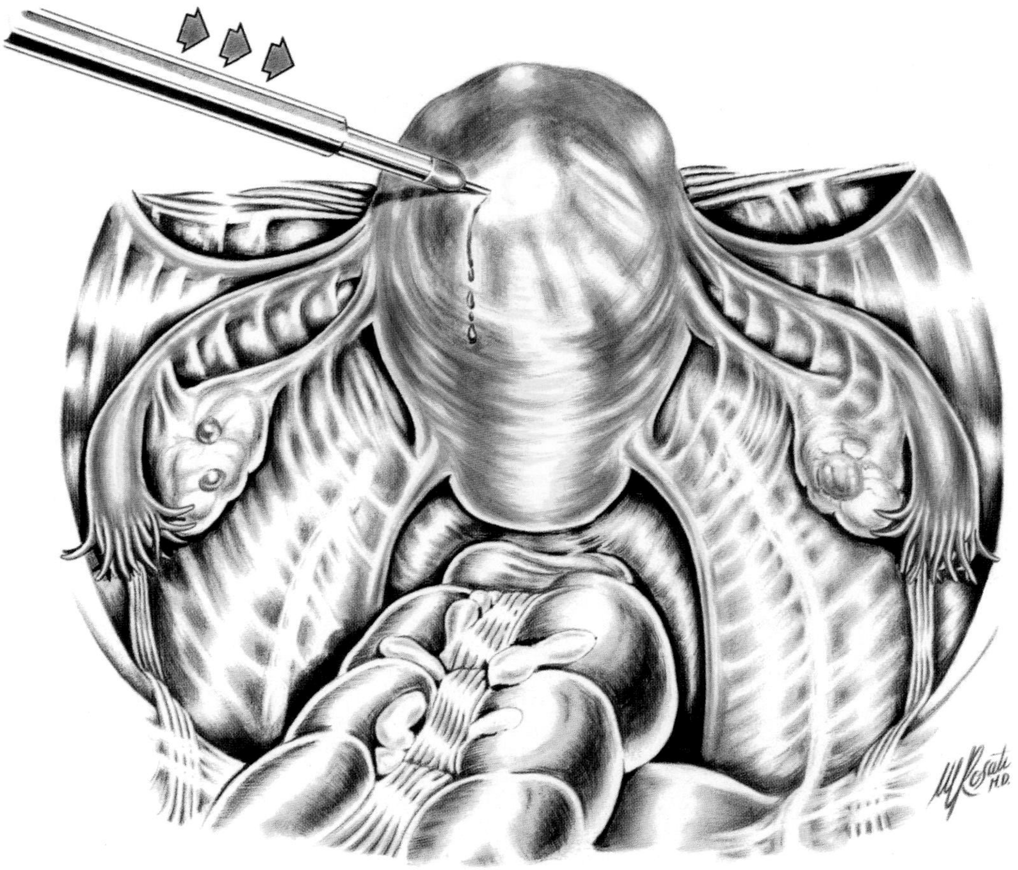

A

Figure 15-2. **A.** Dilute vasopressin is injected into several sites between the myometrium and the myoma. It is essential to be certain that this injection is not intravascular, and the anesthesiologist should be alert for the possibility of acute hypertension.

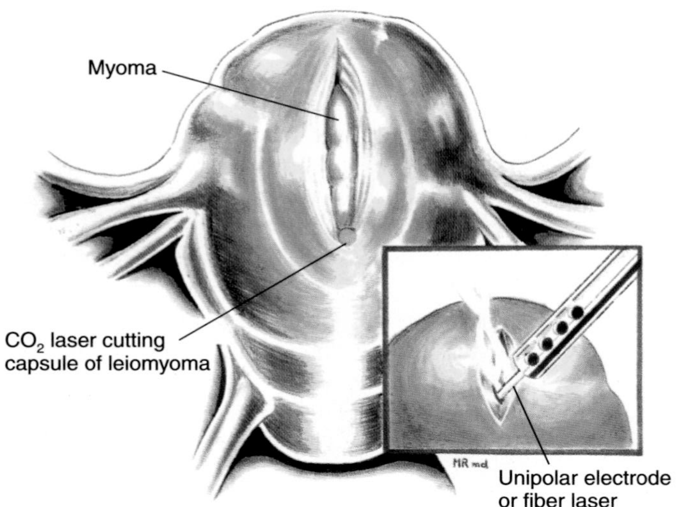

Figure 15-2. (*Continued*) **B.** An incision has been made into the myometrium over the myoma, using a CO_2 laser, fiber laser, or monopolar electrode (*inset*). The incision extends until it reaches the myoma; the myometrium retracts as the tumor becomes visible. **C.** Two grasping toothed forceps hold the edges of the myometrium, and a myoma screw is inserted into the myoma to apply traction.

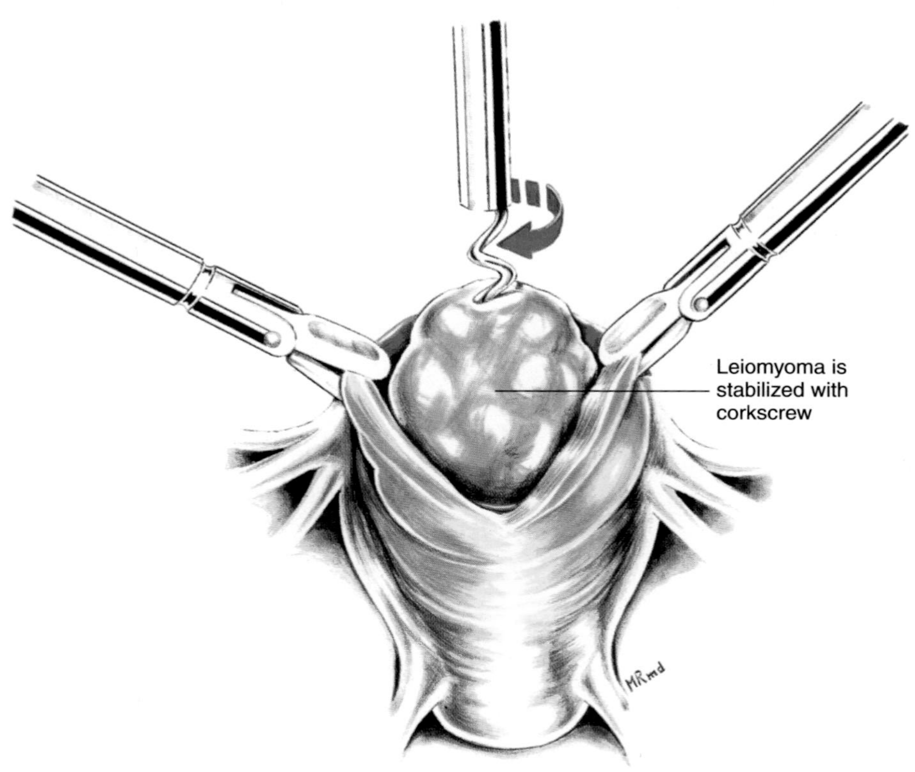

Figure 15-2. (*Continued*) **D.** The suction-irrigator, acting as a blunt dissector, is used as a probe to aid in the enucleation of the tumor. **E.** Myometrial vessels are electrocoagulated as the myoma is removed. After the enucleation process, additional hemostasis is obtained with the bipolar electrode as the exposed myometrial surfaces are irrigated.

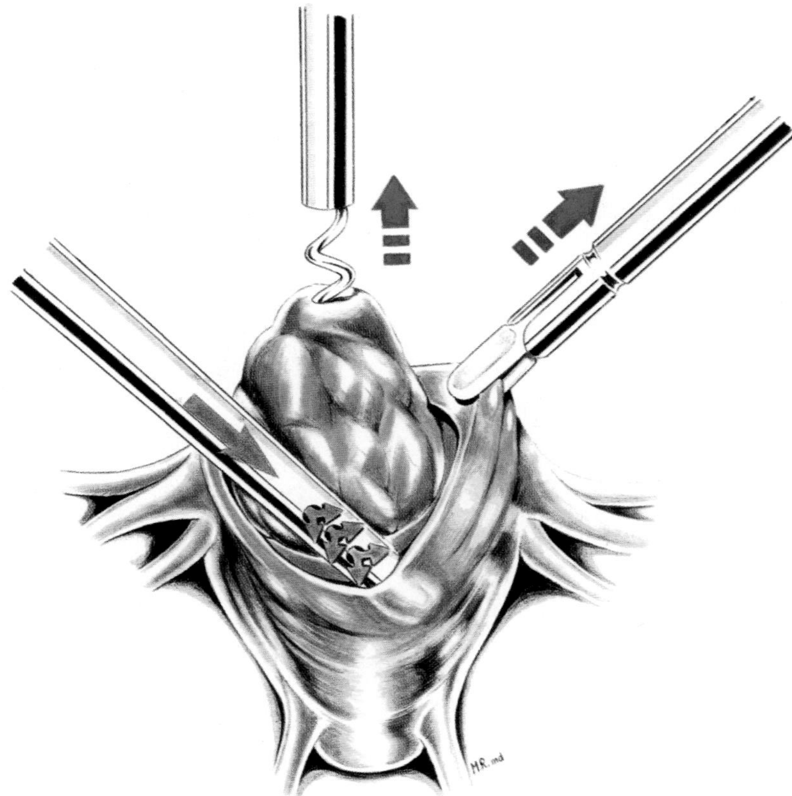

D

Bipolar forceps coagulates small blood vessels

Leiomyoma is removed

E

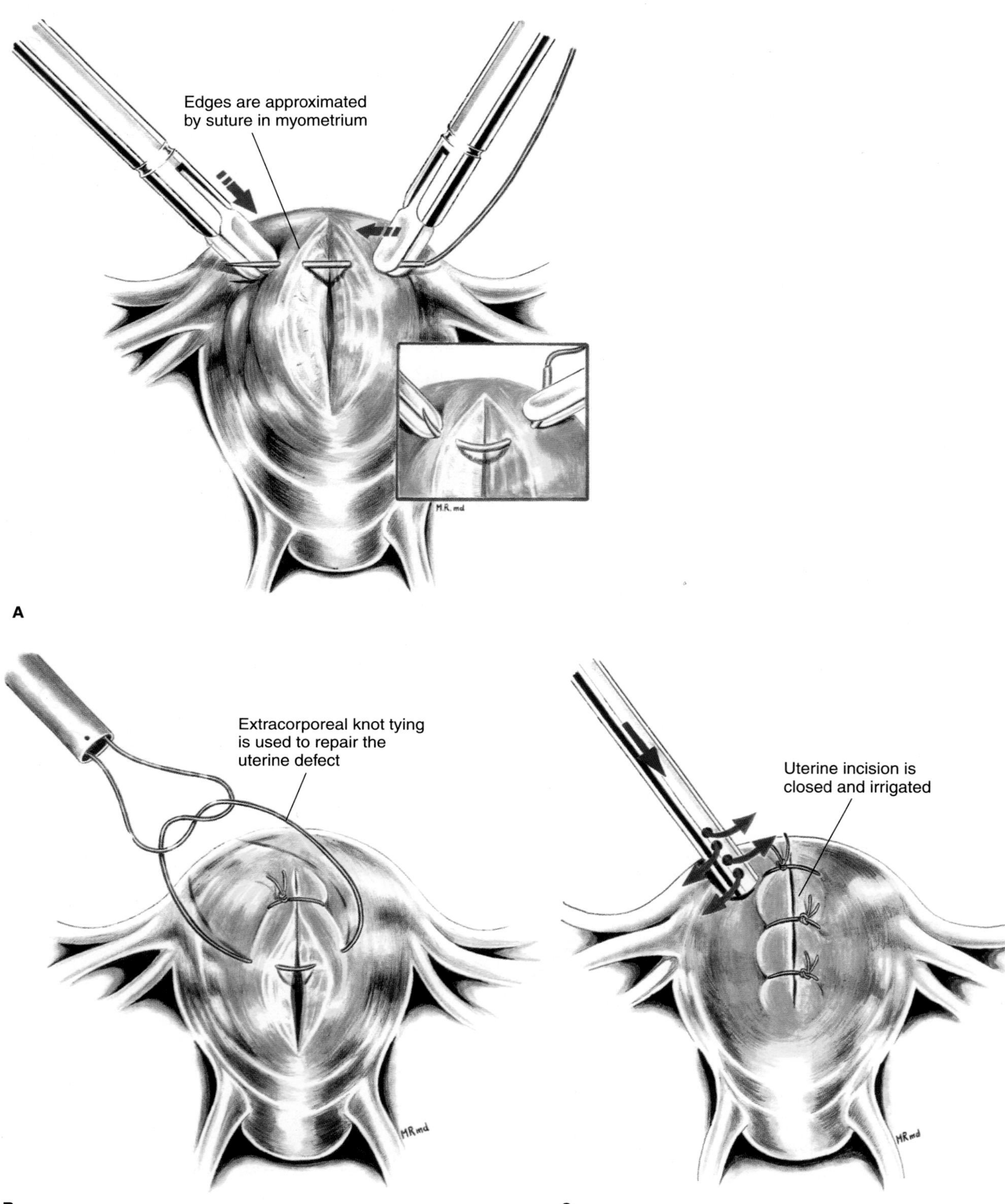

Figure 15-3. **A.** If the myometrial defect is large or deep, the edges are approximated with 4-0 polydioxanone or 1-0 polyglactin suture on a straight or curved needle (*inset*). The suture is brought through the superficial myometrium and serosa in a one-layer closure. **B.** The sutures are applied in 1-cm increments by using extracorporeal or intracorporeal knot-tying techniques. **C.** After the approximation of the uterine wound, the surface is irrigated with warm lactated Ringer's solution to locate any oozing that might require electrocoagulation.

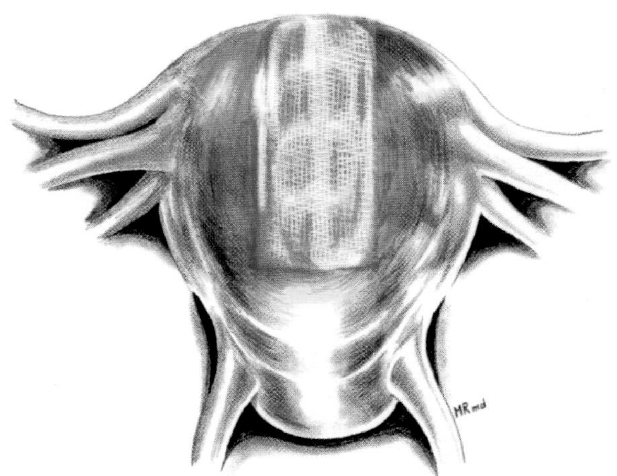

Figure 15-4. The myometrial defect is covered with Interceed.

(Figure 15-4). Spraying 10,000 IU of thrombin over the Interceed contributes to hemostasis. Suturing is limited because of the high incidence of postoperative adhesions (Table 15-2). The defect heals better and with less deformity when the edges are approximated. Even under ideal circumstances, laparoscopic microsurgical closure of the myometrial defect is difficult.

Intraligamentous and broad ligament myomas require careful observation of the course of the ureters and large blood vessels. Depending on the location of the myoma, an incision is made on the anterior or posterior leaf of the broad ligament. The myoma is removed with the techniques described above for subserosal and intramural tumors. Throughout the procedure, the location of the ureters is noted. Hemostasis is obtained with the sutures, clips, or bipolar forceps. None of the available lasers, despite the power setting or focus of the beam, adequately can coagulate bleeding myometrial vessels. A bipolar forceps or argon beam coagulator is excellent for this purpose. The broad ligament and peritoneum are not closed but allowed to heal spontaneously. Drains are used infrequently.

Removal of myomas from the abdominal cavity is a time-consuming procedure, and no methods or instruments are suited ideally for this purpose.

1. A claw-toothed forceps is inserted through a 10-mm sleeve for a myoma <5 cm.
2. A long Kocher clamp is inserted through one suprapubic incision. The midline incision is preferred to avoid injury to the inferior epigastric artery, and this technique is quick. The suprapubic incision often must be extended.
3. Larger myomas can be removed through a posterior colpotomy[9] (Figures 15-5 and 15-6). This approach may increase operative time, infectious morbidity, and the risk of bowel and ureteral injury. In women with concurrent posterior cul-de-sac abnormalities, colpotomy is not safe.
4. Improvements in electronic morcellators have made this task easier. Examples are the 15-mm, 20- & 25-mm morcellators by Gynecare (J&J) & Demm (Wisap).

Patients who attempt a pregnancy after a laparoscopic myomectomy risk a uterine rupture in a subsequent pregnancy[6] because of the difficulties of adequately closing all layers laparoscopically.[7,10] Uteroperitoneal fistulas can occur postoperatively. Postoperative adhesions increase when sutures are placed in the serosal layer.[7,11] One uterine incision is advised for the removal of multiple leiomyomas.

TABLE 15-2. Incidence of Adhesions after Laparoscopic Myomectomy with or without the Use of Sutures

Leiomyoma size	No Suture Used				Suture Used			
	0*	1	2	3	0	1	2	3
<3 cm	18/21	3/21	0/21	0/21	N/A	N/A	N/A	N/A
>3 cm	6	6	6	6	9	9	9	9

*Adhesion score: 0 = no adhesions; grade 1 = filmy and nonvascular; grade 2 = thick and nonvascular; grade 3 = thick, vascular, and bowel.

N/A = suture was not used for myomas <3 cm in size.

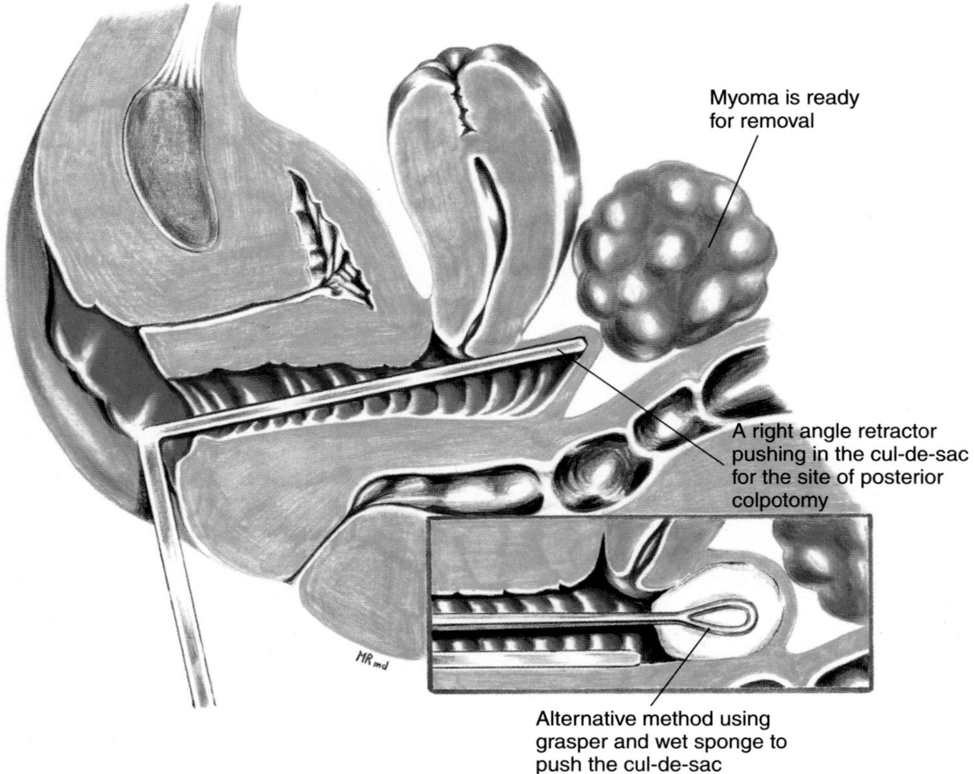

Figure 15-5. Some myomas are removed through the posterior colpotomy. The right-angle retractor pushes the vagina toward the myoma, indicating the site for the vaginal incision. The inset shows the use of a sponge on a sponge stick to accomplish the same purpose.

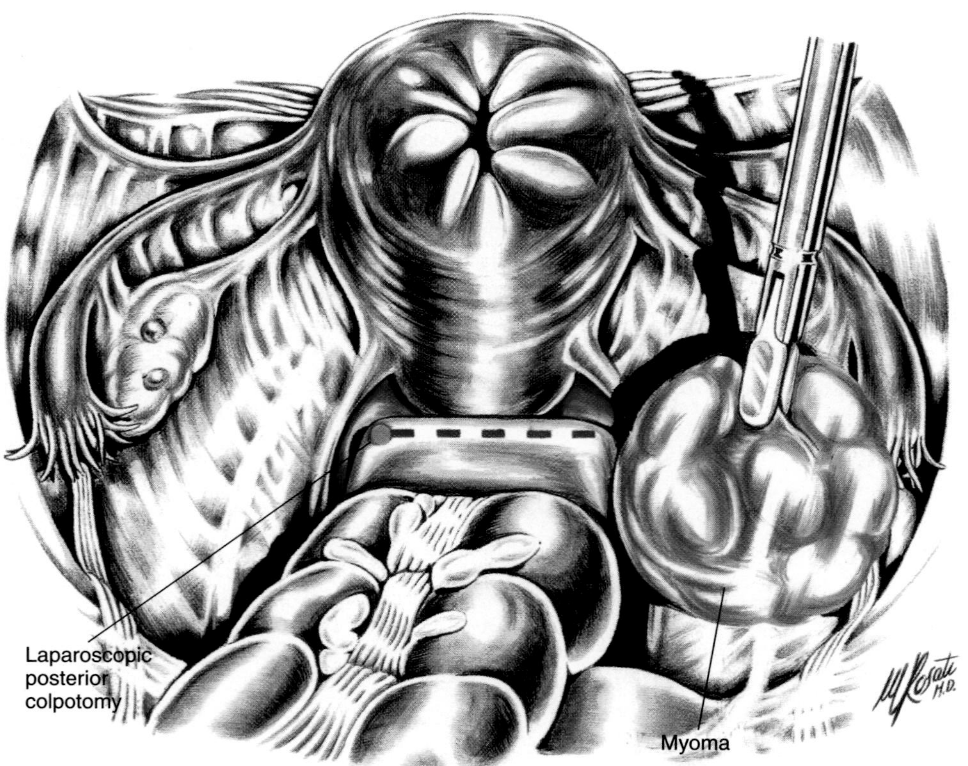

Figure 15-6. Illustration shows the laparoscopic view of the proposed incisional site. The edges of the uterine incision have been approximated without suturing.

Laparoscopically Assisted Myomectomy

Laparoscopically assisted myomectomy (LAM) is a safe alternative to LM. It is less difficult and requires less time to complete. These considerations are summarized in Table 15-3. The decision to do LAM usually is made in the operating room after the diagnostic laparoscopy and treatment of other pelvic abnormalities are completed. The criteria for LAM are a myoma greater than 8 cm, many myomas requiring extensive morcellation, and a deep, large, intramural myoma that requires uterine repair in multiple layers.

A combination of laparoscopy with a 2-4 cm abdominal incision may enable more gynecologists to apply this technique. The conventional uterine suturing in two or three layers reduces the potential for uterine dehiscence, fistulas, and adhesions. Better pelvic exposure during the laparoscopy allows the gynecologist to diagnose and treat associated endometriosis or adhesions.

Three major objectives of LAM are reduction of blood loss, prevention of postoperative adhesions, and maintenance of myometrial integrity. LAM, with morcellation and conventional suturing reduces the duration of the operation and the need for more extensive laparoscopic experience.

Technique

In patients having multiple myomas, the most prominent myoma is injected at its base with 3 to 7 mL of diluted vasopressin. A vertical incision is made over the uterine serosa on to the surface of the tumor and extended until the capsule of the leiomyoma is reached. A corkscrew manipulator is inserted into the leiomyoma and used to elevate the uterus toward the midline suprapubic puncture. With the trocar and manipulator attached to the myoma, this midline 5-mm puncture is enlarged to 4 cm transverse skin incision. After the incision of the fascia transversely, the rectus muscle is divided, using a monopolar electrode. If the inferior epigastric vessels are found, they are coagulated. This approach provides excellent access to the abdominal cavity.

The peritoneum is entered transversely, and the leiomyoma is observed. It is brought to the laparotomy incision by using the corkscrew manipulator to raise the uterus. A corkscrew manipulator is replaced with two Lahey tenacula. The tumor is shelled and morcellated sequentially, and after its complete removal, the uterine wall defect shows through the incision. If uterine size allows, the uterus is exteriorized to complete the repair.

TABLE 15-3. Results of Types of Myomectomy

Studied Parameter	LAM(57) mean ± SEM	LM(64) mean ± SEM	Lap(22) mean ± SEM	P(LM)* P(Lap)†
Leiomyoma weight (g)	247 ± 30.1	58 ± 7.16	337 ± 77.4	P(LM) < 00001 P(Lap) = 0.27
Uterine size (weeks)	12 ± 26	8 ± 14	10 ± 24	
Operative time (min)	127 ± 7.62	136 ± 9.6	134 ± 9.95	P(LM) = 0.36 P(Lap) = 0.59
Blood loss (mL)	267 ± 54.4	143 ± 35.6	245 ± 56.1	P(LM) = 0068 P(Lap) = 0.78
Postoperative hospital stay (days)	1.28	0.91	3.3 ± 0.39	P(LM) = .0141 P(Lap) = .00004
Days to resume normal activity	12.2	11.2	39.2	P(LM) = 0.43 P(Lap) < 0.0001
Days for complete "100%" recovery	23.1	20.9	70.0	P(LM) = 0.41 P(Lap) = 0.0002

*P(LM) compares LAM and LM.

†P(Lap) compares LAM and myomectomy by laparotomy.

When multiple leiomyomas are found, as many of them as possible are removed through one uterine incision. When other myomas are located that cannot be removed through the initial uterine incision, the abdominal 4 cm opening is approximated temporarily with two or three Allis clamps or an inflated latex glove. The laparoscope is reintroduced, the remaining myomas are identified and brought to the level of the abdominal incision. They are removed under laparoscopic control. The uterus is exteriorized through the 4 cm abdominal incision. The myometrium is closed in layers with 2-0 and 0 polydioxanone sutures. The serosa is closed microsurgically with 5-0 sutures. The uterus is palpated to ensure that no small intramural leiomyomas remain. It is returned to the peritoneal cavity. The fascia is closed with a 1-0 polyglactin suture, and the skin is closed in a subcuticular manner. The laparoscope is used to evaluate hemostasis. The pelvis is observed to detect and treat endometriosis and adhesions that may have been obscured previously by myomas. Copious irrigation is used, blood clots are removed, and Interceed is applied over the uterus to help prevent adhesions.

Intraoperatively, injections of dilute vasopressin into the myoma help reduce blood loss. Vertical uterine incisions bleed less than do transverse incisions,[1] and pneumoperitoneum seems to decrease intraoperative bleeding.

Comparison of Results of LAM and LM

While myomectomy is done to preserve fertility, postoperative adhesions can jeopardize this goal. Single, vertical, anterior, and midline uterine incisions cause fewer adhesions.[1] Although sutures predispose patients to adhesions,[12] they often are necessary to close the uterine defect. While several adhesion barriers are available or under development, none are completely effective.[13,14] A prospective, randomized, blinded multicenter study[15] evaluated 127 women undergoing uterine myomectomy with at least one posterior uterine incision ≥ 1 cm in length. Patients were randomized to Seprafilm (HAL-F) Bioresorbable Membrane (Genzyme Corporation, Cambridge, MA) or to no treatment. At second-look laparoscopy, the incidence, measured as the mean number of sites adherent to the uterine surface, was significantly lower in the treated group as were the mean uterine adhesion severity scores and mean area of adhesions. In another study,[16] 50 premenopausal, nonpregnant women who underwent laparoscopic myomectomy were randomized to the control group (25 patients) with surgery alone or to the treatment group (25 patients) including Interceed, an oxidized regenerated cellulose (Ethicon, Somerville, NJ). At second-look laparoscopy 12 to 14 weeks later, 12% (3) of the women in the control group were adhesion free, compared with 60% (15) of those treated with Interceed ($p < 0.05$).

Uterine rupture after myomectomy is rare, accounting for about 2% of all pregnancy-related uterine ruptures.[17] Inadequate myometrial approximation and poor healing predispose patients to uterine rupture.

One hundred forty-three charts from our practice were evaluated. Those patients who had myomectomy by laparotomy (15.3%), laparoscopic myomectomy (44.7%), or laparoscopically assisted myomectomy (39.8%) were included (Table 15-4).[7] The 22 myomectomies by laparotomy were done before the development of LAM. Since LAM replaced myomectomy by laparotomy and patient selection criteria were comparable, the myoma weights of the two groups were similar.

Mean operating times were the same for LM and LAM despite larger myomas, difficult locations of intramural myomas, and adjunctive laparoscopy in the latter group. The leiomyoma weights were greater in the LAM group than in the LM group ($p < 0.05$).

The mean estimated blood loss of the LAM and laparotomy groups was not different. In contrast, blood loss among the LM patients was significantly lower, and this may be attributed to the smaller leiomyomas. In comparing the hospitalization time of the LAM and LM patients, that of the LAM group appeared to be longer (P(LM) = 0.014). This may be explained by the initial reluctance of some physicians to discharge LAM patients on the day of the operation or on postoperative day 1. After the initial 10 to 15 operations, all the women underwent LAM on an outpatient basis. In fact, when the initial 15 cases are removed from the LAM group, the mean hospital stay drops to 1.06 days. This period is not statistically different from that for the LM group.

The comparison of postoperative recovery times shows important distinctions between the LAM and LM groups. Here, despite the differences in size and location of myomas, the recovery time can be compared because of the diverse incisions. The time elapsed before patients resumed work or regular activity was similar ($p > 0.05$). Introducing a 4 cm incision in the LAM group did appear to

TABLE 15-4. Comparison of Hysterectomy, Abdominal Myomectomy, and Laparoscopic Myomectomy for the Management of Symptomatic Leiomyomas

	Hysterectomy	Abdominal Myomectomy	Laparoscopic Myomectomy
Degree of difficulty	Low	Moderate	High
Patient age	>45 years	Childbearing	>45 years
Recurrence (%)	None	10–15	10–15
Blood loss (mL)	<500 mL	Occasionally > 500 mL	<500 mL
Postoperative adhesion formation	Minimal	>30%	>30%
Postoperative hospitalization (days)	3–4	3–4	1–2
Type of myoma	All types	Intramural, subserosal, pedunculated	Subserosal, pedunculated
Uterine rupture	None	1%	Risk of uteroperitoneal fistula

prolong ($p > 0.05$) the subjectively perceived time for the women to achieve 100% recovery.

Previous studies[6,18] underscored the need to decrease the operative time of LM. While myomas less than 8 cm are managed laparoscopically, larger tumors and intramural lesions require prolonged morcellation and laparoscopic suturing of the uterine defect. The largest reported myomas removed by laparoscopy were 15 to 16 cm,[7,18] and one group wrote that 10 cm was its limit.[19] Both laparoscopic morcellation and myometrial suturing are difficult and prolong operations. Hospitalization was much longer for the patients who underwent myomectomy by laparotomy ($p < 0.05$) compared with both the LAM and the LM groups.

Second-look laparoscopies done on postmyomectomy patients who had pedunculated and superficial subserosal myomas without sutures showed complete uterine healing. In contrast, intramural myomas were associated with granulation tissue and indentation of the uterus proportional to the size of the leiomyoma excised unless sutures were used. The use of sutures is associated with more adhesions (Table 15-2).[7]

Most patients are observed in an outpatient unit and discharged the morning after the operation, although some can leave the hospital on the afternoon or evening of the procedure. Women of childbearing age who plan a future pregnancy and require a myomectomy for an intramural tumor should undergo a laparotomy to ensure proper closure of the myometrial incision. A cesarean delivery is safest for such patients. The laparoscopic approach is appropriate for pedunculated or subserosal tumors.

Myolysis

Additional choices for the conservative surgical treatment of myomas include laparoscopic myolysis and cryomyolysis. Laparoscopic myolysis was devised to shrink myomas by coagulating their blood supply. It is proposed as an alternative to myomectomy or hysterectomy in women who do not contemplate future pregnancy. Vilos and coworkers [20] reported that three patients who conceived three months postoperatively, developed a uterine rupture in the third trimester. Cryopmyolysis is an operation in which the size of the tumors is reduced by freezing them.[21] The formation of postoperative adhesions and uterine rupture in the event of a subsequent pregnancy must be discussed with the patient preoperatively.

Uterine Artery Embolization

Embolization of the uterine arteries was described in obstetrics and gynecology initially for the management of severe, uncontrollable uterine bleeding. It involves the catherization of both uterine arteries and the instillation of micro particles of polyvinyl alcohol, and has been used as a primary treatment for myomas. Postoperatively pelvic pain is not uncommon.[22,23] Worthington and coworkers[24] reported that 94% of their patients had relief of pressure related symptoms and reduction in abnormal bleeding was noted in 88% of them. Postoperative sonographic examinations showed a reduction in the uterine volume in 40% to 80% of the women with a mean of 46%. Many more patients must be followed postoperatively for a longer duration before the value of uterine artery empolization for the management of myomas can be ascertained.

Hysterectomy

The number of hysterectomies, a frequently practiced major surgical procedure, varies between different regions and cultures. It reflects differences in health care systems, education, and psychosocial attitudes. The highest rates of hysterectomy are found in the United States and Australia (36% and 40%, respectively),[25-27] and the lowest in France (5.8%) and Italy (5.5%).

Indications

Most hysterectomies are done for leiomyomas, uterine prolapse, endometriosis, and gynecologic cancer.[28] The number of hysterectomies done for endometriosis doubled between 1965 and 1984, exceeding the increase observed for any other indication and probably reflecting an increased recognition of endometriosis. Other indications are abnormal uterine bleeding, pelvic infection and its sequelae, ovarian tumors, and complications of pregnancy. Those indications account for 15 to 21% of hysterectomies.

About 75% of these operations are done abdominally, and 25% vaginally.[28,29] The vaginal procedure is used mainly for uterine prolapse. Other indications depend upon uterine size, coexistent adnexal disease, and the surgeon's skill and preference. Abdominal hysterectomy usually is done for women with significant pelvic disease such as endometriosis and pelvic adhesions that can make a vaginal removal more difficult. (Table 15-5).[30] Compared to those having a vaginal hysterectomy, women having an abdominal operation have more febrile morbidity, receive more blood transfusions,[29,31] and have a longer postoperative hospitalization and convalescence. If more women had a vaginal rather than an abdominal approach, therapeutic, economic, and social benefits would result.[32]

TABLE 15-5. Indications for Hysterectomy

	Abdominal Hysterectomy,%	Vaginal Hysterectomy,%
Leiomyomata	38	1
Uterine prolapse	1	76
Endometriosis	3	0
Abnormal bleeding	13	9
Adenomyosis	9	8
Pelvic pain/adhesions	5	0
Ovarian tumors	10	0
Uterine neoplasia	15	3

Source: Dicker et al.[29]

The route selected depends on the clinical assessment of the pelvic disorder that is based on the medical history, pelvic examination, ultrasound studies, review of prior operative notes, and the surgeon's experience in vaginal surgery.[32] Kovac and coworkers[33] did diagnostic laparoscopy in 46 patients scheduled for abdominal hysterectomy who, on the basis of clinical indicators, were thought to have a serious pelvic abnormality that contraindicated vaginal hysterectomy. Based on the laparoscopic findings, 42 of the 46 women 91% were candidates for vaginal hysterectomy, which was done under the same anesthesia. Since clinical assessment of pelvic disease may not be accurate, laparoscopy can reveal that a vaginal approach is appropriate. For these women, diagnostic or operative laparoscopy provided the benefits of both the vaginal and abdominal approaches without the disadvantages (Table 15-6). In a recent multicenter randomized comparison of 34 women undergoing laparoscopically assisted vaginal hysterectomy (LAVH) and 31 women undergoing abdominal hysterectomy,[34] while the mean operating time was significantly longer for LAVH (179.8 versus 146 minutes), LAVH required a considerably shorter mean hospital stay (2.1 days) and convalescence (28 days) than did abdominal hysterectomy (4.1 days and 38.0 days, respectively). There were no important differences in mean hospital charges, blood loss, or intraoperative complication rates between the study groups. A higher incidence of wound complications in the abdominal hysterectomy group was noted.

A review of the literature reveals many definitions of a laparoscopically assisted hysterectomy. A suggested classification follows:

1. Total laparoscopic hysterectomy (TLH). The hysterectomy is done laparoscopically, the vaginal cuff can be closed laparoscopically or vaginally.
2. Subtotal laparoscopic hysterectomy (SLH). A supracervical hysterectomy is done laparoscopically.
3. Laparoscopically assisted vaginal hysterectomy (LAVH). The hysterectomy starts laparoscopically, but most steps especially the uterosacral and cardinal ligaments are done vaginally.

TABLE 15-6. Advantages and Disadvantages of Abdominal, Vaginal, and Laparoscopically Assisted Vaginal Hysterectomy

	Abdominal	Vaginal	LAVH
Exposure	Excellent	Limited	Excellent
Associated pelvic disease	Easily treated	Reduced access	Easily treated
Incision	Abdominal	Vaginal	Abdominal/vaginal
Hospitalization (days)	3	2–3	1–2
Cost	Average	Average	More expensive
Mortality(%)	30	10	10
Surgical expertise	Average gynecologist	Average gynecologist	Experienced endoscopist
Oophorectomy	Easy	<25%	Easy

Patients who have suspected pelvic endometriosis undergo a diagnostic laparoscopy to inspect the pelvis. Significant pelvic disease is treated endoscopically, and if necessary, adnexectomy is done. The hysterectomy is completed vaginally.[33] Usually, a combined laparoscopic and vaginal approach is used to dissect and remove uterine attachments.[35–40] The extent of laparoscopic and vaginal dissections depends on the gynecologist's preference and experience with laparoscopic and vaginal operations. A more experienced endoscopist can do the entire hysterectomy laparoscopically.[41] However, TLH can be time-consuming, especially if the uterus is more than 16 to 18 weeks of gestational size. Laparoscopic hysterectomy is useful if the vagina is small and narrow and significant infiltrative pelvic endometriosis is present and a vaginal operation would be difficult. Almost all abdominal hysterectomies for endometriosis can be converted to LAVH.[42] Patients who have the indications for traditional vaginal hysterectomy should not undergo LAVH, VALH, or laparoscopic hysterectomy (LH).[43]

Preoperative Evaluation

Routine preoperative tests include a complete blood count with differential, serum electrolytes, bleeding time, and urinalysis. More comprehensive blood studies, thrombin time, partial thrombin time, electrocardiography (ECG), chest x-ray, and endometrial biopsy are done as indicated. A mechanical and antibiotic bowel preparation are advised. Consultations with a urologist, bowel surgeon, and oncologist are sought as necessary. Appropriate informed consent is obtained from the patient after a through explanation of the planned operation, its potential risks and benefits, the possibility of laparotomy, and therapeutic alternatives. After an overnight fast, the patient is admitted to the ambulatory surgical unit the morning of her operation.

A laparoscopic approach allows the treatment of intraabdominal and pelvic disease and the dissection or removal of adnexa. The broad ligament is dissected until the gynecologist feels comfortable converting to a vaginal approach. This varies with the degree of uterine descent and the gynecologist's expertise.

Technique

The patient's initial position is the same as that for standard laparoscopy. The 10-mm trocar is inserted intraumbilically for placement of the operative laparoscope, and two to four accessory trocars are positioned suprapubically. For the vaginal portion, the patient's legs are readjusted to allow vaginal access (Allen Universal stirrups). With an adjustment under the drapes, the legs are flexed and abducted without redraping. Some gynecologists prefer to place the patient's legs in candy-cane stirrups for the vaginal portion.

Every operative laparoscopy begins with exploration of the abdominal and pelvic cavity to assess the extent of disease. Anatomic landmarks, anomalies, distortions, and alterations are identified. The locations of the bladder, ureters, colon, rectum, and major blood vessels are noted. The omentum and small bowel are evaluated for disease and checked for Veress needle or trocar injury.

After the diagnostic portion, the operator uses the CO_2 laser or other cutting instrument and hydrodissection to resect, ablate, or coagulate implants of endometriosis. An electrocoagulator, clips, staplers, or Endoloops (Ethicon) are used to coagulate or ligate large vessels. Monopolar electrodes or fiber lasers or harmonic scalpel also may

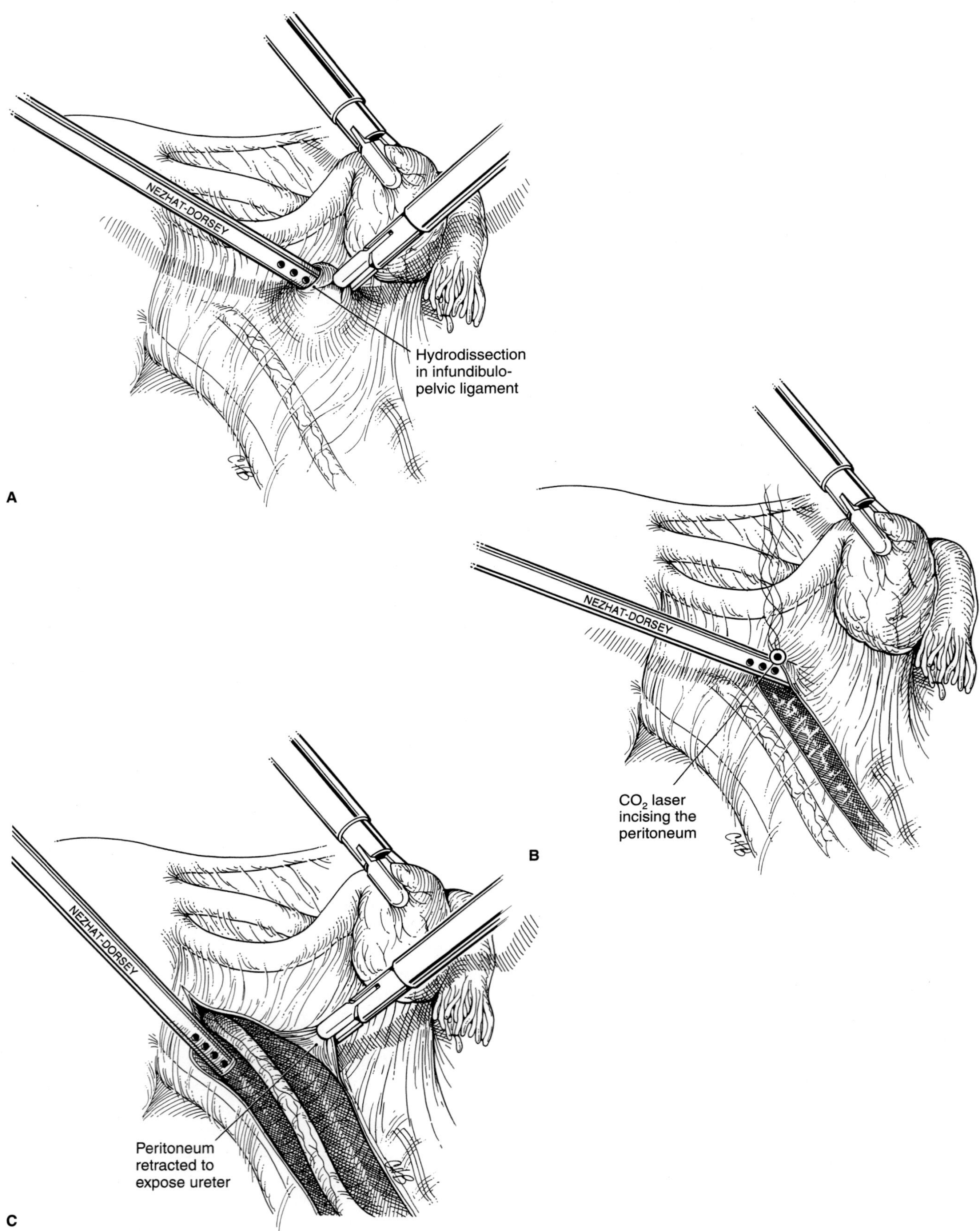

Figure 15-7. **A.** After an opening is made above the ureter in the peritoneum, retroperitoneal hydrodissection is carried out. **B.** Using the suction-irrigator probe as a backstop, an opening is made above the ureter with the CO_2 laser. **C.** The ureter is dissected from the pelvic brim to the back of the bladder by using blunt hydrodissection.

be used or harmonic scalpel.[44] Other instruments include bipolar forceps (middle port), suction-irrigator probe (left), and grasping forceps (right).

The bowel is freed from the pelvic organs to expose the pelvis. Ovaries and tubes are dissected from the cul-de-sac or pelvic side wall, and endometriosis or other abnormalities are treated.

Ureteral evaluation and dissection

The direction and location of both ureters are identified from the pelvic brim to the cardinal ligaments where they are no longer visible. The course of the ureters is marked superiorly with the laser or electrocoagulation so that they can be identified while the broad ligament and adnexa are dissected (Figures 15-7, A, through C). For extensive endometriosis, very wide dissection, as is done during radical hysterectomy, is necessary.[36,38] To identify the ureters at the level of the cardinal ligaments, the peritoneum is opened above or below the ureter and hydrodissection is carried out. A peritoneal incision is made, and the ureter is identified toward its course to the bladder. Small bleeding vessels are coagulated by laser or electrosurgery. If the uterosacral ligaments are dissected, the ureter is retracted laterally and the uterosacral ligaments are dissected at their connection to the back of the cervix. The uterine vessels run superiorly. They are isolated and safely coagulated. When the pelvic anatomy is distorted, it may be safer to do a cystoscopy and place catheters in both ureters for better identification.

Upper broad ligament and adnexa

If adnexectomy is indicated, after electrocoagulation and cutting of the round ligament 2 to 3 cm from the uterus, the infundibulopelvic ligament is coagulated and cut. If the endoscopic linear stapler is used, the adnexa is grasped with forceps. It is retracted medially and caudally to stretch and outline the infundibulopelvic ligament, which is grasped and secured with the stapler. The stapler is not fired until the contained tissue is identified and the ureter's safety is confirmed. Once it is transected, the staple line is examined for placement and hemostasis. After infundibulopelvic ligament transection, the adnexa and uterine fundus are retracted in the opposite direction. Tissue of the upper broad ligament, including the round ligament, is grasped, secured, and cut after safe margins have been established (Figure 15-8A). The infundibulopelvic ligament and the round ligament occasionally are cut with a single staple application (Figure 15-8B).

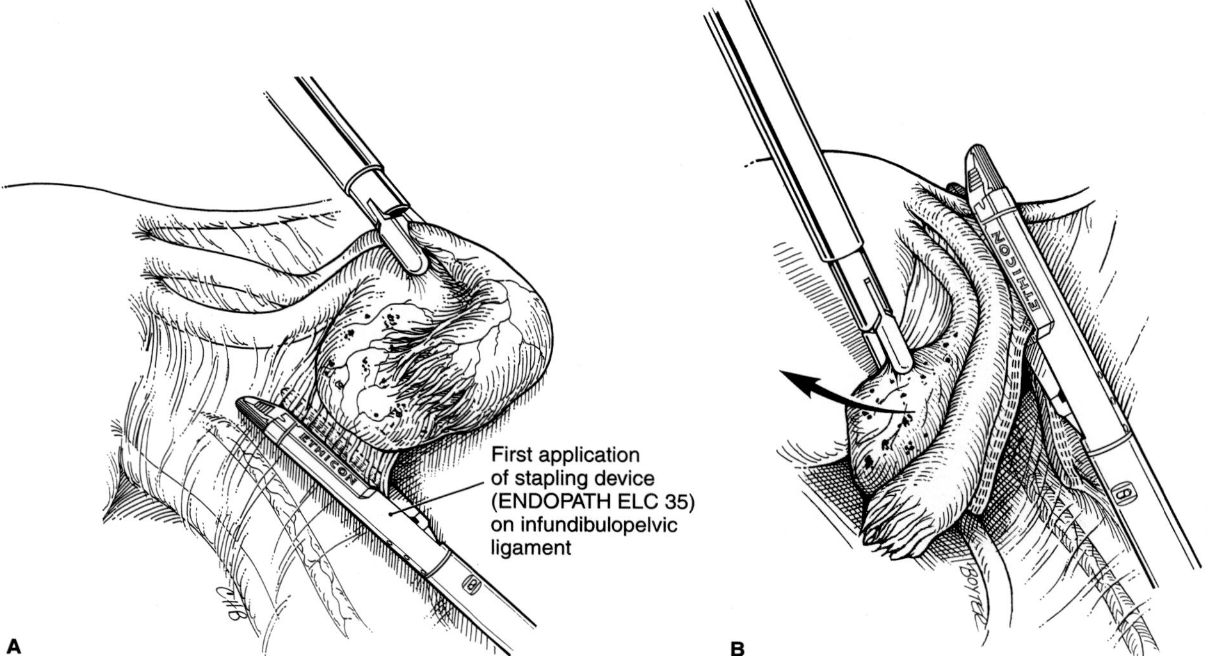

Figure 15-8. **A.** The linear stapler is applied across the infundibulopelvic ligament. Ureteral evaluation before transection of the ligament is very important. **B.** Second application of the stapler across the infundibulopelvic ligament. The round ligament may be included.

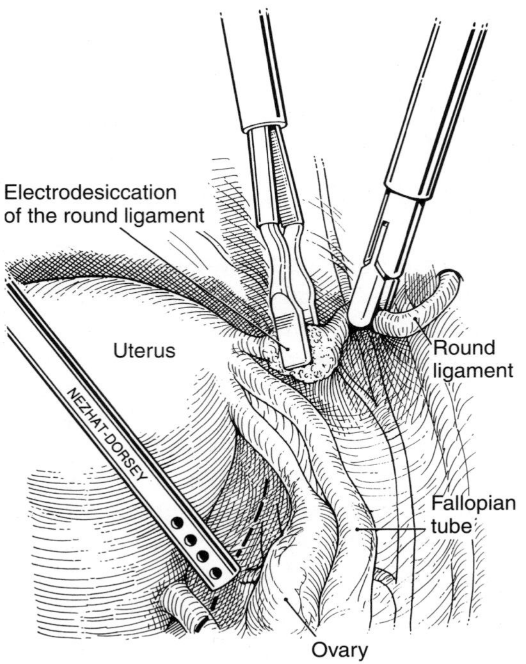

Figure 15-9. The round ligament is coagulated and cut 2 to 3 cm lateral to the uterus.

Development of the bladder flap

If the adnexa are preserved, the round ligament is coagulated and cut approximately 3 cm from the uterus (Figure 15-9). Using hydrodissection, the anterior leaf of the broad ligament is opened toward the vesicouterine fold and the bladder flap is developed (Figure 15-10). The anterior leaf of the broad ligament is grasped with forceps, elevated, and dissected from the anterior lower uterine segment with hydrodissection and the CO_2 laser (Figure 15-11). The utero-ovarian ligament, proximal tube, and mesosalpinx are electrodesiccated and cut, and the posterior leaf of the broad ligament is opened (Figure 15-12). Similarly, the round ligament, fallopian tube, and utero-ovarian ligament can be grasped close to their insertion into the uterus with the endoscopic linear stapler and then secured, stapled, and severed (Figure 15-13, A and B). The distal end of the stapler or bipolar forceps must be kept free of the bladder and ureter.

The uterovesical junction is identified, grasped, and elevated with forceps while being cut with the scissors, laser, or electrode. The bladder pillars are identified, coagulated, and cut. The bladder is dissected from the uterus by pushing downward with the tip of a blunt probe along the vesicocervical plane until the anterior cul-de-sac is exposed completely (Figure 15-14).

In patients who have severe anterior cul-de-sac endometriosis or adhesions or a history of previous cesarean deliveries, sharp dissection of the vesicouterine fold often is necessary. Injecting 5 mL of indigo carmine in the patient's intravenous line can detect bladder trauma. Alternatively, sterile milk, (i.e., infant formula) is instilled through the Foley catheter to detect bladder leaks.

Uterine vessels

After the bladder is dissected from the anterior cervix, the uterine vessels are identified, desic-

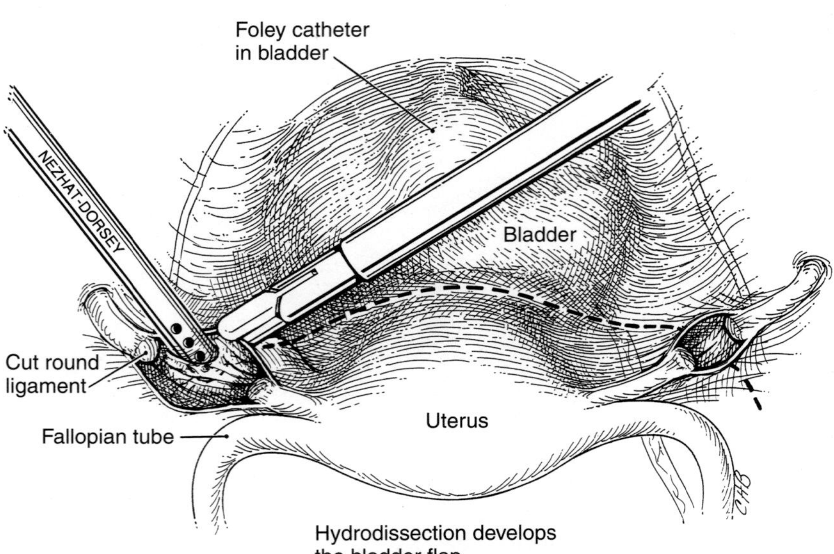

Figure 15-10. While the anterior leaf of the broad ligament is elevated with hydrodissection, the anterior leaf of the broad ligament is opened toward the vesicouterine fold.

Figure 15-11. The bladder is elevated and further separated from the cervix. It is pushed downward, using sharp and blunt dissection and hydrodissection.

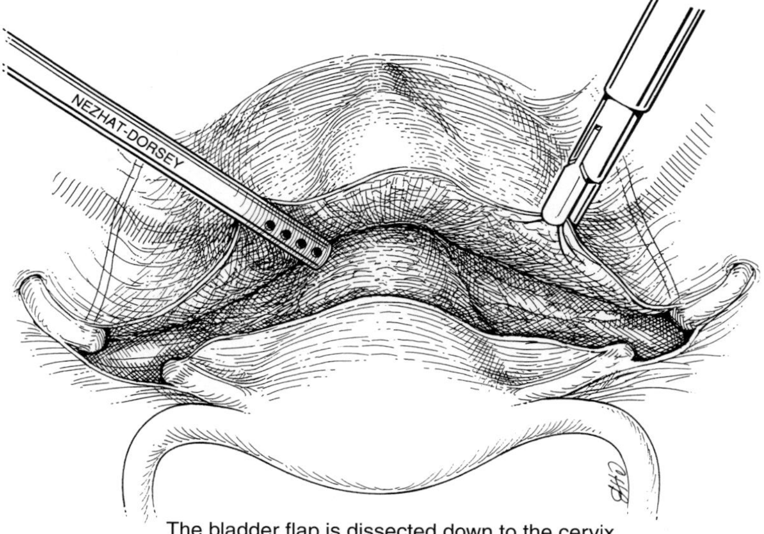

cated and cut to free the lateral borders of the uterus (Figure 15-15). If single clips or linear staplers are used, the vessels are skeletonized to prevent slippage of the clips. As the uterine vessels are grasped and cut, the safety and position of the ureters should be checked. This can be done more easily if they are marked, exposed, or catheterized at the beginning of the procedure. The hysterectomy is completed vaginally or continued laparoscopically.

Cardinal ligament

At the level of the cardinal ligaments, the ureter and the descending branches of the uterine artery are close to one another and the cervix. Therefore,

Figure 15-12. The proximal tube, mesosalpinx, and utero-ovarian ligament are coagulated and cut.

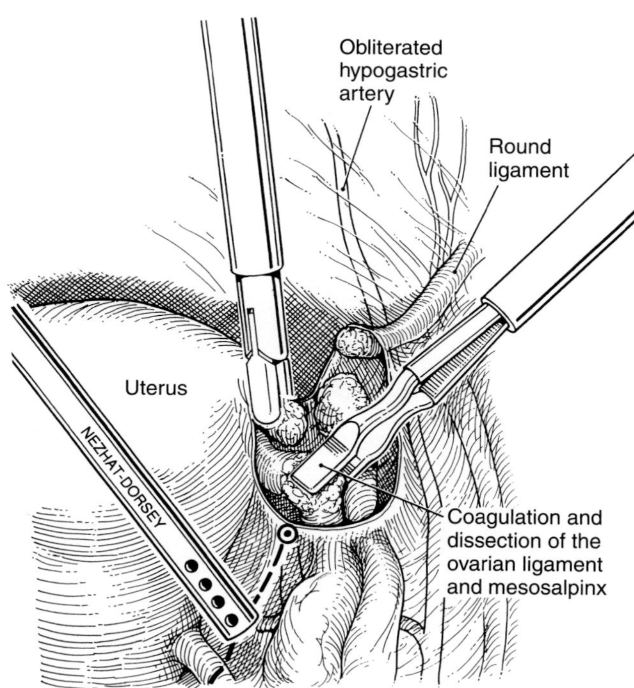

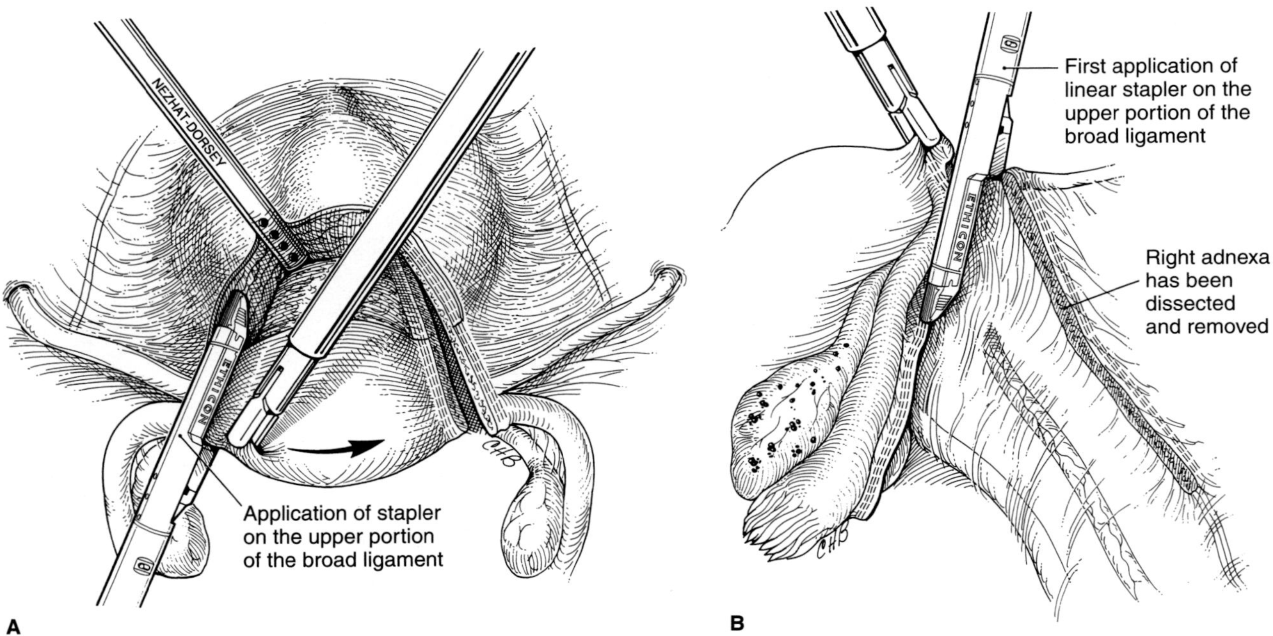

Figure 15-13. **A.** The linear stapler is applied on the upper portion of the broad ligament while preserving the adnexa. **B.** The linear stapler is applied on the upper broad ligament while removing the adnexa.

cardinal ligament dissection must be precise to prevent bleeding and ureteral injury. The linear stapler is used only if the parametrium is dissected with ample margins. The linear stapler is 12 mm wide. Considering the short distance between the cervix and the ureter, the risk of ureteral injury by the stapler increases. Using contralateral retraction of the uterus, the cardinal ligament is dissected to identify tissue planes, vessels, and the ureter. Once the ureter is displaced laterally, the cardinal ligament tissue closest to the cervix is coagulated and transected (Figure 15-16). Alter-

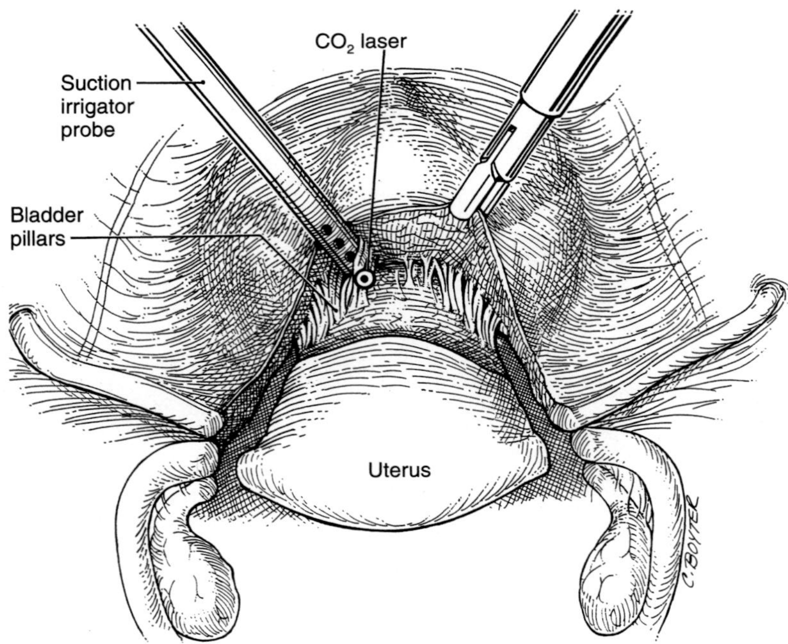

Figure 15-14. The bladder pillars are identified and cut close to the cervix with the CO_2 laser.

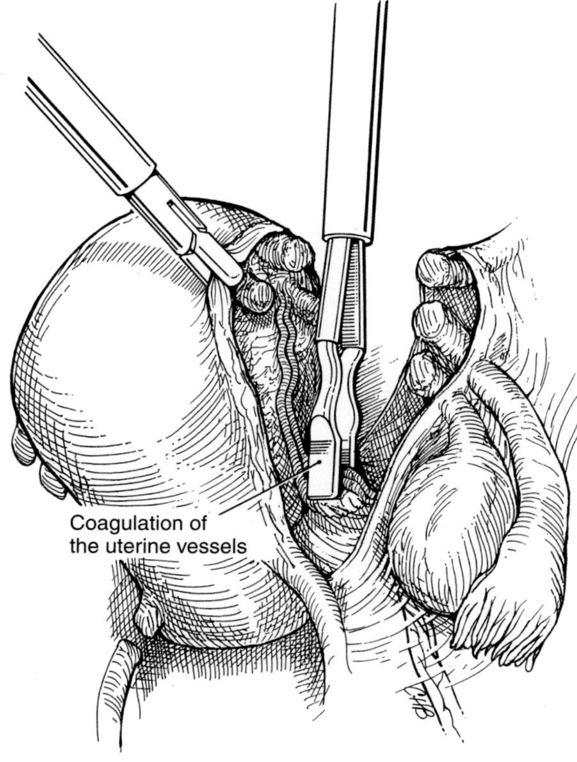

Figure 15-15. While the ureter, is observed the uterine vessels are skeletonized, coagulated, and cut.

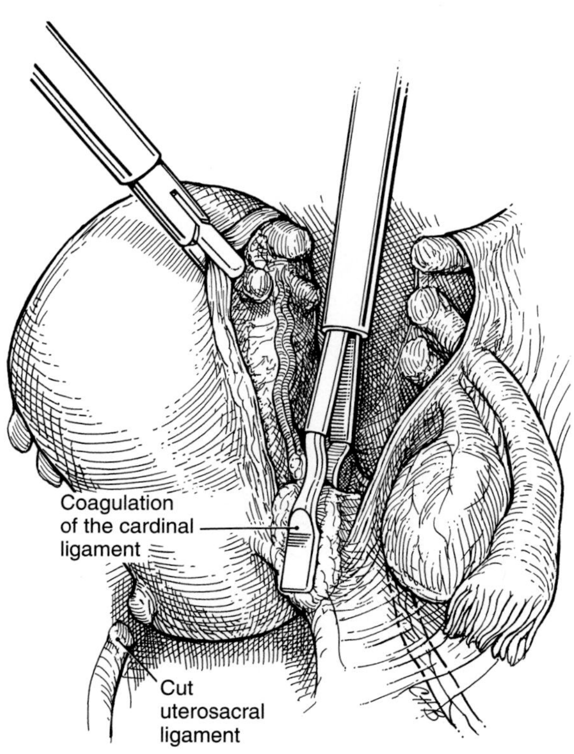

Figure 15-16. The uterus is pulled to the opposite side with a grasping forceps. The ureter must be observed to ensure that it is not damaged by the bipolar forceps during coagulation and cutting of the cardinal ligament.

natively, the linear stapler is applied on both the uterine vessels and the cardinal ligament (Figure 15-17). Harmonic scalpel may be used as an alternative also.

Anterior and posterior culdotomy

A folded wet gauze in a sponge forceps or on the tip of a right-angle Heaney retractor marks the anterior or posterior vaginal fornix. The vaginal wall is tented and transected horizontally (Figures 15-18 and 15-19).

Vaginal portion of hysterectomy

The dissection is extended to the lower uterine segment or to the level of the cardinal ligaments. The laparoscopic portion temporarily ends before or after the anterior or posterior culdotomy. Dissecting and resecting the uterus are done vaginally, using standard techniques. Once the uterus is removed, the vaginal cuff is closed. To ensure support of the vaginal vault, the vaginal angles are attached to the uterosacral and cardinal ligaments with absorbable sutures. The vaginal cuff is closed transversely, and any coexisting cystocele or rectocele is repaired. Once the vaginal part is completed and the cuff is closed, the laparoscopic procedure resumes.

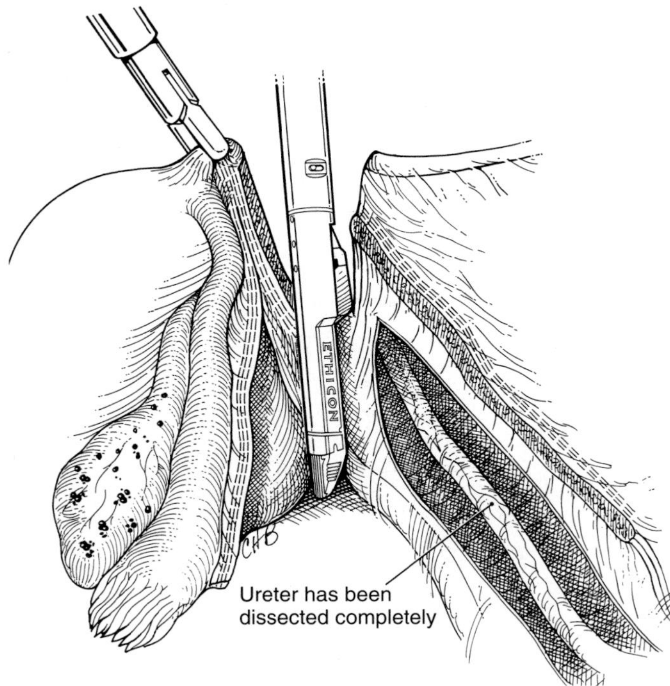

Figure 15-17. The linear stapler is applied across the uterine vessels and cardinal ligament. The ureter is dissected and held away from the stapler jaws.

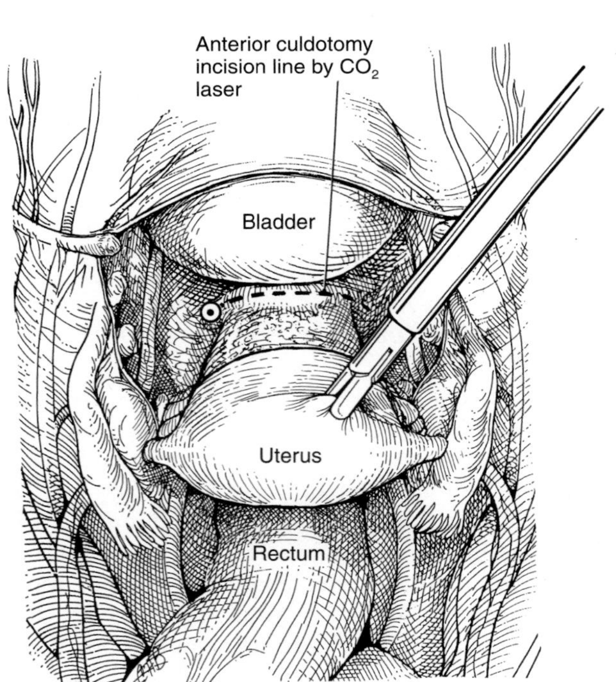

Figure 15-18. The uterus is mobilized, and as it is pushed down, a laparoscopic anterior culdotomy is created by using the CO_2 laser.

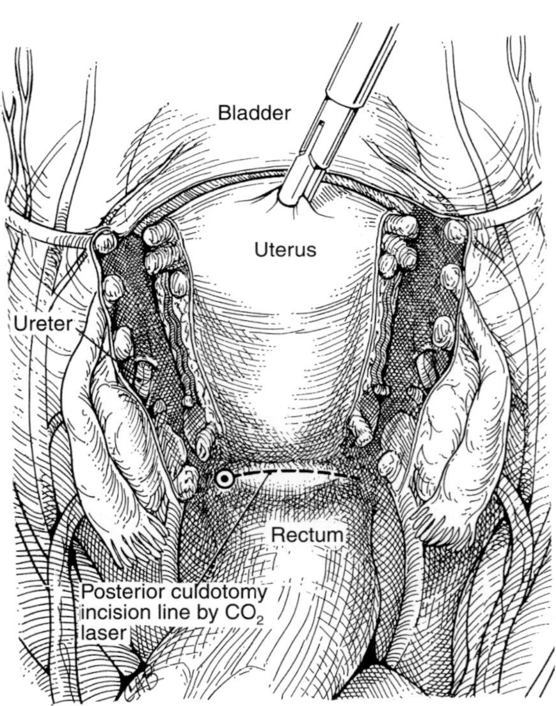

Figure 15-19. The uterus is elevated, and as the assistant identifies the posterior fornix, a laparoscopic posterior culdotomy is done. The gynecologist must select the correct location so that the rectum is not involved.

A comparison of the results of abdominal hysterectomy and those of 10 cases of LAVH was reported in 1992.[37] That report established the validity of LAVH and suggested that it could replace most abdominal hysterectomies for benign lesions. The indications for laparoscopic assisted hysterectomy in this series were similar to those listed for abdominal rather than vaginal hysterectomy. All hysterectomies were completed successfully endoscopically without significant complications. Patients had reduced morbidity, blood loss, postoperative discomfort, hospitalization, and recovery time.

Slightly less optimistic experience with laparoscopic hysterectomy was reported by Bruhat and coauthors[43] in a series of 36 patients. Twenty-seven (75%) were treated successfully by laparoscopy, while nine (25%) were converted to laparotomy. Gynecologists had difficulty achieving hemostasis (six patients) and locating anatomic landmarks (three patients) because of large uteri, myomas, or a long cervix. Nevertheless, the authors concluded that LAVH is an alternative to abdominal hysterectomy in properly selected patients.

Laparoscopic hysterectomy compares favorably with abdominal hysterectomy, offering reduced morbidity, expense, and discomfort. The opposite is true when LAVH is compared to standard vaginal hysterectomy, as reported by Summit and colleagues.[40] Among 56 women scheduled to undergo vaginal hysterectomy in an outpatient setting, 29 were randomized to LAVH and 27 to standard vaginal hysterectomy. In the latter group, all surgical procedures were completed and the patients were discharged within 12 hours of admission. In the LAVH group one patient had a bladder laceration repaired, and the hysterectomy was completed endoscopically. A second patient experienced bleeding from the inferior epigastric vessels. It was not controlled endoscopically, and she underwent exploratory laparotomy with abdominal hysterectomy. When the two groups were compared, the LAVH group required more pain medication, experienced greater blood loss and more intraoperative complications, and incurred higher surgical expenses, a mean of $7,905 compared with $4,891 for the standard vaginal group. These results strongly support the recommendation that LAVH should replace abdominal, not vaginal, hysterectomy.

At our center, 361 women fulfilled the criteria for abdominal hysterectomy but underwent LAVH (172), TLH (176), or SLH (13) from July 1987 through July 1993 (Table 15-7). Bipolar forceps and the CO_2 laser were used for hemostasis and cutting, respectively. Patients who required suturing, staples, or clips for hemostasis or had malignancy were excluded from the study. Preoperative indications for hysterectomy included chronic pelvic pain (116 women), chronic pelvic pain with abnormal uterine bleeding (148 women), abnormal uterine bleeding (40 women), and enlarging leiomyoma (28 women). Other indications were endometrial hyperplasia, cervical dysplasia, pelvic abscess, ectopic pregnancy, and pelvic relaxation (Table 15-8). There were no conversions to laparotomy, although one patient with bowel endometriosis and stricture underwent laparotomy for bowel resection and anastomosis. Intraoperative and pathologic findings are summarized in

TABLE 15-7. Type of Laparoscopic Hysterectomy

		BSO	RSO	LSO
Laparascopically assisted vaginal hysterectomy	24	14	2	3
Vaginally assisted laparoscopic hysterectomy	148	94	12	13
Total laparoscopic hysterectomy	176	114	15	29
Subtotal laparoscopic hysterectomy	13	6	0	1
Total	361	228	29	46

TABLE 15-8. Summary of Women Who Underwent LAVH, TLH, or SLH

Mean age	42.5 (25–72 years)
Gravidity	1.6 (0–7 years)
Parity	1.3 (0–5)
Mean duration of procedure	2.3 hours (55 minutes–6.5 hours)
Uterine size	4–26 weeks' gestational size
Mean uterine weight	178.38 g (36–1530 g)
Average blood loss	73 mL (50–800 mL)
Average hospitalization*	21 hours (20 hours–5 days)
Postoperative full recovery†	3.3 weeks (3 days–13 weeks)
Need for postoperative pain medication‡	3.3 days (0–21 days)

*From termination of procedure until discharge from hospital.

†This information was obtained from office visits, written questionnaires, and telephone interviews.

‡After the patient was discharged from the hospital.

TABLE 15-9. Inoperative and Pathologic Findings in 361 Women

Mild to extensive endometriosis	212
Mild to extensive adhesions	189
Uterine fibroids (uterine size 8–26 weeks)	116
Uterine adenomyosis	119
Endometriomas (5–15 cm in diameter)	22
Endometrial polyp	13
Endometrial hyperplasia	2
Cervical dysplasia	4
Large cornual pregnancy	1
Hydrosalpinx	7
Pelvic abscess	1
Asherman's syndrome	2
Benign cystic teratoma	3
Serous cyst	2
Mucinous cyst	2
Para-ovarian cyst	2

(Table 15-9). Most patients underwent one or more additional procedures (Table 15-10), and the complication rate was 10% (Table 15-11).

Final laparoscopic evaluation

The vaginal cuff is closed from below or above, and pneumoperitoneum is restored. The pelvic and abdominal cavities are evaluated laparoscopically, irrigated, and cleared of blood clots and debris. Bleeding is controlled, and the pelvis is filled with 300 to 500 mL of lactated Ringer's solution before the pedicles and vaginal cuff are evaluated and inspected under low pneumoperitoneal pressure.[39]

TABLE 15-10. Additional Procedures Carried Out with Hysterectomy

Treatment of mild to extensive endometriosis	212
Lysis of mild to extensive abdominal and/or pelvic adhesions	189
Ureterolysis	129
Appendectomy	47
Marshall-Marchetti-Krantz or Burch procedure	43
Moschcowitz procedure	88
Bowel resection	11
Cystocele repair	13
Rectocele repair	24
Enterocele repair	6
Vaginal sacral colposuspension	2
Cholecystectomy	2
Removal of ovarian remnant	4
Removal of pelvic abscess	1

TABLE 15-11. Complications after Hysterectomy in 361 Women

	Number	Incidence per 100 Women
Mortality	0	0.00
Intraoperative		
Vascular		
Inferior epigastric vessel injury	3	0.83
Hemorrhage requiring transfusion	2	0.55
Major blood vessel injury	0	0.00
Gastrointestinal		
Small bowel injury	1	0.27

The vaginal cuff is examined to ensure that no small bowel or omental tissue is included in its closure. At this point, the fluid in the pelvis should be clear and a look at the ureters should confirm normal peristalsis and anatomic integrity. If the stapling device has been used, the stapler line is evaluated for hemostasis under low pneumoperitoneal pressure. To avoid incisional omental or bowel strangulation after the removal of any trocars more than 5 mm in size, the fascia is repaired with delayed absorbable sutures.[45]

Hysterectomy for Extensive Pelvic Endometriosis and Adhesions

In women who have extensive endometriosis, the rectosigmoid colon often is densely adherent to the posterior aspect of the uterus (Figure 15-20). Similarly, if the ovaries are affected by endometriosis and endometriomas, they can become attached to the pelvic side wall. To coagulate the uterine artery, it may be necessary to develop the paravesical space and identify the uterine vessel at its origin from the hypogastric artery. Bipolar forceps, clips, or sutures are used. The rectosigmoid colon is separated from the posterior uterus incrementally, and the bowel endometriosis is resected or vaporized (Figures 15-21 and 15-22). The high-power ultrapulse CO_2 laser is very precise, and with a penetration of only $100\mu m$, the possibility of delayed bowel necrosis is very low. The CO_2 laser is an excellent instrument for the treatment of endometriosis. Hemostasis not obtained with the CO_2 laser is controlled with cautious application of the bipolar electrocoagulator. Endometriosis of the rectum, rectovaginal septum, and uterosacral ligament is treated by vaporization, excision, or a combination, and the posterior cul-de-sac is freed

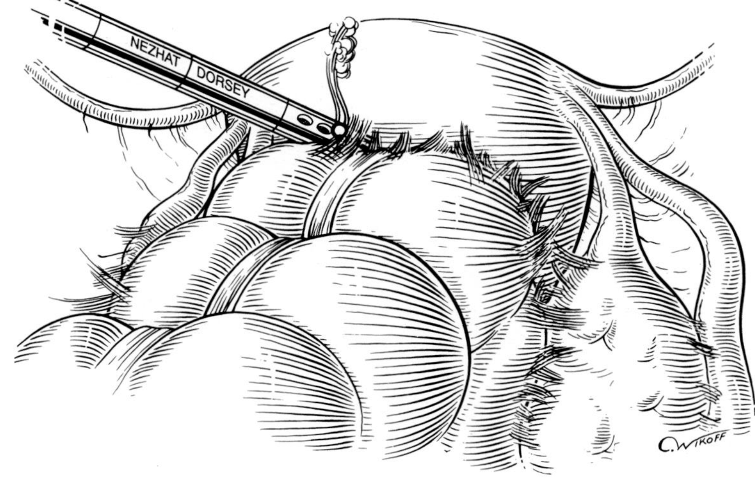

Figure 15-20. Rectosigmoid colon is attached to the posterior aspect of the uterus with dense adhesions and endometriosis. Using the hydrodissection probe and CO_2 laser, the adhesions are lysed and the rectosigmoid colon is separated from the uterus.

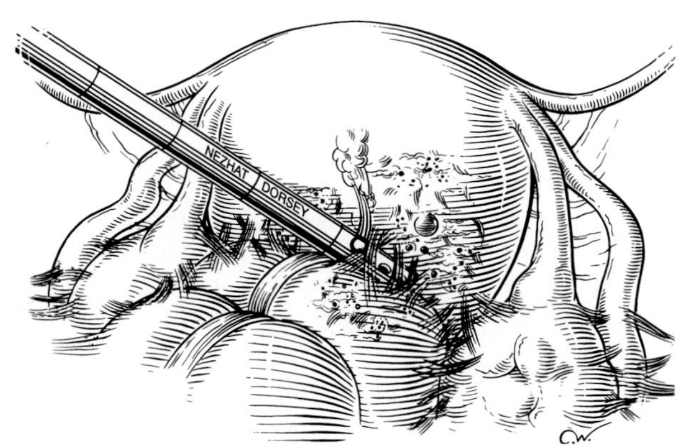

Figure 15-21. The dissection of the rectosigmoid colon is continued.

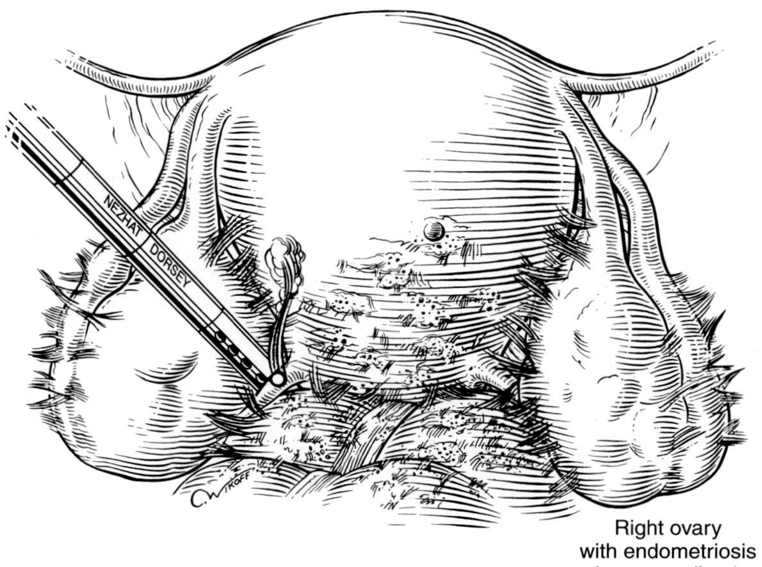

Figure 15-22. The rectum, the back of the cervix, and the uterosacral ligaments are dissected.

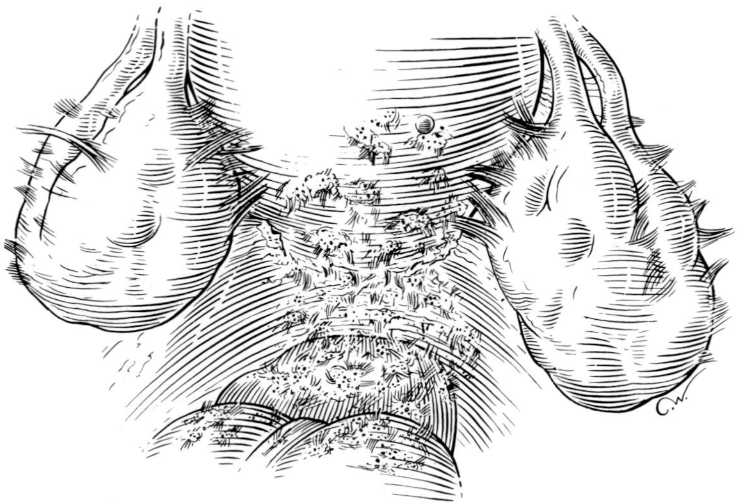

Figure 15-23. The rectosigmoid colon is freed from the posterior aspect of the uterus and cervix.

(Figures 15-23 and 15-24). Bipolar forceps are used to achieve hemostasis. If the endometriosis has penetrated deeply to the bowel muscularis or mucosa and has caused a stricture requiring anterior or complete resection and repair, this procedure is done after the hysterectomy.

The hysterectomy starts with coagulation and transection of the round ligament close to the pelvic side wall (Figure 15-25). The peritoneum is opened, and the paravesical spaces are entered. This technique allows excellent skeletonization of the obliterated hypogastric artery (Figure 15-26).

The bladder serosa is injected with lactated Ringer's solution. The bladder flap is developed with the CO_2 laser and countertraction or any cutting device. After division of scar tissue in the vesicouterine fold, the suction-irrigator probe is used for blunt dissection and mobilization of the bladder. The infundibulopelvic ligaments are

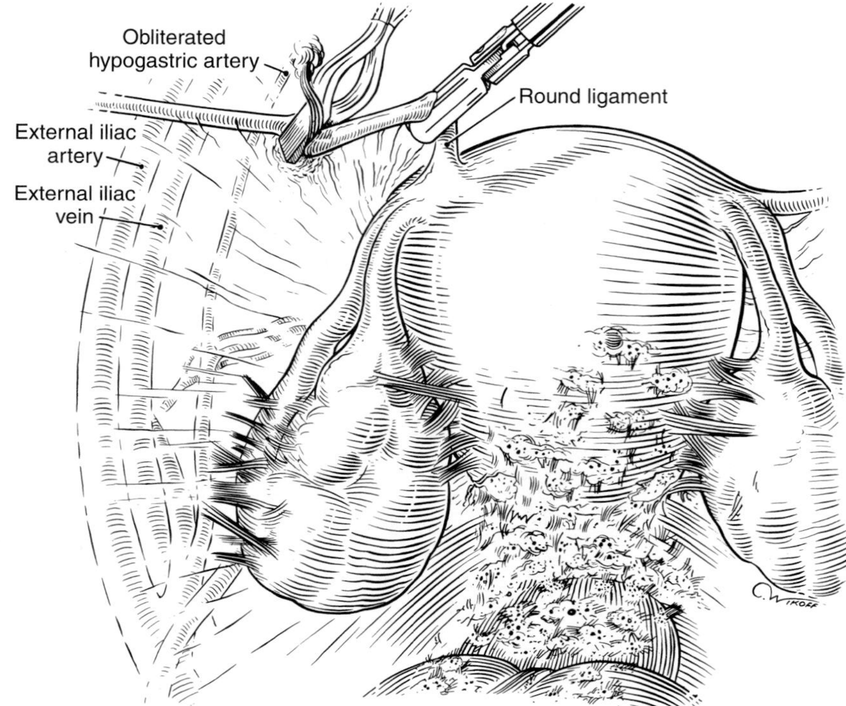

Figure 15-24. While the uterus is pulled to the right, the left round ligament is coagulated close to the pelvic side wall.

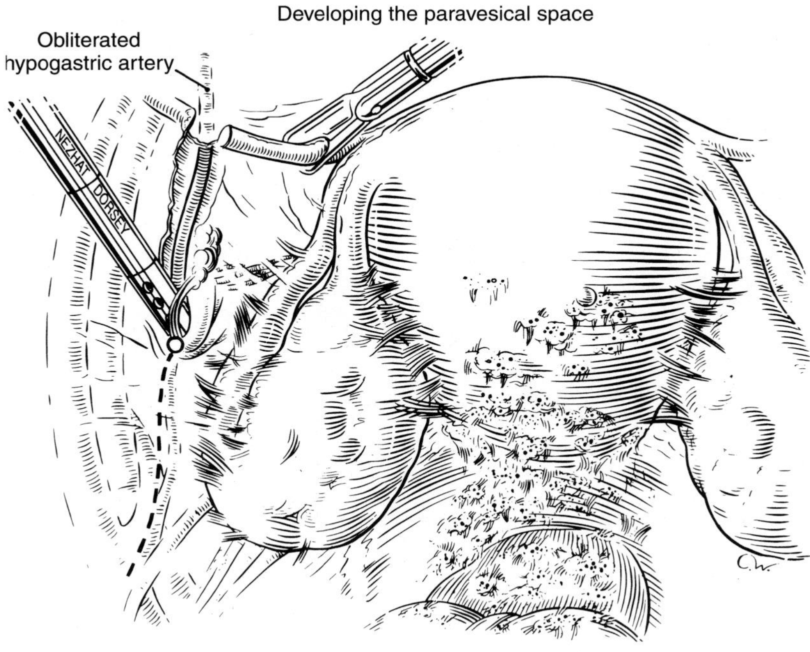

Figure 15-25. The hydrodissection probe is used as a backstop for the CO_2 laser to develop the paravesical space. The gynecologist must be careful to avoid injury to the major pelvic side wall vessels and the ureter.

coagulated with bipolar forceps and transected with the laser (Figure 15-27).

The uterine vessels are retracted medially and removed from the ureter. The anterior parametrium is transected. The ureters are freed from the peritoneum and skeletonized down to the bladder with the suction-irrigator probe and the laser, harmonic scalpel, scissors or electric knife. The uterine vessels are coagulated close to the hypogastric artery (Figures 15-28 and 15-29).

At the level of the cardinal ligaments, the ureter and the descending branches of the uterine artery

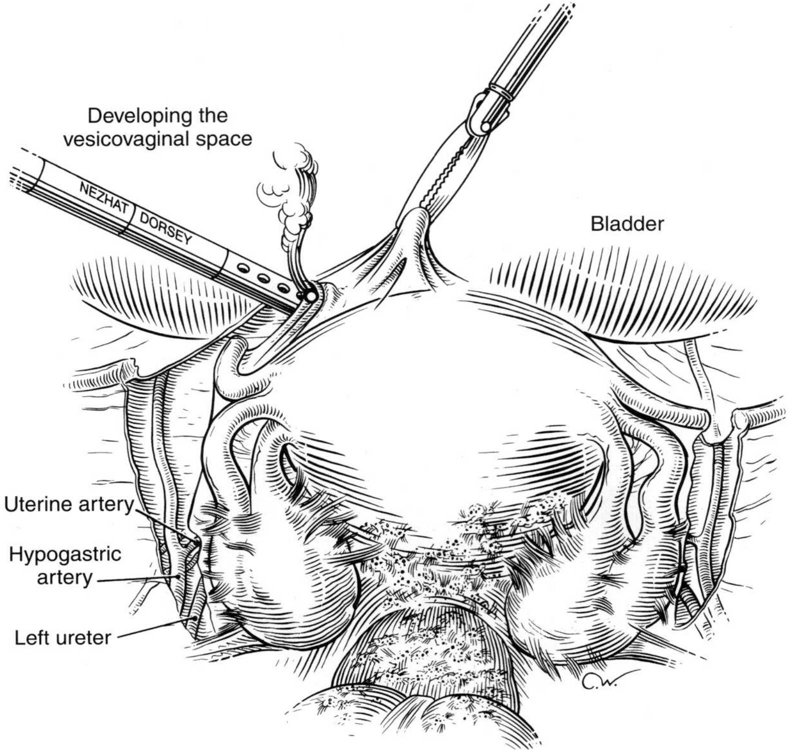

Figure 15-26. The anterior leaf of the left broad ligament is dissected with hydrodissection and the CO_2 laser to develop the vesicovaginal space.

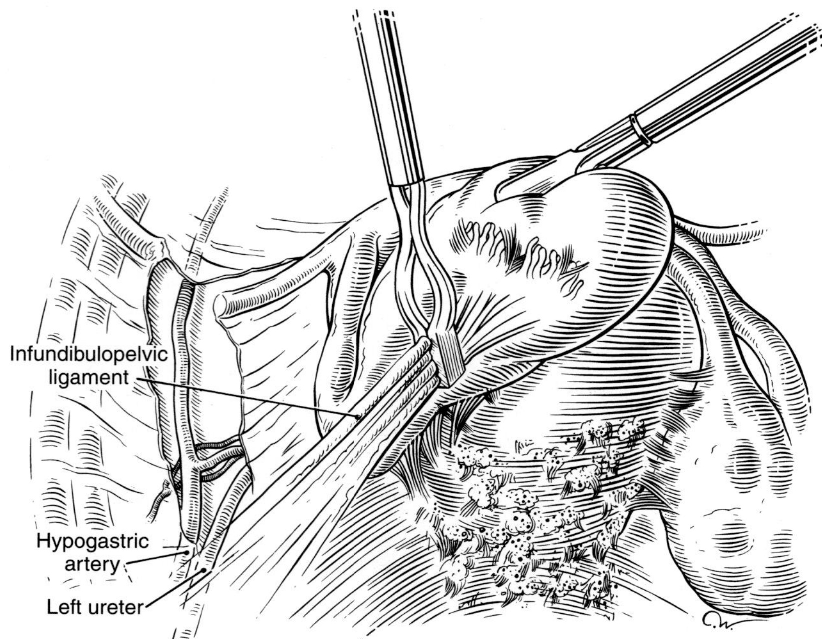

Figure 15-27. The left infundibulopelvic ligament is coagulated close to the ovary with bipolar forceps.

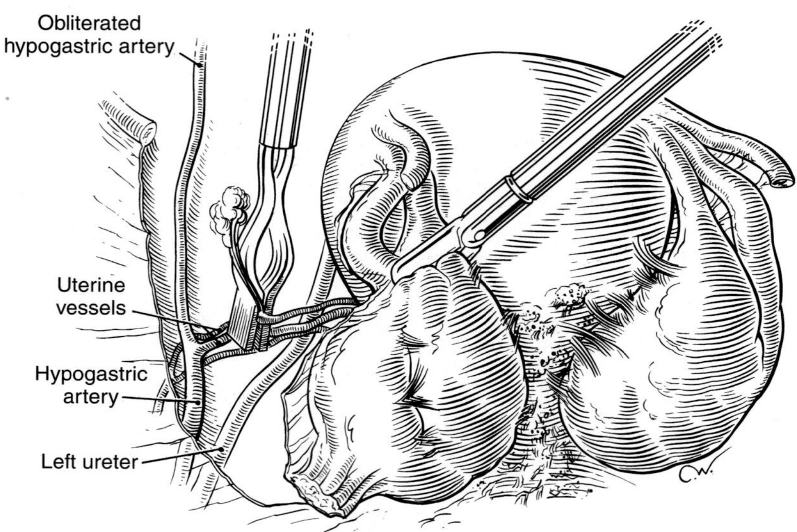

Figure 15-28. The paravesical space is developed, and the uterine vessels are identified. The uterine artery at its origin from the hypogastric artery is coagulated with bipolar forceps. The ureter is observed, and excessive heat avoided to prevent ureteral injury.

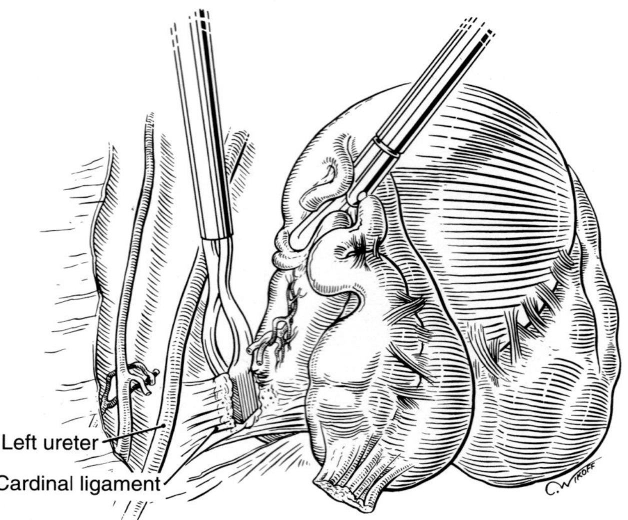

Figure 15-29. While the uterus is pulled to the right, bipolar forceps are used to coagulate the cardinal ligaments close to the cervix. The ureter is distanced from the bipolar forceps.

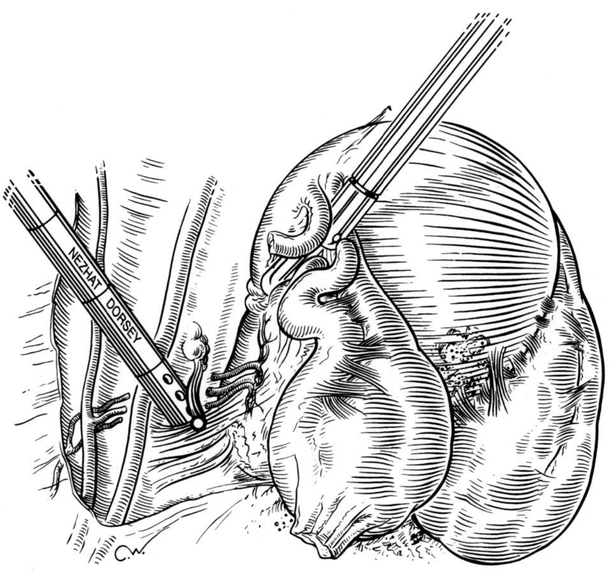

Figure 15-30. The cardinal ligament is dissected with the CO_2 laser.

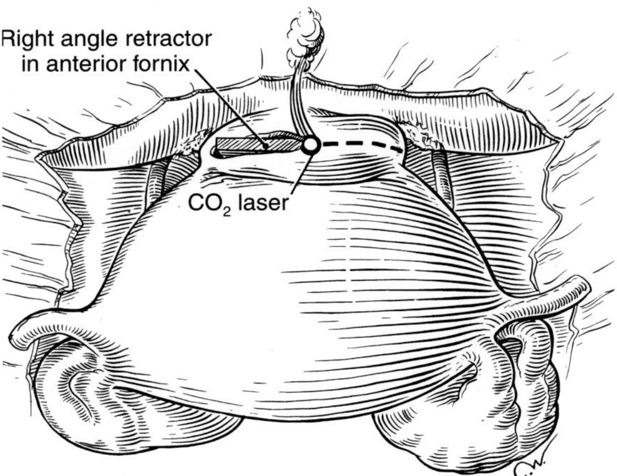

Figure 15-32. An assistant places a right-angle Heaney retractor in the anterior fornix, and the CO_2 laser is used to create an anterior culdotomy.

are close to one another and to the cervix. Therefore, cardinal ligament dissection must be precise to prevent bleeding and ureteral injury. The linear stapler is 12 mm wide, which, considering the short distance between the cervix and the ureter, increases the risk of ureteral injury by the stapler. Using contralateral retraction of the uterus, the cardinal ligament is dissected to identify tissue planes, vessels, and the ureter (Figure 15-30). Once the ureter is displaced laterally, the cardinal ligament tissue closest to the cervix is coagulated and transected. The bladder pillars are transected close to the cervix (Figure 15-31).

After the uterosacral ligaments are dissected, a folded wet gauze in a sponge forceps or the tip of a right-angle Heaney retractor is used to mark the anterior or posterior vaginal fornix. The vaginal wall is tented and transected horizontally with a laser or electrode (Figure 15-32 and Figure 15-33). Bipolar electrocoagulation can be used to control bleeding. The remainder of the procedure is done vaginally.

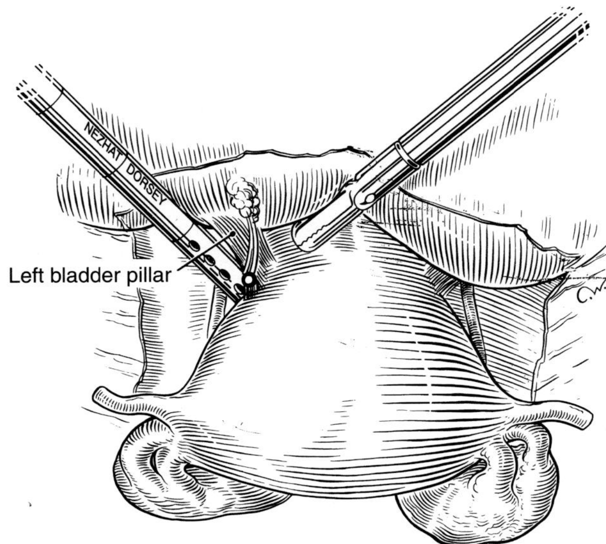

Figure 15-31. The vesicocervical fascia (bladder pillars) is dissected close to the cervix with the CO_2 laser.

Total Laparoscopic Hysterectomy

Role of the laparoscope in assisting vaginal hysterectomy has been described by Semm since 1984.[46,47] Laparoscopic hysterectomy using bipolar electrocautery and the endoscopic stapler were first described in 1989[48] and 1990,[49] respectively.

If TLH is planned, two 4×4 wet sponges are placed in a surgical latex glove and inserted into the vagina to prevent loss of pneumoperitoneum. When contralateral traction is applied to the uterus, the vaginal wall surrounding the cervix is outlined, coagulated with the unipolar scissors or bipolar forceps, and cut circumferentially until the cervix is separated (Figure 15-34). The specimen is pulled to midvagina but not removed to preserve pneumoperitoneum. The vaginal cuff is irrigated and inspected for active bleeding. Once hemostasis is achieved, vaginal angles are sutured to the adja-

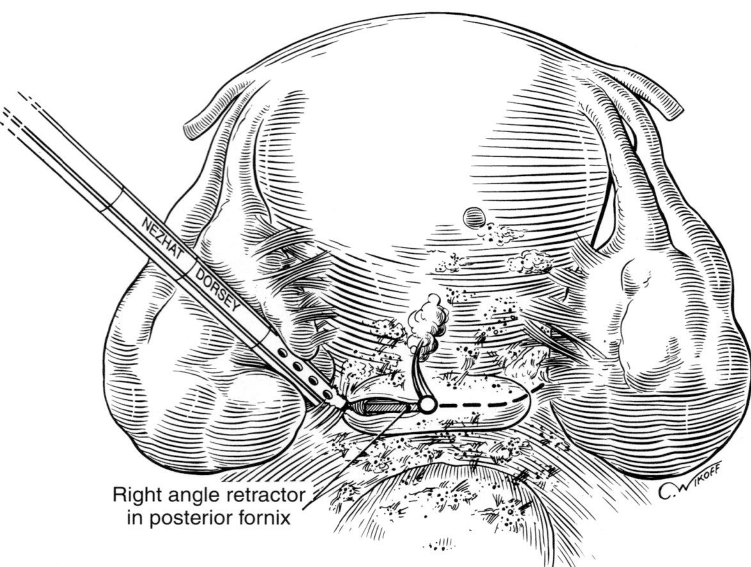

Figure 15-33. A right-angle Heaney retractor helps identify the site for a posterior culdotomy. The CO_2 laser cuts the remainder of the uterosacral and cardinal ligament.

cent cardinal and uterosacral ligaments; care is taken to avoid the ureters. The rest of the vaginal cuff is closed with 0 Vicryl (Ethicon) suture on a straight or curved needle, utilizing extracorporeal knotting (Figures 15-35 and 15-36). Endoscopic suturing is difficult and time-consuming and should be done only in selected cases, such as women with severe vaginal stenosis. Bipolar electrocoagulation should be used cautiously at the vaginal cuff to prevent tissue necrosis and subsequent wound breakdown if sutures are placed in nonviable tissue.

Total laparoscopic hysterectomy is a technically challenging procedure for even the most experienced laparoscopist. Proficiency and comfort in doing the procedure require years of experience. The most difficult aspect of the operation involves ligation and transection of the uterosacral-cardinal ligament complex. This is caused by the close proximity of the bladder, ureters, rectum, and

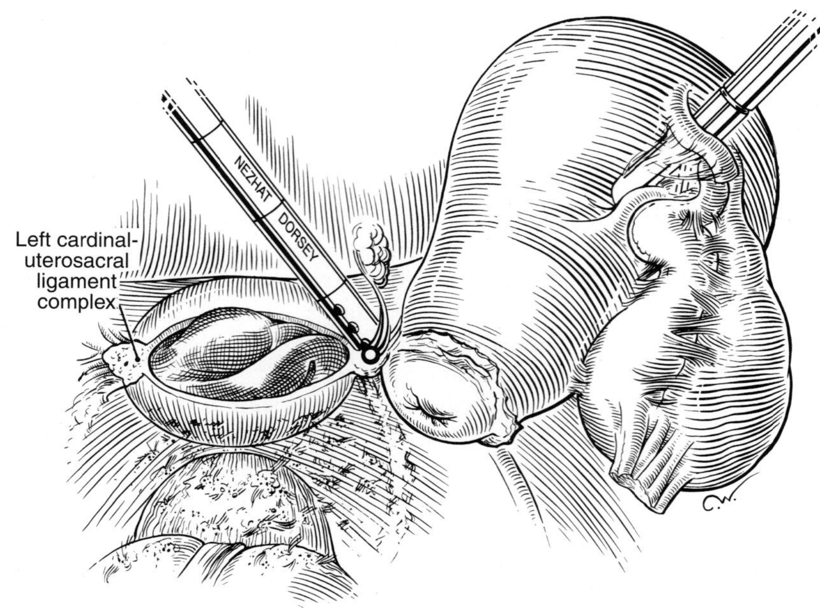

Figure 15-34. After anterior culdotomy and posterior culdotomy are achieved the remainder of the cardinal and uterosacral ligament on each side are dissected. The cervix is amputated from the vagina. The uterus is removed.

Figure 15-35. After the uterus is removed, two sponges are placed in a surgical glove and left inside the vagina to prevent the loss of pneumoperitoneum. The vaginal angles are sutured to the uterosacral-cardinal ligament complex, and the cuff is closed with 0 Vicryl laparoscopic sutures and intracorporeal or extracorporeal knot tying.

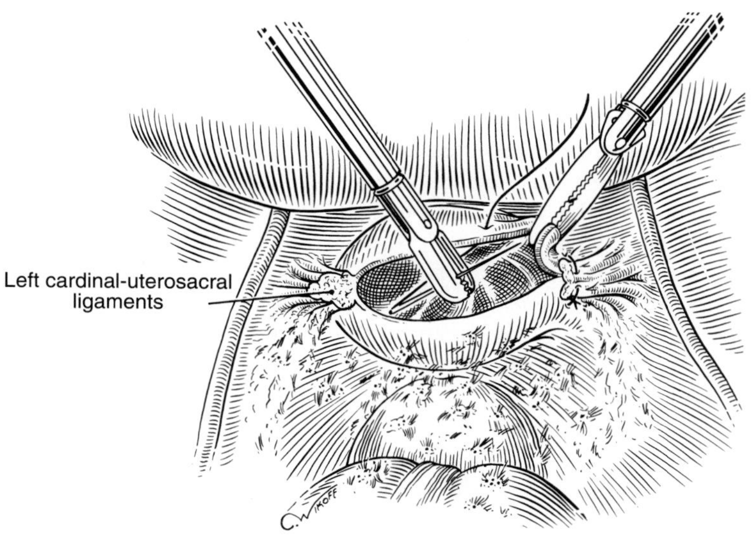

uterine arteries to each other. An expert laparoscopist will be able to place adequate traction on the uterus to avoid injury to these pelvic structures, However, concomitant pelvic disease may distort the anatomy. A rectum that is adherent to the posterior cul-de-sac may be thought to be a thickened uterosacral ligament. A ureter may be mistaken for pelvic vasculature in the case of extensive pelvic adhesions or an anomalous renal system.

In contrast, employing a vaginal approach when ligating the uterosacral-cardinal ligament complex affords the laparoscopist the benefit of tactile inspection of the cervix and vagina using the hands instead of endoscopic instruments. Then the bladder, ureters, and other pelvic structures can be felt more confidently to avoid their injury.

The authors recommend that the role of laparoscopy for hysterectomy should be to visually inspect the pelvis for conditions such as endometriosis and adhesions and to do minimally invasive adnexal surgery. Conversion to vaginal hysterectomy should be undertaken as soon as the laparoscopist is capable and more comfortable in completing the procedure vaginally. Laparoscopic assistance during hysterectomy should be considered a means by which to convert an abdominal hysterectomy to vaginal hysterectomy.

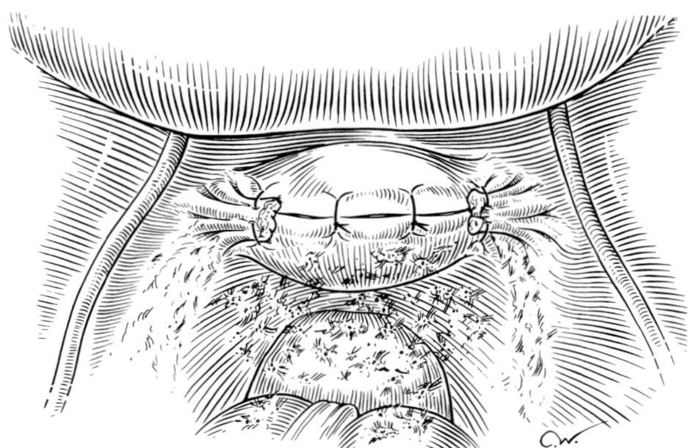

Figure 15-36. The vaginal cuff is repaired laparoscopically. The round ligaments and upper portion of the broad ligaments have been cut and suture ligated.

Moschcowitz procedure

By obliterating the posterior cul-de-sac, this procedure helps prevent enterocele, especially in patients with a deep pelvis. A continuous nonabsorbable or delayed absorbable suture is placed through the various structures of the posterior cul-de-sac, preventing herniation into the rectovaginal space. The suture is started laterally over the periureteral area after the ureter is located. It is passed through the serosa of the rectosigmoid colon posteriorly, the contralateral side to include the opposite periureteral area, and the anterior vaginal wall. When it is tied, the posterior cul-de-sac is obliterated. Injury to the ureter, rectum, and bladder is avoided by meticulous suturing.

Subtotal Laparoscopic Hysterectomy

Supracervical hysterectomy is requested by patients and done by some gynecologists who believe that the cervix affects sexuality and orgasm and helps provide better vaginal support. A comparison[43] of the risks and benefits of subtotal hysterectomy with those of total hysterectomy in women at low risk for cervical cancer revealed the following operative complication rates and ranges for total abdominal hysterectomy and subtotal hysterectomy, respectively: infection 3% (3 to 20%) and 1.4% (1 to 5%), hemorrhage 2% (2 to 15.4%) and 2% (0.7 to 4%), adjacent organ injury 1% (0.7 to 2%) and 0.7% (0.6 to 1%). The study design was a decision analysis and concluded that proposed benefits from subtotal hysterectomy have not been proved. The procedure can be done laparoscopically, but it is difficult to remove the specimen through a small abdominal incision. An electric morcellator is recommended for this purpose. Examples are 15, 20, and 25 mm morcellators by Gynecare (J&J) and Semm (Wisap).

The uterine vessels are coagulated and cut at the level of the cardinal ligaments above the uterosacral ligaments. The uterus is retracted, and its lower segment is amputated with scissors, a unipolar endoscopic electrode, or a laser. After the uterus is transected from the cervix, the uterine manipulator is removed vaginally, the cervical stump is irrigated, and hemostasis is achieved. The endocervical epithelium lining the cervical canal is vaporized or coagulated with the laser or electrosurgery. The rest of the endocervical canal is ablated vaginally to reduce the risk of intraepithelial cervical neoplasia. The cervical stump is closed with interrupted absorbable sutures and covered with peritoneum sewn transversely with either continuous or interrupted sutures. The uterus is morcellated and removed through a 10-20 mm trocar, with an electric morcellator. Peritoneal washing and inspection of the pelvis and abdomen are done at the end of the procedure.

If the vagina was not entered, there are fewer sexual restrictions. These patients are advised of the continued risk of cervical neoplasia and the need for annual examinations and Papanicolaou smears.

Hysterectomy for Large Myomas

The following factors must be considered in selecting patients for this procedure:

1. The patient must have adequate hemoglobin and hematocrit to decrease the possibility of transfusion.
2. GnRH analogs are advisable if the uterus is more than 18 weeks of gestational size.
3. The primary trocar should be inserted between the umbilicus and the xiphoid if the uterus is more than 18 weeks of gestational size. The secondary trocars should be placed nearer to the umbilicus than usual.

A uterus more than 16 weeks' gestational size with multiple, large leiomyomas is more difficult to manipulate laparoscopically. Three and at times four secondary trocars are introduced to provide adequate traction to the uterus if the anatomy is distorted, and ureteral dissection may be recommended in this situation. Although it is possible to completely dissect the uterus laparoscopically, it takes longer and a combination of laparoscopic and vaginal approaches is preferred. If there is a large pedunculated leiomyoma interfering with the exposure and laparoscopic manipulation, myomectomy is done first. The laparoscopic approach is continued until the cardinal ligaments are reached, and the remaining portion of the procedure is completed vaginally. After the uterosacral and cardinal ligaments are ligated and cut vaginally, the uterus is morcellated and removed vaginally.

At our center, the largest uterus removed by us by this method was 29 weeks of gestational size (2394 gs). Currently, 25% of hysterectomies are done vaginally, the least traumatic, safest, and most cost-effective way to remove the uterus. Seventy-five percent of hysterectomies are conducted abdominally. LAVH and LH are excellent alternatives when the standard vaginal approach is contraindicated. Laparoscopic assisted hysterectomy offers many advantages and will become an integral part of gynecologic surgery, replacing the abdominal hysterectomy. Therefore, efforts no longer should be directed toward validating LAVH but toward providing gynecologists with more opportunities for training.

In five reports,[51–55] the complication rate was less than 10% (Table 15-12) and was lower than those from abdominal and vaginal hysterectomy. Although laparoscopic assisted hysterectomy takes longer, this approach tends to cause less postoperative pain, requires less hospitalization, and allows a more rapid recovery. Specific indications and contraindications for LAVH and LH must be established on the basis of outcome data.

TABLE 15-12. Complications of Laparoscopic Hysterectomy

Authors	Cases	Complications No.	Complications percent
Liu[50]	518	30	5.8
Hill et al[51]	220	35	15.9
Jones[53]	252	18	7.1
Nezhat et al[54]	361	40	11.0
Chapron et al[55]	210	21	10.0
Total	1561	144	9.2

Such information is essential for the gynecologist to ascertain the best method for removal of the uterus in each instance.

Classic Intrafascial Supracervical Hysterectomy

Semm[56] described coring the cervix intrafascially without colpotomy by using a calibrated resection tool (CURT) that removes the transformation zone to prevent the subsequent potential development of cervical carcinoma (Figures 15-37 through 15-40). The pelvic floor support is maintained, the ureters are not jeopardized, and sexual function is not compromised. Semm suggested that the classic intrafascial supracervical hysterectomy (CISH) technique should replace total hysterectomy in 80% of patients.[57] It preserves the blood supply to the lower pelvis and prevents subsequent uterine prolapse. Mettler and coworkers[58] described an approach for doing endoscopic intrafascial supracervical hysterectomy using a serrated-edged macromorcellator. When the endoscopic approach for dissection and uterine extraction was used with the morcellator, a colpotomy was avoided. Another modification involved nearly complete excision (95%) of the endocervical mucosa with the calibrated resection instrument. Maintaining the cardinal ligaments provides support to the cervical stump, and the risks of hemorrhage and genitourinary complications are reduced by avoiding dissection of the parametrium at the level of the endocervix.

An evaluation of the efficacy of CISH was ascertained in 90 patients.[59] No major complications occurred even in women who had large myomas. The average operating time was 170 minutes, blood loss was lower than that from conventional hysterectomy, and no procedure was converted to a la-

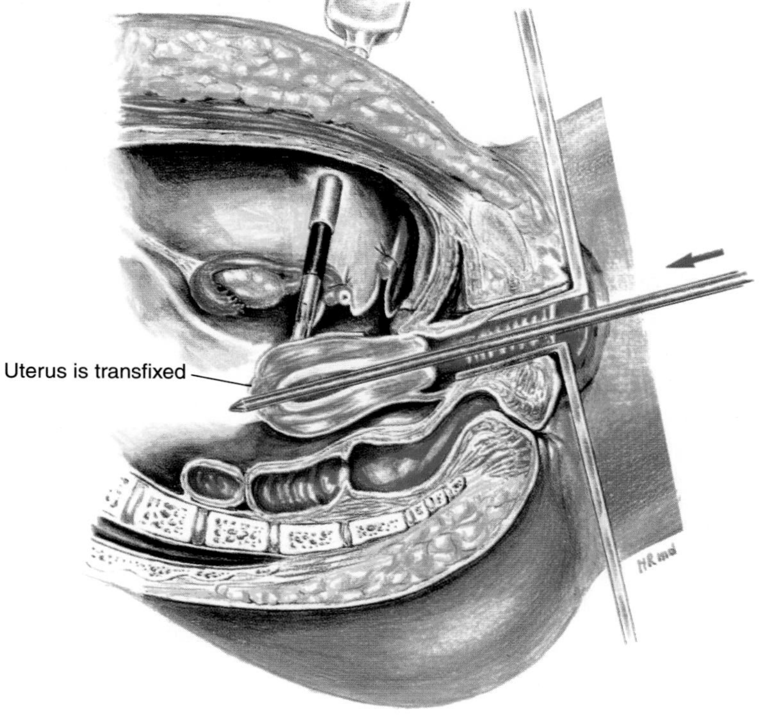

Figure 15-37. The uterus has been transfixed with the CURT instrument. With the CISH procedure, the inner part of the cervix is excised by clockwise rotation of the cutting cylinder of the CURT instrument. The instrument has perforated the fundus.

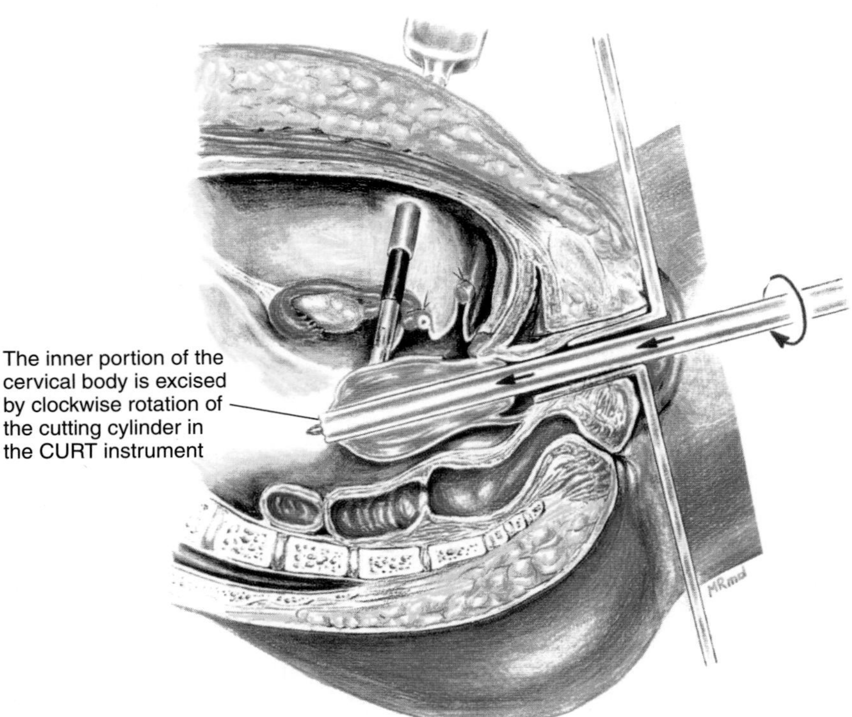

Figure 15-38. The cutting cylinder has removed a portion of the cervix.

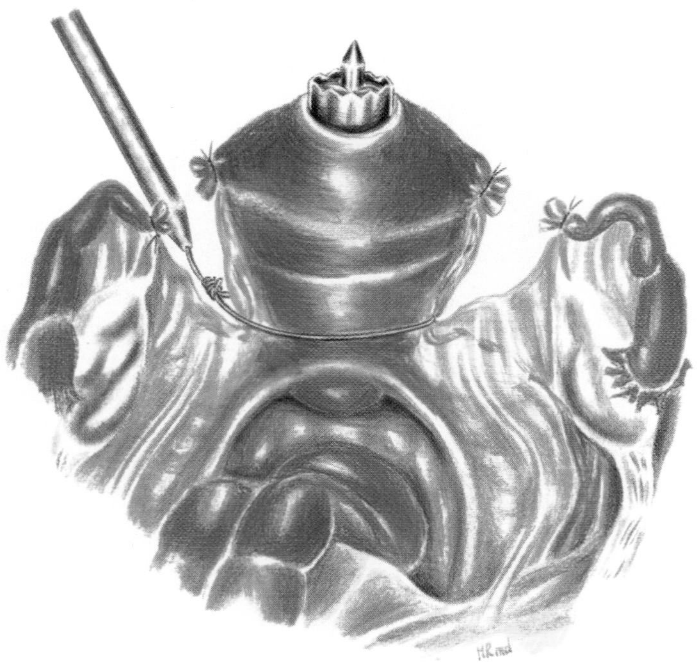

Figure 15-39. **A.** After the uterus has been mobilized, the Roeder loop is placed around the lower uterine segment.

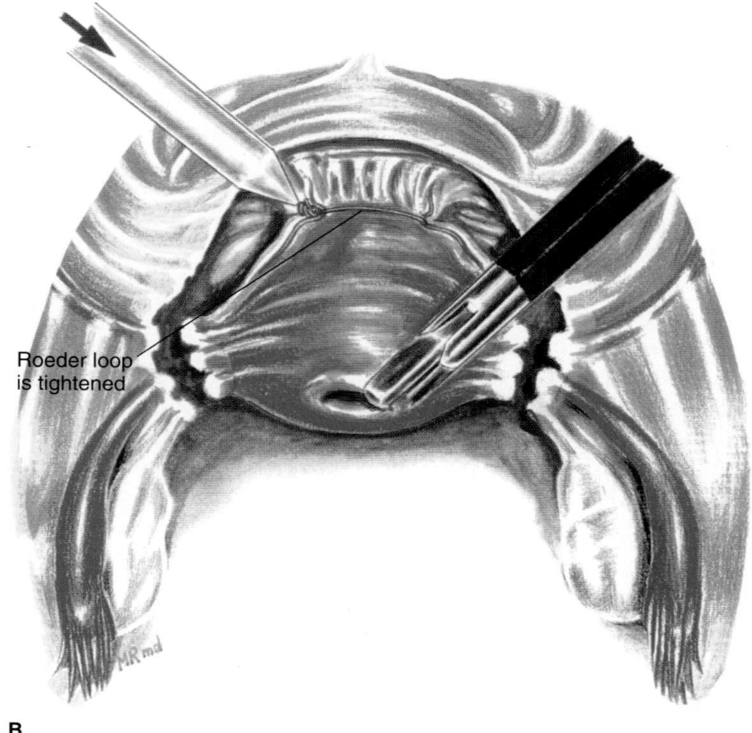

Figure 15-39. (*Continued*) **B.** The loop is tightened around the cervix as the metal cylinder is removed.

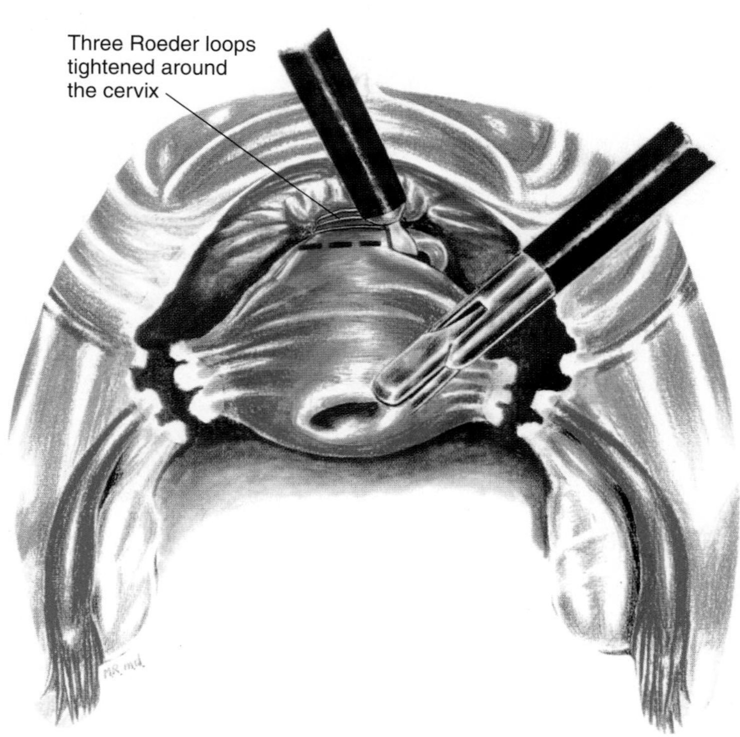

Figure 15-40. The corpus is amputated above the suture, using an electrosurgical knife.

parotomy. Kim and coauthors[60] compared CISH with TLH and LAVH. They found among three groups that CISH resulted in lowest blood loss and the fewest complications and suggested that CISH was preferable for patients with myomas.

Adenomyosis

Adenomyosis is a difficult diagnosis to make preoperatively, and most often the effective treatment is a hysterectomy. Theoretically, if the misplaced endometrial tissue is destroyed, the dysmenorrhea and menorrhagia caused by adenomyosis can be relieved. Since the neodymium-yttrium aluminum garnet (Nd:YAG) laser can penetrate deeply and coagulate large volumes of tissue,[61] it is useful in treating adenomyosis. A preliminary study was conducted in patients who presented with dysmenorrhea and menorrhagia and in whom other causes were excluded by hysteroscopy and laparoscopy. These women did not want future fertility. Pain relief was achieved in 75% of these women by using the following technique.[61]

A green-tinted filter and goggles are added to the operating room setup. A bare Nd:YAG fiber laser set at 50 W is inserted 1 to 1.5 cm into the myometrium repetitively, at 15 to 25 random sites, for 3 to 10 seconds each. The myometrium is approached from both the serosal and endometrial surfaces (Figure 15-41). The fiber is inserted through the hysteroscope for the endometrial approach. Constant laparoscopic surveillance helps prevent perforation or fiber contact with adjacent structures. The same procedure can be done with a 14 to 18-gauge electrosurgical needle.

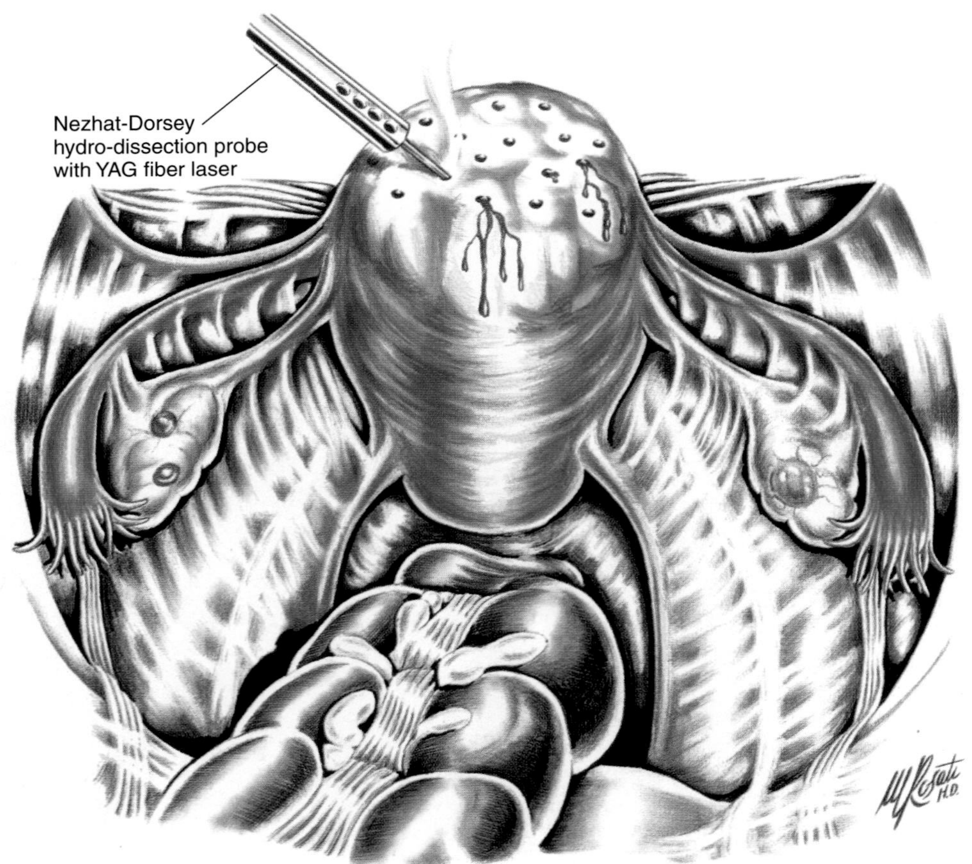

Figure 15-41. Either a fiber laser or an electrosurgical needle is inserted into the tumor for about 2 cm, and the energy is released. The end point in each is the pale appearance of the heated area, indicating the destruction of the juxtaposed blood supply.

Noncommunicating Rudimentary Uterine Horn

Congenital uterine anomalies are caused by failure of müllerian fusion and absorption or development during the eighth week of intrauterine life.[62,63] It is estimated that 20 to 25% of patients with müllerian anomalies have reproductive dysfunction, with the most common being fetal wastage. In patients who have a unicornate uterus, the incidence of spontaneous abortion approaches 50%. Abnormal paramesonephric development can result in a uterus with a unilateral hypoplastic horn. Despite the rudimentary development, the horn may contain functional endometrial glands, and if it is noncommunicating, hematometra or hematosalpinx can result in severe dysmenorrhea.

The high incidence of associated endometriosis is documented in cases of obstructive müllerian anomalies. Removing the obstructed cornu may reduce the incidence or severity of endometriosis. The management of a rudimentary horn involves amputation of the aplastic cornu to avoid associated endometriosis and possible cornual pregnancy.[64,65] Although laparotomy is advocated, Canis and coworkers[66] reported laparoscopic amputation of a rudimentary horn in a patient who presented with a 15-cm endometrioma. Intraoperatively, it was diagnosed as a nondistended, noncommunicating rudimentary uterine horn. Those authors did laparoscopic removal after the diagnosis was confirmed by hysterosalpingography.

Our experience included management of an occluded rudimentary horn severely dilated by hematometra and complicated by a long history of endometriosis.[67] A simultaneous laparoscopic and hysteroscopic evaluation revealed the presence of a rudimentary, noncommunicating horn previously diagnosed as a bicornuate uterus by hysterosalpingography. Removal of the rudimentary horn was done by coagulating and cutting the right round ligament and developing the bladder flap. The right utero-ovarian and broad ligaments and the uterine artery on the right were coagulated and cut. While a colleague was guiding the gynecologist with the hysteroscope, an incision was lengthened by using sequential bipolar electrocoagulation and the CO_2 laser to develop a distinct plane between the two horns. The dilated right horn was amputated at the level of internal cervical os. It was cut in several parts and removed. Five 4-0 polydioxanone sutures closed the muscularis and the serosa of the left uterine horn. Chromopertubation showed left tubal patency and no damage to the left uterine wall. The patient was discharged on postoperative day 1 after an uncomplicated hospital course. Two years later, she was pain-free with regular menses and was planning a pregnancy.

Uterine Suspension

Indications for uterine suspension are limited to dyspareunia secondary to uterine retroversion and retroflexion without other cul-de-sac disease and selected cases of severe endometriosis involving the cul-de-sac and rectum. At laparoscopy, uterine abnormalities can be treated, corrected, and the uterine suspension can be accomplished during the same operation.

Women with dyspareunia secondary to the uterine position will have a retroverted, retroflexed uterus, and palpation of the uterine-cervical junction on vaginal examination will reproduce the pain. Although some authors have advocated the placement of a pessary before attempting to surgically correct the retroversion,[68] others have noted that the dyspareunia was eliminated in the patient but the male partner was disturbed by the pessary during coitus.

Complete or partial relief of dyspareunia[69–71] from laparoscopic uterine suspension has been reported in approximately 90% of patients, but two reports showed no relief.[72,73]

The three most effective operative methods involve the use of fallope rings, ventrosuspension of the round ligament, and the modified Olshausen technique.

Fallope rings

Fallope rings have been used for many years in laparoscopic tubal sterilization. A special instrument fits through a 5-mm accessory trocar sleeve. It simultaneously grasps the tube, retracts it into the instrument, and places a small, tight silicon band around the knuckle of the tube. A similar procedure can shorten the round ligaments (Figure 15-42).[74] It may be necessary to place more than one fallope ring on the round ligaments to achieve the proper tension. Placing the rings on the round ligaments can cause complications such has laceration of the broad ligament or the round ligament. Bipolar electrocoagulation is used for hemostasis.

Ventrosuspension of the round ligament

This procedure involves the placement of two 5-mm suprapubic trocars. Grasping forceps are

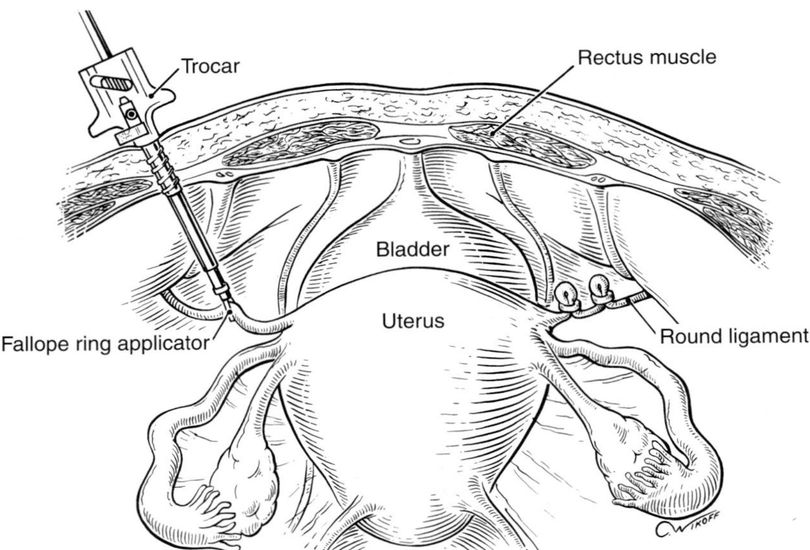

Figure 15-42. The round ligaments are shortened with fallope rings.

introduced into the pelvis through them.[69,75–77] Alternatively, long Kelly clamps also are inserted through suprapubic stab incisions. Both round ligaments are grasped near their midpoint, and the pneumoperitoneum is allowed to escape partially. The knuckle of the round ligament is pulled gently and firmly through the fascial incision (Figure 15-43). The round ligaments are sutured to the rectus fascia with 2-0 Ethibond nonabsorbable sutures. Uterine position is confirmed with the laparoscope, and one must avoid kinking the fallopian tubes.

Potential complications with this procedure include avulsion of the round ligament secondary to an inadequate fascial incision and undue tension or positioning of the round ligaments with a full pneumoperitoneum. The inferior epigastric arteries can

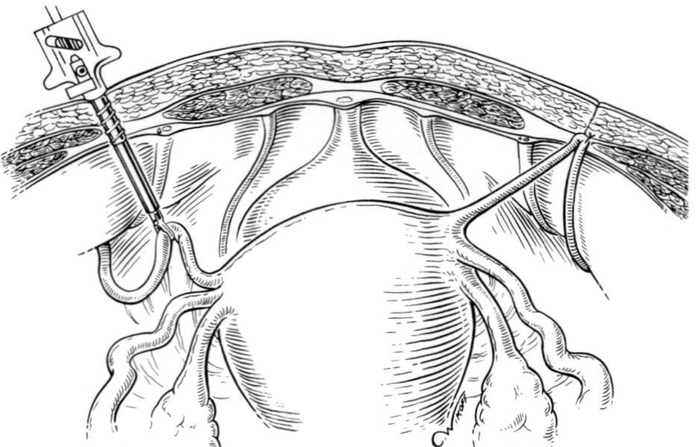

Figure 15-43. The round ligaments at midpoint are pulled through the suprapubic incision and tied to the rectus fascia.

be lacerated during placement of the suprapubic trocars. Although transillumination of the abdomen often helps prevent this complication, it is difficult in obese patients. For most patients, incisional pain and discomfort are managed with mild analgesics and a heating pad. Occasionally, patients who experience more significant postoperative pain from secondary spasms of the recti muscles are relieved with heat, muscle relaxants, and analgesics. Patients are advised to avoid strenuous exercise for 4 to 6 weeks postoperatively.

Modified Olshausen uterine suspension

A delayed absorbable or permanent suture is passed transabdominally at the suprapubic trocar site, using a swaged-on needle. While the round ligament is placed on stretch, several areas are taken where the round ligament enters the inguinal canal moving toward the uterus. Approximately 2 cm from the uterus, the direction of the needle is reversed, and a similar maneuver is done along the length of the round ligament to the inguinal canal. The needle is passed transabdominally. Once both sides are completed, the pneumoperitoneum is decreased and the suture is tied above the fascia (Figure 15-44). The result is a plication of the round ligaments.

This procedure should be considered an alternative to ventrosuspension of the uterus. It is associated with the same risks, except that the risk of round ligament avulsion is lower. This procedure also requires more skill than do others because of the intracorporeal suturing techniques used.

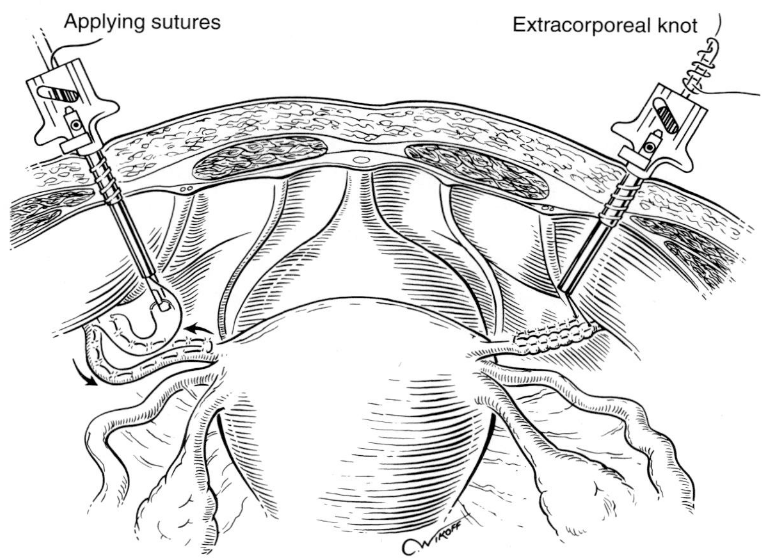

Figure 15-44. Modified Olshausen technique.

References

1. Buttram VC, Reiter RC. Uterine leiomyomata: Etiology, symptomatology, and management. *Fertil Steril* 1981; 36:433.
2. Vollenhoven BJ, Lawrence AS, Healy DL. Uterine fibroids: A clinical review. *Br J Obstet Gynaecol* 1990; 97:285.
3. Cramer SF, Robertson AL, Ziatas NP, et al. Growth potential of human uterine leiomyomas: Some in vitro observations and their implications. *Obstet Gynecol* 1990; 97:393.
4. Freidman AJ, Rein NS, Harrison-Atlas D, et al. A randomized, placebo-controlled, double blind study evaluating leuprolide acetate depot treatment before myomectomy. *Fertil Steril* 1989; 52:728.
5. Lumsden MA, West CP, Baird DT. Goserelin therapy before surgery for uterine fibroids. *Lancet* 1987; 1:36.
6. Fedele L, Vercellmi P, Bianchi S, et al. Treatment with GnRH agonists before myomectomy and the risk of short-term myoma recurrence. *Br J Obstet Gynaecol* 1990; 97:393.
7. Nezhat C, Nezhat F, Silfen SL, et al. Laparoscopic myomectomy. *Int J Fertil* 1991; 36:275.
8. Roemisch M, Nezhat FR, Nezhat A. Pregnancy after laparoscopic myomectomy. *J Am Assoc Gynecol Laparosc* 1996; 3:S42.
9. Davis GD, Hruby PH. Transabdominal laser colpotomy. *J Reprod Med* 1989; 34:438.
10. Nezhat CR, Nezhat F, Bess O, et al. Laparoscopically assisted myomectomy: A report of a new technique in 57 cases. *Int J Fertil Menopausal Stud* 1994, 39(1):39.
11. Harris WJ. Uterine dehiscence following laparoscopic myomectomy. *Obstet Gynecol* 1992; 80:545.
12. Operative Laparoscopy Study Group. Postoperative adhesion development after operative laparoscopy: Evaluation at early second-look procedures. *Fertil Steril* 1991; 55:700.
13. Linsky CB, Diamond MP, DiZerega GS. Effect of blood on the efficacy of barrier adhesion reduction in the rabbit uterine horn model. *Infertility* 1988; 11:273.
14. Bayers SP, Jansen D. Gore-Tex surgical membrane, in DeCherney A, Diamond MP, (eds.,) *Treatment of Post-Surgical Adhesions.* Wiley-Liss, 1990.
15. Diamond MP. Reduction of adhesions after uterine myomectomy by Seprafilm membrance (HAL-F): A blinded, prospective, randomized, multicenter clinical study.Seprafilm Adhesion Study Group. *Fertl Steril* 1996; 66:904.
16. Melis GB, Ajossa S, Piras B, et al. A randomized trial to evaluate the prevention of de novo adhesion formation after laparoscopic myomectomy using oxidized regenerated cellulose (Interceed) Barrier. *J Am Assoc Gynecol Laparosc* 1995; 2:S31.
17. Georgakopoulous PA, Bersis G. Sigmoido-uterine rupture in pregnancy after multiple myomectomy. *Int Surg* 1981; 66:367.
18. Hasson HM, Rotman C, Rana N, et al. Laparoscopic myomectomy. *Obstet Gynecol* 1992; 80:884.
19. Dubuisson JB, Lecuru F, Herve F, et al. Myomectomy by laparoscopy. *Fertil Steril* 1991; 56:827.

20. Vilos GA, Daly LJ, Tse BM. Pregnancy outcome after laparoscopic electromyolysis. *J Am Assoc Gynecol Laparosc* 1998; 5:289.
21. Zreik TG, Rutherford TJ, Palter SF, Troiano RN, Williams E, Brown JM, Olive DL. Cryomyalysis, a new procedure for the conservative treatment of uterine fibroids. *J Am Assoc Gynecol Laparosc* 1998; 5:33.
22. Kuhn R, Mitchell P. Embolic occlusion of the blood supply to uterine myomas: report of 2 cases. *Aust NZ J Obstet Gynecol* 1999; 39:120.
23. Goodwin SC, Walker WJ. Uterine artery empolization for the treatment of uterine fibroids. *Curr Opin Obstet Gynecol* 1998; 10:315.
24. Worthington-Kirsch RL, Popky GL, Hutchins FL Jr. Uterine arterial embolization for the management of Leiomyomas: quality-of-life assessment and clinical response. *Radiology* 1998; 208:625.
25. Selwood T, Wood C. Incidence of hysterectomy in Australia. *Med J Aust* 1978; 2:201.
26. Van Keep PA, Wildemeersch D, Lehert P. Hysterectomy in six European countries. *Maturitas* 1983; 5:69.
27. Porkas R, Hufnagel VG. Hysterectomy in the United States, 1964–84. *Am J Public Health* 1988; 78:852.
28. Bachmann GA. Hysterectomy: A critical review. *J Reprod Med* 1990; 35:839.
29. Dicker RC, Scally MJ, Greenspan JR, et al. Hysterectomy among women of reproductive age. *JAMA* 1982; 248:323.
30. White SC, Wartel LJ, Wade ME. Comparison of abdominal and vaginal hysterectomy: A review of 600 operations. *Obstet Gynecol* 1971; 37:530.
31. Wingo PA, Huezo CM, Rubin GL, et al. The mortality risk associated with hysterectomy. *Am J Obstet Gynecol* 1985; 152:803.
32. Lee NC, Dicker RC, Rubin GL, et al. Confirmation of the preoperative diagnoses for hysterectomy. *Am J Obstet Gynecol* 1984; 150:283.
33. Kovac RS, Cruishank SH, Retto HF. Laparoscopy-assisted vaginal hysterectomy. *J Gynecol Surg* 1990; 6:185.
34. Summitt RL Jr, Stovall TG, Steege JF, Lipscomb GH. A multicenter randomized comparison of laparoscopically assisted vaginal hysterectomy and abdominal hysterectomy in abdominal hysterectomy candidates. *Obstet Gynecol* 1998; 92:321.
35. Nezhat C, Nezhat F, Silfen SL. Laparoscopic hysterectomy and bilateral salpingo-oophorectomy using multifire GIA with standard vaginal hysterectomy in an outpatient setting. *Obstet Gynecol* 1992; 80:895.
36. Nezhat C, Burrell MO, Nezhat FR, et al. Laparoscopic radical hysterectomy with para-aortic and pelvic node dissection. *Am J Obstet Gynecol* 1992; 166:864.
37. Nezhat C, Nezhat F, Gordon S, et al. Laparoscopic versus abdominal hysterectomy. *J Reprod Med* 1992; 37:247.
38. Nezhat CR, Nezhat FR, Ramirez CE, et al. Laparoscopic radical hysterectomy and laparoscopic assisted vaginal radical hysterectomy with pelvic and paraaortic node dissection. *J Gynecol Surg* 1993; 9:105.
39. Nezhat C, Nezhat F, Burrell M. Laparoscopically assisted hysterectomy for the management of a borderline ovarian tumor: A case report. *J Laparoendosc Surg* 1992; 2:167.
40. Summit RL, Stovall TG, Lipscomb GH, et al. Randomized comparison of laparoscopy-assisted vaginal hysterectomy with standard vaginal hysterectomy in an outpatient setting. *Obstet Gynecol* 1992; 80:895.
41. Nezhat C, Nezhat F, Nezhat C. Operative laparoscopy (minimally invasive surgery): State of the art. *J Gynecol Surg* 1992; 8:111.
42. Nezhat F, Nezhat C, Levy JS. A report of laparoscopic injuries and complications over a 10-year period. Presented at the 41st annual clinical meeting of the American College of Obstetricians and Gynecologists, Washington, DC, May 3–6, 1993.
43. Bruhat MA, Mage G, Pouly JL, et al. *Laparoscopic Hysterectomy in Operative Laparoscopy.* New York: McGraw-Hill, 1992.
44. Nezhat C, Nezhat F, Winer W. Salpingectomy via laparoscopy: A new surgical approach. *J Laparosc Surg* 1991; 1:91.
45. Nezhat C, Nezhat F, Bess O, et al. Injuries associated with the use of a linear stapler during operative laparoscopy: Review, diagnosis, management, and prevention. *J Gynecol Surg* 1993; 3:145.
46. Semm K: Operationslehre für endoskopische Abdominalchirugie—operative Pelviskopie, Schattauer, Stuttgart 1984.
47. Semm K: Operative Manual for Endoscopic Abdominal Surgery, Friedrich, ER (Trans. ed) Chicago, Year Book Medical Publishers, 1987 (German: Stuttgart, Schattauer, 1984; Japanese: Tokyo Central Foreign Books, 1986; Chinese: Shanghai, Shanghai Scientific & Technical Publishers, 1988; Italian: Naples, Martinucci, 1988.
48. Reich H, DeCaprio J, McGlynn F. Laparoscopic hysterectomy. *J Gynecol Surg* 1989; 5:213.
49. Nezhat C, Nezhat F, Silfen SL. Laparoscopic hysterectomy and bilateral salpingo-

oophorectomy using multifire GIA surgical stapler. *J Gynecol Surg* 1990; 6:185.
50. Scott JR, Sharp HT, Dodson MK, et al. Subtotal hysterectomy in modern gynecology: A decision analysis. *Am J Obstet Gynecol* 1997; 176:1186.
51. Hill D, Maher PJ, Wood CE, et al. Complications of laparoscopic hysterectomy. *J Am Assoc Gynecol Laparosc* 1994; 1:159.
52. Liu CY. Complications of total laparoscopic hysterectomy in 518 cases. *Gynecol Endosc* 1994; 3:203.
53. Jones RA. Complications of laparoscopic hysterectomy: 250 cases. *Gynecol Endosc* 1995; 4:95.
54. Nezhat F, Nezhat CH, Admon D, et al. Complications and results of 361 hysterectomies performed at laparoscopy. *J Am Coll Surg* 1995; 180:307.
55. Chapron CM, Dubuisson JB, Ansquer Y. Is total laparoscopic hysterectomy a safe procedure? *Hum Reprod* 1996; 11:2422.
56. Semm K. Hysterectomy via laparotomy or pelviscopy: A new CISH method without colpotomy. *Geburtshilfe Frauenheilkd* 1991; 51:996.
57. Semm K. Endoscopic subtotal hysterectomy without colpotomy: Classic intrafascial SEMM hysterectomy: A new method of hysterectomy by pelviscopy, laparotomy, per vagina or functionally by total uterine mucosal ablation. *Int Surg* 1996; 81:362.
58. Mettler L, Semm K, Lehmann-Willenbrock L, et al. Comparative evaluation of classical intrafascial-supracervical hysterectomy (CISH) with transuterine mucosal resection as performed by pelviscopy and laparotomy—our first 200 cases. *Surg Endosc* 1995; 9:418.
59. Kim DH, Lee JC, Bae DH. Clinical analysis of pelviscopic classic intrafascial SEMM hysterectomy. *J Am Assoc Gynecol Laparosc* 1995; 2:289.
60. Kim DH, Bae DH, Hur M, et al. Comparison of classic intrafascial supracervical hysterectomy with total laparoscopic and laparoscopic-assisted vaginal hysterectomy. *J Am Assoc Gynecol Laparosc* 1998; 5:253.
61. Nezhat C, Nezhat F. Videolaseroscopy for the treatment of adenomyosis. Abstract presented at the 19th annual meeting of the American Association of Gynecologic Laparoscopists, Orlando, FL, 1990.
62. Ansbacher R. Uterine anomalies and future pregnancies. *Clin Perinatol* 1983; 10:295.
63. Rock JA, Schlaff WD. The obstetric consequences of uterovaginal anomalies. *Fertil Steril* 1985; 43:681.
64. Buttram VC, Gibbons WE. Müllerian anomalies: A proposed classification. *Fertil Steril* 1979; 32:40.
65. Mattingly RF, Thompson JD, eds. *Surgery for Anomalies of the Müllerian (ducts).* In *Te Londe's Operative Gynecology*, 6th ed. Philadelphia, Lippincott, 1985.
66. Canis M, Wattiez A, Pouly JL, et al. Laparoscopic management of unicornuate uterus with rudimentary horn and unilateral extensive endometriosis: Case report. *Hum Reprod* 1990; 5:819.
67. Nezhat F, Nezhat C, Bess O. Laparoscopic amputation of a non-communicating rudimentary horn after a hysteroscopic diagnosis: A case study. *Surg Laparosc Endosc* 1994; 4:155.
68. Donaldson JK, Sanderlin JH, Harrell WB. A method of suspending the uterus without open abdominal incision. *Am J Surg* 1942; 15:537.
69. Smith DB, Kelsey JF, Sherman RL, et al. Laparoscopic uterine suspension. *J Reprod Med* 1977; 18:98.
70. Paterson MEL, Jordan JA, Logan-Edwards R. A survey of 100 patients who had laparoscopic ventrosuspension. *Br J Obstet Gynaecol* 1978; 85:468.
71. Servy EJ, Aksu MF, Tzingounis VA. Laparoscopic hysteropexy and the position of the fallopian tubes, in Phillips JM (ed.), *Endoscopy in Gynecology.* CA: American Association of Gynecologic Laparoscopists, Department of Publications, 1978.
72. Gleeson NC, Gaffney GM. Ventrosuspension: Five years of practice at the Rotunda Hospital reviewed. *J Obstet Gynecol* 1990; 10:415.
73. Yoon AFE. Laparoscopic ventrosuspension: A review of 72 cases. *Am J Obstet Gynecol* 1990; 163:1151.
74. Massouda D, Ling FW, Muram D, et al. Laparoscopic uterine suspension with fallope rings. *J Reprod Med* 1987; 32:859.
75. Steptoe PC. *Laparoscopy in Gynecology.* London, Livingstone, 1967.
76. Candy JW. Modified Gilliam uterine suspension using laparoscopic visualization. *Obstet Gynecol* 1976; 47:242.
77. Mann WJ, Stenger VG. Uterine suspension through the laparoscope. *Obstet Gynecol* 1978; 51:563.

16

The Role of Laparoscopy in the Management of Gynecologic Malignancy

Most gynecologic oncologists have been hesitant to use operative laparoscopy in the management of gynecologic malignancies. However, an increasing number of surgeons have used advanced operative laparoscopic techniques to evaluate and treat such patients. This endoscopic approach is becoming more prevalent worldwide as studies describe its feasibility and safety. These complex operations should be done in hospitals by surgeons who have the required skills, state-of-the-art equipment, and a well-trained ancillary staff.

Pelvic and abdominal anatomy appear magnified on the video camera and laparoscope. This characteristic potentially improves the identification of subtle findings that may represent metastatic or recurrent cancer. The upper abdomen, surfaces of the liver and diaphragm, the posterior cul-de-sac, broad ligaments, peritoneal surfaces, and the bowel and mesenteric surfaces can be inspected for metastatic lesions. Access to the rectovaginal space is better than it is with laparotomy. Observation of the retroperitoneal spaces, including the paravesical, pararectal, and vesicovaginal spaces, is attainable with laparoscopy. A thorough knowledge of and familiarity with the pelvic anatomy and its relation to adjacent structures are essential for a gynecologist doing laparoscopic pelvic procedures (Figures 16-1 through 16-3).

Additional benefits of laparoscopy in gynecologic oncology include less bleeding from small vessels afforded by pneumoperitoneum, the elimination of large abdominal incisions, early ambulation, a decrease in the length of hospitalization, and more rapid recovery. Patients who need postoperative chemotherapy can start treatment earlier than can those recovering from a laparotomy. Patients requiring postoperative radiation have a reduction in complications secondary to adhesions of the bowel and other peritoneal structures and less of a delay before receiving radiation therapy. Technologic advances such as the development of the carbon dioxide laser and the harmonic scalpel allow disease to be treated precisely and with a greater margin of safety, especially when the pathology is adjacent to blood vessels, bowel, and other vital structures.

Historical Perspectives

Laparoscopic lymphadenectomy for the management of gynecologic malignancies was described by Dargent and Salvat in 1989[1]. Two years later, Querleu and associates[2] reported transperitoneal pelvic lymphadenectomies in 39 patients who had cervical cancer. A radical hysterectomy with para-aortic lymphadenectomy was performed in 1989 and reported in 1991 and 1992.[3,4] Other publications have described laparoscopic lymphadenectomy for cervical, endometrial, and ovarian cancer.[5–12] Chu and associates[13] reported 67 patients who had laparoscopic pelvic and para-aortic lymphadenectomies for cervical cancer. Childers and colleagues[9] described 57 patients with various gynecologic malignancies who underwent para-aortic lymphadenectomies. At the Mount Sinai Medical Center (MSMC) in New York, data have been collected on 94 patients who had laparoscopic lymphadenectomies for various pelvic

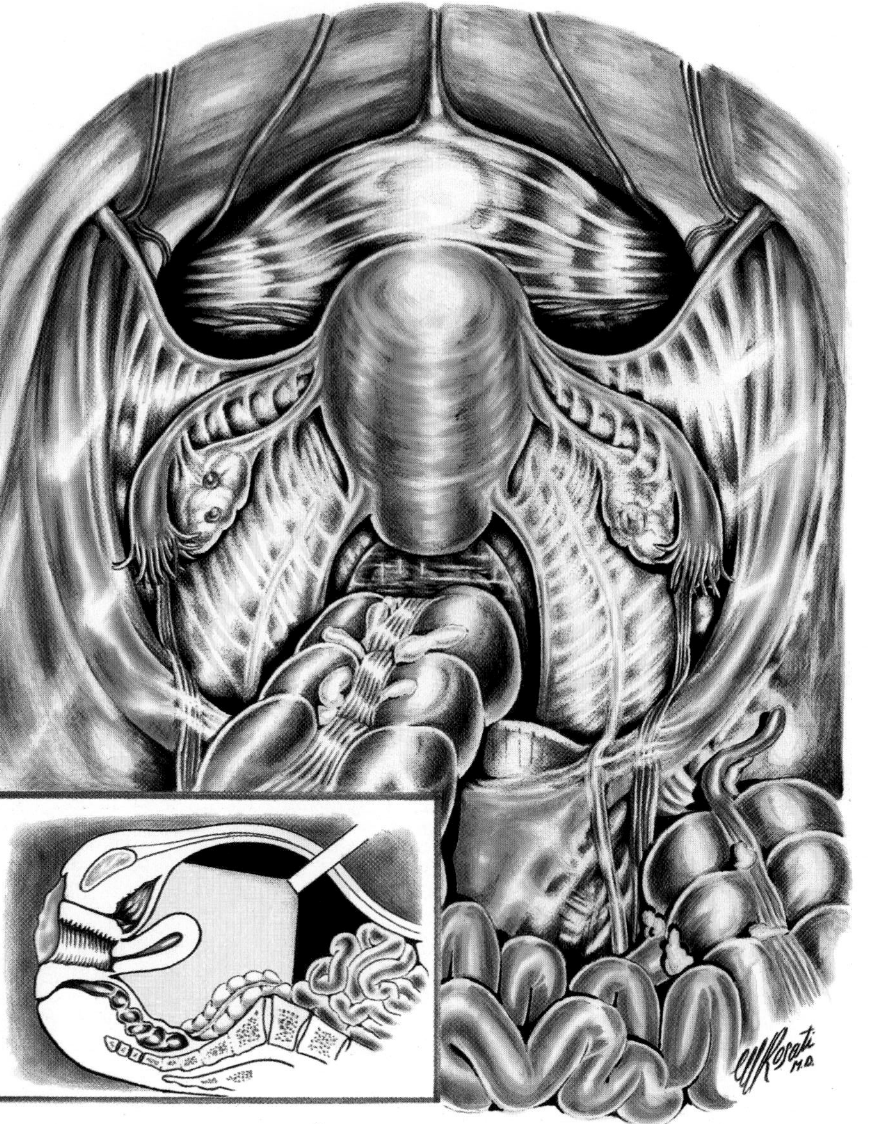

Figure 16-1. A laparoscopic view of the pelvis. The inset shows the effect of the Trendelenburg position.

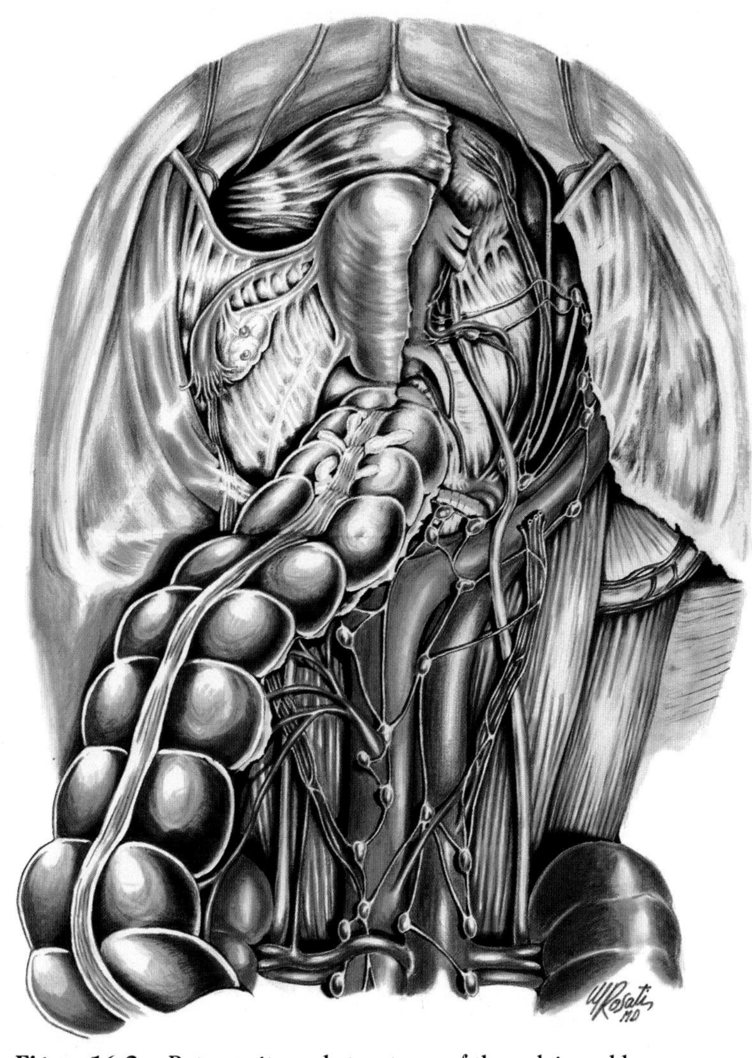

Figure 16-2. Retroperitoneal structures of the pelvis and lower para-aortic areas.

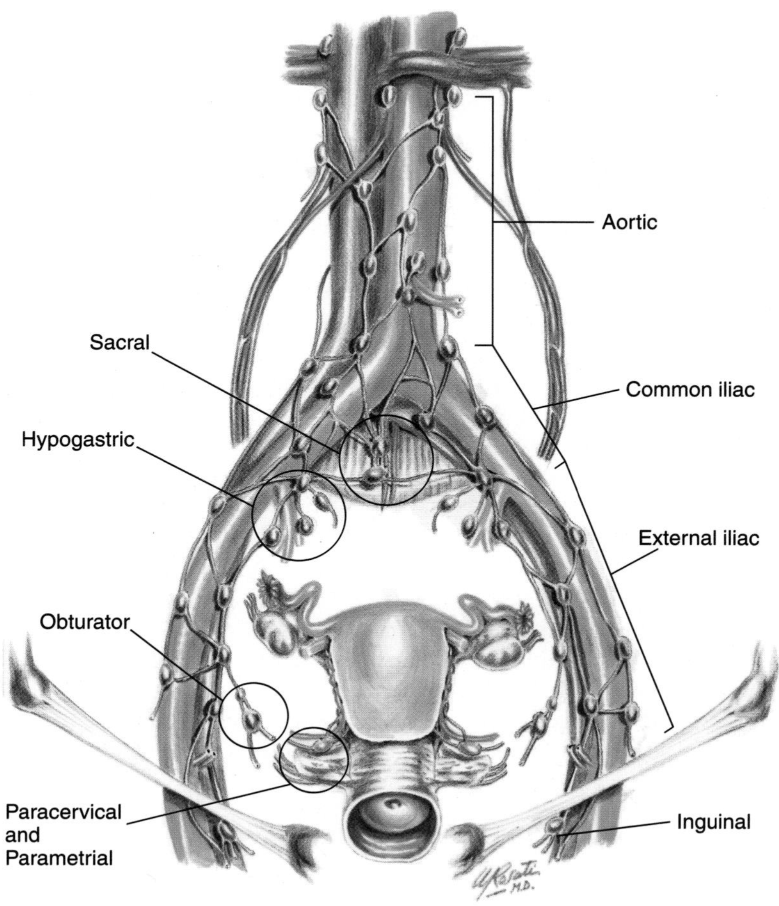

Figure 16-3. The nodal distribution along the para-aortic and pelvic regions.

malignancies. Laparoscopic lymphadenectomies have been done since 1992 for patients with various malignancies.[14] With experience, the yield of pelvic lymph nodes increased to a mean of 19.1 and that of the para-aortic nodes to a mean of 4.1 in the last 2 years of the study. Three patients required conversions to laparotomy: one for a vascular injury to the vena cava, another for a tumor extending to both side walls, and the third for the removal of densely matted lymph nodes. Those procedures were done successfully on patients with a wide variety of body weights, including one who weighed 106.4 kg.

Since 1991, most hysterectomies done at CPS, including radical hysterectomies, have been done by laparoscopy.[15] In 1993, Nezhat and coauthors[10] published a report of 19 patients who underwent total laparoscopic hysterectomy or laparoscopically assisted radical vaginal hysterectomy with pelvic and para-aortic lymph node dissections for cervical cancer. Since then, others have described the successful completion of laparoscopic radical vaginal hysterectomies and laparoscopically assisted radical vaginal hysterectomies.[16,17]

Patients for whom laparoscopic procedures for gynecologic malignancies are contemplated need to be informed that this approach is the state of the art though not universally accepted as the standard of care. Furthermore, laparotomy is a possibility if technical difficulties or complications occur. Intraoperative spread of malignant cells is possible, as it is during a laparotomy, but evidence exists that this does not worsen the prognosis.[18]

Cervical Carcinoma

Laparoscopic Lymphadenectomy

Operative laparoscopy can be useful in the surgical staging of cervical cancer. Para-aortic nodal metastasis has been reported in 5% of women with stage IB, 16% with stage II, and 25% with stage III cancer. Berman and coworkers[19] found that 40 of 47 women with involved para-aortic nodes also had pelvic node metastasis. However, if patients with stage IB cervical cancers have negative pelvic lymph nodes and grossly normal para-aortic nodes, there is no risk of having positive para-aortic nodes.[20] Therefore, there is a trend not to do para-aortic lymphadenectomies routinely in patients with stage IB cervical cancer who have normal-appearing para-aortic lymph nodes with negative pelvic lymph nodes.

If a patient has a normal chest x-ray, computed tomography (CT), and magnetic resonance imaging (MRI), surgical staging by laparoscopy is an option. The purpose of surgical staging is to detect extension of disease to the para-aortic nodes, the incidence of which increases with a higher stage of disease. Clinical staging fails to predict the extension of disease to the para-aortic region in 7% of patients with stage IB disease, 18% with stage IIB, and 28% with stage III.[19] Radiotherapy after transperitoneal lymphadenectomy by laparotomy increases postradiation complications, primarily small bowel obstruction from postoperative adhesions.[21,22] Extraperitoneal dissection significantly decreases this risk to a more acceptable level.[23–25]

There is evidence from porcine models that laparoscopic transperitoneal lymph node dissection leads to decreased postoperative adhesions compared with laparotomy and is equivalent to extraperitoneal lymphadenectomy in terms of postoperative adhesion formation.[26,27] It is assumed that laparoscopic transperitoneal lymphadenectomy will cause less radiation-induced bowel complications than does the traditional transperitoneal technique by laparotomy. Laparoscopic lymphadenectomy is a feasible and preferable procedure for patients in whom surgical staging is required, especially if these women will need postoperative radiation therapy. Access to the rectovaginal space is excellent with laparoscopy, and the vesicovaginal, paravesical, and pararectal spaces are developed easily because of the excellent magnification afforded by videolaparoscopy.

Laparoscopic Radical Hysterectomy

Radical vaginal hysterectomy (Schauta) has a cure rate comparable to that of radical abdominal hysterectomy (Wertheim) for stage IB and IIA cervical cancer.[28] Although the vaginal approach was introduced at the beginning of the twentieth century, it was replaced in the United States by the Wertheim procedure because of the widespread belief in the therapeutic role of lymphadenectomy. Total laparoscopic radical hysterectomy and laparoscopically assisted radical vaginal hysterectomy are feasible alternatives to laparotomy in treating patients who are selected for primary surgical treatment of their disease.[4,10,16,17,29] This includes patients who have at least a stage IA2 lesion and less than stage IIB disease.

Patients with larger lesions have decreased survival and more treatment failures.[30–32] Homesley and colleagues[30] described 45 women who had stage IB disease treated with radiation. They had a 5-year survival of 95% when the tumors were less than 4 cm in size compared with 67% in patients with lesions larger than 4 cm. Van Nagell and associates[33] found a recurrence rate of 11% with radiation and 24% with radical hysterectomy in stage IB patients with lesions larger than 2 cm. Most gynecologic oncologists agree that patients with lesions larger than 4 cm in diameter, stage IB2, have a better prognosis with primary radiation therapy.

Since radiation and surgery have equal cure rates for women with disease less than stage IIB (with the exception of IB2), patients are selected for operation on the basis of the potential benefits and risks of each treatment modality. Radical hysterectomy allows preservation of the ovaries in premenopausal women and postponement of hormonal replacement therapy, and the option of motherhood remains because of advances in reproductive medicine. Intraoperative complications such as ureteral injuries (1 to 2%) and vesicovaginal fistulas (less than 1%) are higher than they are with hysterectomy done for benign disease. The average estimated blood loss is 800 mL and is increased because of the extent of dissection necessary for a radical hysterectomy.[34] The major postoperative complication is bladder dysfunction, specifically inability to void, which can eventually develop to a hypotonic bladder, leading to overflow incontinence. The incidence increases with the extent of the procedure. Fortunately, this complication occurs in only 3% of patients.[35,36]

Laparoscopy and Exenteration

An additional use of operative laparoscopy is to evaluate central pelvic recurrences in patients who are proposed for pelvic exenteration. Typically, these patients frequently have had previous radiation. These women do not need to undergo an exploratory laparotomy when disease is located along the pelvic side wall, an extrapelvic tumor is found, or lymph nodes are malignant. These findings preclude proceeding with the exenterative procedure because of the low likelihood of increased survival. As many as 40 to 63% of scheduled exenterations are terminated although the patient underwent a laparotomy with the accompanying morbidity and long recovery period.[37] A recent series by Plante and Roy[38] of 13 women showed the feasibility of doing operative laparoscopy to reliably evaluate patients for exenteration. Laparoscopy identified a metastatic tumor in 9 of 13 women, and in 4 who underwent laparotomy, no additional disease was found. Laparoscopic evaluation could not be completed in one because of a large myomatous uterus. There were no intraoperative complications. Laparoscopy appears to be safe to evaluate the pelvis effectively and reduce unnecessary laparotomies.

Ovarian Carcinoma

Approximately 80% of women who have ovarian cancer are discovered with advanced disease (stage III or IV), while the remaining patients present with stage I or II disease. Patients who appear to have disease limited to one ovary (stage Ia) require a full surgical staging procedure. This includes aspiration and cytologic assessment of all pelvic and abdominal fluid, pelvic and para-aortic lymph node sampling, infracolic omentectomy, and biopsies of the peritoneum from the cul-de-sacs, paracolic gutters, and diaphragms. One-third of the patients who appear to have disease confined to the ovary are upstaged after a surgical staging procedure. The incidence of positive lymph nodes is as high as 24% in stage I disease.[39] A national cooperative study found that 28% of patients thought to have stage I disease were upstaged after complete surgical staging.[40] Inadequate staging can lead to improper postoperative therapy and a poorer prognosis.

The standard preoperative evaluation includes a history and physical, pelvic examination, a Papanicolaou smear, complete blood count, liver profile, and chest x-ray. Intravenous pyelography, barium enema, colonoscopy, and gastrointestinal series are utilized as indicated by the symptoms and physical exam. Ultrasound can be helpful in evaluating an adnexal mass for cystic and solid components, but the findings are not diagnostic of the malignancy of a mass.[41,42] CT scans are helpful in preoperative planning for patients with an upper abdominal mass or liver metastasis in asymptomatic women and those with normal liver function tests.

The standard therapy for a histologically confirmed ovarian cancer is a cytoreductive operation to eliminate all gross disease. This procedure generally includes a total abdominal hysterectomy and bilateral salpingo-oophorectomy, an infracolic omentectomy, and pelvic and para-aortic lymph node sampling. Multiple retrospective studies have shown that survival is improved if patients have no residual lesions larger than 2 cm in diameter.[43–45] Although no prospective studies randomizing patients to primary surgery or chemotherapy have been conducted, a trial of interval cytoreduction after three cycles of chemotherapy revealed a survival benefit for patients who had an optimal resection of their disease compared with patients who did not.[46]

Laparoscopic Staging

The use of laparoscopy to surgically stage a patient with stage I or II ovarian cancer has been reported.[8, 47–49] Pomel and coworkers[7] described 10 patients who underwent complete surgical staging for presumed stage I ovarian cancer. These procedures included peritoneal washings, peritoneal and ovarian biopsies, infracolic omentectomies, and pelvic and para-aortic lymphadenectomies. A median of six pelvic and eight para-aortic nodes from each homolateral chain was obtained. No intraoperative complications occurred. One patient had a postoperative pulmonary embolism, and another required laparotomy for hemoperitoneum secondary to bleeding from the vaginal cuff (two patients had laparoscopically assisted vaginal hysterectomies).

Childers and colleagues[50] reported 44 ovarian cancer patients having laparoscopic surgical evaluations; 14 of those patients had surgical staging for presumed stage I disease. There were no serious complications, and the average hospital stay was 1.6 days. Among the 14 patients having laparoscopic staging procedures, 8 (57%) were found to have metastatic disease (3 with positive para-aortic lymph nodes). At the Stanford CPS, eight patients with various stages of ovarian cancer underwent laparoscopic procedures.[49] Three patients had initial staging and cytoreduction, three were incompletely staged by laparotomy and underwent laparoscopic stagings, and two had second-look procedures with secondary cytoreduction of residual disease. The mean hospital stay was 2.5 days, with a range of 1 to 6 days. There were no serious intraoperative or postoperative complications. Many surgeons have documented the feasibility of laparoscopic staging of patients who appear grossly to have early-stage ovarian cancer. However, larger studies examining the disease-free interval and overall survival of these patients are necessary to definitively conclude that laparoscopic staging of early-stage ovarian cancer is preferable.

Laparoscopic Technique

For peritoneal cytology, a long suction-irrigator probe is used to obtain washings from the pelvic cavity. Lactated Ringer's solution is used with heparin solution. Once the mass is evaluated and a decision to remove the mass laparoscopically is made, the adnexa is extirpated in the usual fashion. The mass must not be ruptured because such an occurrence can convert a possible stage Ia ovarian carcinoma to stage Ic. If a well-differentiated serous carcinoma is converted to a stage Ic cancer, most oncologists would recommend treatment with chemotherapy. Nevertheless, at least two retrospective studies have shown that patients who are converted intraoperatively do not have a worse prognosis.[18,51] In addition to attempting not to rupture any cystic mass, it is important to remove the adnexal mass or cyst without letting the tissue make contact with the abdominal wall. This is done by removing all possible malignant tissue in a laparoscopic Endobag (Ethicon) or a Cook Endobag. The Cook Endobag is more durable and better for larger masses that require aspiration or morcellation in the bag before removal. Removal of the bag through a posterior colpotomy or minilaparotomy is an option recommended for potential ovarian cancer. A Topel suction-irrigator is a useful suction device that permits the surgeon to pierce and aspirate an ovarian cyst without spillage by doing the aspiration within a wider suction cylinder to create a seal between the cyst wall and the suction device.

Peritoneal biopsies are obtained by using the carbon dioxide laser and hydrodissection, biopsy forceps, and Endoshears or using a combination of sharp dissection with electrocoagulation as needed. Diaphragmatic biopsies are taken very superficially with a biopsy forceps or carbon dioxide laser. Thorough exploration of the diaphragm is obtained but at times may require an additional 5-mm trocar for direct access to accomplish operative laparoscopy in that area. To achieve an infracolic omentectomy, the patient is placed in a straight supine position and the omentum is excised from the inferior margin of the transverse colon, using a harmonic scalpel, a bipolar forceps and Endoshears, a linear stapler, or sutures (Figure 16-4). The harmonic scalpel is superior for omentectomy because of the minimal plume formation, ease and speed of use, and lack of protruding staple edges.

There is concern about abdominal wall metastasis after laparoscopic evaluation for ovarian cancer, though there have been few reports of this occurrence.[52,53] Childers and coworkers[54] noted only 1 instance in 104 cases of laparoscopy for gynecologic malignancies, 80% of which were done for ovarian cancer. The one port site recurrence occurred in a patient with ovarian cancer who underwent a second-look procedure. However, most series on laparoscopic procedures for gynecologic oncology are small and limited in regard to follow-up and survival data. One study retrospectively reviewed the charts of patients with a laparoscopy before primary debulking and found that 7 of those 43 patients had an abdominal wall metastasis at one of the laparoscopic entry sites.[53] Analysis of these data did show a negative effect on survival in the patients with abdominal wall metastasis, although the correlation was not statistically significant. A rat model study suggested that laparoscopy may increase intraperitoneal spread of malignant cells compared with laparotomy.[55] The use of laparoscopy in patients with ovarian cancer, especially with widespread dissemination or ascites, is controversial, and its effect on further metastasis and overall prognosis is unknown.

Second-Look Laparoscopy

Although the indication for second-look operations in patients with ovarian cancer after chemotherapy is debatable, laparoscopy can replace laparotomy safely in most cases. This procedure should be done only in research or protocol situations because there are no data showing that the procedure and the management based on the results of the procedure affect overall survival.[56,57] As many as 50% of patients with negative second-look procedures will have a recurrence.[58,59] Second-look laparoscopy has been used since the late 1970s for patients with ovarian cancer. However, the procedure was associated with a high false-negative rate and complications.[60] Improvements in laparoscopic equipment and skills increased the sensitivity and safety of second-look procedures.

After the abdominal cavity is entered, the pelvic and abdominal cavity is evaluated for any gross disease and peritoneal washings from the pelvis are obtained. A biopsy specimen is taken of suspicious lesions and sent for frozen section. If any lesions are found to be malignant, the procedure is concluded unless the patient has a solitary,

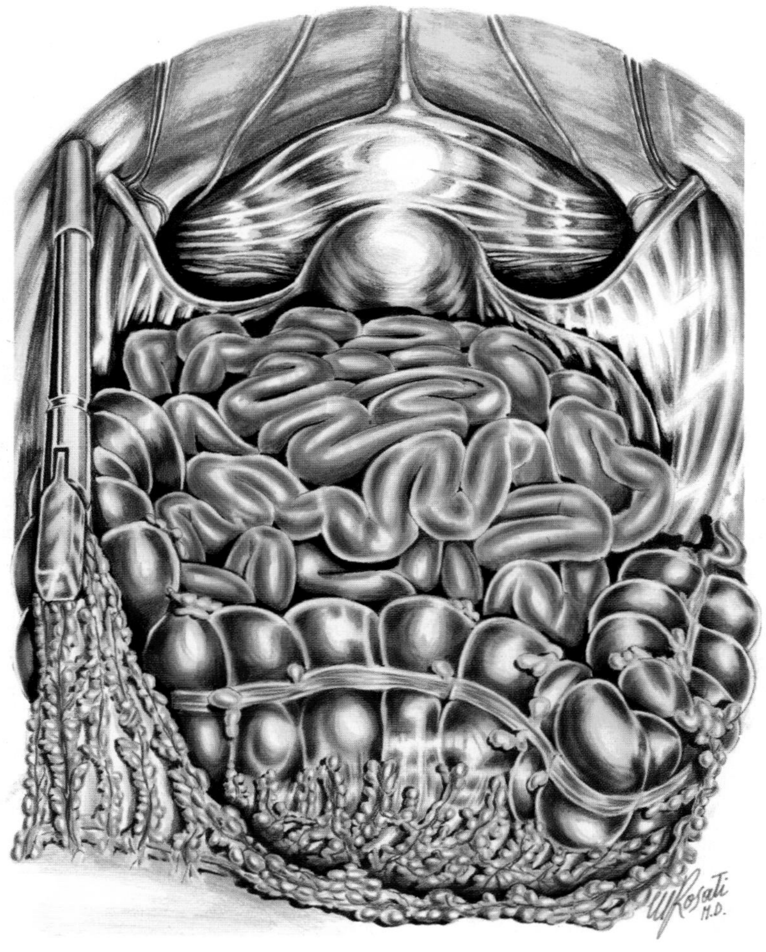

Figure 16-4. The harmonic scalpel, monopolar scissors, bipolar electrosurgery, or stapler can be used to carry out an infracolic omentectomy.

resectable lesion. If no persistent disease is noted, multiple peritoneal biopsies are taken from the pelvis and upper abdomen, including from all adhesions. In general, multiple biopsy specimens are taken from peritoneal surfaces, including the bladder, cul-de-sac, rectum, paracolic gutters, abdominal wall, and round and infundibulopelvic ligaments. If biopsies of lymph nodes and omentectomy were not accomplished previously, these procedures are done at the second-look procedure. Approximately 20 to 30 biopsy specimens should be taken to minimize the chances of missing occult disease.

At the CPS in Atlanta, 19 second-look laparoscopies after a laparotomy for ovarian cancer were carried out. Peritoneal washings, multiple peritoneal specimens from the upper abdomen, and pelvic and para-aortic node samples were obtained. In two patients, a Cavitational Ultrasonic Surgical Aspirator (CUSA) was used for debulking. One bowel perforation occurred that was repaired laparoscopically, and this patient was discharged home without sequelae. All patients were discharged from the hospital within 48 hours. Other authors have described the benefit, safety, and accuracy of laparoscopic second-look procedures.[50,61,62] Abu-Rustum and coauthors[61] described the Memorial Sloan-Kettering experience using laparoscopy to accomplish second-look assessments in 31 patients. After comparing these patients to 70 patients who underwent laparotomy, they noted that there was no difference between the two groups in terms of the number of patients found to have persistent cancer. Seventeen of 31 (54.8%) patients evaluated by laparoscopy had persistent disease, and 43 of 70 (61.4%) patients who had a laparotomy were found to have persistence of their cancer. Furthermore, the mean operating time was significantly shorter with laparoscopy (129 minutes) compared with laparotomy (153 minutes). This difference was significant ($p < 0.01$). Hospital stay and overall hospital charges were both lower among patients having laparoscopy. After a median follow-up of 22 months, no difference in recurrence rates after a negative second-look procedure was found. When second-look reassessments are required, laparoscopy can accomplish this task safely, with efficacy equal to that of laparotomy and with a decrease in hospital stay and costs.[61]

Endometrial Carcinoma

The standard treatment for endometrial cancer is total abdominal hysterectomy, bilateral salpingo-oophorectomy, peritoneal washings, and pelvic and para-aortic lymph node dissection. This type of surgical staging replaced clinical staging in 1988 because of the inaccuracy of clinical staging in patients with early endometrial cancer.[63,66] The use of the laparoscope allows the conversion of abdominal hysterectomies to laparoscopic procedures or laparoscopically assisted vaginal procedures. Most endometrial carcinomas can be staged and managed laparoscopically.[7,67]

Fifteen patients with stage I disease at the CPS in Atlanta and 11 patients at the MSMC had laparoscopic lymphadenectomies. Childers and colleagues[7] reported 53 patients with clinical stage I endometrial cancer who had laparoscopically assisted vaginal hysterectomies. Among the 53 patients, 29 underwent laparoscopic lymphadenectomy because of grade 2 or higher disease or greater than 50% myometrial invasion. In two patients who had indications for laparoscopic lymphadenectomy, obesity (weights of 180 and 250 pounds, respectively) prevented its performance. Two patients had laparotomies because of intraoperative complications (one transected ureter and one cystotomy) related to the laparoscopically assisted vaginal hysterectomy: Estimated blood loss was less than 200 mL, and the average hospital stay was 2.9 days. Although the safety and benefits of laparoscopic lymphadenectomy are documented, its equivalence to laparotomy in terms of recurrence rates and survival remains unproven and is being studied in a randomized trial through the Gynecologic Oncology Group.

In 15 patients with stage I endometrial cancer managed at the CPS, 9 had a laparoscopically assisted vaginal hysterectomy (LAVH) or total laparoscopic hysterectomy, and 6 others required pelvic and para-aortic lymphadenectomy. No intraoperative or postoperative complications occurred. An additional woman with clinical IIIb cancer received preoperative external beam radiotherapy followed by laparoscopic hysterectomy and bilateral salpingo-oophorectomy. Another patient with stage IVb endometrial cancer presented 3 months after laparotomy with a persistent tumor. A laparoscopic attempt at debulking was complicated by an enterotomy and cystotomy; both were repaired at laparotomy. The debulking procedure was completed, and the patient was discharged without complications on postoperative day 7. Chemotherapy was initiated postoperatively, and at 4 years of follow-up, the patient was without evidence of disease.

Lymph Node Dissection

Pelvic and para-aortic lymph node dissection is accomplished after hysterectomy and bilateral salpingo-oophorectomy in patients with endometrial and ovarian carcinomas. However, in patients with a cervical malignancy, the lymph node dissection is done before the radical hysterectomy because the hysterectomy is not done if a patient has lymph node metastasis. Radiation therapy is the procedure of choice.

Pelvic Lymphadenectomy

If a hysterectomy is not necessary or already has been completed, the initial approach is to expose the anterior and posterior leaves of the broad ligament by desiccating and incising the round ligament with bipolar or unipolar electrocoagulation or the harmonic scalpel and cutting the broad ligament in a cephalad fashion lateral and parallel to the infundibulopelvic ligament (Figures 16-5 through 16-7). Development of the paravesical and pararectal spaces is imperative if a radical hysterectomy is to follow. Before proceeding with a pelvic lymph node dissection, creating the avascular paravesical space helps identify the ureter, obturator nerve and vessels, and pelvic vessels. The obliterated hypogastric artery is an important landmark to identify the medial border of the paravesical space. The spaces lateral to this vessel and medial to the external iliac vein and obturator internus muscle are created with blunt and sharp dissection. Electrocoagulation should not be necessary, as this space generally is avascular. Once this space is created, the bony side wall laterally, the levator plate posteriorly, and the obturator nerve and vessels anteriorly should be visible. This optimizes the potential for safely removing the pelvic lymph nodes. Commencing laterally over the psoas muscle and proceeding medially provide a safe approach that avoids the genitofemoral nerve.

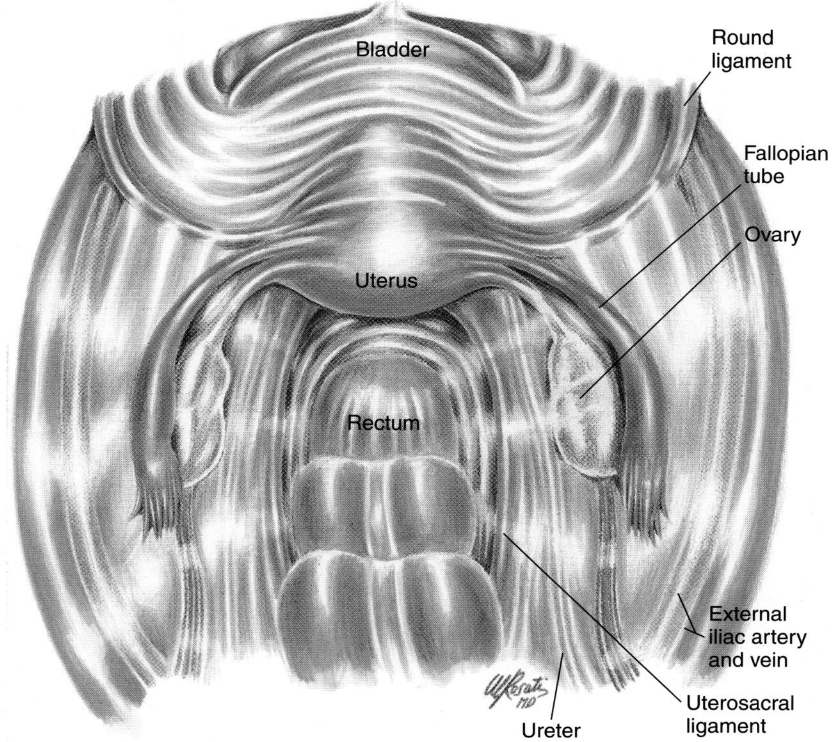

Figure 16-5. The laparoscopic view of the pelvic anatomy before the operation.

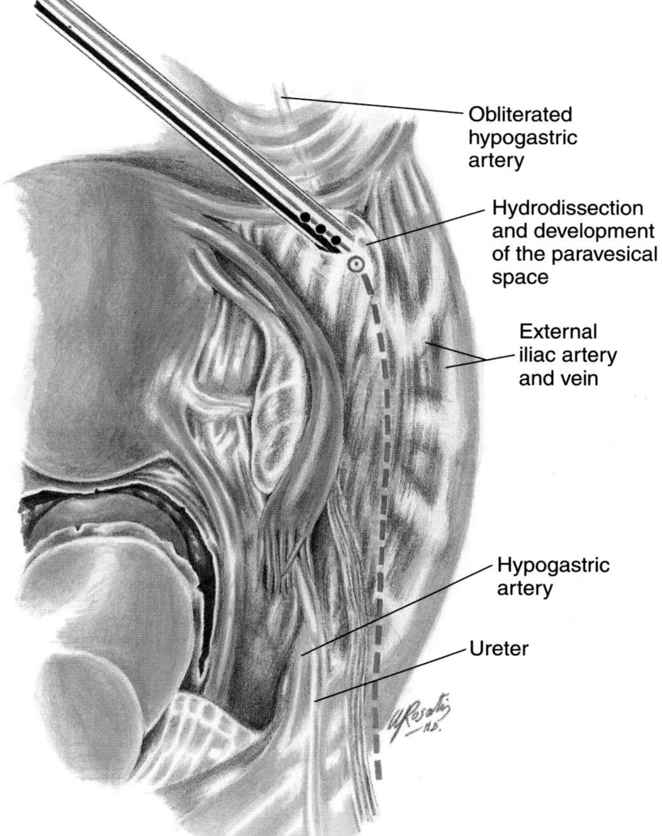

Figure 16-6. An incision is made in the broad ligament lateral or parallel to the infundibulopelvic ligament to develop the paravesical space. The round ligament can be coagulated and cut either before or after this space is developed.

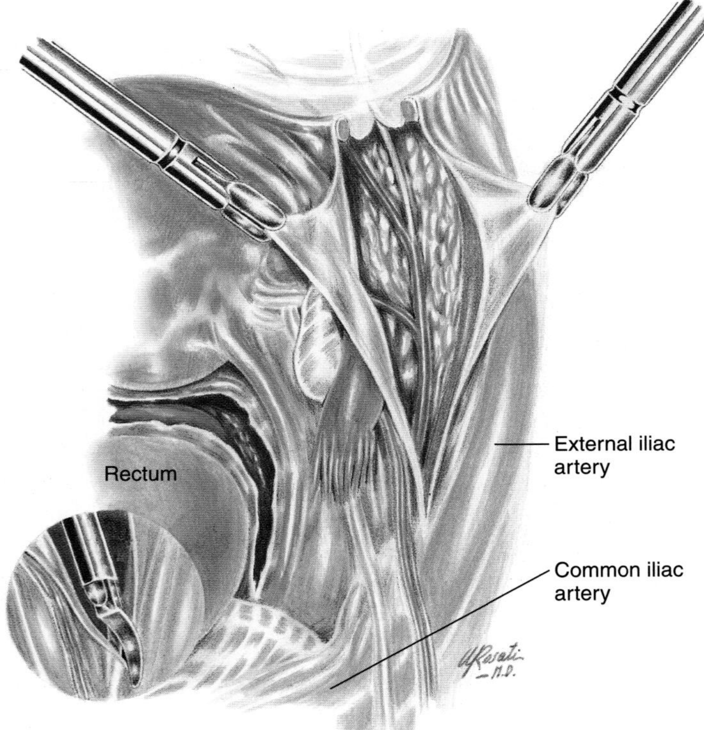

Figure 16-7. Using the suction-irrigator probe, grasper, and scissors, paravesical space is created. It is bordered medially by the obliterated hypogastric artery and laterally by the pelvic side wall.

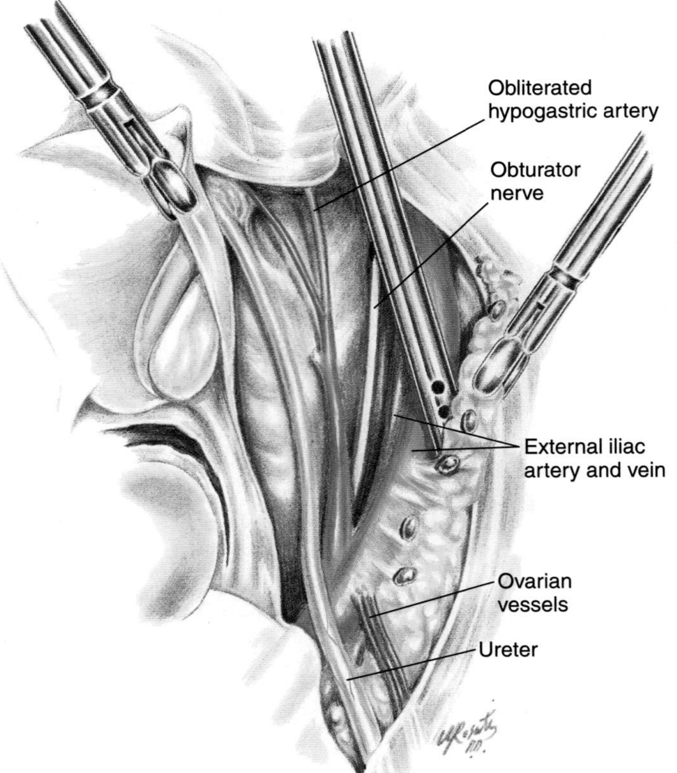

Figure 16-8. The nodes along the external iliac artery and vein are removed to the level of the deep circumflex vein.

The external iliac nodes along the external iliac artery and vein are excised caudally to the level of the deep circumflex iliac vein seen crossing over the distal portion of the external iliac artery (Figure 16-8). The obturator nerve is identified easily by using blunt dissection below and between the obliterated umbilical artery and the external iliac vein. Usually the obturator vessels are posterior to the nerve, but in some instances an aberrant obturator vein arises from the external iliac vein and is anterior to the obturator nerve. The nodal tissue anterior and lateral to the nerve and medial and inferior to the external iliac vein is removed by using blunt and sharp dissection. Venous anastomoses between the obturator and the external iliac veins are observed and saved from injury. The obturator nodal packet is excised caudally down to the pelvic side wall where the obturator nerve exits the pelvis through the obturator canal and cephalad up to the bifurcation of the common iliac artery. Before the removal of each nodal bundle, the pedicle of each one is ligated using electrocoagulation, endoscopic hemoclips, or an Endoloop to prevent lymphocyst formation. The lymph node packets are removed in a bag by pulling the tissue through the largest trocar to avoid contact between the potentially malignant nodes and the abdominal wall (Figures 16-9 and 16-10).

To excise the lymph nodes around the common iliac artery, a plane is created between the posterior peritoneum and the adventitia overlying the common iliac artery. Another option is to extend the dissection over the common iliac vessels when removing the proximal portion of the external iliac nodes. Before the iliac and proximal external iliac nodes are detached, the orientation of the ureter and ovarian vessels crossing the common iliac artery is identified. When one is effecting a left pelvic lymph node dissection, it may be necessary to take down the rectosigmoid colon from the left

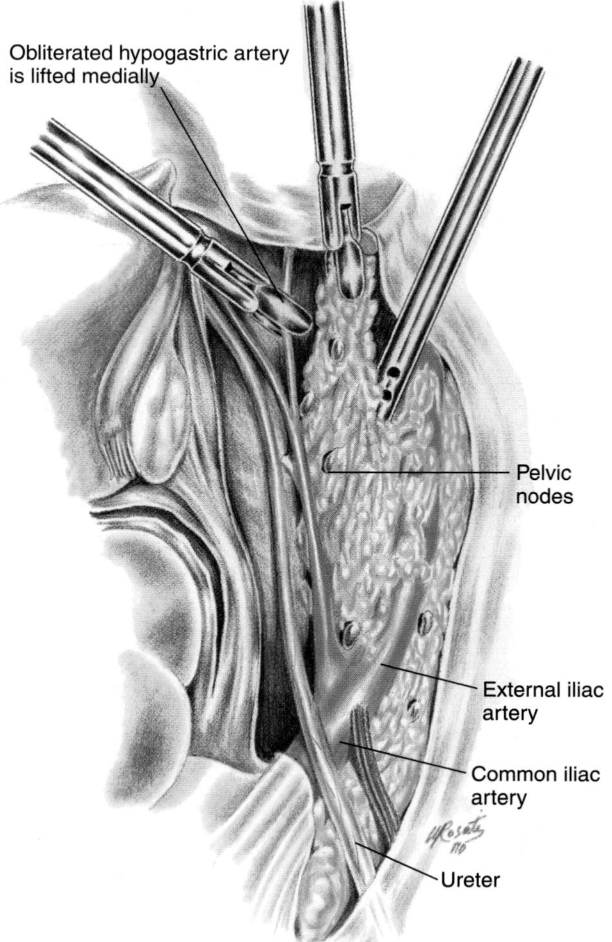

Figure 16-9. Using sharp and blunt dissection, the lymph nodes between the external iliac vessels and the obliterated hypogastric artery are removed. Hemoclips can be used as needed.

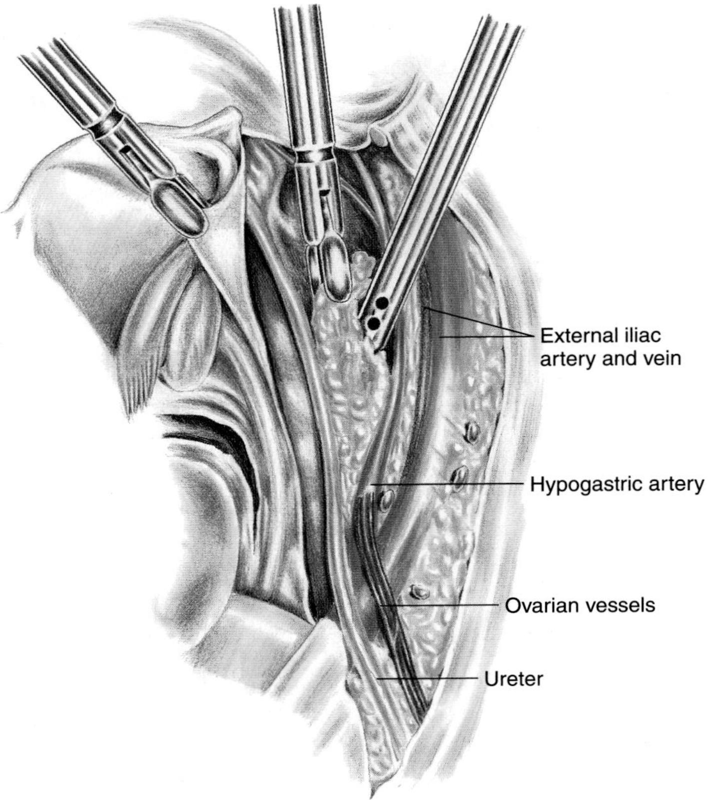

Figure 16-10. The nodes along the hypogastric vessels are excised up to the bifurcation of the common iliac vessels. Caution is necessary to avoid injury to the obturator nerve and hypogastric vein.

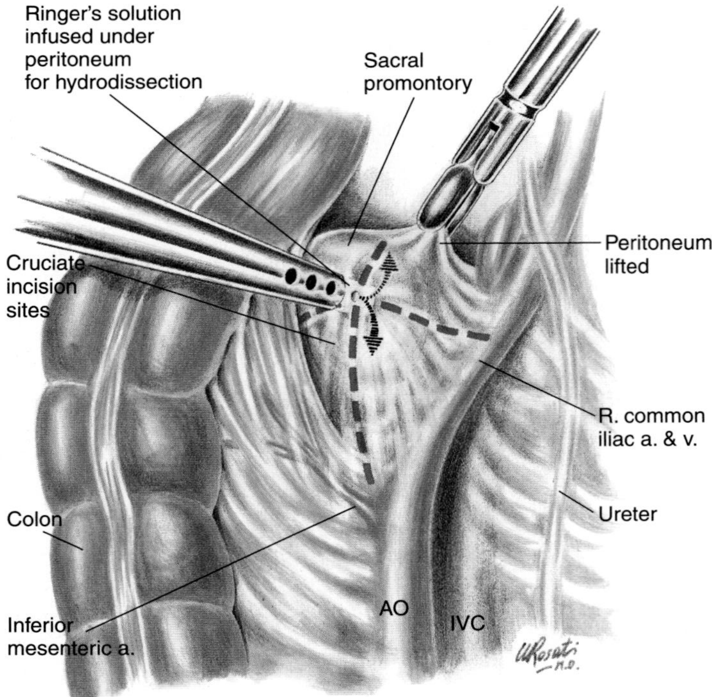

Figure 16-11. The peritoneum over the sacral promontory or lower aorta is incised. The underlying retroperitoneum is developed by using hydrodissection or sharp and blunt dissection.

pelvic side wall to allow for observation of the pelvic vessels. The posterior peritoneum closes spontaneously, and drains are not necessary.

Para-Aortic Lymphadenectomy

The primary trocar is placed through the umbilicus or 2 to 3 cm supraumbilically if a para-aortic lymph node dissection is planned. Depending on the size and anatomy of the patient, the videolaparoscope is placed through the umbilical or suprapubic trocar site. It is easiest to accomplish this procedure with two monitors, each laterally near the patient's sides or shoulders. The patient is in a steep Trendelenburg position (35 to 40 degrees), and it helps to tilt the patient to the left. The bowel is directed toward the upper abdomen and is held in that position with a grasper or laparoscopic fan. The stomach is decompressed with a nasogastric tube, and a preoperative bowel preparation is used, with the patient taking clear liquids for 1 day preoperatively and magnesium citrate the day before surgery. For ovarian cancer, bilateral lymph nodes up to the level of the renal vessels are removed. Patients with endometrial and cervical cancer have lymph nodes removed up to the level of the inferior mesenteric artery.

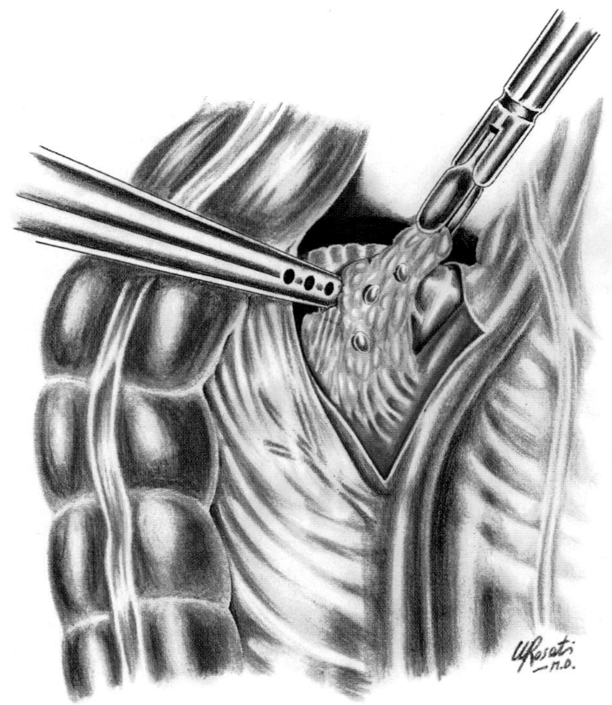

Figure 16-12. Fibrofatty and nodal tissue overlying the sacral promontory are removed. This tissue can contain hypogastric nerves. The left common iliac vein must be observed before commencing this dissection.

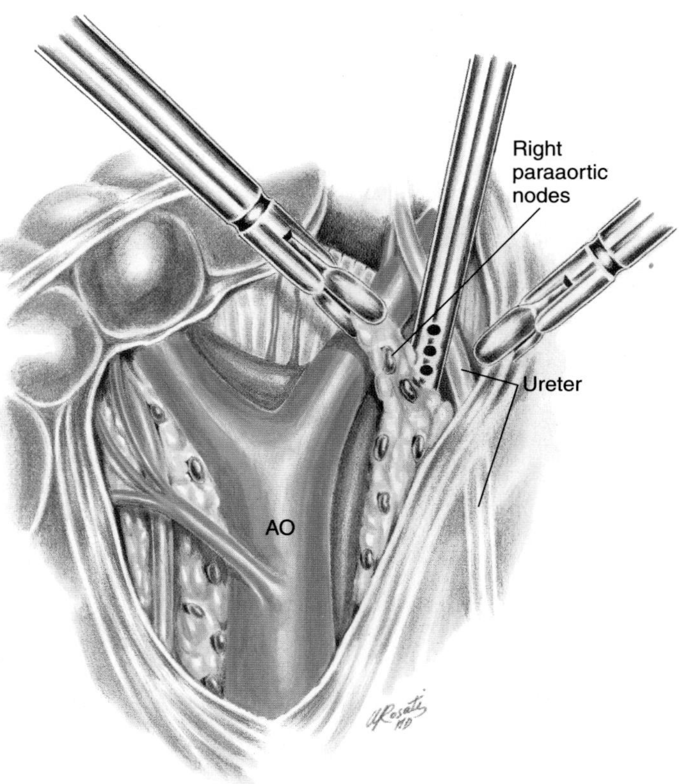

Figure 16-13. The nodal tissue along the aorta (AO) and vena cava is removed above the level of the inferior mesenteric artery. The right ureter must be seen and constantly retracted laterally.

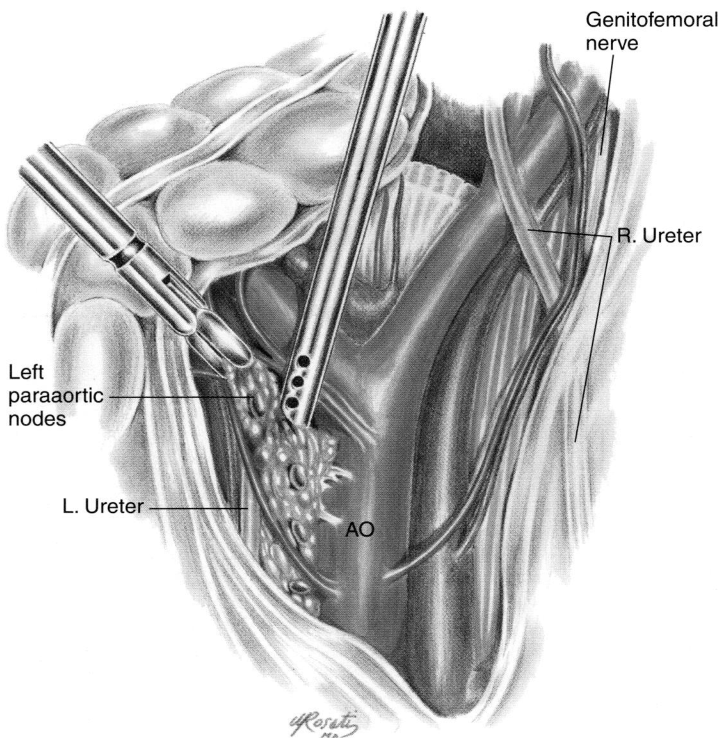

Figure 16-14. The lymph nodes along the left side of the aorta are removed from above the inferior mesenteric artery to below the left common iliac artery.

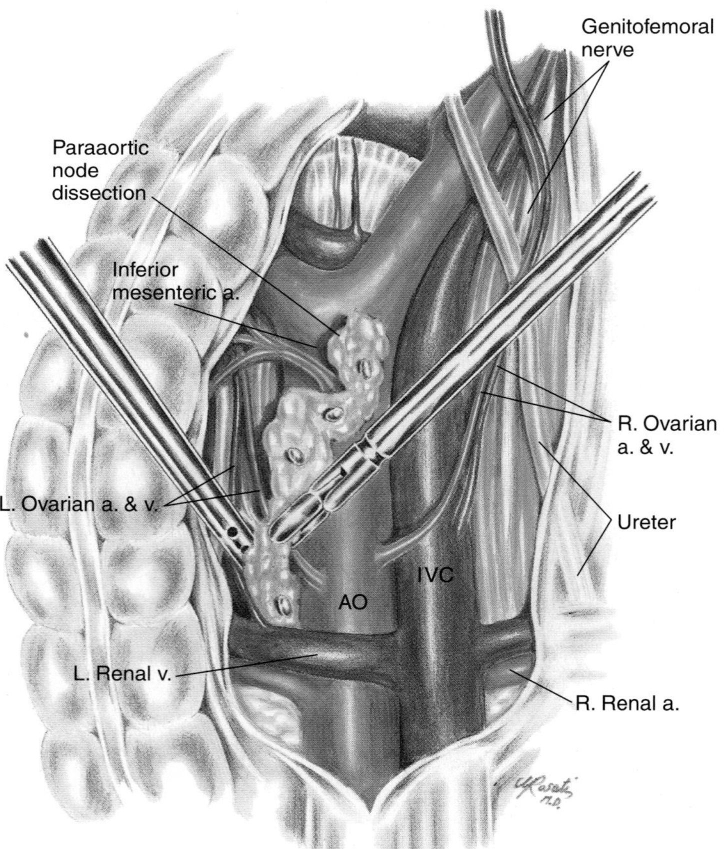

Figure 16-15. In patients who have ovarian carcinoma, the para-aortic nodes are excised to the level of the left renal vein and right ovarian vein.

There are several ways to begin the dissection: incising the peritoneum overlying the aorta, opening the peritoneum over the sacral promontory, and extending the incision overlying the common iliac artery toward the aorta (Figure 16-11). Next the retroperitoneal space is developed by infusing this space with lactated Ringer's solution (hydrodissection) or using blunt and sharp dissection to develop the space lateral to the aorta. Before cutting, it is essential to identify the ureter, separate it from the underlying tissue, and retract it laterally. The nodal tissue overlying the aorta, right common iliac artery, and sacral promontory is removed laterally toward the psoas muscle (Figure 16-12). This maneuver allows the nodal tissue anterior to the vena cava to be detached. The dissection is continued cephalad to the level of the inferior mesenteric artery, removing all lymphatic and fatty tissue anterior to and between the aorta and inferior vena cava (Figure 16-13). It is important to identify the ureter along the inferior border of the dissection and the transverse duodenum along the superior margin of the dissection. Perforating vessels, especially from the vena cava, are electrocoagulated or ligated with hemoclips.

The removal of the left para-aortic nodes can be more difficult because of the location of the sigmoid colon. Caution is necessary to avoid injuring the inferior mesenteric artery, ovarian vessels, and ureter. The left common iliac vein lies at the bifurcation of the aorta. Gentle manipulation is mandatory to avoid vascular injuries, especially before clear observation of the major vessels in the para-aortic region. The dissection proceeds from the aorta laterally toward the left psoas muscle, excising the lymph nodes cephalad to the level of the inferior mesenteric artery and caudad to the level of the left common iliac artery (Figure 16-14). This allows the surgeon to dissect laterally in a plane that is beneath the inferior mesenteric artery and the mesentery of the sigmoid colon.[8] It is important not to dissect laterally until the adventitia of the aorta is incised to prevent entering the wrong plane.

In ovarian cancer, the para-aortic lymphadenectomy is extended to the level of the left renal vein and right ovarian vein (Figure 16-15). This is especially difficult in obese patients. The vena cava and aorta are separated from the transverse duodenum by blunt and sharp dissection. On the right side, the dissection continues to the origin of the ovarian vein from the vena cava. On the left side, the operation proceeds to the level where the left renal vein drains into the vena cava. The ovarian vessels are ligated, if necessary, to prevent bleeding. After the lymphadenectomy is completed, evaluation of the area with decreased pneumoperitoneal pressure is done to ensure adequate hemostasis. As with pelvic lymphadenectomy, the peritoneum is not closed and drains are not placed. Interceed can be applied to decrease postoperative adhesions (Figure 16-16).[17]

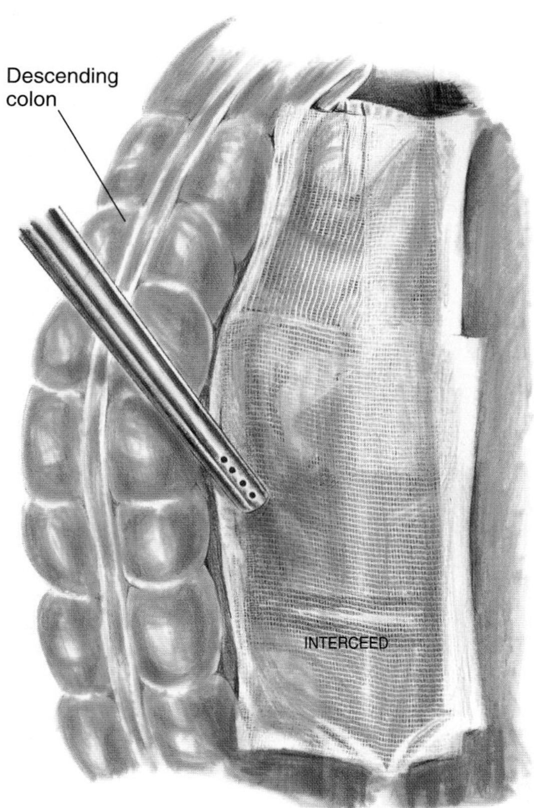

Figure 16-16. Interceed is applied to cover the openings in the peritoneum.

Laparoscopically Assisted Radical Vaginal Hysterectomy

The pelvic lymphadenectomy is carried out first. If any nodes are positive, the hysterectomy is not done. In patients with stage IB1 or smaller lesions, para-aortic lymph node dissection is not required as long as the pelvic lymph nodes are normal and no suspicious para-aortic nodes are found.[21,68] The paravesical and pararectal spaces were created during the pelvic lymph node dissection (Figures 16-17 and 16-18). The round ligament that was cut

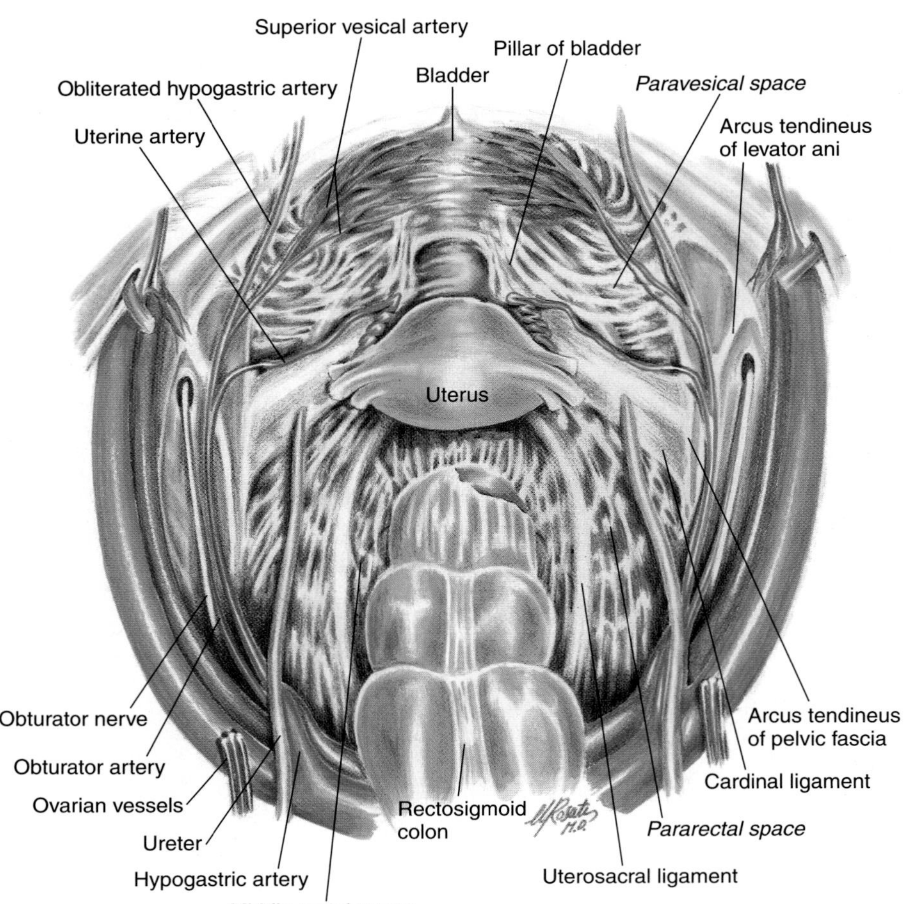

Figure 16-17. The anatomic structures of the paravesical and pararectal spaces.

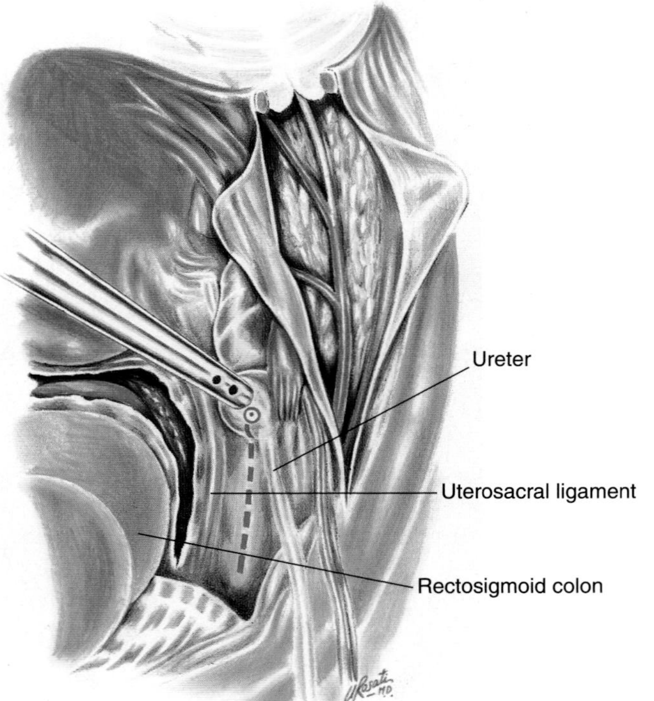

Figure 16-18. The space lateral to the ureter and medial to the hypogastric artery is opened after the peritoneum over the ureter has been incised.

Figure 16-19. The uterine vessel is ligated or coagulated at its origin from the anterior division of the hypogastric artery.

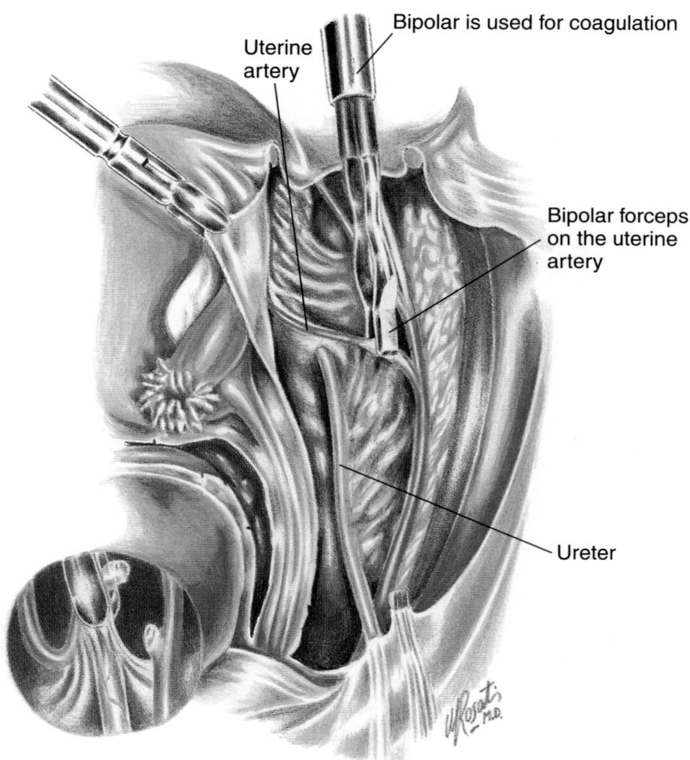

to develop the pelvic retroperitoneal spaces is ligated close to the pelvic side wall. The uterine artery is located by finding the obliterated hypogastric artery and tracing it proximally until the uterine vessels are reached or clipped. The uterine vessels are skeletonized, desiccated, and cut just medial to their origin from the anterior division of the hypogastric artery (Figure 16-19). The medial pedicle of the uterine vessels is grasped and pulled anteriorly to assist in the unroofing of the vesicouterine ligament (the "web") above the ureter (Figure 16-20). Additional vessels between the

Figure 16-20. The vesicouterine ligament (the web) above the ureter is unroofed by pulling the uterine pedicle anteriorly and cutting the ligament.

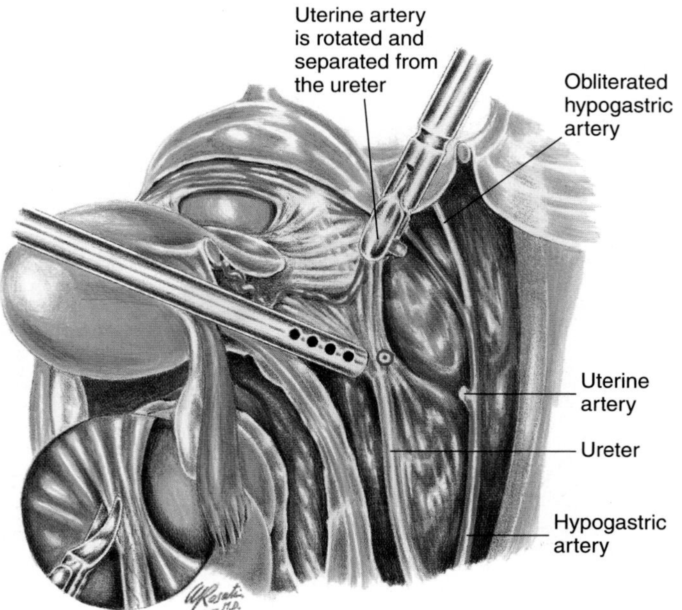

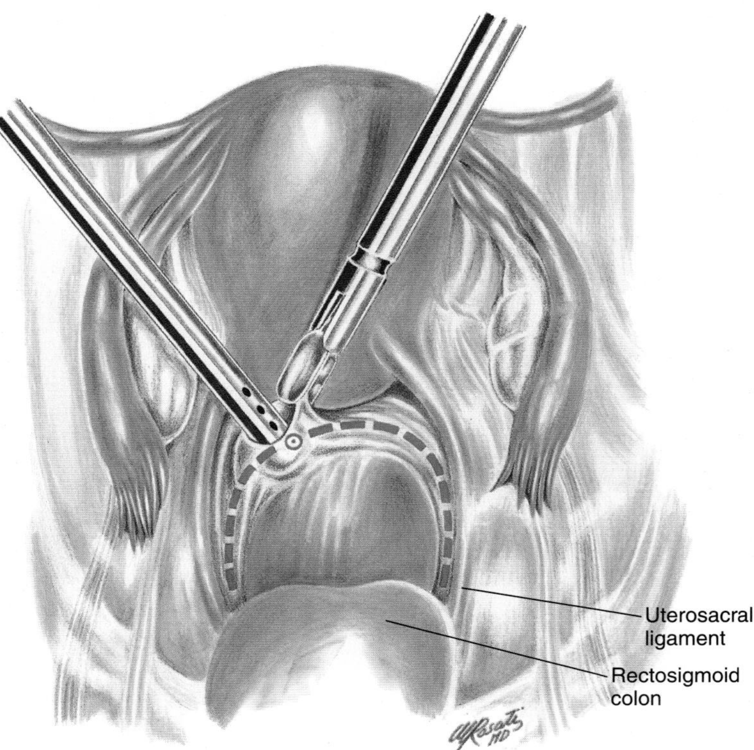

Figure 16-21. While an assistant does a rectovaginal examination, an incision is made between the uterosacral ligaments at the junction of the posterior aspect of the cervix and vagina. The rectum is pushed off the posterior vagina by using sharp and blunt dissection.

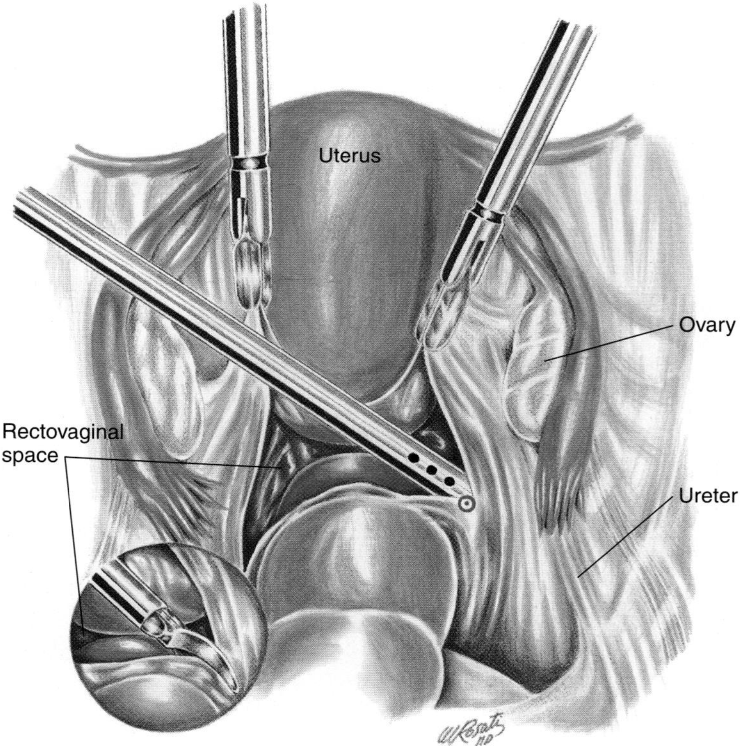

Figure 16-22. Blunt and scissors (*inset*) dissection are used to further develop the rectovaginal space.

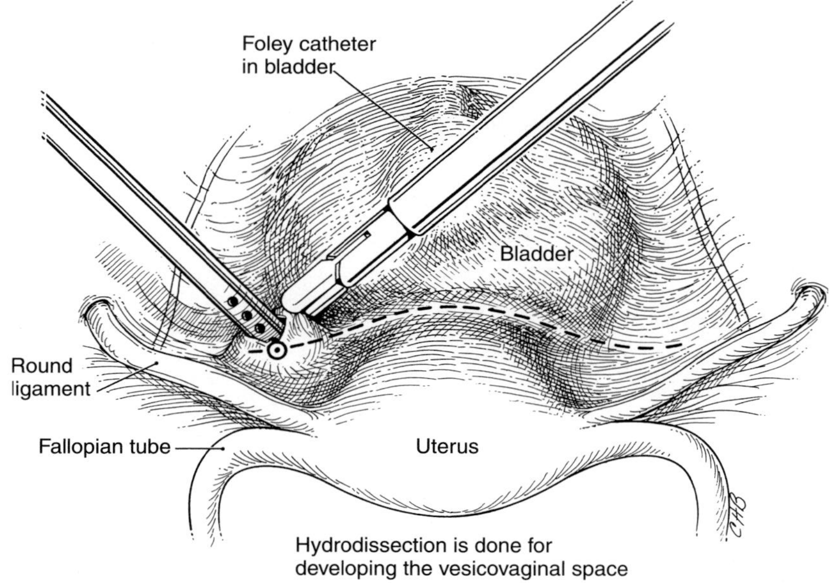

Figure 16-23. The anterior leaf of the broad ligament is elevated with grasping forceps, and hydrodissection is carried out. An incision is made toward the bladder, using sharp and blunt dissection.

uterine artery and the underlying ureter are ligated during this portion of the procedure. The rectovaginal space is dissected while an assistant delineates the rectum and vagina by carrying out a rectovaginal digital exam (Figures 16-21 and 16-22). The cul-de-sac is incised and the rectum is pushed from the posterior vaginal wall by using the CO_2 laser, blunt dissection, and hydrodissection to a level 4 to 5 cm below the cervix. The vesicovaginal space is developed by sharp dissection or the CO_2 laser after the bladder space has been injected with lactated Ringer's solution. Once this space is formed, the bladder is pushed off of the cervix and the upper third of the vagina by using a grasper or the suction-irrigator (Figures 16-23 and 16-24). The anterior vesicouterine ligament is divided by using the CO_2 laser or electrocoagulation and sharp dissection. The ureters are freed from the posterior leaf of the broad ligament and skeletonized down to the bladder. Infundibulopelvic or utero-ovarian ligaments, depending on the patient's menopausal status, are ligated with the bipolar forceps or the endoscopic stapler at this point or at the beginning of the procedure.

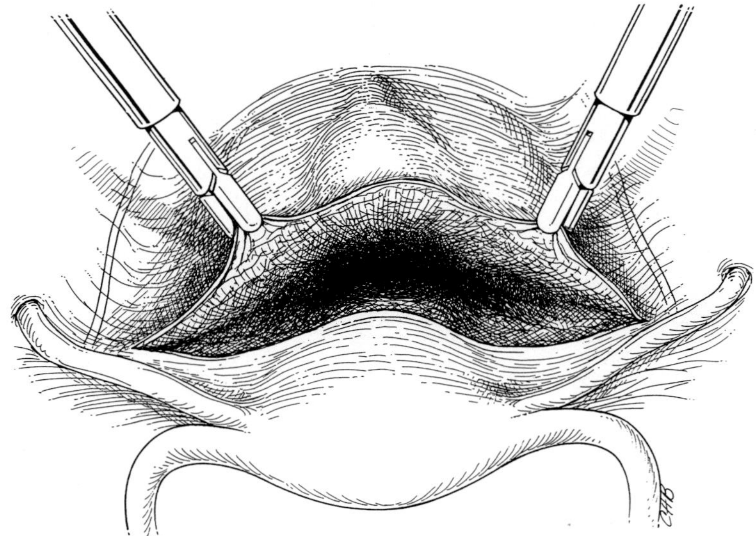

Figure 16-24. The bladder flap is held with grasping forceps and blunt, sharp and hydrodisection were used for further development of the vesicovaginal space.

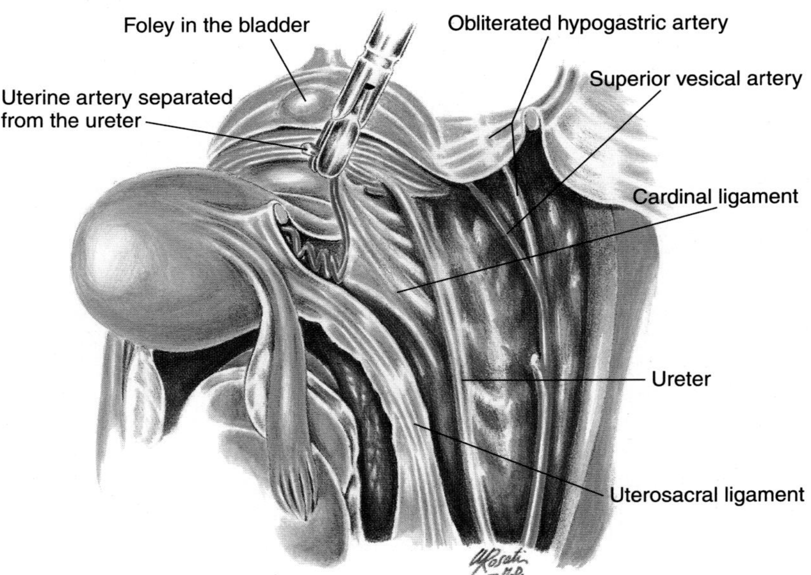

Figure 16-25. The ureter has been mobilized laterally out of the ureteric tunnel.

The uterosacral and cardinal ligaments and remaining parametria are desiccated with bipolar forceps or a harmonic scalpel and sequentially transected using sharp dissection or the endoscopic staplers (Figures 16-25 through 16-27). The line of transection is made lateral to the cervix, with the distance being dependent on the size of the lesion and the requirement to remove the tumor with at least 1 cm of normal parametria surrounding it. A type III radical hysterectomy

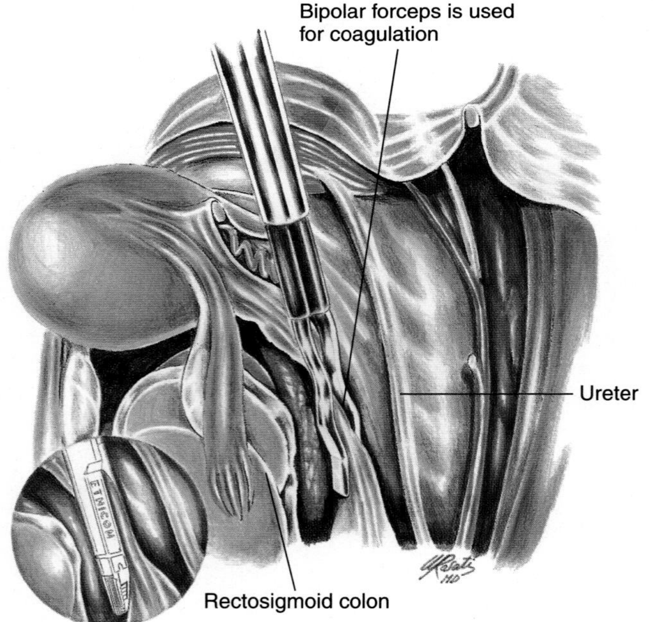

Figure 16-26. The uterosacral ligaments are coagulated; staplers and the harmonic scalpel are equally effective.

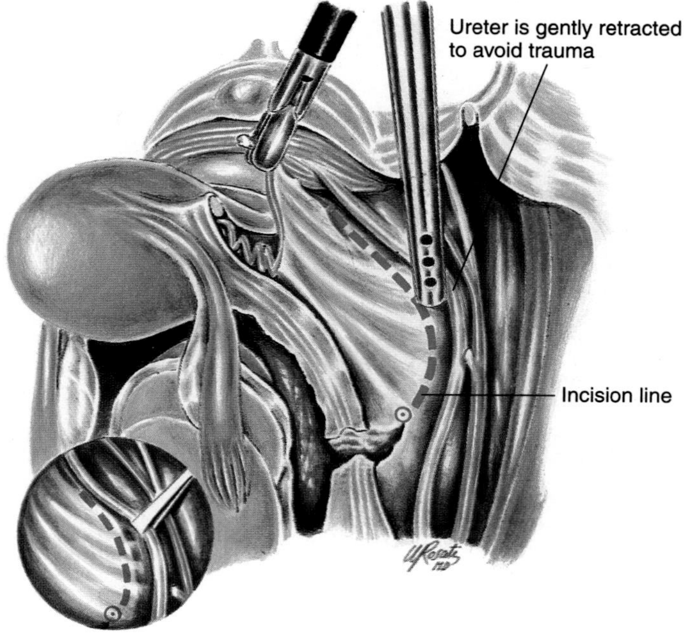

Figure 16-27. The cardinal ligament or parametrium is cut laterally, with the ureter retracted to avoid injury.

includes transecting the uterosacral and cardinal ligaments as laterally as possible for patients with a stage Ib lesion. With a stage Ia2 tumor, a type II or modified radical hysterectomy is carried out. The latter is less extensive than a radical hysterectomy and involves transecting the uterosacral and cardinal ligaments at the midpoint between their lateral attachments and uterine insertions (Figures 16-28 and 16-29). For stage IB1 or smaller lesions, a 2-cm parametrial border lateral to the cervix is sufficient. The vaginal dissection occurs approximately 2 to 3 cm below the cervix.

The vagina is entered anteriorly and posteriorly using the CO_2 laser after a sponge on a ring forceps is placed in the vagina to push the walls of the vagina anteriorly and posteriorly and help

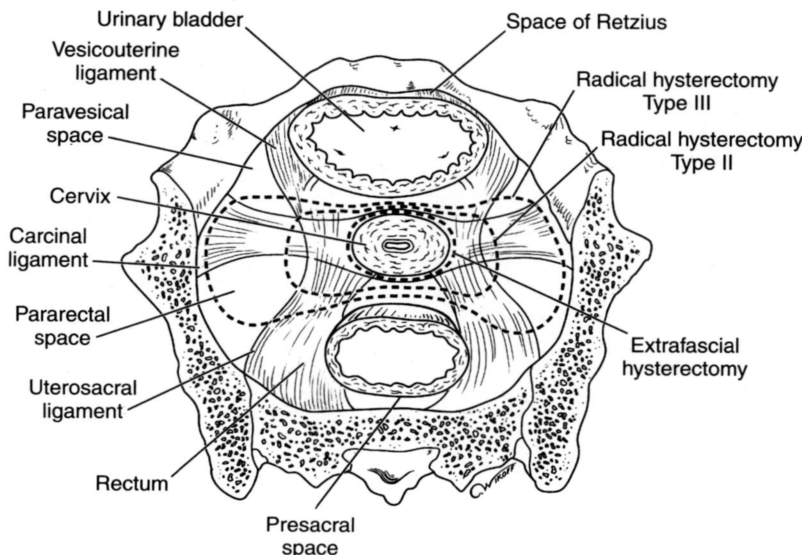

Figure 16-28. A schematic representation of the anatomic areas and sites of division of the cardinal and uterosacral ligaments for type II and type III radical hysterectomies.

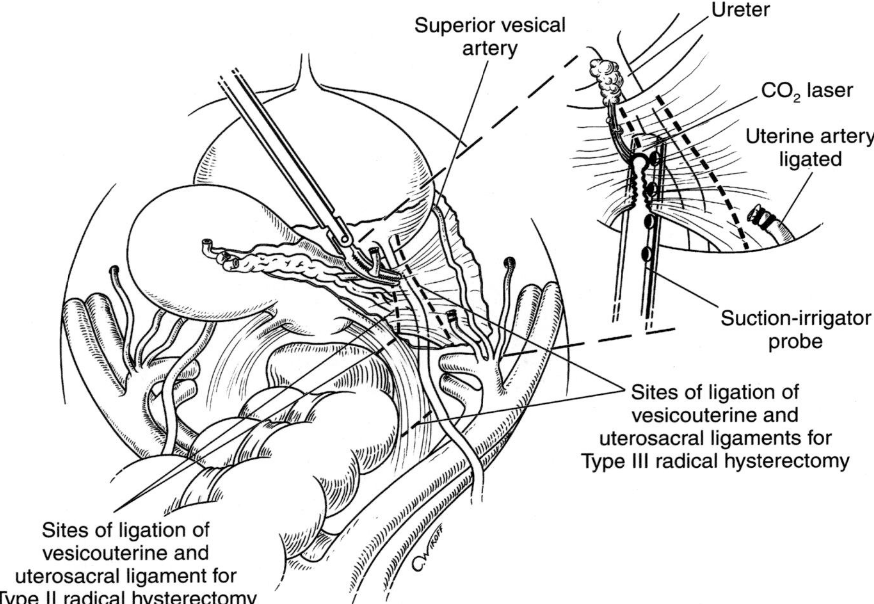

Figure 16-29. After the ureter has been dissected and mobilized laterally, the sites for ligation of the vesicouterine and uterosacral ligaments are seen.

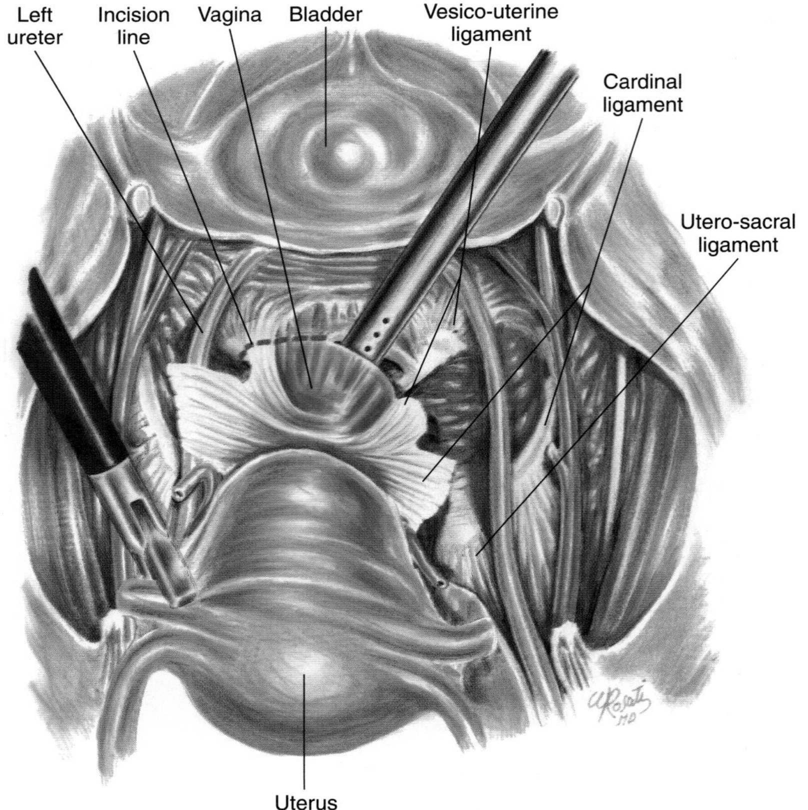

Figure 16-30. The vagina has been opened anteriorly and posteriorly using the laser, electrosurgical scissors, or harmonic scalpel.

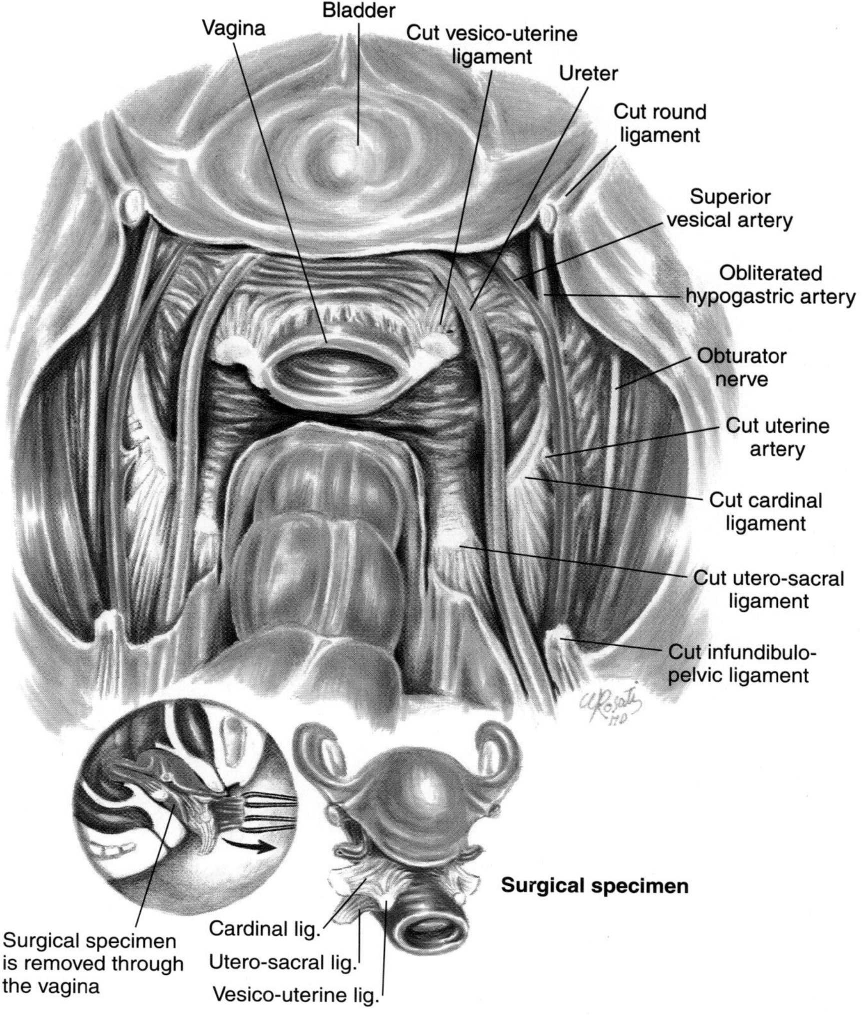

Figure 16-31. The vagina has been incised circumferentially, and the specimen has been removed abdominally. The inset shows its removal vaginally.

the surgeon know when the vagina has been entered (Figure 16-30). The procedure is completed vaginally or laparoscopically by incising the vagina circumferentially around the cervix, removing approximately 3 cm of the upper vagina (Figure 16-31). Residual cardinal ligaments are mobilized anteriorly and posteriorly and divided 2 cm lateral to the cervix. The uterus is removed through the vagina, and the vault is closed vaginally or laparoscopically with sutures. A urethral or suprapubic catheter is placed and kept in place for a minimum of 7 days. No retroperitoneal drains are required. Interceed is applied to descrease the formation of postoperative adhesions (Figure 16-32).

There are many variations of this operation, with the main difference being the amount of the procedure that is done laparoscopically. Some physicians carry out the laparoscopic portion to include uterine dissection to the cardinal ligaments, separation and ligation of the uterine vessels at their origin, medial displacement of the ureters, and pelvic lymphadenectomy. The rest is completed vaginally, using the Schauta technique. Other gynecologists do a radical vaginal hysterectomy, using the laparoscope only for the pelvic lymphadenectomy and to create the paravesical and pararectal spaces. The remainder of the procedure, including the removal of the ureter from the vesicouterine ligament, is done vaginally. The choice of a procedure is based on the experience and skill of the surgeon.

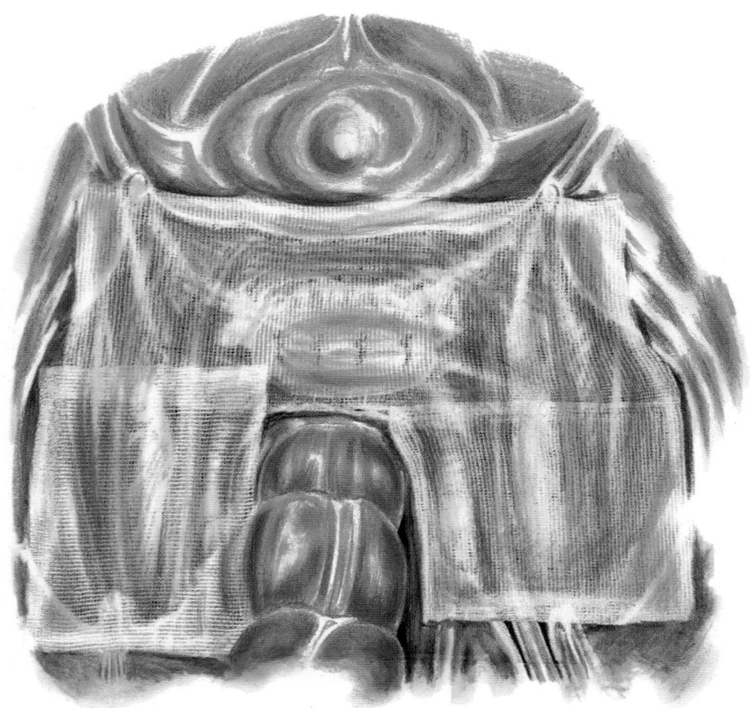

Figure 16-32. Interceed has covered the denuded areas in the pelvis.

Conclusions

Operative laparoscopy has many potential uses in gynecologic oncology, including laparoscopic lymphadenectomy, laparoscopically assisted vaginal hysterectomy, second-look laparoscopy, and laparoscopically assisted radical vaginal hysterectomy or total laparoscopic radical hysterectomy. When these procedures are done laparoscopically, many patients have shorter hospitalization and recovery periods. If continuing reports reveal the feasibility, safety, diagnostic accuracy, and treatment equivalence of these operations, wider acceptance and interest in this useful surgical approach modality probably will develop.

References

1. Dargent D, Salvat J. *Lienvahissement ganglionnaire pelvien*. Paris: MEDSI, 1989.
2. Querleu D, Leblanc E, Catelain B. Laparoscopic pelvic lymphadenectomy. *Am J Obstet Gynecol* 1991; 164:579.
3. Nezhat C, Nezhat F, Silfen SL. Videolaseroscopy: The CO_2 laser for advanced operative laparoscopy. *Obstet Gynecol Clin North Am* 1991 Sep; 18(3):585-604.
4. Nezhat C, Burell MO, Nezhat FR, et al. Laparoscopic radical hysterectomy with paraaortic and pelvic node dissection. *Am J Obstet Gynecol* 1992; 166:864.
5. Childers JM, Hatch K, Surwit EA. The role of laparoscopic lymphadenectomy in the management of cervical carcinoma. *Gynecol Oncol* 1992; 47:38.
6. Fowler JR, Carter JW, Carlson R, et al. Lymph node yield from laparoscopic lymphadenectomy in cervical cancer: A comparative study. *Gynecol Oncol* 1993; 51:187.
7. Childers JM, Brzechffa PR, Hatch KD, et al. Laparoscopically assisted surgical staging of endometrial cancer. *Gynecol Oncol* 1993; 51:33.
8. Pomel C, Provencher D, Dauplat J, et al. Laparoscopic staging of early ovarian cancer. *Gynecol Oncol* 1995; 58:301.
9. Childers JM, Hatch KD, Tran A, et al. Laparoscopic paraaortic lymphadenectomy in gynecologic malignancies. *Obstet Gynecol* 1993; 82:741.
10. Nezhat CR, Nezhat FR, Ramirez CE, et al. Laparoscopic radical hysterectomy and laparoscopic assisted vaginal radical hysterectomy

with pelvic and paraaortic node dissection. *J Gynecol Surg* 1993; 9:105.
11. Querleu D. Laparoscopic paraaortic node sampling in gynecologic oncology: A preliminary experience. *Gynecol Oncol* 1993; 49:24.
12. Canis M, Mage G, Wattiez A, et al. La chirurgie endoscopique a-t-elle une place dans la chirurgie radicale du cancer du col uterin? *J Gynecol Obstet Biol Reprod* 1990; 19:921.
13. Chu KK, Chang SD, Chen FP, et al. Laparoscopic surgical staging in cervical cancer—preliminary experience among Chinese. *Gynecol Oncol* 1997; 64:49.
14. Dottino PR, Tobias DH, Beddoe AM, et al. Laparoscopic lymphadenectomy for gynecologic malignancies. *Gynecol Oncol* 1999; 73:383.
15. Nezhat C, Nezhat F, Silfen SI. Videolaseroscopy: The CO_2 laser for advanced operative laparoscopy. *Obstet Gynecol Clin North Am* 1991; 18:585.
16. Roy M, Plante M, Renaud MC, et al. Vaginal radical hysterectomy versus abdominal radical hysterectomy in the treatment of early-stage cervical cancer. *Gynecol Oncol* 1996; 62:336.
17. Schneider A, Possover M, Kamprath S, et al. Laparoscopy-assisted radical vaginal hysterectomy modified according to Schauta-Stoeckel. *Obstet Gynecol* 1996; 88:1057.
18. Dembo AJ, Davy M, Stenwig AE. Prognostic factors in patients with stage I epithelial ovarian cancer. *Obstet Gynecol* 1990; 75:263.
19. Berman M, Keys H, Creasman W, et al. Survival and patterns of recurrence in cervical cancer metastatic to perioaortic lymph nodes: A Gynecologic Oncology Group study. *Gynecol Oncol* 1984; 19:8.
20. Patsner B, Sedlacek TV, Lovecchio J. Paraaortic node sampling in small (3-cm or less) stage 1b invasive cervical cancer. *Gynecol Oncol* 1992; 44:53.
21. Piver MS, Barlow JJ, Krishnamsetty R. Five-year survival (with no evidence of disease) in patients with biopsy-confirmed aortic node metastasis from cervical carcinoma. *Am J Obstet Gynecol* 1981; 193:575.
22. Wharton JT, Jones HW III, Day TG, et al. Preirradiation celiotomy and extended field irradiation for invasive carcinoma of the cervix. *Obstet Gynecol* 1977; 49:333.
23. Ballon SC, Berman ML, Lagasse LD, et al. Survival after extraperitoneal pelvic and paraaortic lymphadenectomy and radiation therapy in cervical carcinoma. *Obstet Gynecol* 1981; 57:90.
24. Twiggs LB, Potish RA, George RJ, Adcock LL. Pretreatment extraperitoneal surgical staging in primary carcinoma of the cervix uteri. *Surg Gynecol Obstet* 1984; 158:243.
25. Weiser EB, Bundy BN, Hoskins WJ, et al. Extraperitoneal versus transperitoneal selective paraaortic lymphadenectomy in the pretreatment surgical staging of advanced cervical carcinoma (a Gynecologic Oncology Group study). *Gynecol Oncol* 1989; 33:283.
26. Fowler JM, Hartenbach EM, Reynolds HT, et al. Pelvic adhesion formation after pelvic lymphadenectomy: Comparison between transperitoneal laparoscopy and extraperitoneal laparotomy in a porcine model. *Gynecol Oncol* 1994; 55(1):25.
27. Chen MD, Teigen GA, Reynolds HT, et al. Laparoscopy versus laparotomy: An evaluation of adhesion formation after pelvic and paraaortic lymphadenectomy in a porcine model. *Am J Obstet Gynecol* 1998; 178(3):499.
28. Massi G, Savino L, Susini T. Schauta-Amreich vaginal hysterectomy and Wertheim-Miegs abdominal hysterectomy in the treatment of cervical cancer. A retrospective analysis. *Am J Obstet Gynecol* 1993; 168:928.
29. Canis M, Maye G, Wattiez A, et al. Vaginally assisted laparoscopic radical hysterectomy. *J Gynecol Oncol* 1992; 8:103.
30. Homesley HD, Raben M, Blake DD, et al. Relationship of lesion size to survival in patients with stage IB squamous cell carcinoma of the cervix uteri treated by radiation therapy. *Surg Gynecol Oncol* 1980; 150:529.
31. Perez CA, Gribsby PW, Nene SM, et al. Effect of tumor size on the prognosis of carcinoma of the uterine cervix treated with irradiation alone. *Cancer* 1992; 69:2796.
32. Eifel PJ, Morris M, Wharton JT, Oswald MJ. The influence of tumor size and morphology on the outcome of patients with FIGO stage IB squamous cell carcinoma of the uterine cervix. *Int J Radiat Oncol Biol Phys* 1994; 29:9.
33. Van Nagell JR Jr, Rayburn W, Donaldson ES, et al. Therapeutic implications of patients of recurrence in cancer of the uterine cervix. *Cancer* 1979; 44:2354.
34. Boyce J, Fruchter R, Nicastri A. Prognostic factors in stage I carcinoma of the cervix. *Gynecol Oncol* 1981; 12:154.
35. Hatch K, Hems CW. Cancer of the cervix surgical treatment, in Blackledge GRP, Jordan JA, Shingleton HM, eds., *Textbook*

of Gynecologic Oncology London: Saunders, 1991.
36. DiSaia PJ, Creasman WT. Invasive Cervical Cancer, in *Clinical Gynecologic Oncology*, 5d ed. St. Louis: Mosby, 1997.
37. Miller B, Morris M, Rutledge F, et al. Aborted exenteration procedures in recurrent cervical cancer. *Gynecol Oncol* 1993; 50:94.
38. Plante M, Roy M. Operative laparoscopy prior to a pelvic exenteration in patients with recurrent cervical cancer. *Gynecol Oncol* 1998; 69:94.
39. Chen SS, Lee L. Incidence of paraaortic and pelvic lymph node metastasis in epithelial ovarian cancer. *Gynecol Oncol* 1983; 16:95.
40. Young RC, Decker DG, Wharton JT, et al. Staging laparotomy in early ovarian cancer. *JAMA* 1983; 250:3072.
41. Van Nagell JR Jr, DePriest PD, Puls LE, et al. Ovarian cancer screening in asymptomatic postmenopausal women by transvaginal sonography. *Cancer* 1991; 68:458.
42. Nezhat F, Nezhat C, Welander CE, Benigno B. Four ovarian cancers diagnosed during laparoscopic management of 1011 women with adnexal masses. *Am J Obstet Gynecol* 1992; 167:790.
43. Vogl SE, Pagano M, Kaplan BH, et al. Cisplatin based combination chemotherapy for advanced ovarian cancer: High overall response rate with curative potential only in women with small tumor burdens. *Cancer* 1983; 51:2024.
44. Neijt JP, ten Bokkel Huinink WW, van der Burg MEL, et al. Long-term survival in ovarian cancer: Mature data from the Netherlands Joint Study Group for Ovarian Cancer. *Eur J Cancer* 1991; 27:1367.
45. Omura GA, Bundy BN, Berek JS, et al. Randomized trial of cyclophosphamide plus cisplatin with or without doxorubicin in ovarian carcinoma: A Gynecologic Oncology Group study. *J Clin Oncol* 1989; 7:457.
46. Van der Burg MEL, van Lent M, Buyse M, et al. The effect of debulking surgery after induction chemotherapy on the prognosis in advanced epithelial ovarian cancer. *N Engl J Med* 1995; 332:629.
47. Querleu D. Laparoscopic paraaortic node sampling in gynecologic oncology: A preliminary experience. *Gynecol Oncol* 1993; 49:24.
48. Querleu D, LeBlanc E. Laparoscopic infrarenal paraaortic lymph node dissection for restaging of carcinoma of the ovary or fallopian tube. *Cancer* 1994; 73(5):1467.
49. Amara DP, Nezhat C, Nelson NR, et al. Operative laparoscopy in the management of ovarian cancer. *Surg Laparosc Endosc* 1996; 6(1):38.
50. Childers JM, Lang J, Surwit E, Hatch KD. Laparoscopic surgical staging of ovarian cancer. *Gynecol Oncol* 1995; 59:25.
51. Hreshchyshyn MM, Park RC, Blessing JA, et al. The role of adjuvant therapy in Stage I ovarian cancer. *Am J Obstet Gynecol* 1980; 138:139.
52. Gleeson NC, Nicosia FV, Mark JE, et al. Abdominal wall metastases from ovarian carcinoma after laparoscopy. *Am J Obstet Gynecol* 1993; 169:522.
53. Kruitwagen RF, Swinkels BM, Keyser KG, et al. Incidence and effect on survival of abdominal wall metastases at trocar or puncture sites following laparoscopy of paracentesis in women with ovarian cancer. *Gynecol Oncol* 1996; 60(2):233.
54. Childers JM, Aqua KA, Surwit EA, et al. Abdominal-wall tumor implantation after laparoscopy for malignant conditions. *Obstet Gynecol* 1994; 84(5):765.
55. Canis M, Botchorishvili R, Wattiez A, et al. Tumor growth and dissemination after laparotomy and CO_2 pneumoperitoneum: A rat ovarian cancer model. *Obstet Gynecol* 1998; 92:104.
56. Freidman JB, Weiss NS. Second thoughts about second-look laparotomy in advanced ovarian cancer. *N Engl J Med* 1990; 322:1079.
57. Rubin SC, Hoskins WJ, Hakes TB, et al. Recurrence after negative second-look laparotomy for ovarian cancer: Analysis of risk factors. *Am J Obstet Gynecol* 1988; 159:1094.
58. Berek JS, Hacker NF, Lagasse ID, et al. Second-look laparotomy in stage III epithelial ovarian cancer: Clinical variables associated with disease status. *Obstet Gynecol* 1984; 64:297.
59. Schwartz PE, Smith JP. Second-look operation in ovarian cancer. *Am J Obstet Gynecol* 1980; 138:1124.
60. Bagley CM, Young RC, Schein PS, et al: Ovarian cancer metastatic to the diaphragm frequently undiagnosed at laparotomy: A preliminary report. *Am J Obstet Gynecol* 1973; 116:247.
61. Abu-Rustum NR, Barakat RR, Siegle PL, et al. Second-look operation for epithelial ovarian cancer: Laparoscopy or laparotomy? *Obstet Gynecol* 1996; 88:549.

62. Nicoletto MO, Tumolo S, Talamini R, et al. Surgical second look in ovarian cancer: A randomized study in patients with laparoscopic complete remission in a Northeastern Oncology Cooperative Group-Ovarian Cancer Cooperative Study. *J Clin Oncol* 1997; 15(3)994.
63. Lotocki RJ, Copeland LJ, DePetrillo AD, et al. Stage I endometrial adenocarcinoma: Treatment results in 835 patients. *Am J Obstet Gynecol* 1983; 146:141.
64. Coweles TA, Magrina JF, Materson BJ, Capen CV. Comparison of clinical and surgical staging in patients with endometrial carcinoma. *Obstet Gynecol* 1985; 66:413.
65. Boronow RC, Morrow CP, Creasman WT, et al. Surgical staging in endometrial cancer: Clinicopathologic findings of a prospective study. *Obstet Gynecol* 1984; 63:825.
66. Creasman WT, Morrow CP, Bundy BN, et al. Surgical pathologic spread patterns of endometrial cancer. *Cancer* 1987; 60:2035.
67. Nezhat C, Nezhat F, Gordon S, et al. Laparoscopic versus abdominal hysterectomy. *J Reprod Med* 1992; 37:247.
68. Hackett TE, Olt G, Sorosky J, et al. Surgical predictors of para-aortic metastases in early-stage cervical carcinoma. *Gynecol Oncol* 1995; 59:15.

17

Presacral Neurectomy and Uterosacral Transection and Ablation

Presacral Neurectomy

Introduction

Dysmenorrhea that is severe enough to limit social activities afflicts more than 18 million women in the United States. Surgical management of dysmenorrhea has been reviewed by Fontaine and Hermann.[1] In 1899, Jaboulay[2] described severance of sacral sympathetic afferent fibers using a posterior extraperitoneal approach, and in the same year, Ruggi[3] described resections of the utero-ovarian plexus to relieve dysmenorrhea. Leriche[4] advocated periarterial sympathectomy of the internal iliac (hypogastric) arteries, and Cotte[5] reported excellent results after transection of the superior hypogastric plexus. Cotte claimed that his technique was simpler and as effective as the Leriche operation. Other surgical procedures have been reported.[6,7] Cotte did the first "presacral neurectomy" in 1924. He emphasized that only nerve tissue within the interiliac triangle should be removed and that resection of all nerve elements within the triangle was essential. Both measures tend to maximize effectiveness and minimize complications. In the absence of precise physiologic data concerning the presacral nerve (superior hypogastric plexus of Hovelacque), it is difficult to explain the successful results obtained with presacral neurectomy.[8]

The introduction of nonsteroidal anti-inflammatory drugs, oral contraceptives, danazol, and gonadotropin-releasing hormone (GnRH) analogs since the 1960s significantly reduced interest in presacral neurectomy for dysmenorrhea. However, it has been shown that medical treatment of dysmenorrhea fails in 20 to 25% of patients. For this reason, presacral neurectomy remains a useful alternative for women who are not responsive to medical therapy. Because of advances in minimally invasive operations, there is renewed interest in neurectomy for the treatment of disabling pelvic pain. It is possible to successfully treat most patients who complain of midline pelvic pain with medication or laparoscopic presacral neurectomy.

Anatomy

Pain impulses from the cervix, the body of the uterus, and the proximal fallopian tube are transmitted through afferent fibers that accompany sympathetic nerves into the spinal cord at the thoracic and lumbar levels. The sympathetic nerves that emerge from the uterus pass through the uterosacral ligament along the cardinal ligament to join the pelvic plexus. Parasympathetic fibers from S-1 through S-4 travel with the phrenic nerve through the pelvic plexuses (Frankenhauser's ganglia) lateral to the cervix to reach the bladder, rectum, and uterus.

The presacral nerve is a plexus of nerves known as the superior hypogastric plexus. Elaut,[9] Davis,[10] Labate,[11] and Curtis and associates,[12] among others, reported anatomic observations of this plexus based on cadaver dissections. The variable anatomic findings emphasize the differences surgeons encounter. In some dissections, one-third to two-thirds of the fibers were observed left of the midline; the rest were in central locations. In 8 to 15%, the mesocolon was over the triangle, making neurectomy difficult or impossible. Findings of a single nerve were reported in 8 to 13% of dissections.[11] Labate did 75 dissections and described a plexus in 84%, parallel nerve trunks in 8%, and single nerves in 8%. In 27 presacral neurectomies, Black[13] found three (11.1%) single nerves and 23 (85.2%) plexiform elements. Davis[6] reported an accessory ureter lying on the midline in one instance during 20 presacral neurectomies.

Within the interiliac trigone, the common iliac artery and ureter are on the right and the common iliac vein is on the left. The inferior mesenteric, superior hemorrhoidal, and midsacral arteries are in the center of the prelumbar space. This trigone is defined caudally by the sacral promontory and laterally by the common iliac arteries; the superior edge of the triangle is delineated by the aortic bifurcation. Centrally and to the left, multiple nerve fibers, sometimes in bundles, run caudally from the aortic plexus above and through the interiliac trigone to form the superior hypogastric plexus. These fibers, representing the presacral nerve, are buried in loose areolar tissue. They display no particular patterns and vary among individuals. To the left and right of the trigone, both ureters are identified before they transect the nerve bundle. The left ureter is more difficult to see because it lies under the rectosigmoid and mesocolon.

Indications

Presacral neurectomy is indicated for patients who have disabling midline dysmenorrhea and pelvic pain and have not responded to appropriate and adequate medication. The success rate is difficult to predict, although the operation is likely to relieve pain in 50 to 75% of patients.

Presacral neurectomy does not alleviate adnexal pain because ovarian innervation originates from the ovarian plexus, a meshwork of nerve fibers that arise from the aortic and renal plexuses and accompany the ovarian artery throughout its course.

Primary dysmenorrhea or dysmenorrhea caused by endometriosis may be an indication for endoscopic corrective procedures followed by presacral neurectomy. In most patients, dyspareunia is decreased and chronic pain is alleviated.

Technique

After associated pelvic abnormalities have been treated, the steep Trendelenburg position is used and the patient is tilted slightly to the left. The aortic bifurcation, the common iliac arteries and veins, the ureters, and the sacral promontory are identified; the peritoneum overlying the promontory is elevated with grasping forceps, and a small opening is made with the CO_2 laser or scissors or any other cutting modality (Figure 17-1). Through

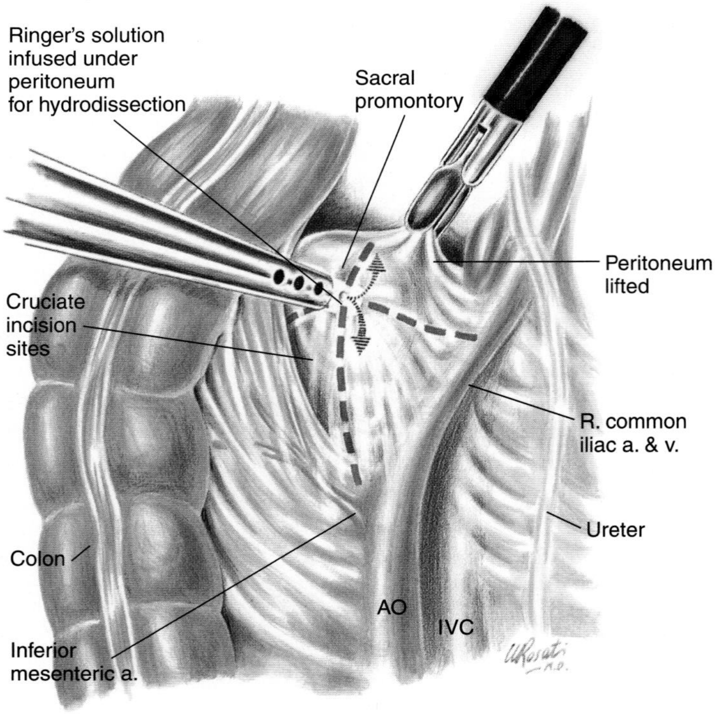

Figure 17-1. The peritoneum over the promontory is elevated with grasping forceps, and a small opening is made with the CO_2 laser, knife electrode, or scissors. The suction-irrigator is inserted, and the peritoneum is elevated with hydrodissection. The peritoneum is incised horizontally and vertically, and the opening is extended cephalad until the bifurcation of the aorta is seen.

this opening, the suction-irrigator is inserted, and the peritoneum is elevated by hydrodissection. The peritoneum is incised horizontally and vertically, and the opening is extended cephalad to the aortic bifurcation (Figure 17-2). Bleeding from the peritoneal vessels is controlled with the bipolar electrocoagulator. Retroperitoneal fatty tissue is removed before the hypogastric plexus is reached. Hemostasis is obtained with bipolar electrocoagulation.

The nerve plexus is grasped with an atraumatic forceps. Using blunt and sharp dissection, the nerve fibers are skeletonized, coagulated, and excised (Figure 17-3). All the nerves that lie within the boundaries of the interiliac triangle are removed, including any fibers entering the area from under the common iliac arteries (Figure 17-4). The retroperitoneal space is irrigated, and bleeding points are coagulated. Sutures are not required. Excised tissue is sent for histologic confirmation of nerve removal. At second-look laparoscopy, the presacral area appears to be healed; usually no small bowel is attached to this area. If a mesocolon detachment is required at the initial procedure, the mesocolon usually reattaches itself to the presacral area. The mesocolon does not cover the sacral promontory in most patients. When the mesocolon covers the sacral promontory, the procedure is more difficult and the surgeon must avoid injuring the inferior mesenteric artery and its branches.

Results

The most favorable results reported with presacral neurectomy described only a 2% failure rate in 1500 selected patients.[14] Meigs[15] studied 20 women who had primary dysmenorrhea and noted relief in 17 (85%). Black[16] reviewed 2516 patients and noted 70% with relief, 19% improved, and 11% unimproved. Polan and DeCherney[17] reported in 1980 that 14 of 20 patients (70%) were relieved of pain after presacral neurectomy. In the control group, 14 of 54 (26%) showed significant pain relief. Lee and colleagues[7] found a 74% success rate, 14% partial cures, and a 12% failure rate.

Perez[18] studied 25 patients and concluded that 96% of them had pain relief. On a scale of 1 to 10, the preoperative mean pain score was 8.4, while the postoperative mean was 2.2. Tjaden and coauthors[19] initiated a randomized, prospective study to ascertain the efficacy of presacral neurectomy. The study was terminated by the monitoring committee after the 6-week review because it was deemed unethical to deny patients with midline dysmenorrhea the relief provided by presacral neurectomy. Of the 26 patients, 17 had a presacral neurectomy. Fifteen of the 17 (88%) noted relief, while 2 (12%) had no improvement. In nine patients who did not undergo presacral neurectomy, the pain persisted. In 1992, Nezhat and Nezhat[20] completed a 1-year follow-up on 52

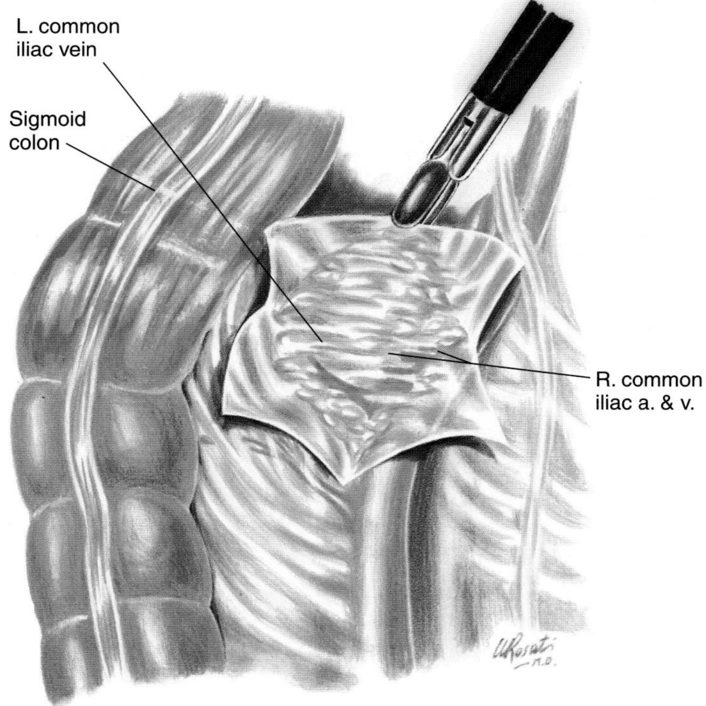

Figure 17-2. Retroperitoneal fatty tissue is removed before the hypogastric plexus is reached. Hemostasis is achieved with bipolar electrocoagulation.

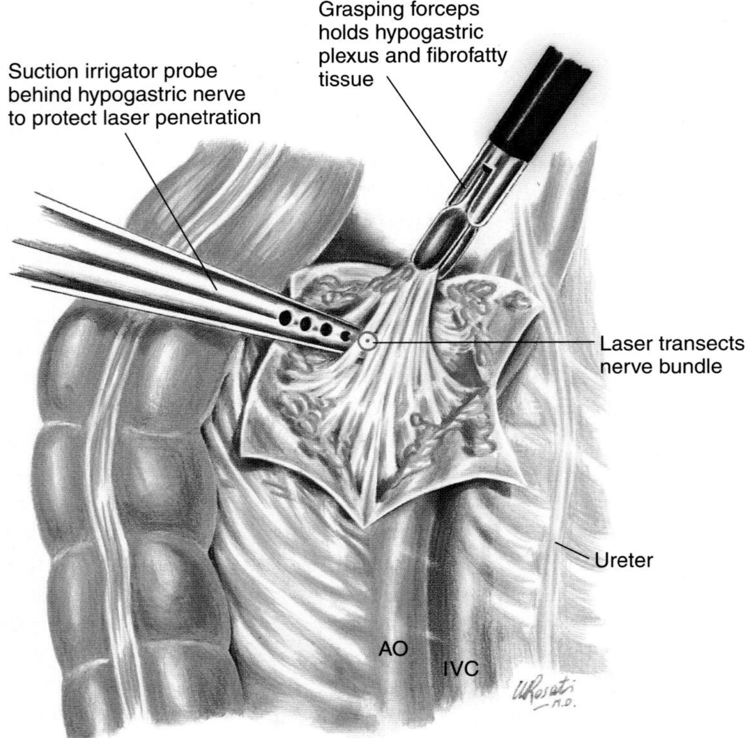

Figure 17-3. The plexus of nerves is grasped with atraumatic forceps. The nerves are skeletonized, coagulated, and excised. Nerves that lie within the boundaries of the interiliac triangle are removed along with fibers entering the area from underneath the common iliac arteries.

women who received laparoscopic presacral neurectomy for dysmenorrhea that were not responsive to medical treatment. The severity of endometriosis varied among these patients from minimal to severe: Thirty-one had minimal, 13 mild, 5 moderate, and 3 severe endometriosis. Forty-eight of the 52 (92.3%) reported relief of dysmenorrhea, including 27 (51.2%) who reported complete pain relief. Of the 27 patients reporting complete pain relief, 16 (59%), 6 (22%), 3 (11%), and 2 (8%) had minimal, mild, moderate, and severe endometriosis, respectively.

Chen and coworkers[21] reported on 67 patients with primary dysmenorrhea and a poor response to previous medical treatment. The patients were divided into two groups. Thirty-three had laparoscopic presacral neurectomy, and 34 had laparoscopic uterine nerve ablation. The reported efficacy of the two procedures was identical after 3 months but the efficiency of the laparoscopic presacral neurectomy was significantly better than that of laparoscopic uterine nerve ablation after 12 months. The authors concluded that presacral neurectomy was preferable to uterine nerve ablation for long-term relief of primary dysmenorrhea. Those authors[22] also reported a retrospective review of 655 patients who had laparoscopic conservative surgery and laparoscopic presacral

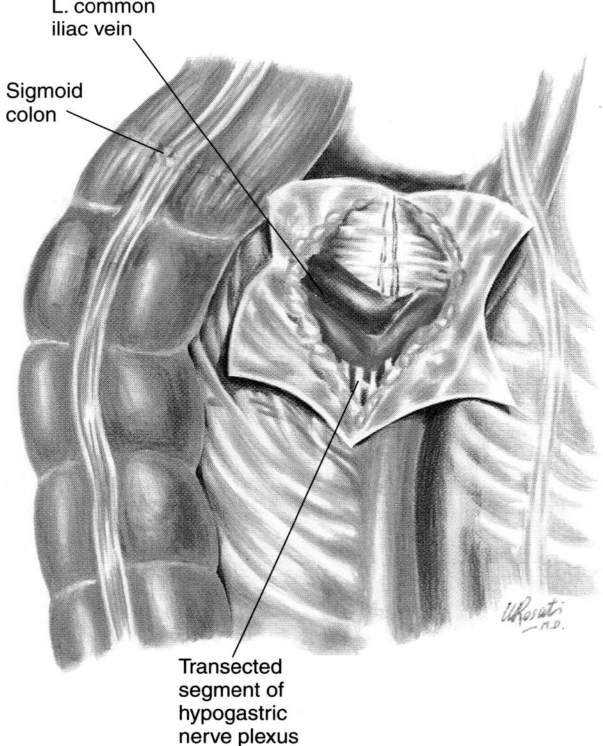

Figure 17-4. Transected segments of the pelvic nerve. Sutures are not required to close the defect. The excised tissue is sent for histologic examination.

neurectomy. Of the 655 patients, 527 (80%) reported significant alleviation of pain. Cure was obtained in 22 (52%) of 42 patients with adenomyosis, 75 (73%) of 103 with moderate to severe endometriosis with dysmenorrhea, 123 (75%) of 164 with minimal to mild endometriosis with dysmenorrhea, 64 (77%) of 83 with primary dysmenorrhea, and 84 (62%) of 135 with chronic pelvic pain.

Nezhat and coworkers[23] evaluated long-term decrease of pain achieved by laparoscopic presacral neurectomy. One hundred seventy-six women underwent presacral neurectomy combined with treatment of endometriotic lesions. More than a 50% alleviation of pain was reported by 69.8%, 77.3%, 71.4%, and 84.6% for patients with endometriosis in stage I, II, III, and IV, respectively, using the revised classification of the American Fertility Society (Table 17-1). The long-term outcome of laparoscopic presacral neurectomy is satisfactory in most patients, and the stage of endometriosis is not related directly to the degree of pain improvement achieved.

Complications

Bleeding is the most important intraoperative complication of presacral neurectomy. The middle sacral vessels are in the midline between the "presacral nerve" and the periosteum of the sacral promontory. Usually, the nerve is dissected anterior to the vessels and ligation is not necessary. Hemostasis is obtained by ligation or coagulation. However, an injury to the common iliac vein or vena cava can require an immediate laparotomy.

Ureteral injury, urinary urgency, and poor bladder emptying are potential complications. Meigs[15] noted urinary urgency in some patients that persisted for 7 years postoperatively and persistent constipation in 32% of patients Black[16] reported the need for catheterization in 13 of 26 patients postoperatively: 4 for 1 day, 6 for 2 days, and 1 each for 3, 5, and 6 days. In a discussion at the end of Black's 1964 paper, Raney noted three complications: one patient with transient "poor bladder emptying" and permanent constipation and painless labor in two patients who, unwarned by labor pains, delivered at home. In the same discussion, Pratt remarked that he had cared for one woman who developed intermittent ileal obstruction because of adhesions involving the fifth lumbar vertebra just above the sacral promontory after presacral neurectomy. Lee and associates[7] noted similar complications in 4% of 50 patients. Eight (18%) of 45 patients who benefited from presacral neurectomy had a return of lateral pain within 19 months. Jones and Rock[24] cited vaginal dryness that usually resolved within 6 months as a complication in 10 to 15% of patients. Lee and associates[7] noted one acute operative complication involving an estimated 1500 mL blood loss from a damaged presacral vein. Davis[6] recognized a vascular injury to the left common iliac vein that was repaired. Cotte[14] reported one instance of damage to the left ureter among 1500 operations and noted postoperative bleeding in four other patients. Two required a second operation and repair of the posterior peritoneum; the other two cases, which involved subperitoneal blood infiltrating the posterior rectal areas, resolved spontaneously.

TABLE 17-1. Pain Reduction after Laparoscopic Presacral Neurectomy by Stage of Endometriosis

	Degree of Improvement				
	>80%	50–80%	<50%	None	No Response
Pelvic pain					
Stage I (n = 53)	18 (34.0)	19 (35.8)	10 (18.9)	5 (9.4)	1 (1.9)
Stage II (n = 22)	13 (59.1)	4 (18.2)	3 (13.6)	2 (9.1)	0
Stage III (n = 7)	2 (28.6)	3 (42.9)	1 (14.3)	1 (14.3)	0
Stage IV (n = 13)	8 (61.5)	3 (23.1)	2 (15.4)	0	0
Total (n = 95)	41 (43.2)	29 (30.5)	16 (16.8)	8 (8.4)	1 (1.1)
Dysmenorrhea					
Stage I (n = 53)	12 (22.6)	16 (30.2)	14 (26.4)	5 (9.4)	6 (11.3)
Stage II (n = 22)	10 (45.5)	5 (22.7)	3 (13.6)	2 (9.1)	2 (9.1)
Stage III (n = 7)	2 (28.6)	3 (42.7)	0	2 (28.6)	0
Stage IV (n = 13)	7 (53.8)	2 (15.4)	1 (7.7)	1 (7.7)	2 (15.4)
Total (n = 95)	31 (32.6)	26 (27.4)	18 (18.9)	10 (10.5)	10 (10.5)

Wetherell[25] did not find a mortality in the American literature after removal of the superior hypogastric plexus. Bonica[26] tabulated 165 operations from six authors and found no mortality among four of them. Fontaine and Herrmann[1] reported a fatality in one patient that occurred on the second postoperative day. Cerebral edema was found at autopsy. Cotte[8] described two patients who died from acute pulmonary complications.

Chen and coworkers[27] reported four cases of chylous ascites after laparoscopic presacral neurectomy. This rare complication is caused by intraoperative injury of the retroperitoneal lymphatic plexus. Of the four injuries, two were treated successfully with bipolar cauterization. One was managed by compression with Gelfoam, and closure of the peritoneum was achieved by laparoscopic suturing. The fourth patient had persistent chylous leakage from the drainage tube. This complication was resolved by conservative management, removal of the drainage tube, and a low-fat diet.

Uterosacral Transection and Ablation

Uterosacral transection was developed and popularized as an alternative to presacral neurectomy with Doyle's vaginal approach[28] involving transection of the uterosacral ligaments. Doyle's results were as good as those obtained with presacral neurectomy. Lichten and Bombard[29] reported relief of incapacitating primary dysmenorrhea in 9 of 11 (81%) patients who underwent uterosacral nerve transection but no cure in the control group who had only a diagnostic laparoscopy. However, 1 year later, fewer than half the patients who originally experienced improvement were pain-free. Gurgan and colleagues[30] reported that 17 of 23 patients had alleviation of dysmenorrhea. The subjects quantified their pain preoperatively and postoperatively; the mean preoperative score was reduced by 33%. In a similar study, Sutton[31] reported a 63% reduction in the intial average score. Uterosacral transection should be done as a secondary procedure that can provide partial or temporary relief of central dysmenorrhea. It also should be used in conjunction with nonsteroidal anti-inflammatory analgesics.

A standard three-puncture technique is suggested. The procedure is done by placing the uterosacral ligaments on stretch by anteverting the uterus with the uterine manipulator. The CO_2 laser (40 to 60 W) or another cutting instrument is employed to transect the ligaments at their insertion into the cervix, using a vertical motion from medial to lateral (Figure 17-5). Transection at this location maximizes the number of nerve fibers transected because the fibers disperse as they pass along the uterosacral ligaments. However, this segment of the uterosacral ligament is closest to the uterine vessels and ureter. The suction-irrigator

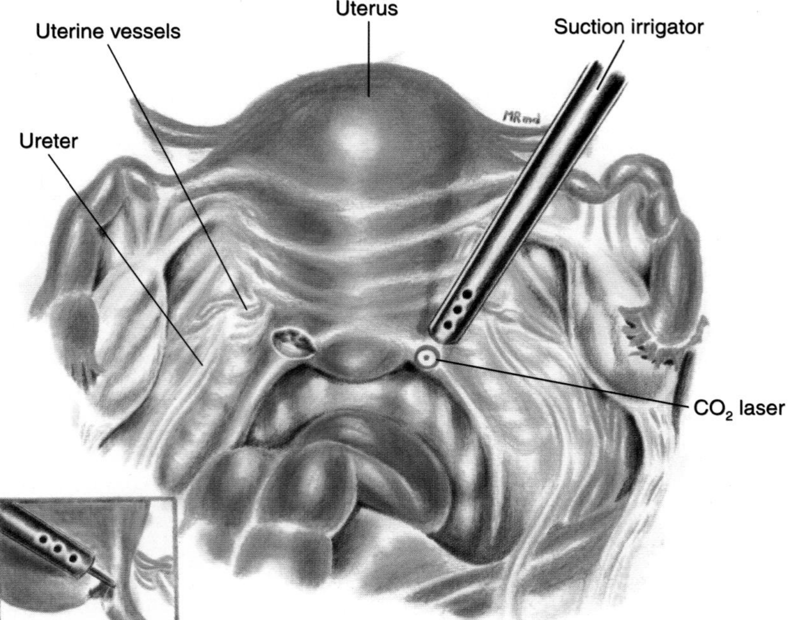

Figure 17-5. The CO_2 laser or a needle electrode (inset) transects the ligaments and their insertion into the uterus. The depth of the incision should be examined frequently because the goal is to transect these ligaments completely.

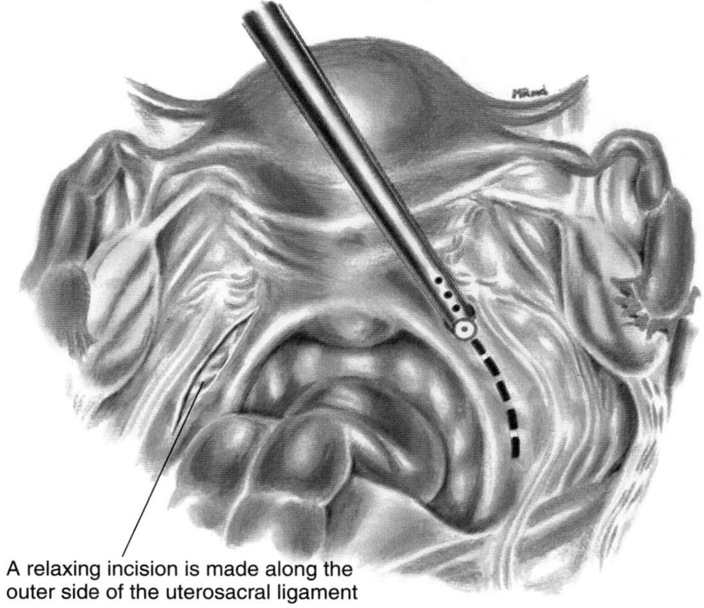

Figure 17-6. If the ureter is close to the uterosacral ligament, a "relaxing" incision is made along the outer side of the ligament. The ureter is retracted laterally before the ligament is transected. Occasionally the rectum may appear similar to these ligaments.

serves as a backstop to make the uterosacral ligament more prominent and protect the ureter. The depth of the incision should be examined frequently, because the goal is complete transection of the uterosacral ligament (Figure 17-6). Blood vessels run along the medial aspect of the uterosacral ligament, and bleeding in this area must be controlled carefully because of the proximity of the ureter and rectum. Some gynecologists also vaporize a path along the base of the cervix between the uterosacral ligaments. If the uterosacral ligaments are difficult to identify, uterosacral transection is not recommended. When the uterosacral ligament is cut, a blood vessel inside it tends to bleed. To ascertain if this has occurred, uterine traction should be released and pneumoperitoneum should be decreased.

The direction of the ureter should be identified from the pelvic brim to the bladder because ureteral injury is a serious complication associated

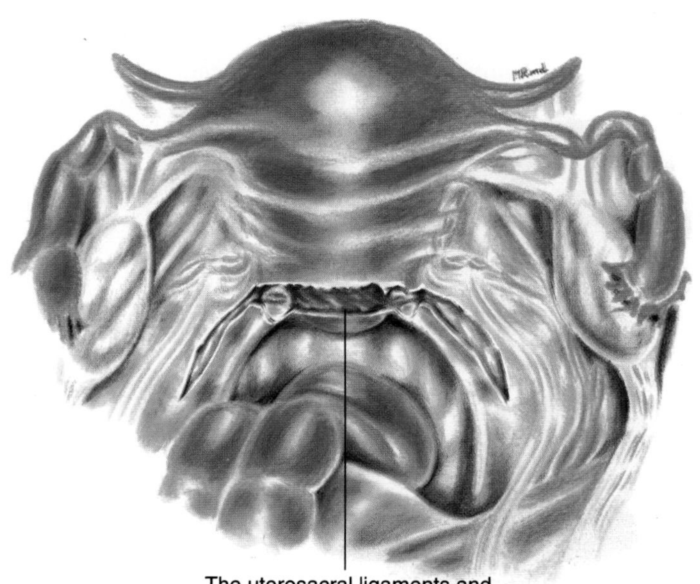

Figure 17-7. The ligaments have been transected with ablation of the contained nerves.

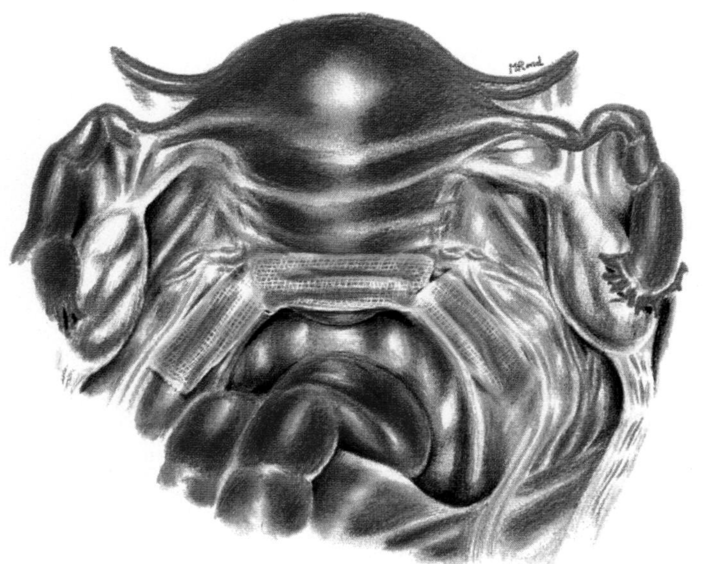

Figure 17-8. Interceed is placed over the areas of transection.

with this procedure.[32] There is usually a distance of 2 to 3 cm between the ureter and the uterosacral ligaments. However, this proximity varies. If the ureter is close to the uterosacral ligament, a "relaxing" incision is made along the outer side of the uterosacral ligament (Figure 17-7). Interceed is placed over the transected area (Figure 17-8). The ureter is retracted laterally before the ligament is transected.

If uterosacral transection is unsuccessful, it is presumed that interruption of the nerve fibers was incomplete or the nerves regenerated. Lichten[33] reported that repeating the procedure did not relieve dysmenorrhea, implying that the course of the nerve fibers in these individuals may not be normal. Several patients with failed uterosacral transection obtained relief from a subsequent presacral neurectomy.[18] Complications can cause loss of uterine support, adhesions, and ureteral transection. These procedures benefit women with midline pelvic pain because adnexa are innervated mostly by nerve fibers traversing the infundibulopelvic ligaments. The difference in innervation accounts for the anatomic and physiologic differences between lateral pain and midline pain.

Summary

Laparoscopic presacral neurectomy is an effective, safe operation for patients who have incapacitating central dysmenorrhea that is not relieved by medication. The procedure is empirical, since success rates are not predictable. Complications and mortality rates have been minimal. Unsuitable patients and incomplete neurectomy because of neurologic variability or failure to remove all nerve tissue within the Cotte triangle are the most common reasons for poor results.

References

1. Fontaine R, Herrmann LG. Clinical and experimental basis for surgery of pelvic sympathetic nerves in gynecology. *Surg Gynecol Obstet* 1932; 54:133.
2. Jaboulay M. Le traitement de la navralgie pelvienne par a paralysie du sympathetique sacre. *Lyon Med* 1899; 90:102.
3. Ruggi G. Della sympathectamia al collo ed ale adome. *Policinico* 1899; 1:193.
4. Leriche R. Resultant eloigne cinq ans at demi d'une sympathectomie de deux ateres hypogastriques pour dysmenorrhee douloureuse. *Lyon Ch* 1927; 24:360.
5. Cotte MG. Sur le traîtement des dysmenorrhees rebelles par la sympathectomie hypogastrique periaterielle ou la section du nerf presacre. *Lyon Med* 1925; 135:153.
6. Davis AA. The technique of resection of the presacral nerve (Cotte's operation). *Br J Surg* 1933; 20:516.
7. Lee RB, Stone K, Magelssen D, et al. Presacral neurectomy for chronic pelvic pain. *Obstet Gynecol* 1986; 68:517.
8. Cotte MG. Resection of the presacral nerve in the treatment of obstinate dysmenorrhea. *Am J Obstet Gynecol* 1937; 33:1030.

9. Elaut L. Surgical anatomy of the so-called presacral nerve. *Surg Gynecol Obstet* 1933; 57:581.
10. Davis AA. Discussion on sympathectomy for dysmenorrhea. *Proceedings of the Royal Society of Medicine* 1934; 27:258.
11. Labate JS. The surgical anatomy of the superior hypogastric plexus—"presacral nerve." *Surg Gynecol Obstet* 1938; 67:199.
12. Curtis AH, Anson BJ, Ashley FL, et al. The anatomy of the pelvic autonomic nerves in relation to gynecology. *Surg Gynecol Obstet* 1942; 75:743.
13. Black WT. Presacral neurectomy for dysmenorrhea and pelvic pain *Am Surg* 1936; 75:743.
14. Cotte MG. Technique of presacral neurectomy. *Am J Surg* 1949; 78:50.
15. Meigs JV. Excision of the superior hypogastric plexus (presacral nerve) for primary dysmenorrhea. *Surg Gynecol Obstet* 1939; 68:723.
16. Black WT. Use of presacral neurectomy in the treatment of dysmenorrhea—a second look after 25 years. *Am J Obstet Gynecol* 1964; 89:16.
17. Polan ML, DeCherney A. Presacral neurectomy for pelvic pain in infertility. *Fertil Steril* 1980; 34:557.
18. Perez JJ. Laparoscopic presacral neurectomy: Results of the first 25 cases. *J Reprod Med* 1990; 5:625.
19. Tjaden B, Schlaff WD, Kimball A, et al. The efficacy of presacral neurectomy for the relief of midline dysmenorrhea. *Obstet Gynecol* 1990; 76:89.
20. Nezhat C, Nezhat F. A simplified method of laparoscopic presacral neurectomy for the treatment of central pelvic pain due to endometriosis. *Br J Obstet Gynaecol* 1992; 99:659.
21. Chen FP, Chang SD, Chu KK, et al. Comparison of laparoscopic presacral neurectomy and laparoscopic uterine nerve ablation for primary dysmenorrhea. *J Reprod Med* 1996; 41:463.
22. Chen FP, Soong YK. The efficacy and complications of laparoscopic presacral neurectomy in pelvic pain. *Obstet Gynecol* 1997; 90:974.
23. Nezhat CH, Seidman D, Nezhat F, et al. Long-term outcome of laparoscopic presacral neurectomy for the treatment of central pelvic pain attributed to endometriosis. *Obstet Gynecol* 1998; 91:701.
24. Jones HW, Rock JA. *Reparative and Constructive Surgery of the Female Generative Tract*. Baltimore and London: Williams & Wilkins, 1983.
25. Wetherell FS. Relief of pelvic pain by sympathetic neurectomy. *JAMA* 1933; 101:1255.
26. Bonica JJ. *The Management of Pain*, 2d ed. Philadelphia: Lea & Febige, 1990.
27. Chen FP, Lo TS, Soong YK. Management of chylous ascites following laparoscopic presacral neurectomy. *Hum Reprod* 1998; 13:880.
28. Doyle EB. Paracervical uterine denervation by transection of the cervical plexus for the relief of dysmenorrhea. *Am J Obstet Gynecol* 1955; 70:11.
29. Lichten EM, Bombard J. Surgical treatment of primary dysmenorrhea with laparoscopic uterine nerve ablation. *J Reprod Med* 1987; 32:37.
30. Gurgan T, Urman B, Asku T, et al. Laparoscopic CO_2 laser uterine nerve ablation for treatment of drug resistant primary dysmenorrhea. *Fertil Steril* 1992; 58:422.
31. Sutton C. Laser uterine nerve ablation, in Donnez J, ed., *Laser Operative Laparoscopy and Hysteroscopy*. Leuven: Nauwelaerts, 1989.
32. Nezhat C, Nezhat F. Laparoscopic repair of resected ureter during operative laparoscopy to treat endometriosis: A case report. *Obstet Gynecol* 1992;80: 543.
33. Lichten E. Three years experience with L.U.N.A. *Am J Gynecol Health* 1989; 3:9.

18

Laparoscopic Urethral Suspension, Sacral Colpopexy, Repair of Cystourethrocele and Vesicovaginal Fistula

Retropubic Urethral Suspension

Urinary incontinence is becoming more prevalent as the population ages,[1,2] with 20 to 40% of women having this complaint.[1-4] The psychologic status of these patients improves significantly after a successful surgical cure.[5] Despite more than 160 different corrective operations, an optimal approach has not been demonstrated.[6]

Retropubic urethropexy[7-9] has produced excellent results with relatively few complications. Although needle urethropexy[10-14] is a shorter operation and is less invasive, it is not as effective and is associated with more complications.[15-18] Tanagho's modification of the Burch procedure[19] has succeeded in curing patients with pure genuine urinary stress incontinence (GUSI) and an intact urethral sphincter.[19-23] Laparoscopic bladder neck suspension has been carried out with good results.[24-26]

Laparoscopic retropubic urethral suspension is an outpatient procedure that potentially provides a long-term solution for this condition. The advantages include excellent exposure and access to the retropubic space because of videolaparoscopic magnification, enhancing the surgeon's ability to place the sutures precisely. The improved exposure allows proper support and avoids urethral obstruction and compression. Laparoscopic retropubic colposuspension (Burch method) has produced good results with relatively few complications.

Preoperative Evaluation

The workup should include a history and physical examination and gynecologic and neurologic examinations. Attempts should be made to evaluate and correct factors that contribute to urinary incontinence. Office tests include stress test (lithotomy and standing), the Q-tip test, urinalysis, urine culture and sensitivity, and blood chemistry analysis.[27] Multichannel urodynamic evaluation in the lithotomy and standing positions is done with an emphasis on voiding time, voiding volume, and postvoid residual urine volume.[28-30] Additional tests include a waterfill cystometrogram with continuous urethral pressure monitoring and subtracted rectal and abdominal pressures. GUSI is diagnosed by a positive stress test in the absence of simultaneous detrusor contractions or pressure equalization on the stress urethral closure pressure profile. Patients are encouraged to keep 24- to 48-hour symptom diaries.

Operative Technique

After induction of general endotracheal anesthesia, the patient is placed in Allen stirrups, which permit the assistant to do a vaginal examination. A Foley catheter is placed. A 10-mm operative videolaparoscope is introduced infraumbilically, and three 5-mm accessory cannulas are inserted (Figure 18-1). The middle cannula is 5 to 6 cm above the pubic symphysis, and the other two cannulas are 7 to 8 cm above the pubic symphysis lateral to the

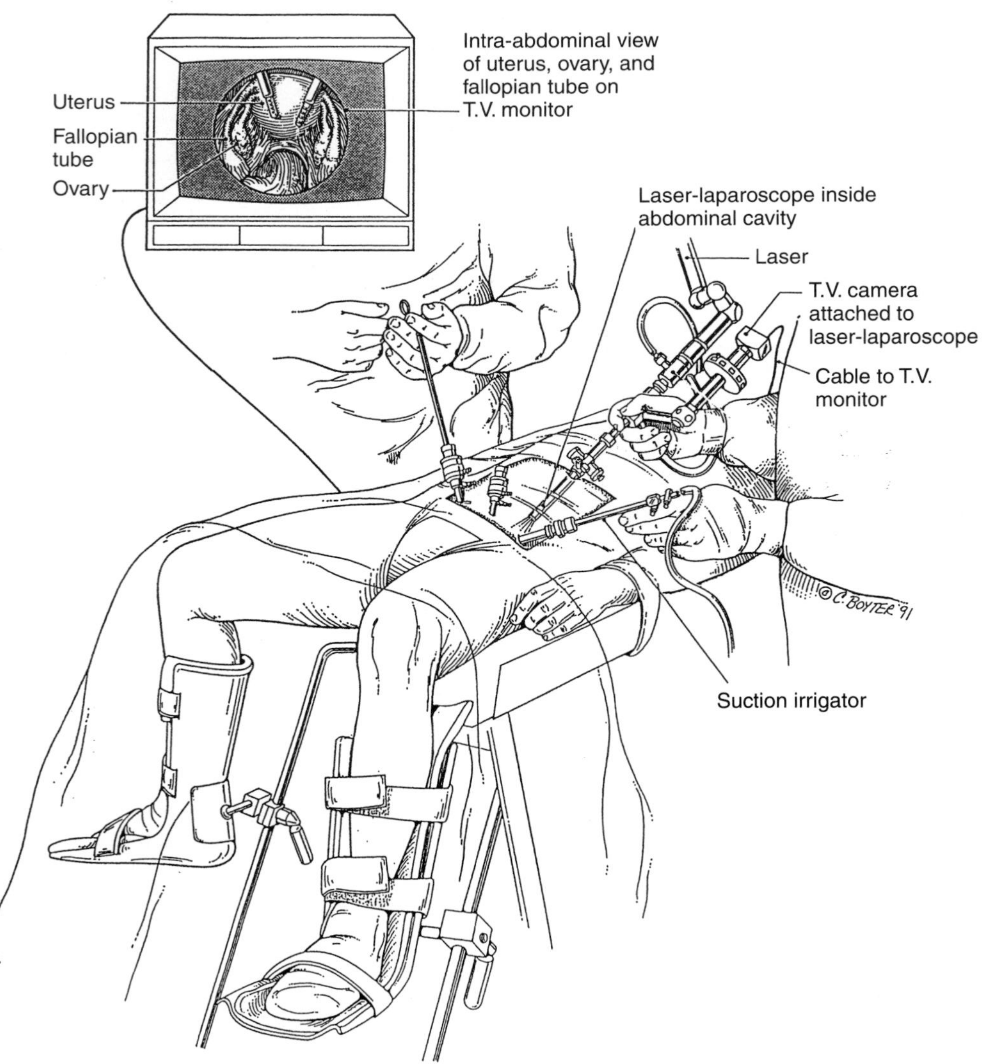

Figure 18-1. Room setup and location of the suprapubic incisions.

umbilical ligaments, avoiding injury to the inferior epigastric vessels. The carbon dioxide (CO_2) laser is placed through the operative channel of the 10-mm laparoscope and used as a long knife. A suction-irrigator, a grasping forceps, a needle holder, and a bipolar electrocoagulator are introduced through the accessory cannulas.

The intraperitoneal cavity is inspected to detect any pelvic abnormalities that require surgical treatment. Intially, indicated gynecologic procedures are done. After the ureters are identified, a culdoplasty is carried out if indicated. The enterocele sac is excised, and a laparoscopic purse-string suture (1-0 polybutilate-coated polyester) is used, beginning at the bottom of the cul-de-sac and exercising care to incorporate the posterior wall of the vagina, the peritoneum laterally at the left and right pararectal areas, and shallow bites of serosa over the anterior rectosigmoid colon. In patients who have undergone previous hysterectomy, remnants of uterosacral ligaments are included in the suture. Closure of the cul-de-sac should leave no defect that could result in bowel entrapment.

The transperitoneal technique is one of the procedures that can be used to enter the space of Retzius. The anterior abdominal wall peritoneum 5 to 7 cm above the pubic symphysis is pulled down with grasping forceps placed through a lateral accessory cannula (Figure 18-2). A transverse incision is made with the CO_2 laser, scissors, or harmonic scalpel caudal to the midsuprapubic cannula above the pubic symphysis on the peri-

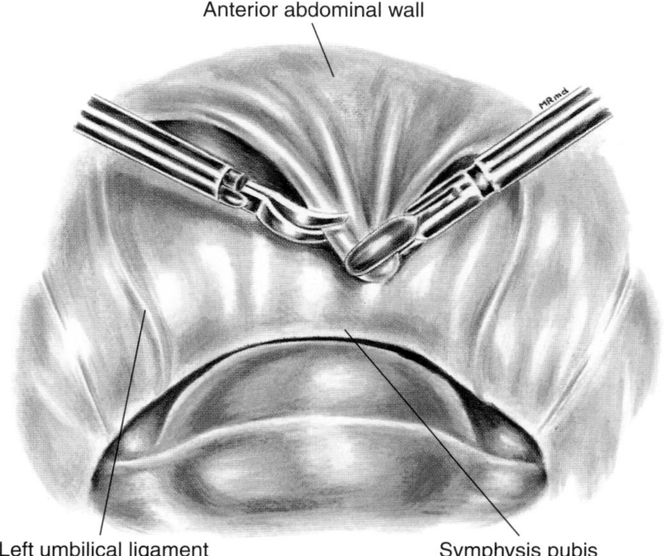

Figure 18-2. An incision is made in the peritoneum 5 to 7 cm above the symphysis pubis.

toneum between the two umbilical ligaments. The midline cannula entry and anatomic landmarks, including the round ligament from the internal ring, are used to avoid injury to the bladder. The retropubic space is dissected bluntly with hydrodissection or any of the above-mentioned instruments (Figure 18-3). The incision should remain close to the back of the pubic bone to drop the anterior bladder wall, vaginal wall, and urethra downward. Dissection is limited over the urethra in the midline to approximately 2 cm lateral to the urethra to protect its delicate neuromusculature. An assistant does a vaginal examination with one finger on each side of the catheterized urethra, elevating the lateral vaginal fornix. The overlying fibrofatty tissue is cleared from the anterior vaginal wall under videolaparoscopic magnification. Beginning laterally, the bladder is dissected medially from the paravaginal fascia. The thin-walled venous plexus is identified and protected from trauma. Pneumoperi-

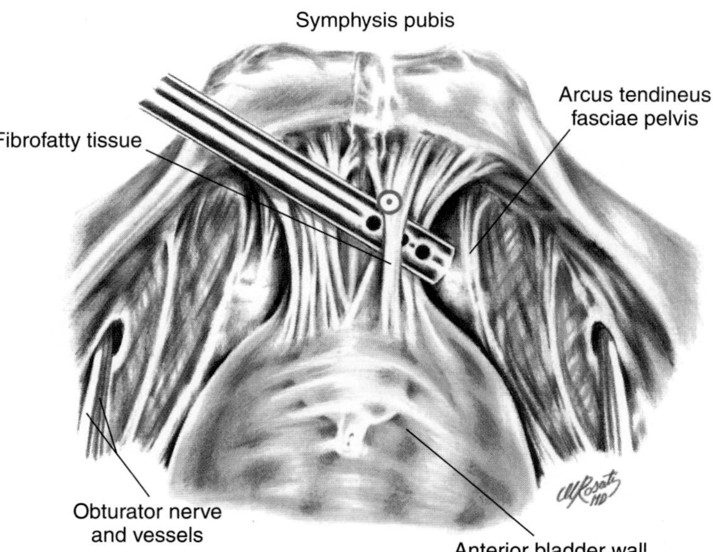

Figure 18-3. The space of Retzius is developed with blunt and sharp dissection of fibrofatty tissue. Care is taken to avoid periurethral neurovascular injury.

toneal pressure and the coagulating effect of the cutting instrument, such as a harmonic scalpel, help control bleeding from small vessels.

Balloon dissector

The balloon dissector (General Surgical Innovations, Inc., Portola Valley, CA) consists of a cannula, a guide rod, and a balloon system. The dissector is inserted through a 1-cm infraumbilical incision. It is advanced between the rectus muscle and the anterior surface of the posterior rectus sheath to the pubic symphysis. The external sheath of the dissector is removed, and the balloon is inflated with approximately 750 mL of saline solution. During inflation, the balloon unrolls sideways and exerts a perpendicular force that separates tissue layers. Blunt dissection of the connective tissues is propagated as the balloon expands. When the maximal volume is reached, the balloon is deflated and removed through the incision. The dissected space is insufflated with CO_2 at a pressure of 8 to 10 mm Hg. The predefined shape of the balloon, its nonelastomeric material, and the incompressible character of the saline ensure a large, relatively bloodless working space of predictable size and shape. The space is adequate for identifying pertinent landmarks and for unencumbered manipulation of endoscopic surgical instruments.

Preperitoneal approach

The preperitoneal technique for access to the space of Retzius employs the patient positioning and trocar placement described above. To begin dissection of the space, the midsuprapubic cannula is withdrawn into the preperitoneal area and a 16-gauge laparoscopic needle is inserted through it. Approximately 30 to 50 mL of dilute vasopressin (20 U in 60 to 100 mL of lactated Ringer's solution) is injected subperitoneally in the lower anterior abdominal wall above the bladder to decrease oozing. The needle is replaced with a suction-irrigator probe by injecting 300 to 500 mL of lactated Ringer's solution or normal saline at a pressure of 300 mm Hg to form a subperitoneal space in the anterior abdominal wall. The laparoscope is retracted from the abdominal cavity and directed toward the newly created subperitoneal space in the anterior abdominal wall. A long hydrodissection probe is inserted through the space under direct observation, and the space is expanded further, using hydrodissection. The laparoscope is advanced into this space, which is insufflated with CO_2. The lateral suprapubic trocars are retracted to the pneumosubperitoneal space. Blunt or sharp dissection may be required to lyse adhesions that remain after hydrodissection. The pubic symphysis and Cooper's ligaments can be seen. The patient is placed in a deep Trendelenburg position and rotated to the left to facilitate left-handed suture placement.

Experience with this technique in 10 patients resulted in good outcomes.[31] The technique has several advantages over transperitoneal and balloon dissection.[32] Extension of the peritoneal incision is avoided, eliminating repair and minimizing the risks of bowel herniation and adhesions. The danger

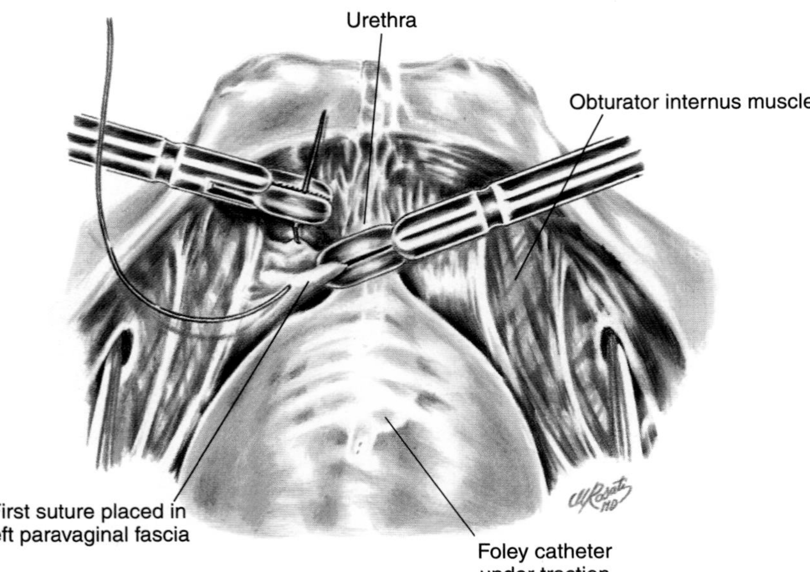

Figure 18-4. A no. 0 Ethibond (Ethicon) suture is placed 1 to 1.5 cm from the urethra. The assistant's finger in the vagina is used to elevate the paraurethral fascia and guide the surgeon.

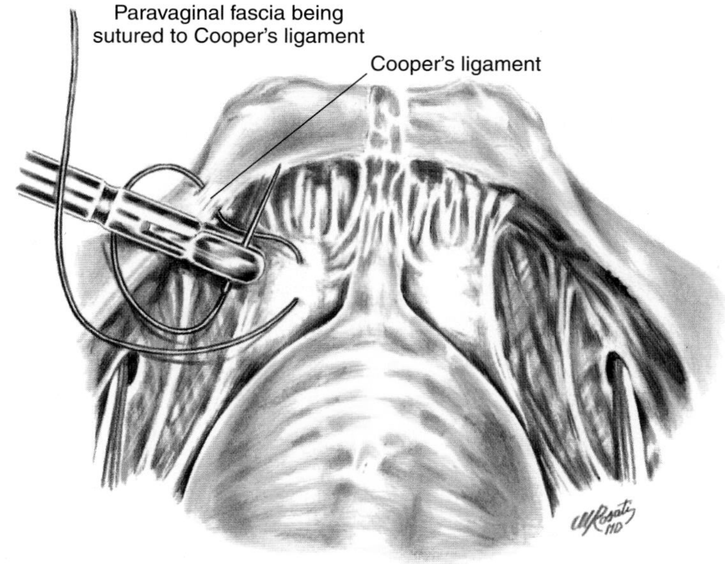

Figure 18-5. The suture is passed through Cooper's ligament in the Burch procedure.

of trauma to the thin-walled venous plexus in this area during blunt or sharp dissection is minimized.

The balloon dissector is an effective alternative to manual dissection of the space of Retzius[32] but is more costly to use. The balloon should be inserted between the rectus muscle and the anterior surface of the posterior rectus sheath. It may be advanced inadvertently into an incorrect plane. The predefined shape of the balloon and its nonelastomeric material can force dissection that is less dependent on anatomic planes.

After dissection of the space of Retzius by any of the routes mentioned above is complete and the paravaginal fascia is identified, using an atraumatic grasping forceps, the paravaginal fascia is elevated and a 1-0 polybutilate-covered polyester endoscopic (Ethibond) suture on a tapered 2.2-cm straight or curved needle is placed at the level of the urethrovesical junction, approximately 1 to 1.5 cm from the urethra (Figure 18-4). The assistant's finger is used as a guide, and traction on the bulb of the Foley catheter facilitates the placement of the suture. The suture is inserted perpendicular to the vaginal axis to include approximately 1 to 2 cm of tissue (the complete vaginal fascia) but not the vaginal mucosa and is fixed to the Cooper's ligament (Figures 18-5 through 18-7). The sutures are tied intracorporeally or extracorporeally with

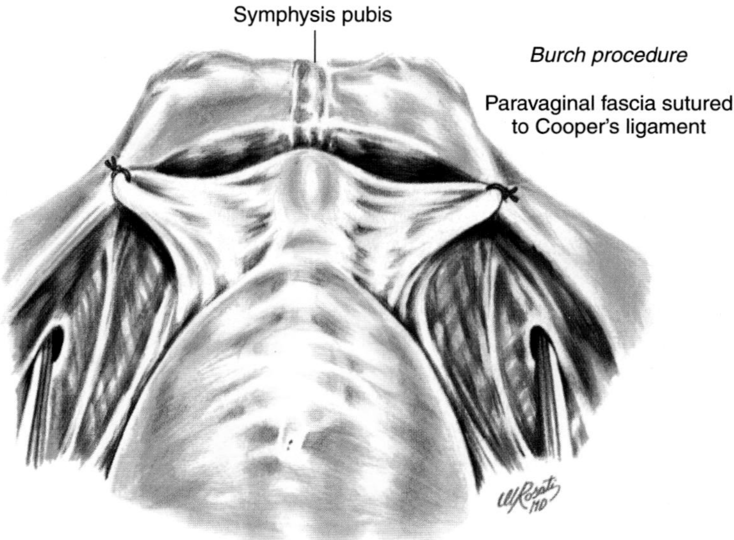

Figure 18-6. The suture is tied extracorporeally or intracorporeally to elevate the urethrovesical angle.

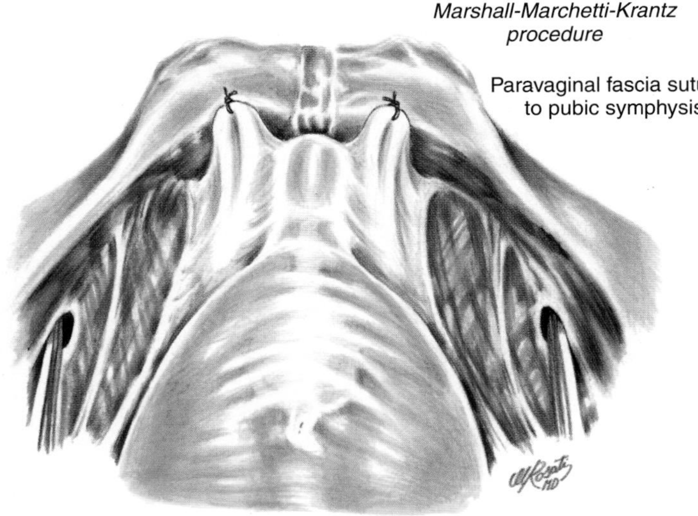

Figure 18-7. The paravaginal fascia is sutured to the symphysis pubis in the Marshall-Marchetti-Krantz procedure.

help from an assistant, who lifts the vagina upward and forward. Direct observation allows the surgeon to gauge the tension in the vaginal wall while tying the sutures. The urethra is observed to ensure that it is not compressed against the pubic bone. Suturing is repeated on the opposite side to create a platform on which the bladder neck rests while cinching is avoided. If the suspension is judged inadequate by visual inspection, manual elevation, or cystoscopy, a second set of sutures is placed cephalad along the base of the bladder.

Cystoscopy is accomplished to ensure that no suture material is in the bladder and to assess the urethrovesical junction angle and urethral patency. Pneumosubperitoneal pressure is decreased, and the retropubic space is observed for bleeding. Hemostasis is achieved with the bipolar electrocoagulator. The laparoscope is withdrawn from the space of Retzius into the abdomen. No drain is used, and the peritoneal defect is closed with an absorbable suture if needed. The laparoscope is removed from the abdomen, and the procedure is complete. The transurethral Foley catheter is left in place for 2 or 3 days, or the patient is instructed on self-catheterization. Patients should receive perioperative intravenous antibiotic prophylaxis followed by a course of oral antibiotics for 5 days or until self-catheterization is discontinued when post voiding residuals are less than 100 mL. Postoperative osteitis pubis after this procedure is a concern,[31] but that complication has not occurred in the authors'[32] series.

In 62 operations, one bladder perforation occurred during bladder dissection and entry into the space of Retzius. It was repaired laparoscopically in one layer, using 0 polyglactin interrupted sutures. One patient, who also had an oophorectomy, developed an incisional hernia at the site of the midline suprapubic cannula, although the fascia had been repaired with one interrupted absorbable suture. Another patient who was unable to void postoperatively required self-catheterization for 10 days. Nine women had dysuria without infection that resolved with phenazopyridine hydrocholride (Pyridium) treatment. During the 8- to 30-month follow-up, all patients reported relief of stress incontinence. Subjective success was ascertained by a questionnaire on urinary leakage and the absence of a need to wear pads (none were required). Objective success was assessed by comparison of pre- and postoperative symptom diaries, postvoid residual volume, urethrovesical junction angle as detected by catheter and Q-tip placement, bladder support, and a negative standing stress test.[32]

Although the principles of an abdominal approach are followed, the disadvantages of a laparotomy incision are avoided. Elevation of the bladder neck depends on the scarring of the perivesical tissue to the pubic symphysis or pelvic side wall, not on the two periuretheral sutures as in a needle procedure. GUSI can be corrected laparoscopically with comparable results. Such an approach appears to be less traumatic and invasive, with decreased operative and postoperative recovery times and less morbidity.

Sacral Colpopexy

Vaginal vault prolapse occurs whenever the apex of the vagina descends below the introitus, turning the vagina inside out. It is uncommon in the United States, affecting between 900 and 1200 women annually.[33] The approaches to the treatment of vaginal vault prolapse include the use of a pessary, vaginal reconstruction, and vaginal closure. For the obliterative approach, patient selection criteria should include the patient's physiologic age, sexual desires, general health status, and symptoms. Total colpocleisis is not an option for sexually active women.

The goal of vaginal vault suspension is to correct all anatomic defects, maintain or restore normal bowel and bladder function, and restore a functioning vagina. Transvaginal sacrospinous vault suspension and needle urethropexy can result in a satisfactory outcome in most operations.[34] The vaginal route can be used in women whose preference or medical disorders contraindicate the abdominal approach. However, studies have shown a 33% rate of recurrent prolapse associated with sacrospinous fixation and transvaginal needle suspension.[40] The probability of an optimal surgical outcome is twice as great with a transabdominal operation.

Among the proposed surgical techniques to prevent and correct this condition is abdominal sacral colpopexy utilizing the interposition of a synthetic suspensory hammock between the prolapsed vaginal vault and the anterior surface of the sacrum.[35–37] However, this technique usually requires a midline abdominal incision, abdominal packing, and extensive bowel manipulation. It has a potential for infection, wound separation or dehiscence, and ileus or bowel obstruction.[42] To minimize these drawbacks, sacral colpopexy can be carried out laparoscopically.

Patient evaluation and preparation for the endoscopic procedures should focus on the degree of prolapse and associated rectocele, cystourethrocele, and incontinence. Preoperative mechanical and antibiotic bowel preparation is essential.

Technique

After the introduction of the operative laparoscope and ancillary 5-mm suprapubic trocars, the patient is placed in a Trendelenburg position and tilted to the left. After evaluation of the peritoneal cavity and completion of other indicated procedures, the vaginal vault is elevated by a sponge on a ring forceps.[38] The vaginal apex is prepared by removing the peritoneum and connective tissue until the vaginal fascia and scar are seen (Figure 18-8). The bladder is dissected from the anterior vaginal wall and the rectum is dissected from the posterior vaginal wall so that approximately 4 cm of the vaginal vault is exposed. If the vagina is opened because of hysterectomy or partial vaginectomy, pneumoperitoneum is maintained by placing an inflated surgical glove (Ceana glove) in the vagina.

Repair of an enterocele is achieved laparoscopically by excising the sac and using a modified Moschcowitz procedure (Figure 18-9). The rectosigmoid colon is pushed to the left side to expose the sacral area. The posterior parietal peritoneum

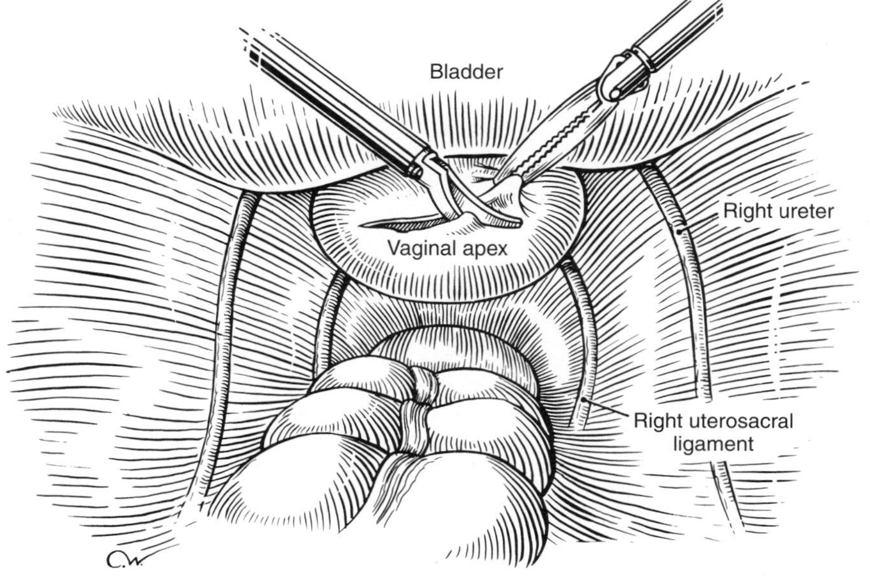

Figure 18-8. The vesical peritoneum over the vaginal apex is incised, and the vaginal apex is cleaned.

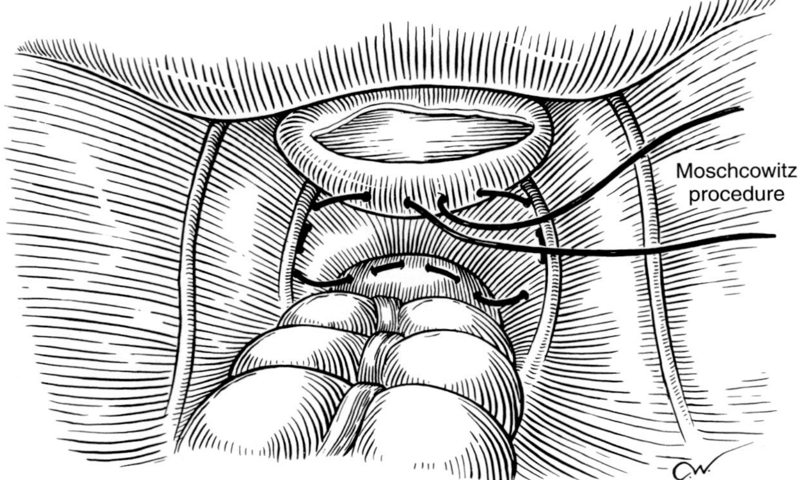

Figure 18-9. The posterior cul-de-sac is obliterated with the Moschcowitz procedure, using a nonabsorbable suture.

at or below the sacral promontory is lifted with grasping forceps and incised to the level of the third and fourth sacral vertebrae (S3 to S4), and the anterior sacral fascia is exposed. The peritoneal incision is extended from the right pararectal area downward toward the vagina through the presacral space (Figure 18-10). The right ureter, internal iliac artery and vein, descending colon, and presacral vessels are identified.

A 2.5- by 10 mm piece of Mersilene or Gore-Tex (W.L. Gore and Associates, Inc., Phoenix, AZ) mesh is rolled and introduced into the abdomen through the 10-mm suprapubic port. Three to five 0 Ethibond sutures (Ethicon, Inc., Somerville, NJ) are placed in a single row in the posterior vaginal wall apex (excluding the vaginal mucosa) from one lateral fornix to the other. Each suture is placed through one end of the mesh and tied loosely (Figure 18-11).

Other supportive measures in the lower vagina, such as anterior and posterior colporrhaphy, may be necessary for the lower and middle third of the vagina. If required, partial vaginectomy is accom-

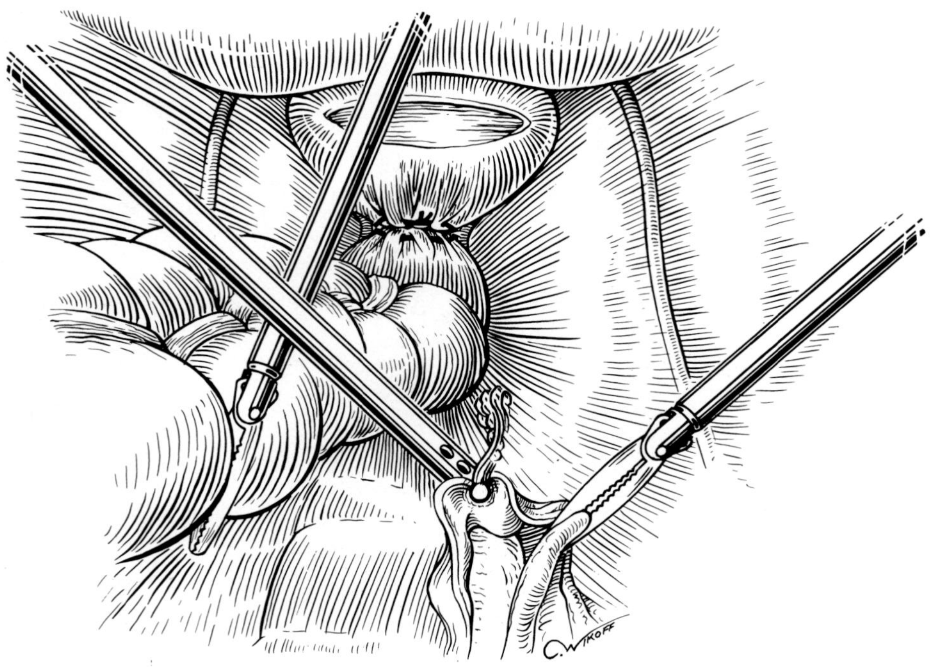

Figure 18-10. Using hydrodissection and the CO_2 laser, the right pararectal and presacral spaces are developed.

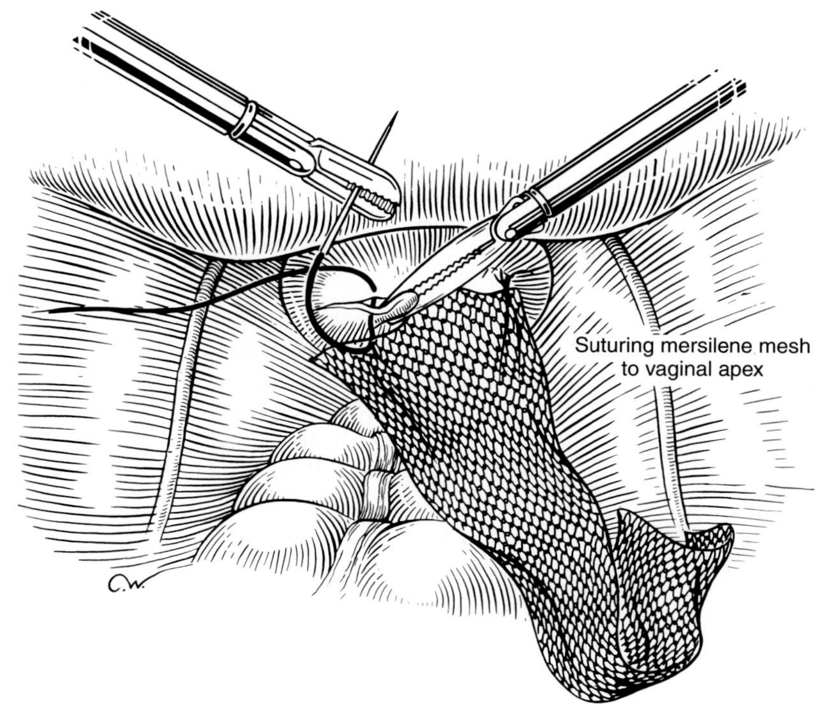

Figure 18-11. The Mersilene mesh is tied very loosely to the vaginal apex.

plished. The mesh is sutured to the posterior vaginal wall with a nonabsorbable suture and placed intraperitoneally before the vaginal cuff is closed with delayed absorbable sutures.

The mesh is adjusted to hold the vaginal apex in the correct anatomic position without being tight. Two permanent sutures or staples are placed in the longitudinal ligaments of the anterior surface of the sacrum, approximately 1 cm apart in the midline over S3–S4 (Figure 18-12). The peritoneum is

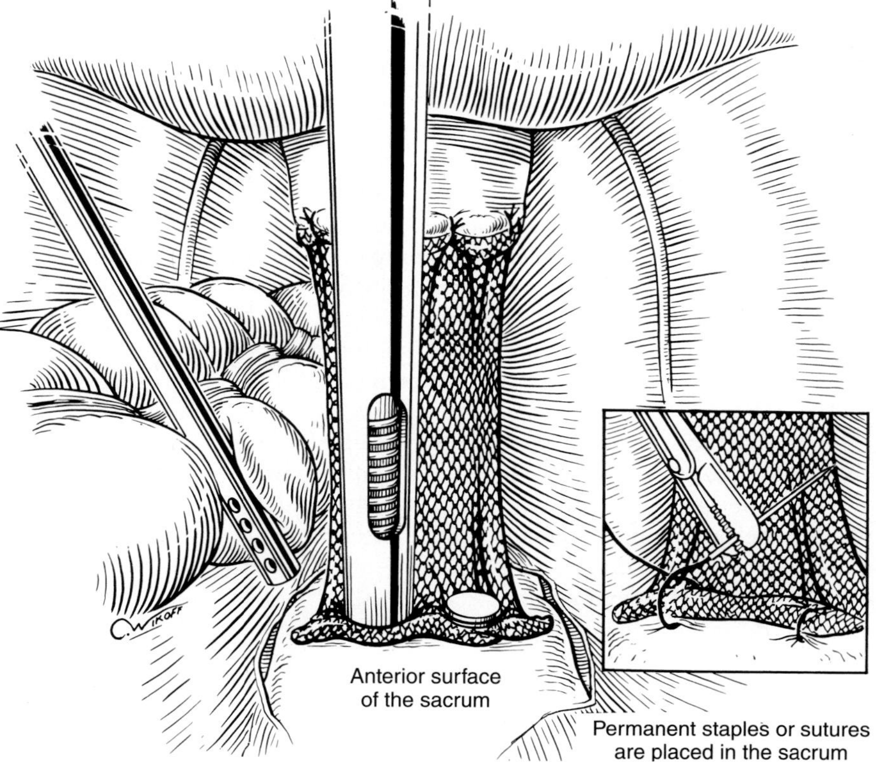

Figure 18-12. Two permanent sutures or staples are placed in the presacral ligament approximately 1 cm apart in the midline over the third and fourth sacral vertebrae. The inset shows a close-up view of the suturing technique. Sutures or staples can be used to retroperitonealize the mesh.

sutured over the graft from the sacrum toward the vagina. Usually, only a small segment of the graft cannot be covered. The serosa of the tail of the bladder (posterior peritoneal fold) and the superficial serosa of the sigmoid colon are used to cover the exposed mesh completely. If indicated, laparoscopic urethropexy is carried out.

Postoperatively, the patient is instructed to limit her activity, avoid intercourse for 6 weeks, and avoid strenuous exercise and heavy lifting for 2 months. Diet is advanced as tolerated, and a mild laxative is prescribed to prevent constipation.

In 15 women, 1 patient had substantial bleeding during the application of presacral staples to anchor the mesh to the sacrum and required laparotomy. The patients were followed for 3 to 40 months, and all indicated complete relief of their symptoms, with excellent vaginal vault support and no coital difficulty.[45]

Repair of Cystourethrocele

Prolonged, bothersome vaginal protrusions and pelvic pressure that worsens with ambulation and daily activity are common symptoms in women who have vaginal prolapse. Other symptoms include difficulty walking, voiding, or defecating; urinary incontinence; recurrent mucosal irritation; ulceration; and coital difficulty. Improvement of the quality of life is achievable in certain patients with behavioral modification and nonsurgical vaginal devices.

Paravaginal repair is required when cystourethrocele results from a separation of the pubocervical fascia from its lateral attachment to the pelvic side wall. If this defect is accompanied by GUSI, the paravaginal repair almost always will correct the problem.[39]

Dissection during anterior colporrhaphy splits the vaginal muscularis, and vaginal repair involves plication of the muscularis and adventitia in the midline and can pull the lateral attachments farther from the pelvic side wall. Paravaginal repair restores the lateral attachments to the pelvic side wall at the linea alba. Reported failure rates range from 0 to 20% for anterior colporrhaphy and from 3 to 14% for paravaginal repair.[40]

Four different pubocervical fascial defects can cause cystocele. Distinguishing these defects is important, as each type requires a different operative procedure.

1. The paravaginal defect results from detachment of the pubocervical fascia from its lateral attachment to the fascia of the obturator internal muscle at the level of the arcus tendineus fascia of the pelvis.[41–44] This is the most common cause of cystourethrocele. The repair consists of reestablishing the lateral pelvic side wall attachments of the pubocervical fascia and restoring the stability of this "hammock" by correcting the fundamental anatomic defect.
2. The transverse defect is caused by transverse separation of the pubocervical fascia from the pericervical ring into which the cardinal and uterosacral ligaments insert. The base of the bladder herniates into the anterior vaginal fornix and forms a cystocele without displacing the urethra or urethrovesical junction.
3. The midline or central defect results from a break in the central portion of the hammock between its lateral, dorsal, or ventral attachments.
4. With the distal defect, the distal urethra becomes avulsed or separated from its attachment to the urogenital diaphragm as it passes under the pubic symphysis.

Technique

Many operations have been described to correct loss of pelvic support. The abnormalities are identified, and the operation is planned with the intention of correcting each defect to achieve the optimal outcome.[35] The patient should be able to tolerate general anesthesia, increased intraabdominal pressure, and the Trendelenburg position.

The principles of the transabdominal approach used at laparotomy are employed during laparoscopy. This technique has evolved as an alternative in reconstructive pelvic operations.[36,37] Laparoscopy involves a smaller incision, eliminates the need for abdominal packing, causes less manipulation of the viscera, affords a better view of the pelvis, and allows precise hemostasis.

The patient is given intravenous antibiotics prophylactically. After induction of general endotracheal anesthesia and placement, a 10- to 11-mm umbilical trocar is inserted. Three lower abdominal 5-mm ancillary trocars also are placed; two are lateral to the epigastric vessels at the level of the iliac crest, and one is in the midline 5 cm above the pubic symphysis. The patient is put in the Trendelenburg position and tilted to the left to shift the bowel away from the operating field. After evaluation of the peritoneal cavity and completion of other indicated procedures, the pelvic reconstruction can proceed. The retropubic space is entered and dissected. The pubic symphysis, obturator foramen, and obturator neurovascular bundle are identified. The paravaginal defect (the lateral vaginal sulci) can be seen detached from the arcus tendineus fascia.

The bladder is mobilized medially, and the pubocervical fascia is exposed. The ischial spine can be located digitally by placing the operator's fingers inside the vagina while viewing through the laparoscope. During mobilization of the bladder, the lateral superior sulcus of the vagina is lifted by the assistant's fingers in the vagina to facilitate dissection.

Separation of the lateral sulcus from the pelvic side wall can be seen laparoscopically. Permanent sutures (2-0 prolene) are used to attach the superior lateral sulcus of the vagina to the arcus tendineus fascia (white line). The superior lateral sulcus of the vagina is elevated with the assistant's fingers in the vagina. Beneath the prominent paraurethral vascular plexus, the vagina is sutured to the linea alba of the pelvic side wall.

The paraurethral vascular plexus runs longitudinally along the axis of the vagina and is electrodesiccated before the placement of sutures. Otherwise, bleeding can occur if the plexus is penetrated by the needle. Such bleeding invariably stops when the suspension sutures are tied. To avoid bleeding, the first paravaginal suspension stitch should be placed close to the ischial spine. Figure-of-eight sutures are used for the suspension stitches to obtain good hemostasis and suspension. After placement of the first stitch, additional sutures are placed through the vaginal sulcus with its overlying fascia and the arcus tendineus fascia ventrally toward the pubic symphysis. The last stitch should be as close as possible to the pubic ramus.

Before this first suture is placed, the gynecologist should identify the ischial spine by vaginal palpation and by viewing through the laparoscope to avoid injuring the pudendal vessels and nerve. The initial stitch is placed through the linea alba approximately 1 to 1.5 cm ventral to the ischial spine.[38] Frequent vaginal examinations are done while suturing to assist the proper placement of the stitches, assess the adequacy of suspension, and establish anterior support. The procedure is completed by bladder neck suspension.

Vesicovaginal Fistula Repair

Vesicovaginal fistulas are treated with different surgical techniques, depending on their cause and location.[45] Small vesicovaginal fistulas that are not responsive to nonsurgical management usually are repaired easily.[46] The edges of the fistula are removed, and the defect is closed. Latzko's technique is used commonly[47] for fistulas that are surrounded by severe fibrosis and close to the bladder neck or urethral meatus. Lee and coworkers[48] recommended an abdominal approach for fistulas in the upper part of a narrow vagina, multiple fistulas, those associated with other pelvic abnormalities, and fistulas close to the ureter. A combined abdominal and vaginal approach is used in some instances.[49]

Technique

The basic principles for repair include adequate exposure, excision of fibrous tissue from the edges of the fistula, approximation of the edges without tension, the use of suitable suture material, and efficient postoperative bladder drainage.[50]

A 10-mm infraumbilical incision is made for the insertion of the operative laparoscope coupled with the CO_2 laser. Three 5-mm trocars are inserted in the lower abdomen for the suction-irrigator probe, grasping forceps, and bipolar forceps.[24] A simultaneous cystoscopy is done, and both ureters are catheterized to aid in their identification and protection during excision and closure of the fistula. A ureteral catheter is pulled through the fistula into the vagina to facilitate identification during excision.

A digital rectovaginal examination is carried out to exclude rectal involvement. An opening is made in the vagina, avoiding the bladder and rectum, and an inflated glove in the vagina helps maintain pneumoperitoneum. The anterior vaginal wall is elevated with a grasping forceps, and the fistula is identified with the previously inserted catheter, which also delineates the posterior bladder wall. The bladder is filled with water, and a cystotomy is made above the fistula, using the CO_2 laser. The water is evacuated as the bladder is distended by the pneumoperitoneum from

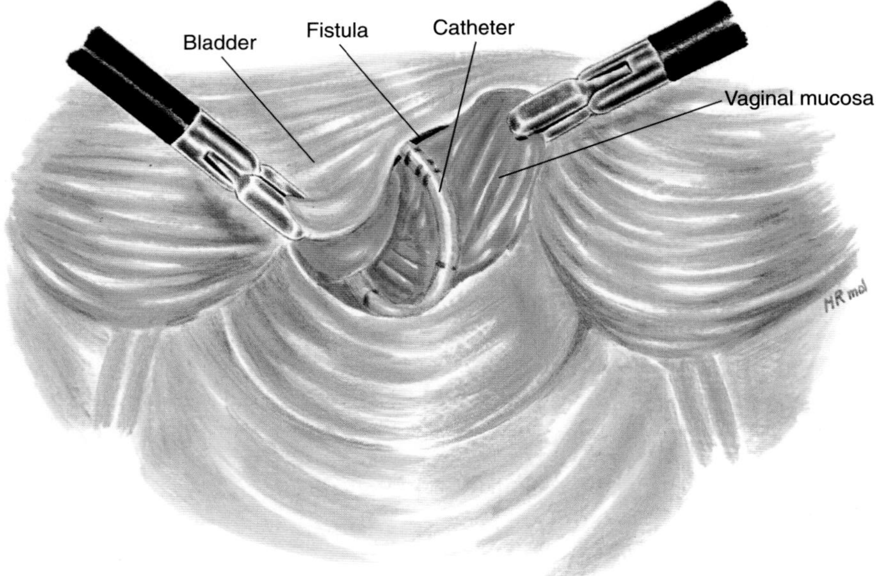

Figure 18-13. The fistula tract, vesicovaginal space, and ureters are observed laparoscopically.

the cystotomy. The fistula tract, vesicovaginal space, and ureters are observed laparoscopically (Figures 18-13 and 18-14). The vesicovaginal space is developed laparoscopically with the CO_2 laser and hydrodissection. The bladder is freed posteriorly from the vaginal wall. The fistula is identified, held with a grasping forceps, and excised (Figure 18-15). Adequate bladder dissection and mobilization are essential to eliminate tension upon suturing.

Initially, the vaginal wall opening of approximately 1.5 cm is closed with one layer of interrupted polyglactin suture (Figure 18-16). Then the vesical defect is repaired in one layer with interrupted 1-0 Endoknot polyglactin sutures (Ethicon), using extracorporeal knotting. Defects in the vagina and bladder are closed separately. Hemostasis in the vesicovaginal space and fistula area is essential. A peritoneal flap is obtained superior and lateral to the bladder dome, close to the round ligament and diverted toward the bladder base. The flap is used to separate the vesicovaginal space. It is secured with two interrupted polyglactin sutures. The dissected peritoneal area heals secondarily. No intraperitoneal drainage is used. After the procedure, a suprapubic or transurethal catheter is inserted and ureteral catheters are removed.

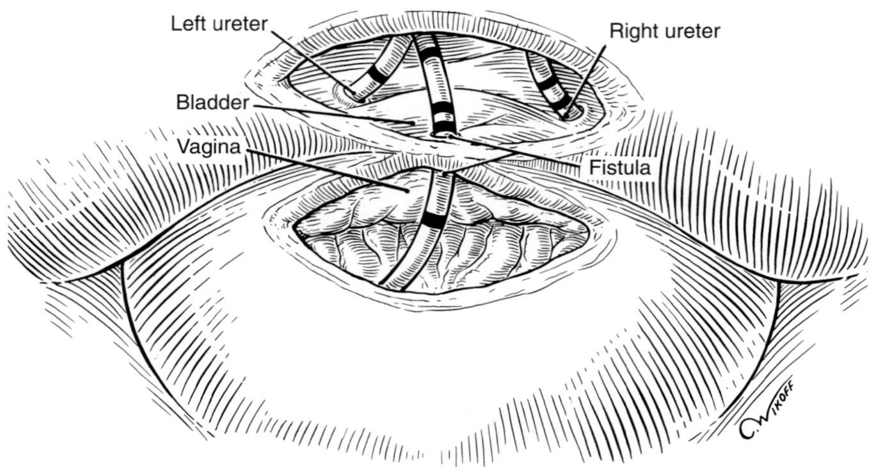

Figure 18-14. The bladder has been freed posteriorly from the vaginal wall.

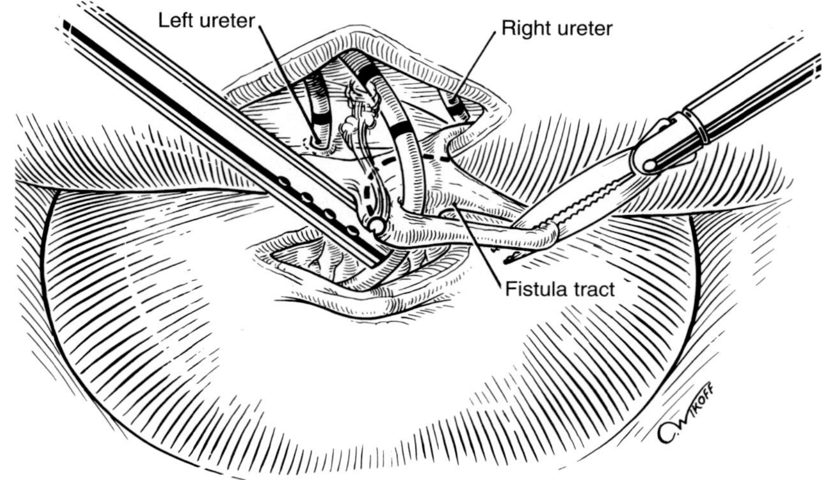

Figure 18-15. The bladder fistula is identified, and excised with the CO_2 laser.

Results

Laparoscopic repair of a vesicovaginal fistula in two patients was reported. After a laparoscopic excision of an ovarian remnant, a 45-year-old patient developed a posterior vesicovaginal fistula in the upper third of the vagina that failed to resolve with prolonged bladder drainage.[51] A vaginal approach was not appropriate because of the complexity, location, and condition of the defect. The morning after the repair of the fistula, the patient was discharged. Prophylactic antibiotics and estrogen were prescribed, and on postoperative day 10, the Foley catheter was removed. A cystogram was done, and no evidence of the fistula was seen. The patient was cured. A 48-year-old woman had a history of multiple previous abdominal operations. After a total abdominal hysterectomy with bilateral salpingo-oophorectomy and an inadvertent cystotomy, she developed a vesicovaginal fistula. After the repair, she was cured.

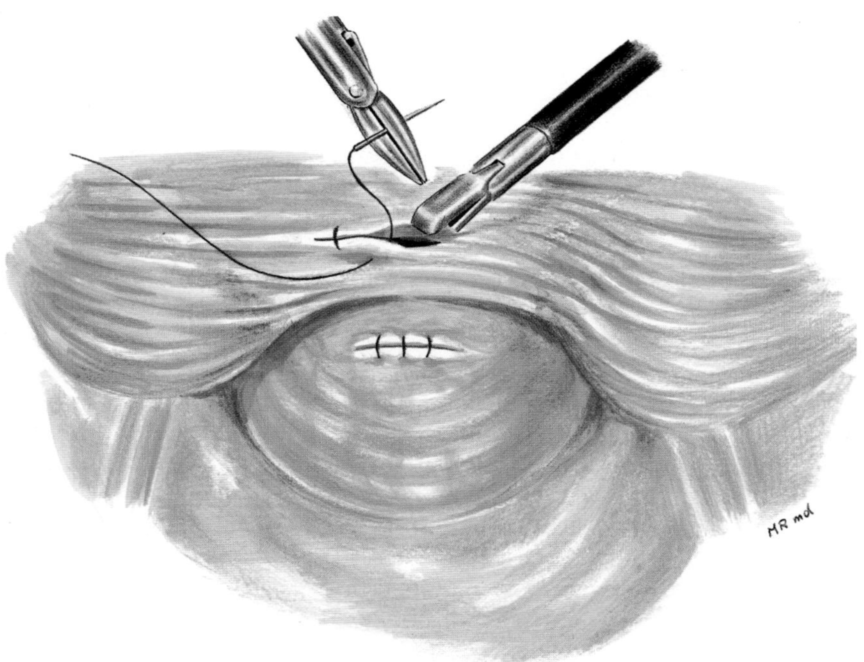

Figure 18-16. The vaginal wall repair is complete, and the bladder opening repair is in progress.

References

1. Thomas TM, Plymat DR, Blannin J, et al. Prevalence of urinary incontinence. *Br Med J* 1980; 281:1243.
2. Diokno AC, Brock BM, Brown MD, et al. Prevalence of urinary incontinence and other urological symptoms in the noninstitutionalized elderly. *J Urol* 1986; 136:1022.
3. Yarnell JW, St. Leger AS. The prevalence, severity and factors associated with urinary incontinence in a random sample of the elderly. *Age Aging* 1979; 8:81.
4. Holst K, Wilson PD. The prevalence of female urinary incontinence and reasons for not seeking treatment. *N Z Med J* 1988; 101:756.
5. Rosenzweig BA, Hischke MD, Thomas S, et al. Stress incontinence in women: Psychological status before and after treatment. *J Reprod Med* 1991; 36:835.
6. Horbach NS. Genuine SUI: Best surgical approach. *Contemp Obstet Gynecol* 1992; 37:53.
7. Marshall VF, Marchetti AA, Krantz KE. The correction of stress incontinence by simple vesicourethral suspension. *Surg Gynecol Obstet* 1941; 88:509.
8. Burch JC. Cooper's ligament urethrovesical suspension for stress incontinence. *Am J Obstet Gynecol* 1968; 100:764.
9. Stanton SL. Colposuspension, in Stanton SL, Tanagho E, eds., *Surgery of Female Incontinence*, 2d ed. New York: Springer-Verlag, 1986.
10. McGuire EJ, Lytton B. Pubovaginal sling procedure for stress incontinence. *J Urol* 1978; 119:82.
11. Pereyra AJ, Lebherz TB. Combined urethrovesical suspension and vaginourethroplasty for correction of urinary stress incontinence. *Obstet Gynecol* 1967; 30:537.
12. Raz S. Modified bladder neck suspension for female stress incontinence. *Urology* 1981; 17:82.
13. Hohnfellner R, Petrie E. Sling procedures in surgery, in Stanton SL, Tanagho E, eds., *Surgery of Female Incontinence*, 2d ed. New York: Springer-Verlag, 1986.
14. Gittes RF, Loughlin KR. No incision pubovaginal suspension for stress incontinence. *J Urol* 1987; 138:568.
15. Bhatia NN, Bergman A. A modified Burch versus Pereyra retropubic urethropexy for stress urinary incontinence. *Obstet Gynecol* 1985; 66:255.
16. Mundy AR. A trial comparing the Stamey bladder neck suspension procedure with colposuspension for the treatment of stress incontinence. *Br J Urol* 1983; 33:687.
17. Green DF, McGuire EJ, Lytton B. A comparison of endoscopic suspension of the vesical neck versus anterior urethropexy for the treatment of stress urinary incontinence. *J Urol* 1986; 136:1205.
18. Karram MM, Bhatia NN. Transvaginal needle bladder neck suspension procedures for stress urinary incontinence: A comprehensive review. *Obstet Gynecol* 1989; 73:906.
19. Tanagho EA. Colpocystourethropexy: The way we do it. *J Urol* 1976; 116:751.
20. Bergman A, Ballard C, Koonings P. Primary stress urinary incontinence and pelvic relaxation: Prospective randomized comparison of three different operations. *Am J Obstet Gynecol* 1989; 161:97.
21. Bergman A, Ballard C, Koonings P. Comparison of three different surgical procedures for genuine stress incontinence: Prospective randomized study. *Am J Obstet Gynecol* 1989; 160:1102.
22. Penttinen J, Kindholm EL, Kaar K, et al. Successful colposuspension in stress urinary incontinence reduces bladder neck mobility and increases pressure transmission to the urethra. *Acta Gynecol Obstet* 1989; 224:233.
23. Van Geelen JM, Theeuwes AGM, Eskes TKAB, et al. The clinical and urodynamic effects of anterior vaginal repair and Burch colposuspension. *Am J Obstet Gynecol* 1989; 159:137.
24. Nezhat CH, Nezhat F, Nezhat C. Operative laparoscopy (minimally invasive surgery): State of the art. *J Gynecol Surg* 1992; 8:111.
25. Vancaille TG, Schuessler W. Laparoscopic bladder neck suspension. *J Laparoendosc Surg* 1991; 1:169.
26. Nezhat CH, Nezhat F, Nezhat CR, Rottenberg H. Laparoscopic retropubic cystourethropexy. *J Am Assoc Gynecol Laparosc* 1994; 1(4):339.
27. Walters M, Shields L. The diagnostic value of history, physical examination and the Q-tip cotton swab test in women with urinary incontinence. *Am J Obstet Gynecol* 1988; 159:145.
28. Hilton P, Stanton SL. A clinical and urodynamic assessment of the Burch colposuspension for genuine stress incontinence. *Br J Obstet Gynaecol* 1983; 90:934.
29. Bergman A, Bhatia NN. Uroflowmetry for predicting postoperative voiding difficulties in

women with SUI. *Br J Obstet Gynaecol* 1985; 92:835.

30. Bhatia NN, Bergman A. Use of preoperative uroflowmetry and simultaneous urethrocystometry for predicting risk of prolonged postoperative bladder drainage. *Urology* 1986; 28:440.
31. Nezhat CH, Nezhat F, Seidman DS, et al. A new method for laparoscopic access to the space of Retzius during retropubic cystourethropexy. *J Urol* 1996; 155:1916.
32. Nezhat CH, Nezhat F, Nezhat CR, Rottenberg H. Laparoscopic retropubic cystourethropexy. *J Am Assoc Gynecol Laparosc* 1994; 1:339.
33. Dunton JD, Mikuta J. Post-hysterectomy vaginal vault prolapse. *Postgrad Obstet Gynecol* 1988; 8:1.
34. Sze EH, Miklos JR, Partoll L, et al. Sacrospinous ligament fixation with transvaginal needle suspension for advanced pelvic organ prolapse and stress incontinence. *Obstet Gynecol* 1997; 89:129.
35. Arthur HG, Savage D. Uterine prolapse and prolapse of vaginal vault treated by sacral hysteropexy. *J Obstet Gynaecol Br Emp* 1957; 64:355.
36. Randall CL, Nichols DH. Surgical treatment of vaginal inversion. *Obstet Gynecol* 1971; 38:327.
37. Symmonds RE, Williams TJ, Lee RA, Webb MJ. Posthysterectomy enterocele and vaginal vault prolapse. *Am J Obstet Gynecol* 1981; 140:852.
38. Nezhat C, Nezhat F, Gordon S, Wilkins E. Laparoscopic versus abdominal hysterectomy. *J Reprod Med* 1992; 37:247.
39. Richardson AC. How to correct prolapse paravaginally. *Contemporary Ob/Gyn* 1990; 35:100.
40. Weber AM, Walters MD. Anterior vaginal prolapse: Review of anatomy and techniques of surgical repair. *Obstet Gynecol* 1997; 89:311.
41. Richardson AC, Lyon JB, Williams NL. A new look at pelvic relaxation. *Am J Obstet Gynecol* 1976; 126:568.
42. Richardson AC, Lyon JB, Williams NL. Treatment of stress urinary incontinence due to paravaginal fascial defect. *Obstet Gynecol* 1981; 57:357.
43. Baden WF, Walker TA. Urinary stress incontinence: Evolution of paravaginal repair. *Female Patient* 1987; 12:89.
44. Liu CY. Laparoscopic cystocele repair: Paravaginal suspension, in Liu CY, ed. *Laparoscopic Hysterectomy and Pelvic Floor Reconstruction*. Cambridge, MA: Blackwell, 1996.
45. Drutz HP. Urinary fistulas. *Obstet Gynecol Clin North Am* 1989; 16:11.
46. Falk HC, Orkin LA. Nonsurgical closure of vesicovaginal fistulas. *Obstet Gynecol* 1957; 9:538.
47. Latzko W. Behandlund Hochsitzender Blasen und Mastdarmscheidenfisteln nach Uteruseztipation mit hohom Schedienverschluss. *Zentralbl Gynakol* 1914; 38:904.
48. Lee RA, Symmonds RE, William TJ. Current status of genitourinary fistula. *Obstet Gynecol* 1988; 72:313.
49. Taylor JS, Hewson AD, Rachow P. Synchronous combined transvaginal repair of vesicovaginal fistulas. *Aust N Z J Surg* 1980; 50:23.
50. Moir JC. Principles and methods of treatment of vesicovaginal fistulae, in *The Vesicovaginal Fistula*. London: Bailliere, Tindall, and Cassell; 1967; 52.
51. Nezhat CH, Nezhat F, Nezhat LC, Rottenberg H. Laparoscopic repair of a vesicovaginal fistula: A case report. *Obstet Gynecol* 1994; 83:899.

19

Appendectomy

As gynecologic and general surgeons do more endoscopic procedures, the advantages of laparoscopic appendectomy should be considered. Semm did a laparoscopic appendectomy in 1980.[1] The completion of more than two dozen prospective randomized trials shows that the laparoscopic technique produces better outcomes for patients with suspected acute appendicitis, than does conventional open appendectomy.[2,3]

This chapter describes the value of laparoscopy in the diagnosis of appendicitis, discusses the indications for laparoscopic appendectomy, and illustrates the techniques.

Why Laparoscopy?

Acute appendicitis can be difficult to diagnose in women because many gynecologic disorders cause symptoms and signs indistinguishable from those of appendicitis.[4] The type and location of pain or discomfort associated with ovulation, ovarian cysts, endometriosis, salpingitis, and urinary tract disorders cannot be differentiated easily from those of acute appendicitis. In the general population, 15 to 20% of appendixes removed by laparotomy for suspected appendicitis show no abnormality compared with 30 to 45% in young women.[5] Accurate diagnosis and prompt management help prevent complications from perforation, including significant postoperative morbidity and an increased risk of tubal infertility.[6–8] The diagnosis of acute appendicitis is difficult in women of childbearing age. In young women who complain of right lower abdominal pain, laparoscopy can give a precise diagnosis and reduce the rate of unnecessary appendectomies. Laine and associates[9] did a randomized study to compare laparoscopic and open appendectomy in 50 young female patients with suspected acute appendicitis. They reported that the diagnosis was established accurately in 96% of the patients in the laparoscopic group and 72% in the open group. There were 11 (44%) unnecessary appendectomies in the open group but only 1 (4%) in the laparoscopic group. The impact of laparoscopic appendectomy on the incidence of histologically normal appendixes recently was evaluated by Barrat and associates[10] who found that in 930 patients operated on using the classic McBurney approach, the incidence of histologically normal appendixes was 25.1%. The incidence was only 8.2% in 290 patients who underwent laparoscopic exploration, with an appendectomy carried out if there were macroscopic abnormalities. The risk of false positives and false negatives was approximately 10%. The diagnostic difficulties usually occurred in the initial phase of the disease with acute mucosal involvement in a morphologically normal appendix. Those authors concluded that laparoscopy reduced the number of histologically normal appendixes compared with a laparotomy. This was achieved by not removing macroscopically normal appendixes. A small proportion (5 to 10%) could be patients with early appendicitis with only mucosal involvement. Moberg and coauthors[11] summarized the results of diagnostic laparoscopy in 1043 patients with symptoms and signs of acute appendicitis. They showed that diagnostic laparoscopy is safe and can be recommended in patients with suspected acute appendicitis, particularly in women. Their data also suggested that a macroscopically normal-looking appendix need not be removed.

Reiertsen and coworkers[12] did a randomized controlled trial with sequential design of laparoscopic and conventional appendectomy in 272 patients with suspected appendicitis. They found that the risk of unnecessary appendectomy was significantly lower after laparoscopy and concluded that an initial laparoscopy may reduce the rate of errors.

The sequelae from appendectomies by laparotomy that reveal a normal appendix usually are not serious, although a 1 to 17% morbidity rate from such operations has been reported.[2,13] These observations and concern about postoperative adhesions have increased the use of laparoscopy for the diagnosis of the cause of pelvic and abdominal pain before definitive therapy.[14–16] In a patient with suspected appendicitis, laparoscopy can reduce the need for laparotomy because the surgeon can inspect the peritoneal cavity and pelvis thoroughly with the laparoscope and avoid even a McBurney or small laparotomy incision.[17,18] However, observation of the entire appendix by laparoscopy is possible in only 90 to 95% of patients.[19] In addition, some visually normal appendixes have been removed in which histologic examination revealed acute or chronic inflammation.[16,20] In a series of 100 incidental appendectomies, 52 appendixes were normal, 28 had adhesions, 14 showed foci of endometriosis, 4 showed focal chronic inflammation, 1 contained a benign mucocele, and 1 had a carcinoid.[2] These findings demonstrate the potential yield of appendiceal disease associated with a grossly normal appendix. A similar abnormality rate was reported by Krone[21] in his series of 1718 incidental appendectomies: 21.4% were normal, but 65.1% showed evidence of chronic disease and 5.6% had a carcinoid, a mucocele, or endometriosis. Women with chronic right lower quadrant pain also have a high rate of gross or microscopic appendiceal abnormalities. In a series of 62 laparoscopic appendectomies done for acute and chronic pain,[22] 38 were associated with entrapping adhesions, 12 showed evidence of chronic inflammation, and 5 were involved with endometriosis. Only seven were normal. Of the 55 patients with predominantly right lower quadrant or flank pain, 53 had complete or significant pain relief on long-term follow-up (1 to 6 years). In addition, in a patient who has chronic right lower quadrant pain and no obvious appendiceal abnormality, prophylactic laparoscopic appendectomy should be considered. The procedure eliminates the chance of missing early appendicitis or other appendiceal abnormalities. Prolonging laparoscopy for 4 to 21 minutes to carry out an appendectomy imposes minimal stress to the patient.[2]

Incidental Appendectomy by Laparoscopy

Prophylactic laparoscopic appendectomy is relatively easy and safe. It is similar in principle to appendectomy by laparotomy. With the expansion of laparoscopic procedures, the transition from laparoscopic diagnosis to laparoscopic appendectomy is logical. Removal of a normal-appearing appendix while operating for suspected acute appendicitis has been the standard of care. It has been suggested that the introduction of operative laparoscopy should not alter this practice. Others contend that a normal-looking appendix may be left in place.[11,12] Laparoscopy can prevent unnecessary appendectomies.[9,12] Laparoscopic removal of the normal appendix caused no increase in morbidity or length of hospitalization compared with diagnostic laparoscopy.[23] This observation shows the cost-effectiveness of laparoscopic appendectomy in terms of preventing missed and future appendicitis. Incidental laparoscopic appendectomy may be the preferred treatment option.

The appendix may be a cause of chronic pelvic pain. The laparoscopic appearance of chronic or recurrent appendicitis was studied prospectively in 42 women with long-term or recurrent lower abdominal pain.[24] Appendectomy was done when at least two of the following pathologic changes were present at diagnostic laparoscopy: vascular injection of appendiceal peritoneum, periappendiceal adhesions, and induration of the appendix. During a mean observation of 13 months, 74% of women had no abdominal pain, 12% had partial relief in a mean of 15 months of observation, and 12% experienced no change in abdominal pain. New laparoscopic techniques with associated local anesthesia and conscious sedation allow operative laparoscopic procedures to be achieved while the patient is awake. Such evaluation of the appendix with intraoperative patient feedback concerning the presence and absence of pain allows more accurate diagnosis of chronic appendicitis during conscious pain mapping.[25]

Prophylactic antibiotics are administered preoperatively to patients who complain of right lower quadrant pain. The operation is carried out under general anesthesia. Appendectomy is advisable after other laparoscopic procedures have been completed. Copious irrigation is advisable to minimize bacterial contamination.

After the pelvis is inspected, the appendix is identified, mobilized, and examined. Periappendiceal or

Figure 19-1. After the pelvis is inspected and the other pelvic abnormalities have been treated, the appendix is identified, mobilized, and examined.

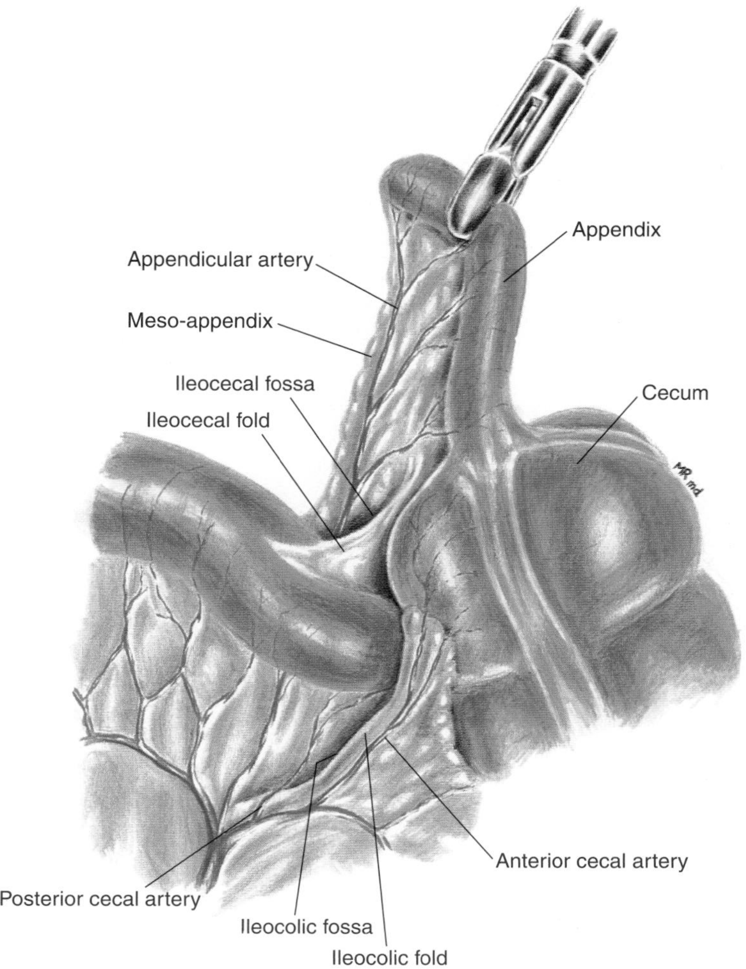

pericecal adhesions are lysed, using the laser or scissors, because adequate mobilization and good exposure are essential, particularly if the appendix is adherent to the pelvic side wall or is retrocecal. The mesoappendix is coagulated with bipolar forceps or clipped and cut with laparoscopic scissors or a laser to skeletonize the appendix (Figures 19-1, 19-2, A and B, and 19-3). Fecal contents are milked toward the tip of the appendix by using a grasper over an area 2 cm from the cecum. Two Endoloop sutures (Ethicon) are passed sequentially through one of the 5-mm suprapubic trocar sleeves and looped around the base of the appendix next to each other (Figure 19-4). A third Endoloop suture is applied 5 mm distal to the first two sutures. Hulka tubal clips (used for tubal sterilization) also can be used to secure the proximal and distal portions of the appendix.[14,26] The appendix is cut between the two sets of sutures, using the laser or laparoscopic scissors (Figure 19-5). The luminal portion of the appendiceal stump is seared with the CO_2 laser, povidone-iodine (Betadine) solution may be applied, and the tissues are irrigated copiously with lactated Ringer's solution (Figure 19-6). A purse-string or Z-suture can be placed in the cecum to bury the appendiceal stump,[27] although there appears to be no advantage to its invagination.[28] Countersinking the stump does not guarantee that adhesions or complications will be avoided. If the stump is to be buried, a polydioxanone Endosuture (Ethicon) is used with two needle holders or graspers inserted through the suprapubic trocar sleeves. The stump is invaginated with a grasper, and the purse-string suture is tied, using an instrument-tying method or extracorporeal suturing. A significant difference was found in the incidence of postoperative small bowel obstruction when invagination was compared with stump ligation. In the invagination group, there were six instances of bowel obstruction (1.6%), while the stump ligation group included only one patient who became

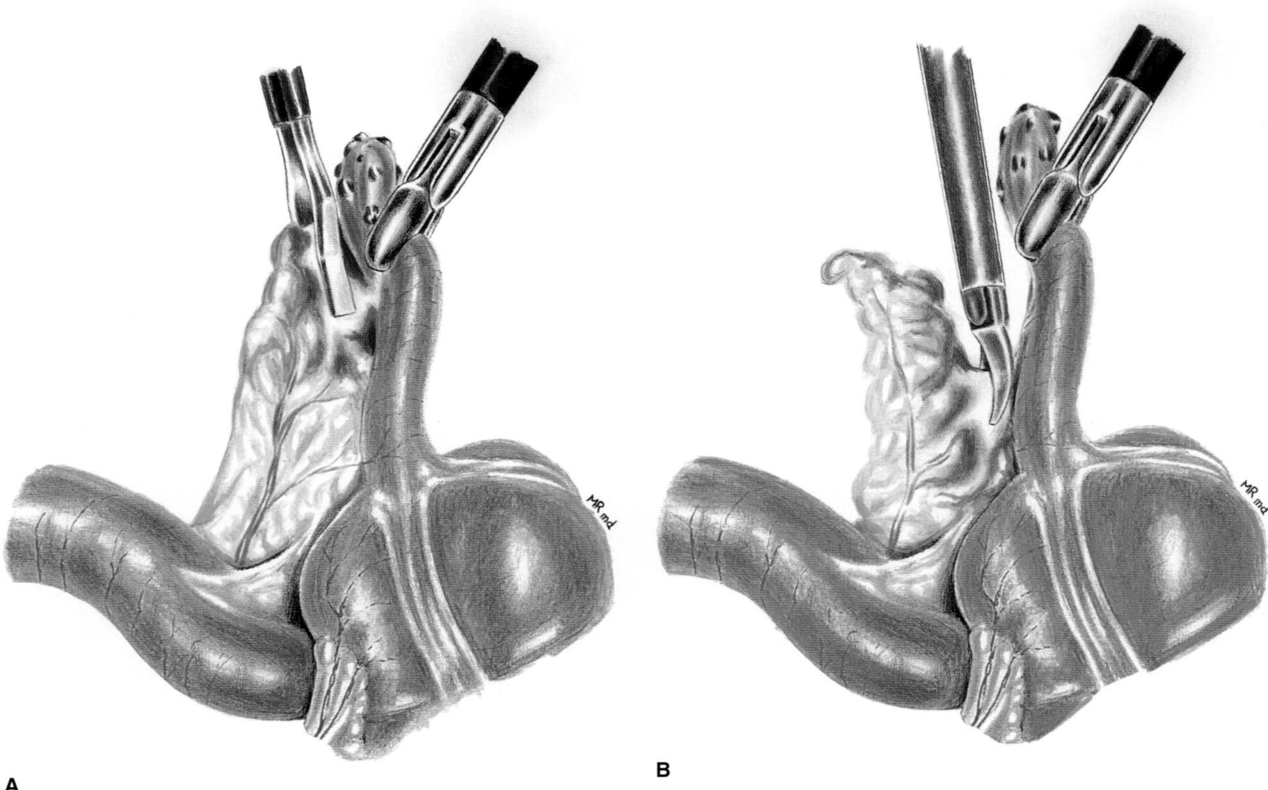

Figure 19-2. **A.** The mesoappendix is coagulated with bipolar forceps. **B.** It is cut with scissors or a laser to skeletonize the appendix.

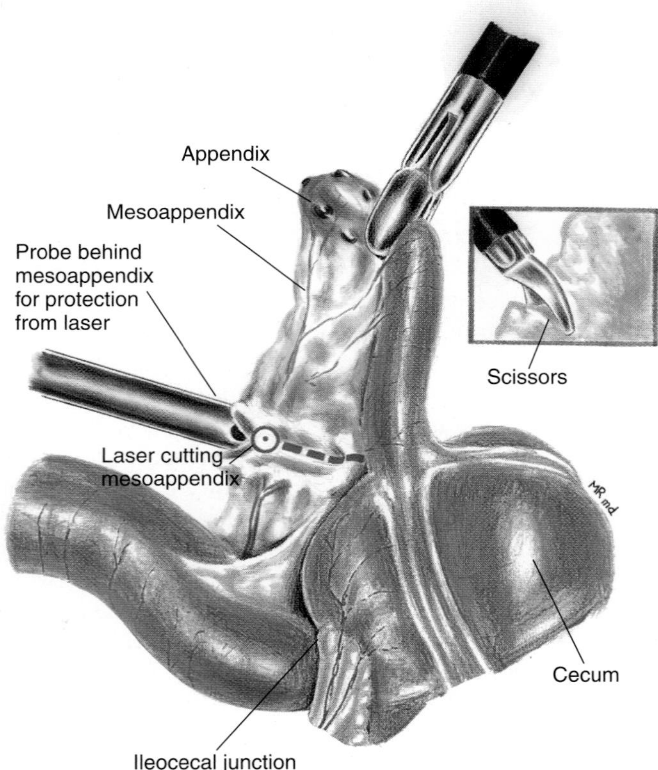

Figure 19-3. Alternatively, the base of the mesoappendix can be cut with the CO_2 laser or a scissors *(inset)*. The tip of the appendix contains endometrial implants.

Figure 19-4. After the fecal contents have been "milked" out by using a grasper over an area 2 cm from the cecum, two Endoloop sutures are passed sequentially through one of the 5-mm trocar sleeves around the base of the appendix close to each other. A third Endoloop suture is applied 5 mm distal to the first two sutures.

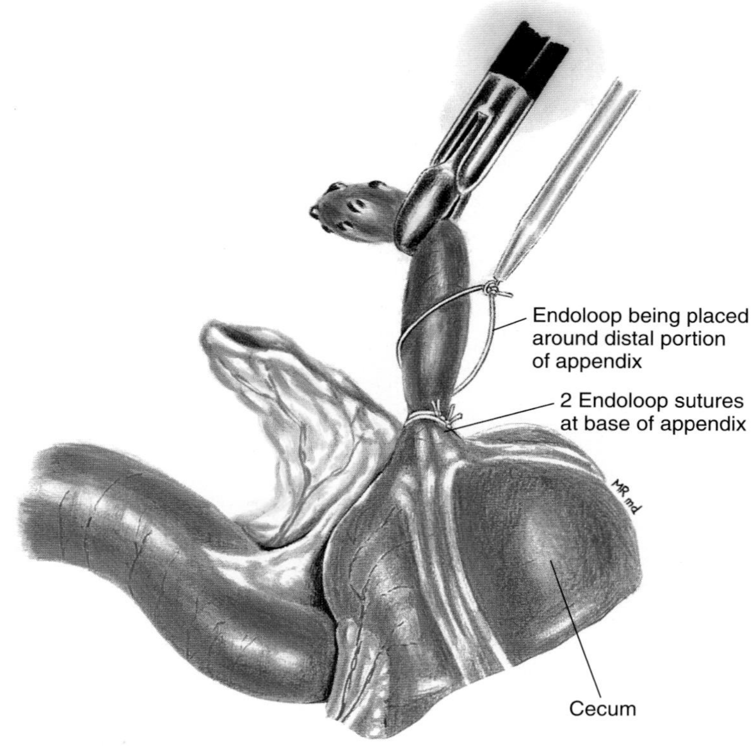

Figure 19-5. The appendix is cut between two sets of sutures, using either the laser or laparoscopic scissors.

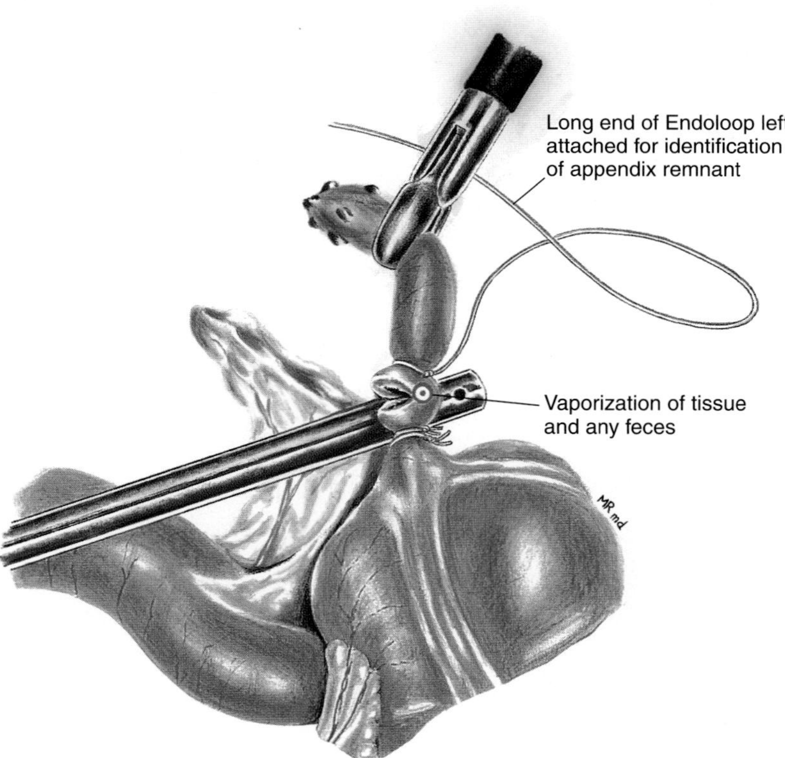

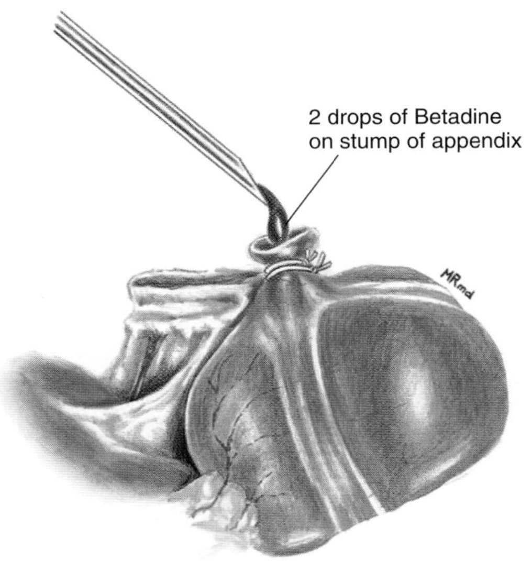

Figure 19-6. The luminal part of the stump is seared with either the laser or electrosurgery, Betadine is applied, and the tissue is irrigated copiously with lactated Ringer's solution.

obstructed postoperatvely (0.3%). This difference in complications may be related to the high incidence of adhesions found in more than 70% of patients with purse-string or Z-suture placement.[20] Simple ligation simplifies the technical procedure and shortens the operating time. It produces no deformation of the cecal wall that might arouse suspicion of a neoplasm in subsequent contrast radiography.

An Endoloop suture can be placed around the distal tip of the appendix as a substitute for a grasping instrument during initial mobilization and excision of the appendix. Once the appendix is free, the suture is used to pull the appendix into a 5- or 10-mm accessory trocar sleeve. The trocar sleeve is removed from the suprapubic incision with the appendix contained within it. Endobags (Ethicon) that minimize contact between contaminated tissue and the pelvis are available. Traction on the purse string of the bag allows it to be drawn through a small skin incision without contaminating it. The appendix also can be removed from the abdomen with long grasping forceps placed through the operating channel of the laparoscope. However, this method contaminates both the graspers and the operating channel.

Stapling devices make laparoscopic appendectomy easier and faster. The multifire stapler is introduced through a 12-mm suprapubic midline incision and applied directly across the entire mesoappendix and appendix. In a single motion, the entire appendix and its mesoappendix are clipped and cut (Figure 19-7). The stapler's

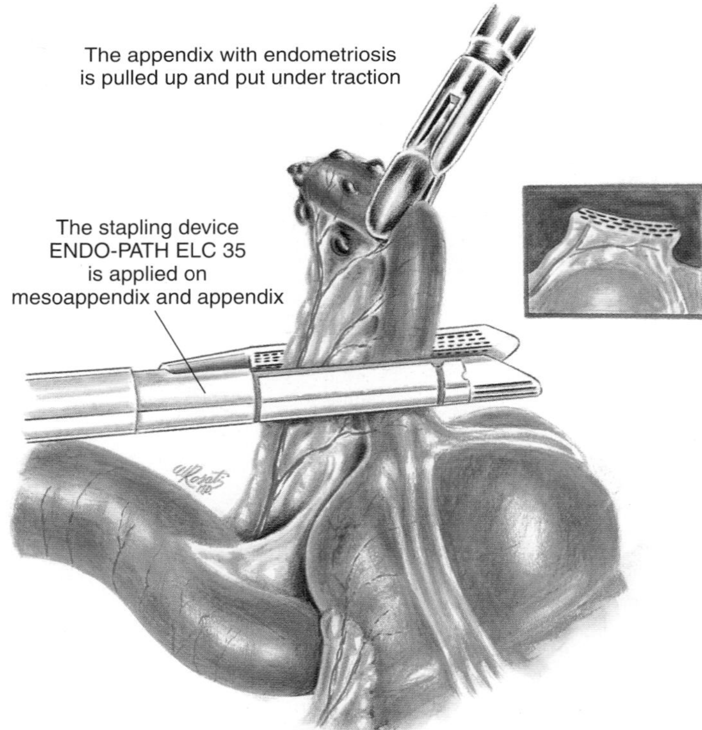

Figure 19-7. The multifire stapler is inserted through a 12-mm trocar sleeve and applied directly across the mesoappendix and appendix. In a single motion, the entire appendix and the mesoappendix are clipped and cut. The appendix can be removed from the abdomen with long grasping forceps placed through the trocar sleeve. The trocar sleeve is removed with the appendix contained within it. Alternatively, an Endobag can be used as the receptacle for the detached appendix. Inset shows the line of staples.

operation should not be hindered by contact with surrounding tissue, and the cecum must be free from attachments. Appendiceal contents do not leak intraperitoneally, and the larger trocar sleeve allows easier removal of the separated appendix. Two disadvantages to the stapling device are its cost and the need to use a 12-mm trocar.

Patients are discharged on the same day or after an overnight stay. They should avoid solid food for 24 hours. In a series of 100 patients at the Center for Special Pelvic Surgery, all were discharged within 24 hours, although 7 remained overnight because of their own preference or a delayed surgery.[2] Although the procedure has a favorable cost-benefit ratio, complications include stump blowout, wound infection, hemorrhage, and postoperative ileus.[29,30] Laparoscopic appendectomy can be achieved safely by using instruments smaller than 3 mm that leave practically no scars.[31] This technique may appeal to pediatric surgeons[32] and possibly be of value in the office setting with local anesthesia and conscious sedation.[25]

The diagnosis of acute appendicitis is difficult in pregnant women, and diagnostic laparoscopy may allow a timely diagnosis. Laparoscopic appendectomy can be achieved safely during pregnancy.[33,34]

Laparoscopic Appendectomy for Appendicitis

The procedure is similar to an incidental appendectomy except that the appendix is edematous and possibly more fragile. The presence of gross inflammation, ease of excision, and absence of abscess formation influence the decision to do an appendectomy. Two or three accessory trocars are required, with the laparoscope in the umbilical position. Adhesions are lysed with the laser or scissors so that the appendix is mobile. In removing the appendix at its base, a sufficient stump is left to prevent spillage of luminal contents from the pedicle. An alternative procedure[26] is to place Hulka clips on the base of the inflamed appendix and then control the blood supply in the mesoappendix with electrocoagulation, hemaclips, or a multifire stapling device. If an inflamed appendix is removed laparoscopically, a larger trocar may be needed to ease its removal[35] and the operative site is irrigated copiously.

A retrocecal appendicitis makes laparoscopic appendectomy more difficult. Gotz and coworkers[36] noted that complications requiring laparotomy (including bleeding, adhesions, and an abnormal position of the appendix) occurred early in their series of 388 patients with appendicitis who had a laparoscopic appendectomy. These findings prompted them to emphasize the significant learning curve and the long period needed to become proficient in laparoscopic appendectomy for a ruptured appendix, in the presence of extensive adhesions, or if the appendix is relatively inaccessible. Laparoscopically assisted appendectomy has been described for cases in which the proper endoscopic instruments and sutures are unavailable.[35] The laparoscope facilitates the definitive diagnosis of appendicitis, and a grasper is passed through an accessory trocar located over McBurney's point. The tip of the appendix is grasped and then pulled from the trocar insertion along with the trocar sleeve and grasper. Routine appendectomy can be done through a small abdominal incision. The procedure usually requires 5 to 20 minutes but takes longer if the appendix is ruptured or an abscess is present.

Laparoscopic appendectomy appears to be as safe as open appendectomy and seems to have the advantage of allowing a quicker recovery.[37] A meta-analysis that included multiple randomized controlled trials found that laparoscopic appendectomy reduced the time to full recovery by 5.5 days, reduced postoperative pain at 24 hours, and decreased the absolute risk for wound infection by 3.2%.[3] There was no difference between the two techniques in regard to length of hospitalization, readmission rate, and intraabdominal abscess formation. The longer operative time for the laparoscopic approach had been attributed to the learning curve associated with the procedure and was not found to increase morbidity.[38] The operating time was increased on average by 17 minutes.[25] Moberg and Montgomery[39] suggested that at the price of a longer operation, the laparoscopic technique offered significant benefits over the conventional approach. Decreased trauma, better diagnostic accuracy, and superior cosmetic results were achieved.

Laparoscopic appendectomy has been associated with higher hospital costs. In 1997, the average total charge for an open appendectomy was $9,670 while that for a laparoscopic appendectomy was $11,290.[40] However, laparoscopic appendectomy offers significant cost savings for working patients.[41,42]

References

1. Litynski GS. Kurt Semm and the fight against skepticism: Endoscopic hemostasis, laparoscopic appendectomy, and Semm's impact on the "laparoscopic revolution." *J Soc Laparoendosc Surg* 1998; 2:309.
2. Nezhat C, Nezhat F. Incidental appendectomy during videolaseroscopy. *Am J Obstet Gynecol* 1991; 165:559.
3. Garbutt JM, Soper NJ, Shannon WD, et al. Meta-analysis of randomized controlled trials comparing laparoscopic and open appendectomy. *Surg Laparosc Endosc* 1999; 9:17.
4. Bongard F, Landers DV, Lewis F. Differential diagnosis of appendicitis and pelvic inflammatory disease: A prospective analysis. *Am J Surg* 1985; 150:90.
5. Condon RE: Appendicitis, in Sabiston DG, ed., *Textbook of Surgery*, 13th ed. Philadelphia: Saunders, 1986.
6. Mueller BA, Daling JR, Moore DE, et al. Appendectomy and the risk of tubal infertility. *N Engl J Med* 1986; 315:1506.
7. Geerdsen J, Hansen JB. Incidence of sterility in women operated on in childhood for perforated appendicitis. *Acta Obstet Gynecol Scand* 1977; 56:523.
8. Powley PH. Infertility due to pelvic abscess and pelvic peritonitis in appendicitis. *Lancet* 1965; 1:27.
9. Laine S, Rantala A, Gullichsen R, Ovaska J. Laparoscopic appendectomy—is it worthwhile? A prospective, randomized study in young women. *Surg Endosc* 1997; 11:95.
10. Barrat C, Catheline JM, Rizk N, Champault GG. Does laparoscopy reduce the incidence of unnecessary appendicectomies? *Surg Laparosc Endosc* 1999; 9:27.
11. Moberg AC, Ahlberg G, Leijonmarck CE, et al. Diagnostic laparoscopy in 1043 patients with suspected acute appendicitis. *Eur J Surg* 1998; 164:833.
12. Reiertsen O, Larsen S, Trondsen E, et al. Randomized controlled trial with sequential design of laparoscopic verus conventional appendicectomy. *Br J Surg* 1997; 84:842.
13. Chang FC, Hogle HH, Welling DR. The fate of the negative appendix. *Am J Surg* 1973; 126:752.
14. Leahy PF: Technique of laparoscopic appendectomy. *Br J Surg* 1989; 76:616.
15. Paterson-Brown S, Thompson JN, Eckersley JRT, et al. Which patients with suspected appendicitis should undergo laparoscopy? *Br Med J* 1988; 296:1363.
16. Whitworth CM, Whitworth PW, Sanfilippo J, et al. Value of diagnostic laparoscopy in young women with possible appendicitis. *Surg Gynecol Obstet* 1988; 167:187.
17. Deutsch AA, Zelikovsky A, Reiss R. Laparoscopy in the prevention of unnecessary appendectomies: A prospective study. *Br J Surg* 1982; 69:336.
18. Leape LL, Ramenofsky MD. Laparoscopy for questionable appendicitis—can it reduce the negative appendectomy rate? *Ann Surg* 1980; 191:410.
19. Nowzaradan Y. Laparoscopic appendectomy for acute appendicitis: Indications and current use. *J Laparoendosc Surg* 1991; 7:247.
20. Schrieber JH. Early experience with laparoscopic appendectomy in women. *Surg Endosc* 1987; 1:211.
21. Krone HA. Preventive appendectomy in gynecologic surgery: Report of 1718 cases. *Geburtshilfe frauenheilkd* 1989; 49:1035
22. Bryson K: Laparoscopic appendectomy. J Gynecol Surg 1991; 7:93
23. Greason KL, Rappold JF, Liberman MA. Incidental laparoscopic appendectomy for acute right lower quadrant abdominal pain: Its time has come. *Surg Endosc* 1998; 12:223.
24. Popp LW. Gynecologically indicated single-endoloop laparoscopic appendectomy. *J Am Assoc Gynecol Laparosc* 1998; 5:275.
25. Almeida OD Jr, Val-Gallas JM, Rizk B. Appendectomy under local anaesthesia following conscious pain mapping with microlaparoscopy. *Hum Reprod* 1998; 13:588.
26. Schultz LS, Pietrafitta JJ, Graber JN, et al. Retrograde laparoscopic appendectomy: Report of a case. *J Laparoendosc Surg* 1991; 1:111.
27. Semm K. Endoscopic appendectomy. *Endoscopy* 1983; 15:59.
28. Engstrom L, Fenyo G. Appendectomy: Assessment of stump invagination versus simple ligation: A prospective, randomized trial. *Br J Surg* 1985; 72:971.
29. Fisher KS, Ross DS. Guidelines for therapeutic decision in incidental appendectomy. *Surg Gynecol Obstet* 1990; 171:95.
30. Nezhat C, Baggish M, Nezhat F. Operative gynecology (minimally invasive surgery): State of the art. *J Gynecol Surg* 1992; 8:111.
31. Gagner M, Garcia-Ruiz A. Technical aspects of minimally invasive abdominal surgery

performed with needlescopic instruments. *Surg Laparosc Endosc* 1998; 8:171.

32. Schier F. Laparoscopic appendectomy with 1.7-mm instruments. *Pediatr Surg Int* 1998; 14:142.
33. Nezhat FR, Tazuke S, Nezhat CH, et al. Laparoscopy during pregnancy: A literature review. *J Soc Laparoendosc Surg* 1997; 1:17.
34. Thomas SJ, Brisson P. Laparoscopic appendectomy and cholecystectomy during pregnancy: Six case reports. *J Soc Laparoendosc Surg* 1998; 2:41.
35. Fleming JS. Laparoscopically directed appendicectomy. *Aust N Z Obstet Gynecol* 1985; 25:238.
36. Gotz F, Pier A, Bacher C. Modified laparoscopic appendectomy in surgery: A report on 388 operations. *Surg Endosc* 1990; 4:6.
37. Hellberg A, Rudberg C, Kullman E, et al. Prospective randomized multicentre study of laparoscopic versus open appendicectomy. *Br J Surg* 1999; 86:48.
38. Tarnoff M, Atabek U, Goodman M, et al. A comparison of laparoscopic and open appendectomy. *J Soc Laparoendosc Surg* 1998; 2:153.
39. Moberg AC, Montgomery A. Appendicitis: Laparoscopic versus conventional operation: A study and review of the literature. *Surg Laparosc Endosc* 1997; 7:459.
40. Mushinski M. Laparoscopic and open appendectomies—average charges. *Stat Bull Metrop Insur Co* 1999; 80:23.
41. Wagaman, R, Williams RS. Conservative therapy for adnexal torsion. A case report. *J Reprod Med* 1990; 35(8):833.
42. Heikkinen TJ, Haukipuro K, Hulkko A. Cost-effective appendectomy: Open or laparoscopic? A prospective randomized study. *Surg Endosc* 1998; 12:1204.

20

Complications

Despite the degree of caution used, complications occur during operative laparoscopy. Since sequelae can result from even relatively easy procedures, a surgeon must be able to recognize them promptly and carry out proper management. The risks increase with the complexity of the procedure, the relative inexperience of the surgeon, and deviation from standard technique. As laparoscopic operations become more complex, the ability to handle them endoscopically becomes important.

Diagnostic laparoscopy and laparoscopic tubal sterilization involve few risks. The rate of intraoperative and postoperative complications is less than 1% (Table 20-1). Most reports are from large practices with experienced gynecologists,[1] surveys of American Association of Gynecologic Laparoscopists (AAGL) members,[2–6] and tertiary referral clinics.[7]

The intraoperative and postoperative complication rates in 361 women who underwent laparoscopic hysterectomy for benign pathologic conditions were evaluated.[8] The overall complication rate for hysterectomy carried out by laparoscopy was 11.1%. Most of the complications were minor, including cystitis (1.66%), transient high fever (1.39%), abdominal wall ecchymosis (1.12%), and pneumonia and bronchitis (1.12%). There was no correlation between the type of laparoscopic hysterectomy and the complication rate. Complication rates associated with laparoscopic hysterectomy compare favorably with published complication rates for vaginal and abdominal hysterectomy.[9]

While most gynecologists are taught traditional operations under supervision during residency, advanced laparoscopic procedures often are learned in clinical practice. The learning curve for laparoscopic operations is lengthy. The risk of complications is greatest early in a surgeon's experience and increases when new techniques or equipment is utilized. In 17,521 diagnostic and operative procedures done at seven centers, a complication rate of 3.2 per 1000 was found (Table 20-2).[10] The rate for diagnostic and minor procedures was 1.1 per 1000, and it was 5.2 per 1000 for major and advanced operations. Laparotomies were done for hemorrhage in 17 instances and for visceral injuries in 40 patients. One fatality was reported. Three national surveys conducted in the Netherlands,[11] France,[12] and Finland[13] included, respectively, 25,764, 29,966, and 70,607 laparoscopic procedures. The total complication rates were 5.7,[11] 4.6,[12] and 3.6[13] per 1000 procedures. Laparotomy was needed in 3.3 per 1000 operations.

Prevention

Avoiding complications is the best form of prevention. Thorough preoperative evaluation, consultation, and proper patient selection help lessen the possibility of injury and subsequent legal action. A successful operation depends on the gynecologist's familiarity with normal and abnormal anatomy, a thorough evaluation of abnormal findings, meticulous dissection and vaporization, familiarity with instruments and energy sources, training under the supervision of a qualified surgeon, and a properly trained operation room (OR) staff and assistant.

Soderstrom and Butler[14] reported that the complication rate for laparoscopic sterilization was highest among physicians who had done fewer

TABLE 20-1. Major Complications per 1000 Operative Laparoscopy Procedures

Intestinal	1.1–2.6
Bladder	0.2–1.7
Ureteral	0.1–1.4
Vascular	0.4–2.5
Laparotomy	3.3

Source: Jansen et al.,[11] Chapron et al.,[12] Harkki-Siren and Kurki.[13]

than 100 procedures. It requires 4 to 7 years to gain adequate laparoscopic skills by doing several procedures each week with gradually increasing levels of complexity.[15]

TABLE 20-3. Relative Contraindications to Laparoscopy

- Generalized peritonitis
- Hypovolemic shock
- Intestinal obstruction
- Class IV cardiac disease
- Large pelvic or abdominal mass
- Intrauterine pregnancy >16 wks
- Pelvic abscess
- Multiple prior abdominal surgical procedures
- Diaphragmatic hernia
- Chronic pulmonary disease
- Extremes of body weight

Contraindications

In some patients, laparoscopy may not be appropriate (Table 20-3). However, improvement in laparoscopic skills and experience, combined with the availability of the proper instruments, has reduced the number of conditions that are considered absolute contraindications for laparoscopy. These conditions include obesity,[16,17] severe adhesions,[18] previous abdominal operations,[19] cancer,[20–22] abdominal hernia,[23] pregnancy,[24] hypovolemic shock,[25] and bowel perforation with generalized peritonitis.[26–29]

In patients who have generalized peritonitis, the bowel frequently is matted and adherent to the abdominal wall. However, laparoscopic treatment of generalized peritonitis secondary to perforated sigmoid diverticulitis has been a safe alternative to conventional operations.[26,27] Laparoscopy was found to be safe and effective in the diagnosis and treatment of patients with peritonitis.[28] Laparoscopic treatment was practical in a patient who had an appendicular and gastroduodenal perforation.[29] Hemoperitoneum in an unstable patient has been considered a contraindication because the bleeding source may be difficult to find and treat laparoscopically. However, laparoscopy offers many theoretical advantages for the immediate diagnosis and management of a patient presenting with hemodynamic instability and suspected active intraabdominal bleeding caused by an ectopic pregnancy.[25] These features include superior observation of the entire abdominal cavity, decreased intraabdominal bleeding because of compression by the creation of a pneumoperitoneum, and ability to control the source of bleeding effectively with minimal tissue damage. Thus, it seems appropriate when an optimal set-up is available, to diagnose and treat suspected intraabdominal bleeding caused by ectopic pregnancies or a bleeding hemorrhagic corpus luteum.

Intestinal obstruction and bowel distention are associated with an increased risk of perforation. Although laparoscopy is less invasive than laparotomy and often is the better of the two approaches, bowel obstruction not relieved by conservative decompression techniques may require laparotomy.

Patients with class IV cardiac disease have a high risk of cardiac arrhythmias and failure as a result of Trendelenburg positioning, even for relatively short procedures. Anesthesia for laparoscopic cholecystectomy may be achieved safely in elderly American Society of Anesthesiology classification (ASA) class III patients with increased cardiac risk.[30] Laparoscopic cholecystectomy appears to be safer than open cholecystectomy in all

TABLE 20-2. Complications of Gynecologic Laparoscopy

Laparoscopic Procedures	No. of Procedures	Laparotomies for Complications	Rate/1000
Diagnostic	4130	7	1.7
Minor	4213	2	0.5
Major extensive adhesiolysis	1910	16	8.4
Other	6370	24	3.8
Advanced	898	8	8.9

eligible patients, especially elderly individuals and patients in higher ASA classes.[31,32]

Procedural Failures

It is better to complete a procedure by laparotomy than to risk injury to the patient or be forced to proceed with an emergency laparotomy because of a complication. This deviation from the surgical plan raises concerns about the adequacy of the presurgical evaluation, the patient's consent, and the surgeon's skill.

The possibility of complications is increased during the insertion of the Veress needle and primary and secondary trocars in patients with multiple previous laparotomies, those with a body mass index >30, and very thin patients. Bowel preparation is recommended if there is a risk of bowel injury. Veress needle and trocar insertion is modified in the presence of a large pelvic mass.

The most critical point of laparoscopy is abdominal cavity entry of the Veress needle and the primary and secondary trocars. In a series of 2324 laparoscopies, there were more complications from Veress needle and trocar insertion than from the actual operative procedures.[33] Another study suggested that about half the complications occur during the insertion of the Veress needle and laparoscopic trocars .[34]

The frequency of adhesions between the abdominal wall and the underlying omentum and bowel was assessed in 360 women undergoing operative laparoscopy after a previous laparotomy.[35] Patients with prior midline incisions had more adhesions than did those with prior Pfannenstiel incisions. Patients with midline incisions carried out for gynecologic indications had more adhesions than did those with all types of incisions done for obstetric indications. Adhesions to the bowel were more common after midline incisions above the umbilicus. Twenty-one women had direct injury to adherent omentum and bowel during the laparoscopic procedure. Intraabdominal adhesions between the abdominal scar and the underlying viscera are a common consequence of laparotomy. When patients undergo laparoscopy after a previous laparotomy, the presence of adhesions between the old scar and the bowel and omentum must be considered.

Veress Needle

Intraabdominal placement of the Veress needle is required to establish a pneumoperitoneum. Since the Veress needle is inserted "blindly," it can enter inappropriate spaces or puncture organs. Further instillation of CO_2 under pressure through the Veress needle can create serious complications.

Prevention of complications

Factors increasing the risk of perforation or laceration include bowel adhesions, lateral displacement of the needle during its insertion, too steep an insertion angle, and uncontrolled, sudden entry. The patient must be in a horizontal position so that the sacral promontory and sacral curve are identified easily. A premature Trendelenburg position should be avoided.

When an upper abdominal site is used to establish a pneumoperitoneum, the needle can puncture the pleural cavity, stomach, liver, or spleen. The stomach becomes distended after prolonged manual ventilation with a mask or when endotracheal intubation is difficult. The stomach can be punctured even with umbilical placement of the Veress needle. A distended stomach displaces the transverse colon toward the lower abdomen and increases the probability of an intestinal puncture (Figure 20-1). A nasogastric tube lessens the risk of gastric distention. An overdistended bladder also is at risk for injury. Routine placement of a Foley catheter before the procedure should eliminate the risk of inadvertent vesical injury.

Recognition

Veress needle injuries generally are not apparent until CO_2 insufflation or after the insertion of the laparoscope. Abnormally high insufflation pressures are encountered if the needle is misplaced. During the initial examination of the pelvis, one should survey the middle and upper abdomen for signs of needle-induced trauma, such as hematomas, needle trauma, and collections of gas.

Management

Puncture of a hollow viscus with the Veress needle generally requires examination of the puncture site to look for a bleeding vessel or leakage from the viscus. If the needle punctures the viscus, repair is indicated. The route of repair depends on the organ involved (small or large bowel, bladder, stomach, or major blood vessels), the nature of the leaking fluid, and the operator's skill. Many injuries require immediate laparotomy for repair and copious irrigation of the abdomen, whereas some surgeons can repair injuries laparoscopically.

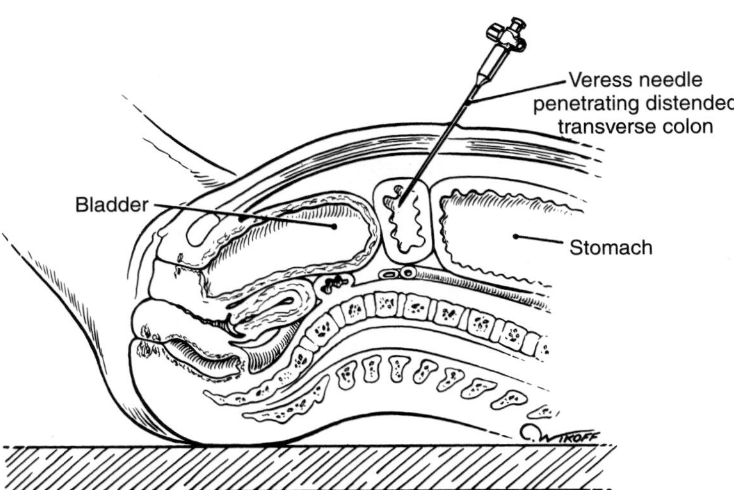

Figure 20-1. A distended stomach can displace the transverse colon toward the lower abdomen, increasing the possibility of puncture of the colon.

Postoperatively, the patient is instructed to call the physician if there is increasing abdominal pain or fever.

Establishing a Pneumoperitoneum

Complications developing as a result of insufflating a space other than the abdominal cavity vary, depending on the perforated structure and the amount of CO_2 instilled.

Prevention

Placement of a Foley catheter preoperatively virtually eliminates the risk of a vesical injury. Aspiration facilitates early recognition of stomach or bowel penetration, but this method is fallible. Stomach or bowel insufflation is suspected if there is asymmetric abdominal distention, belching, or passing of flatus. If these signs develop, the gas is allowed to escape. Once a proper pneumoperitoneum is established, the laparoscope is inserted and the suspected perforation site is examined.

If a large vessel entry is not noticed on insertion of the Veress needle, intravascular insufflation with CO_2 may lead to a gas embolism and even death.[36] This event usually occurs in patients with a previous abdominal or pelvic surgical history.[37] Transuterine insufflation is associated with a risk of gas embolism.[38] Gas embolism initially presents as cardiorespiratory distress with cardiac bradycardia or arrhythmia and an associated classic "mill wheel" murmur. Sudden bilateral mydriasis is the earliest neurologic sign.[37] Once it is recognized, the patient needs to be placed in the left lateral decubitus position for a possible immediate cardiac puncture to release the gas.[38]

Recognition

Signs of potential complications include elevated CO_2 filling pressures; continued liver dullness after the instillation of 1 L of CO_2; subcutaneous crepitation; belching or passing of flatus; asymmetric abdominal distention; hematuria or air bubbles in the Foley catheter line; a sudden drop in blood pressure, tachycardia, or cardiac arrest; and difficulty in ventilating the patient.

However, the absence of these signs does not confirm proper placement. Preperitoneal placement of the Veress needle with sufficient insufflation of CO_2 leads to the disappearance of liver dullness. If the Veress needle enters the bowel, the condition may not be recognized immediately because the bowel's large capacity allows low filling pressures. Even though the needle is placed correctly, the increased abdominal pressure and peritoneal irritation associated with the instillation of CO_2 can cause bradycardia and hypotension. These signs respond readily to supportive measures.

Treatment

When the initial flow rate or intraabdominal pressure is high, elevating the abdominal wall can correct the placement of the needle, particularly if initially it was placed within the omentum. If the pressure does not fall immediately to normal levels, the needle is withdrawn and examined to confirm that the spring action of the device works properly and no tissue is occluding the tip. If a second placement attempt fails, consideration is given to insertion of the needle at another site, open laparoscopy, or direct trocar entry.

The most common extraperitoneal site insufflated is the preperitoneal space. If this is recognized early, the CO_2 line is disconnected and the gas is allowed to escape. The needle is removed and reinserted with attention to the "pop" that occurs as the needle pierces the peritoneum. If this is not recognized early and enough gas is instilled, the preperitoneal gas collection will be discovered after trocar placement and insertion of the laparoscope. The spiderweb appearance of the tissue becomes apparent, and gas is allowed to escape before the surgeon attempts to reinsert the needle. Preperitoneal insufflation can extend to the mediastinum and endanger cardiac function. If this occurs, the laparoscopy is stopped and the gas is allowed to escape.

Pneumo-omentum is a common, benign occurrence unless a vessel is lacerated. Omental trauma from the needle is associated with higher than normal filling pressures. Slight withdrawal of the needle or traction on the abdominal wall releases the omentum. Since this occurs frequently, the omentum and other structures in the path of the needle and trocars are examined at initial exploration of the pelvis to search for laceration of omental vessels. If a large vascular injury is missed on insertion of the Veress needle, intravascular insufflation with CO_2 can cause a gas embolism and mortality.

Primary Trocar Injuries

Punctures or lacerations of pelvic structures during trocar insertion are potentially serious because of the large diameters of trocars.

Prevention

An adequate pneumoperitoneum provides a safe distance between the anterior abdominal wall and the pelvic viscera, but trocar injuries can result from poor technique or adherent bowel (Figure 20-2).[39] Excessive force while inserting the trocar can be caused by an inadequate umbilical incision, scar tissue, or a dull trocar. Uncontrolled sudden entry of the trocar, its lateral displacement during insertion, and too steep an angle for placement increase the risk of injury. Even with meticulous technique, abdominal wall bleeding, hollow viscus perforation, blood vessel laceration, and liver and spleen injury can occur. The use of a minilaparoscope allows the gynecologist to observe and carry out adhesiolysis at the entry site before the insertion of an umbilical cannula. Minilaparoscopy reduced serious vascular or visceral injury from the insertion of the primary cannula in patients who had had previous pelvic and abdominal operations.[40]

The trocar should be pyramidal-tipped and sharp to penetrate muscle and fascia. Establishing a large pneumoperitoneum and elevating the abdominal wall to increase the distance between the abdominal wall and the viscera decrease the chance of intestinal and vascular injury. The syringe test can indicate the presence of adhesions. Nezhat and coworkers[41] showed that direct insertion of the umbilical trocar without prior pneumoperitoneum is safe. The benefits of direct trocar insertion have been demonstrated by several authors.[41–43] The operating time was reduced; in tubal ligations, there was less gas inflated and the duration of exposure of the patient to the gas and anesthesia was lessened.

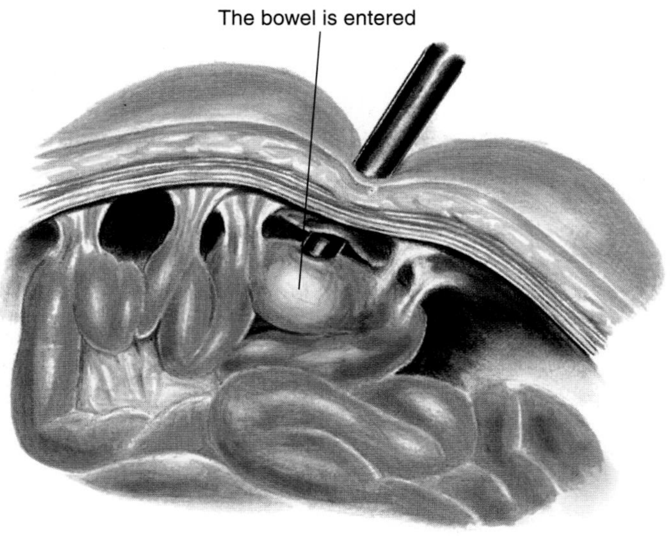

Figure 20-2. The trocar has penetrated the adherent bowel.

Woolcott[44] reviewed the records of 6173 laparoscopies that used the technique of direct insertion of the umbilical trocar and insufflation of carbon dioxide under vision. He found that there were four perforating bowel injuries (0.06%) that required laparotomy (two small intestine, two large intestine). Three of the four patients who had bowel injury had undergone prior abdominal operations and had midline vertical subumbilical incisions. There were no instances of major vascular injury or gas embolus necessitating operative or resuscitative measures. Woolcott concluded that bowel or vessel perforation rates (requiring laparotomy or resuscitation) were 1 in 1000 regardless of whether the method of gaining peritoneal access was the open (Hasson) technique, Veress needle insufflation, or direct trocar insertion. The latter method may reduce the risk of gas embolism by insufflating only after intraperitoneal replacement has been confirmed; it allows immediate recognition and rapid treatment of major blood vessel lacerations, which is crucial in reducing laparoscopy-associated mortality. A large retrospective French study[45] evaluated the incidence of serious trocar accidents in 103,852 laparoscopic operations involving almost 390,000 trocars. The results identified seven perioperative deaths (mortality, 0.07 per 1000) arising almost exclusively from vascular injuries. The open insertion of the first trocar appeared to be the best means of preventing these accidents. Each method has advantages and disadvantages and similar morbidity when done by experienced operators with appropriate indications.

The disposable trocar with its sharp tip and spring-loaded safety shield should allow a controlled entry and decrease the risk of injury to intraabdominal structures.[46] However, no large-scale clinical trial has established its advantages, and the unexpected ease of insertion could result in accidental damage. One study compared patients treated in a nonrandomized design with either sharp cutting single-use trocars or cone-shaped noncutting reusable trocars.[47] The data suggested that patients treated with a sharp trocar tip had more trocar-related bleeding events at the insertion site in the abdominal wall than did those treated with the conic tip design. The relative risk of vessel injury was increased by the use of pyramidal-tipped trocars compared with conical-tipped trocars, especially when larger-diameter trocars were used.[48]

The first trocar is inserted with the patient in a horizontal position because a premature Trendelenburg position can alter the relation of the sacral promontory and sacral hollow. The abdominal wall is elevated on both sides of the umbilicus with towel clips. As the trocar is inserted, it is advanced toward the sacral hollow to provide the greatest distance between the trocar tip and solid tissue. With this technique, the bowel slides away from the advancing trocar.

In an obese patient, the trocar is angled almost perpendicular to the skin so that the distance between the sacral promontory, blood vessels, and trocar is large. In thin patients, the distance between the anterior abdominal wall and sacral promontory is small (Figure 20-3). The force required to introduce the trocar often is less than anticipated and so a controlled, angle entry is essential.

In a prospective study[49] the cephalocaudal relationship among the umbilicus, aortic bifurcation, and iliac vessels was measured during laparoscopy in 97 patients. The distance from the aortic bifurcation relative to the umbilicus was assessed in both the supine and Trendelenburg positions with a marked suction-irrigator probe. Patients were stratified into three groups on the basis of body mass index (kg/m^2). The position of the aortic bifurcation ranged from 5 cm cephalad to 3 cm caudal to the umbilicus in the supine position and from 3 cm cephalad to 3 cm caudal in the Trendelenburg position. In the supine position, the aortic bifurcation was located caudal to the umbilicus in only 11% of patients compared with 33% in the Trendelenburg position. This difference was significant for the total study population and for the nonoverweight group. In both positions, no correlation was found between the distance from the aortic bifurcation to the umbilicus and body mass index. Mean $\pm$SD distance of the aortic bifurcation from the umbilicus in the supine position was 0.1 ± 1.2 cm for the nonoverweight group, 0.7 ± 1.5 cm for the overweight group, and 1.2 ± 1.5 cm for the very overweight group. Respective values in the Trendelenburg position were 1.0 ± 1.1, -0.4 ± 1.2, and -0.2 ± 1.3 cm. The common iliac artery was caudal to the umbilicus in four women. The space between common iliac arteries always was occupied, at least partly, by the left common iliac vein and was filled completely in 19 women (28%). The cephalocaudal relationship between the aortic bifurcation and the umbilicus varies widely and is not related to body mass index in anesthetized patients. Regardless of body mass index, the aortic bifurcation more likely is located caudal to the umbilicus in the Trendelenburg position compared with the supine position. The presumed location of the aortic bifurcation can be misleading during

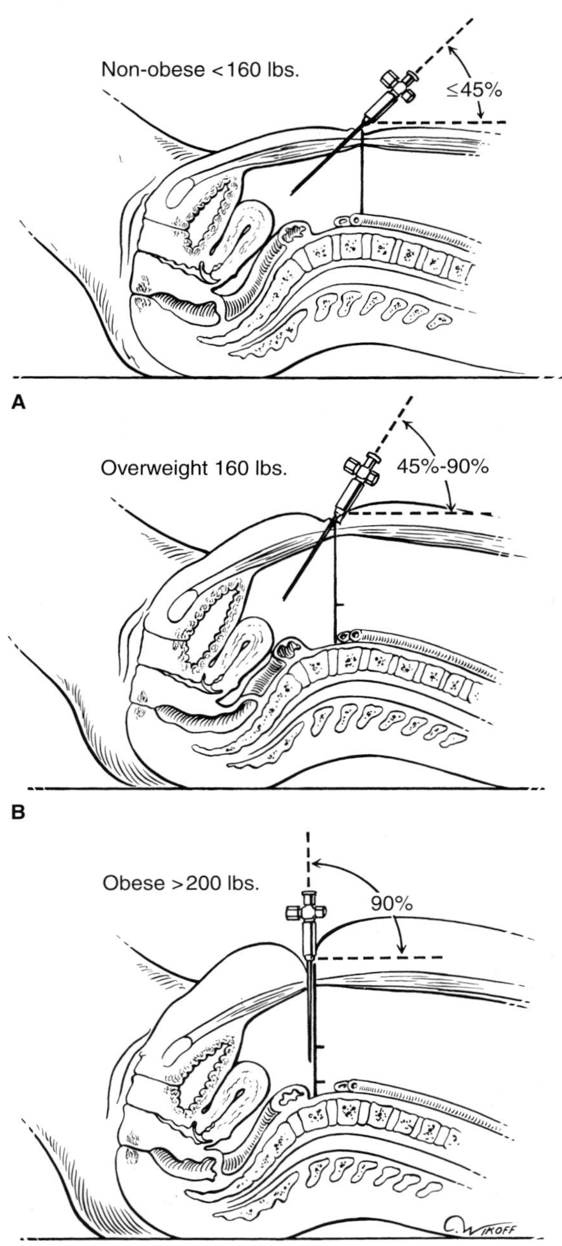

Figure 20-3. Angles of the Veress needle and umbilical insertion of the trocar. **A**. Nonobese patient. **B**. Overweight patient. **C**. Obese patient.

Veress needle or primary cannula insertion, and a more reliable guide is necessary for this procedure to avoid major retroperitoneal vascular injury.

A distended bowel increases the risk of trocar injury. This condition can be iatrogenic, resulting from intraluminal placement of the Veress needle. The surgeon may be unaware of this complication because the filling pressure of the small bowel is the same as that of the abdominal cavity.

Recognition

When the trocar is removed, signs of complications requiring immediate evaluation are bleeding from the trocar sleeve or a fecal odor. Insertion of the laparoscope allows assessment of the injury. If the laparoscope enters the bowel lumen, the instrument is left in place to prevent the escape of bowel contents and help locate the injury (Figure 20-2). In the presence of excessive bleeding, immediate laparotomy is indicated.

Treatment

See "Bleeding" and "Bowel Injuries," below.

Accessory Trocar Injuries

Prevention

Intraabdominal injury is less likely to occur during insertion of accessory trocars because they are inserted under direct observation. The structures most frequently injured are the inferior epigastric vessels that run lateral to the rectus muscles.[11] The most common complication of multipuncture operative laparoscopy is inferior epigastric vessel injury. Two methods are utilized to avoid injuring these vessels. First, the position of the superficial vessels often can be ascertained with transillumination of the abdominal wall, particularly in thin women. Second, the courses of the inferior epigastric vessels are seen through the parietal peritoneum laparoscopically. As the trocar is advanced through the abdominal wall, the direction of the trocar is altered to avoid laceration of those vessels.

Quint and colleagues[50] did a prospective study to ascertain the efficacy of transillumination for locating abdominal wall vessels before trocar placement during laparoscopy. They showed that in women of normal weight, a single vessel could be seen approximately 5 cm from the midline in >90% of the patients and a second vessel could be seen approximately 8 cm from the midline in 51%. The more medial vessels did not correlate with the course of the inferior epigastric vessels seen laparoscopically. The ability to see vessels was decreased significantly by the patients' weight but not by skin color. Superficial abdominal wall vessels were located by transillumination in most women of normal weight regardless of skin color, but this technique is less useful in overweight and obese women. However, the deep (inferior) epigastric vessels cannot be located effectively by transillumination, and other techniques should be used to minimize the risk of injury to those vessels.

Second, the course of the inferior epigastric vessels can be seen through the parietal peritoneum laparoscopically. As the trocar is advanced through the abdominal wall, the direction of the trocar can be altered to avoid laceration.

Despite these safeguards, the inferior epigastric vessels can be injured intraoperatively. Inferior epigastric injury was the most common complication of laparoscopically assisted vaginal hysterectomy in an AAGL survey.[4] Retroperitoneal bleeding may spread and accumulate before it is recognized. Significant damage to large retroperitoneal blood vessels may not be apparent during laparoscopy.[51] This injury occurs mostly in thin patients and those who have had abdominal surgery or have lax abdominal walls.

Long procedures are associated with moving, dislocating, and enlarging the trocar sleeve. Inserting clamps and other instruments through accessory trocar incisions or enlargement of the incision to remove large tissue pieces can damage these vessels. The risk of complications increases if the trocar is not aimed toward the sacral hollow; it may go down the pelvic side wall or puncture the posterior peritoneum. In inserting the accessory trocars, sudden, uncontrolled entry or the use of excessive force can result in laceration of the bladder, uterus, or bowel.

Recognition

If a vessel is damaged, the surgeon may notice blood running down the cannula or the formation of an abdominal wall hematoma. Trocar sleeves can tamponade bleeding from a small laceration that does not become apparent until the trocar sleeve is removed. Profuse bleeding from the incisional site or significant local swelling can be observed postoperatively.

Injuries to iliac vessels are associated with profuse hemorrhage or a rapidly enlarging retroperitoneal hematoma, both of which require immediate laparotomy. Retroperitoneal bleeding can spread and accumulate before it is recognized. This injury mostly occurs in thin patients, those who have had abdominal operations, and those with lax abdominal walls.

Uterine lacerations are not life-threatening, and the bleeding usually is controlled easily. Bladder injury can occur if that organ is displaced because of a previous laparotomy or if an accessory trocar is placed less than 4 cm above the pubic symphysis.

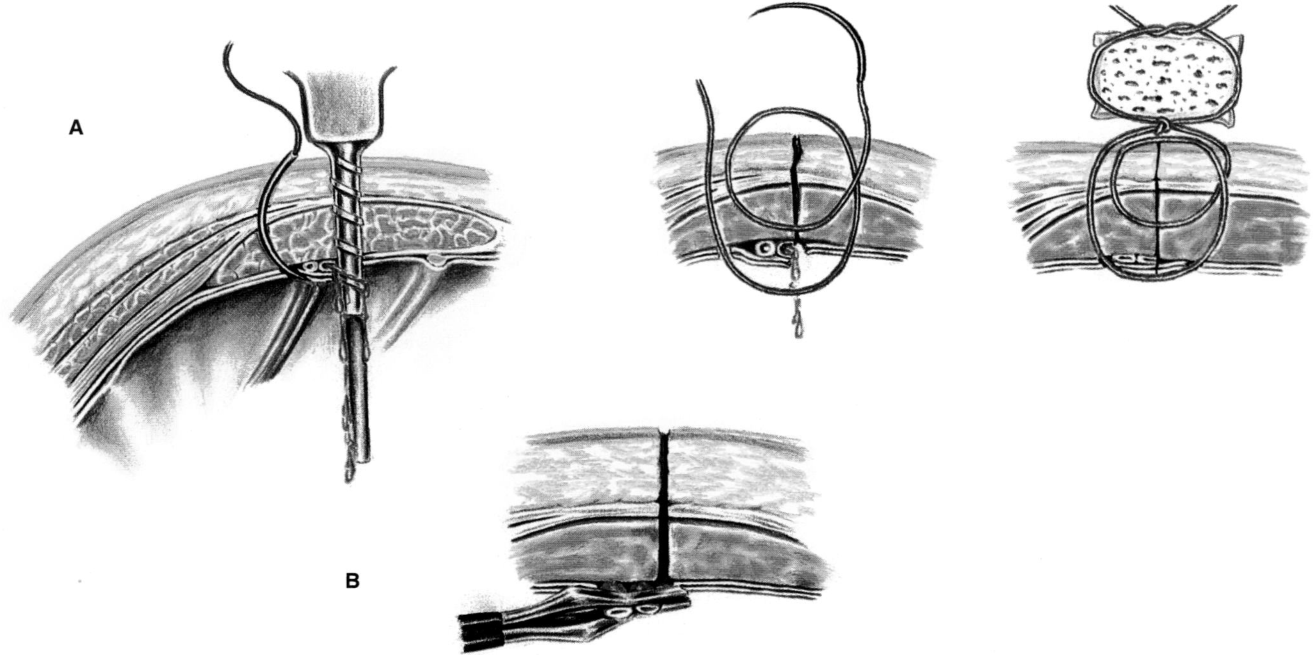

Figure 20-4. Methods to control bleeding from the inferior epigastric vessel. **A**. A figure-of-eight suture is placed on either side of the trocar and tied above the incision. **B**. Bipolar forceps is introduced through the opposite trocar sleeve, and the vessel is coagulated.

Management

Bleeding from an inferior epigastric artery can be controlled by sutures, electrocoagulation, or pressure. With the trocar in place, using 0 absorbable suture on a CT-1 needle, a figure-of-eight is placed on either side of the trocar. Alternatively, a straight needle can be passed transabdominally on the distal side of the trocar and pulled through the abdominal wall again, using laparoscopic forceps. The suture is tied within the trocar incision and buried beneath the skin (Figure 20-4, A). The suture is removed within 24 hours postoperatively. Control of inferior epigastric artery hemorrhage caused by cannula injury from percutaneous transabdominal placement of polypropylene sutures allows the procedure to be completed with the cannula in place.[52] However, cutaneous necrosis requiring debridement and delayed primary closure may occur if the sutures are not removed less than 24 hours postoperatively. If these two methods fail to control bleeding, the trocar incision is extended and a grasping forceps is used to apply pressure to the inferior epigastric artery to help find the bleeding point. Sutures are applied. A blunt instrument placed through a contralateral accessory trocar can be used to apply pressure to the bleeding point. Bipolar forceps are applied at the source of the bleeding (Figure 20-4B). Finally, an expandable trocar can be placed and used to apply pressure at the site from the skin and parietal surfaces or the bleeding sistes can be tied with Carter-Thomason, Valley or J needles.

Anesthesia

Increased intraabdominal pressures caused by the pneumoperitoneum, absorption of CO_2 gas or fluid, and the Trendelenburg position concern anesthesiologists. A vasovagal reaction and cardiac arrhythmias developing from CO_2 absorption are avoided by administering atropine preoperatively. Difficulties in ventilation result from a steep Trendelenburg position, high intraabdominal pressures, and obesity. The risk of carbon monoxide poisoning caused by smoke generated by laser and bipolar electrosurgery during prolonged laparoscopic operations was studied.[53] A decrease in carboxyhemoglobin concentrations was found intraoperatively. The carboxyhemoglobin level was increased at the end of the operation in one woman. In one patient, the levels exceeded 1% (1.33%), well below the human threshold tolerance level of 2%. Carbon monoxide (CO) poisoning is not associated with even prolonged laparoscopy. This observation was attributed to high-flow carbon dioxide insufflation and intensive evacuation of intraabdominal smoke that minimizes exposure to CO and active elimination of CO by controlled ventilation with high oxygen concentrations.

Fluid overload and high-molecular-weight dextran used as a distention medium for hysteroscopy are circumvented by accurately measuring input and output. Pulmonary edema is a rare complication of absorbing crystalloid irrigating fluid during laparoscopy.[54] Lavage with large volumes of room-temperature irrigation fluid can be associated with hypothermia, and so the fluid should be warmed or a heating blanket should be used. The use of warmed irrigation fluid decreased the drop in core temperature associated with laparoscopy.[55]

Reconditioning laparoscopic gas by filtering, heating, and hydrating the gas may reduce or eliminate laparoscopically-induced hypothermia, shortening recovery room length of stay and reducing postoperative pain.[56] Warming the insufflation gas reduced the postoperative intraperitoneal cytokine response.[57] However, the heat-preserving effect of humidified gas insufflation during prolonged laparoscopic procedures has been questioned.[58]

Arrhythmias, including junctional rhythm, bradycardia, bigeminy, and asystole, have been associated with CO_2 insufflation of the abdomen. Bradycardia results from pressure on the peritoneum with an increased vagal response.

Electrosurgical Injuries

Improper use of electrosurgery during a procedure, unfamiliarity with the equipment, and the use of incompatible components contribute to many injuries. The first response to electrosurgical equipment failure should never be to increase the current. Since equipment malfunction is rarely the sole reason for injury, each component is checked systematically to localize the problem. Even properly functioning equipment can result in injury. Attempts to control a bleeding vessel with the bipolar forceps can damage nearby structures if the surgeon fails to identify them. While some injuries are evident intraoperatively, others become clinically apparent postoperatively.

When unipolar current is used, the grounding pad must be applied. One should not use mixed trocars (half plastic and half metal) that will result in undesired capacitation and contribute to burns.

Energy sources used without proper understanding and caution can cause significant vascular injury.[59]

Bleeding

Uncontrolled bleeding and hemorrhage are the cause of most emergency laparotomies.[60,61] Bleeding occurs during sharp dissection of adhesions, transection of vessels during laser excision or dissection (the laser effectively coagulates very small vessels), uterosacral ablation, and rough handling of tissues. Lacerations of the oviduct, mesosalpinx, and infundibulopelvic ligament can bleed profusely. Distorted anatomy is an important compounding factor in many cases of major retroperitoneal vascular injury.[58]

When pressure gradients return to normal, bleeding into the retroperitoneal space may begin, eventually leading to hematoma and hypovolemic shock.[52] All exposed vessels should be evaluated at the end of the procedure with the patient supine and intraabdominal pressure reduced. Blood clots in the pelvic side wall should be evacuated before complete hemostasis is confirmed.

An injury to the hypogastric artery was managed laparoscopically with bipolar electrodesiccation.[62] Those authors did three laparotomies to control bleeding after the treatment of dense adhesions in their first 2000 operations but only one in the last 5000. The adequacy and safety of laparoscopic control of major vessel bleeding should be investigated further, and consultation with a vascular surgeon should be considered in all cases.[59]

Unipolar and bipolar electrocoagulators, vasopressin, clips, sutures, and loop ligatures should be available to control bleeding. The choice of methods depends on the surgeon's preference. Pressure allows evacuation of blood and reduces blood loss until the necessary equipment is placed in the abdomen. Most bleeding is controlled with bipolar forceps. Fine bipolar forceps are employed near the fallopian tube to lessen thermal damage and subsequent adhesions.

Uterine Injuries

Complications involving the uterus include cervical lacerations or uterine perforation from sounding the uterus and the use of a uterine dilator or uterine manipulator. Cervical lacerations are treated with pressure from a sponge stick or are sutured. Bleeding from uterine perforations is controlled with bipolar electrocoagulation or observed. Since a CO_2 laser beam can lacerate the uterine serosa, the uterus cannot be used as a backstop.

Bladder Injuries

Vesical injury is rare and occurs in patients who have had laparotomies[63] or whose bladders are not empty. Under these conditions, trocars, uterine anteverters, and blunt instruments can perforate or lacerate the bladder and electrosurgery and lasers can cause thermal injury. Certain laparoscopic procedures increase the risk of vesical injury.

Prevention

The Veress needle can perforate a distended bladder. A misplaced Rubin's cannula can perforate the vagina and bladder with upward pressure.[64] Insertion of accessory trocars can injure a full bladder or one with distorted anatomy from a previous pelvic operation, endometriosis, or adhesions. Coagulation or laser ablation of endometriosis implants or adhesiolysis in the anterior cul-de-sac can predispose a patient to bladder injury unless hydrodissection or a backstop is used with the CO_2 laser. During laparoscopic hysterectomy (LH) or laparoscopically assisted vaginal hysterectomy (LAVH), the bladder can be lacerated or torn if blunt dissection is used to free it from the pubocervical fascia, particularly in women with prior cesarean delivery, severe endometriosis, or lower segment myomas. Also, a vesical injury can occur while entering and dissecting the space of Retzius before laparoscopic bladder neck suspension.

To prevent injuries, a Foley catheter is placed to drain the bladder. The position of the bladder should be assessed during the initial examination with the laparoscope. If the boundaries of the bladder are not clear, particularly when the pelvic anatomy is distorted, the bladder should be filled with 350 mL of normal saline to delineate its position. When one is doing an LH or LAVH, the assistant should push the uterus up during bladder dissection.

Recognition

Signs of intraoperative bladder injury include the following:

1. Air is seen in the urinary catheter and bag during insufflation.

2. The bladder appears to be pushed by the accessory trocar as the trocar is advanced through the abdominal wall.
3. Hematuria develops during the procedure.
4. Urine drainage is noted from the accessory trocar incision.
5. The amount of urine obtained during catheterization is less than anticipated.
6. Leakage of indigo carmine is seen from the injured site.
7. Suprapubic bruising.
8. Mass in the abdominal wall or pelvis.
9. Abdominal swelling.
10. Azotemia or peritonitis.

Since trocar injury often involves entry and exit punctures, locating both is important. Some bladder complications become apparent postoperatively, particularly those caused by electrocoagulation. If a vesical injury is suspected, a retrograde cystogram may reveal the defect.

Management

Small holes in the bladder generally heal without sequelae. Trocar injuries to the bladder dome require closure followed by urinary drainage for 5 to 7 days. Drainage promotes healing, encourages spontaneous closure, and reduces further complications. Lacerations may require a laparotomy, although some laparoscopists repair the laceration laparoscopically. Care should be used when doing an LH or LAVH, and the assistant should push the uterus up during bladder dissection.[8]

One report described the laparoscopic closure of intentional or unintentional bladder lacerations during operative laparoscopy in 19 women.[65] The defect was repaired laparoscopically in one layer using interrupted absorbable polyglycolic suture (17 patients) or polydioxanone suture (2 patients) and followed by 7 to 14 days of transurethral drainage. Complications were limited to one vesicovaginal fistula that required reoperation. After 6 to 48 months of follow-up, all the patients were well with a good outcome. Since urinary bladder injury is one of the most common complications associated with LAVH, laparoscopists are becoming more familiar with laparoscopic management of urinary bladder injury.[66] An experienced laparoscopic surgeon may elect in selected cases of bladder injury to repair the laceration laparoscopically.

Ureteral Injuries

Prevention

Knowledge of the ureter's path through the pelvis and the vulnerable points are the key to preventing injuries. The intrapelvic segment of the ureter is near the broad ligament, ovaries, and uterosacral ligaments, and injuries occur in those areas (Table 20-4).[67] The ureter is at risk during laparoscopic surgery when the cardinal ligament is dissected and divided below the uterine vessels.[68] Endometriosis and severe pelvic adhesions can thicken the peritoneum, obscuring the location of the ureter, especially near the uterosacral ligaments.[69]

Laparoscopic placement of transmural sutures at the bladder neck also has been reported to lead to entrapment of the intramural portion of the ureter.[70] Ureteral injury can occur in the course of sharp dissection of an ovary adherent to the pelvic side wall; uterosacral transection; ligation, transection, and coagulation of the uterine arteries; removal of endometriotic implants or fibrosis from the ureter;[71–73] and attempts to control bleeding vessels.

To prevent such injuries, the ureter must be identified before irreversible action is taken. Precise and continuous attention to the location of the ureter will reduce the incidence of complications. Methods to protect the ureter include using hydrodissection and resecting affected peritoneum.[74] A small opening is made in the peritoneum, and 50 to 100 mL of lactated Ringer's solution is injected along the course of the ureter. This displaces it laterally, providing a plane for

TABLE 20-4. Laparoscopic Procedures Associated with Increased Risk of Ureteral Injury

Infundibulopelvic ligament/ovarian fossa
Oophorectomy
Pelvic side wall adhesions
Presacral neurectomy
Endometriosis ablation
Severe bowel adhesions
Ureteric canal
Uterosacral nerve transection
Uterosacral plication
Hysterectomy
Cardinal ligament
Hysterectomy
Vaginal cuff closure
Bladder neck suspension

safe ablation of endometriotic implants, lysis of adhesions, or resection of involved peritoneum (Figure 20-5). Fluid absorbs laser energy and decreases the risk of thermal damage to underlying tissue.[75] This procedure is applicable if the peritoneum is not adherent to the underlying ureter. During uterosacral transection, a backstop is placed between the lateral aspect of the uterosacral ligament and the ureter. Before the bipolar forceps is used during an adnexectomy, the infundibulopelvic ligament is put under traction to identify the ureter and avoid thermal damage. No prospective study has substantiated the routine use of preoperative intravenous pyelography to prevent ureteral injury. In selected patients, it can help diagnose ureteral obstruction and allow appropriate surgical planning. In patients who have severe endometriosis and adhesions the ureters are difficult to see; ureteral catheters may be useful. Lighted ureteral catheters are available and are supposed to provide a visual road map of the ureter during laparoscopy.[76] The prophylactic use of ureteral catheters, including the use during laparoscopy of lighted catheters, is safe and technically simple. Ureteral catheters enhance identification of ureters and facilitate ureteral dissection.[77] However, prophylactic ureteral catheters did not reduce the rate of ureteral injury.[78] The routine use of ureteric catheters at laparoscopic hysterectomy may result in unnecessary complications.[79] As long as surgical techniques meticulously avoid ureteral injury, routine catheterization during laparoscopic hysterec-

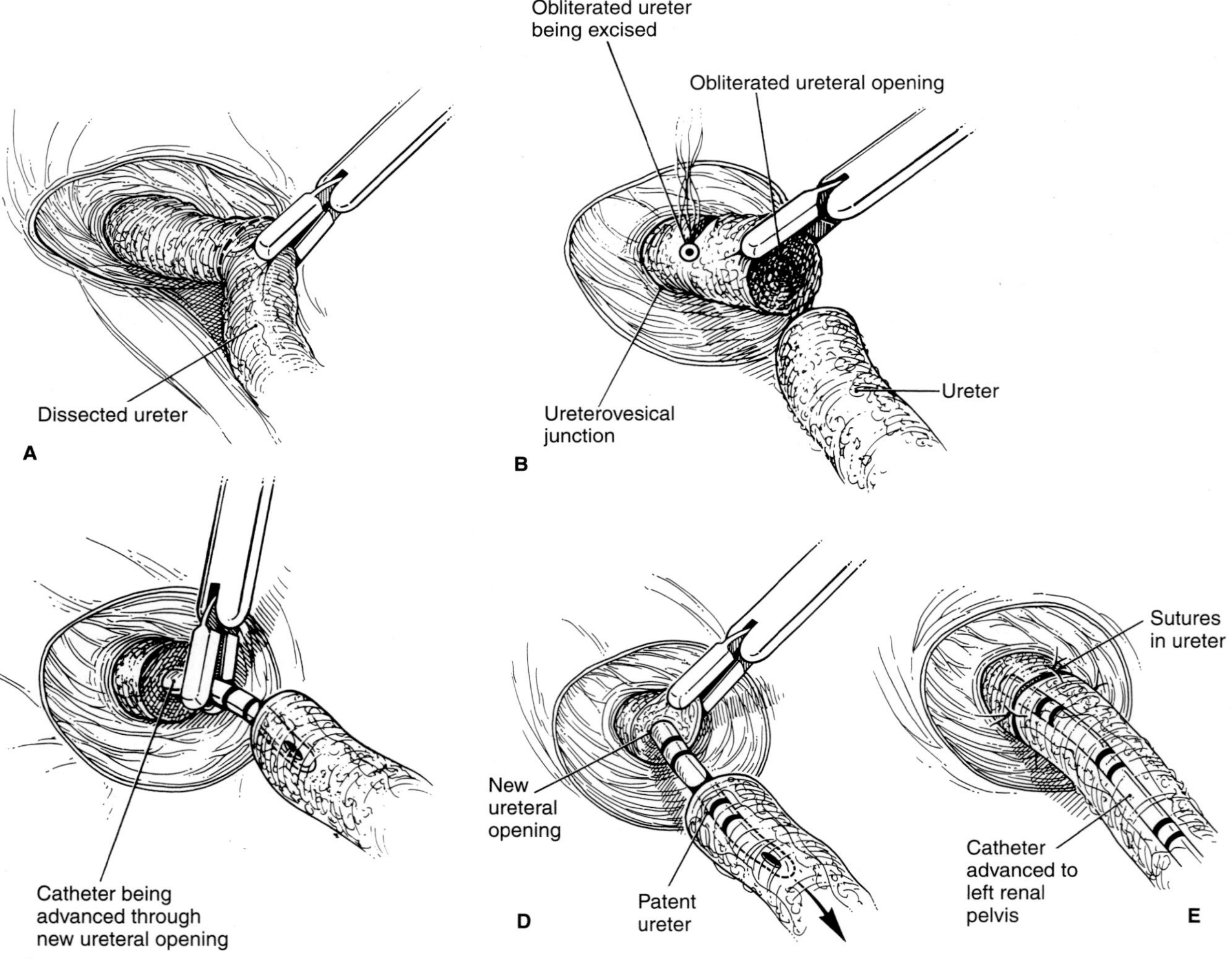

Figure 20-5 **A.** A uterolysis is done. The involved endometriosis is dissected and pulled medially. **B.** The obliterated portion of the ureter is excised. **C.** Under cystoscopic guidance, a 7 French ureteral catheter is passed through the uterovesical junction. **D.** The catheter is advanced through the proximal part of the ureter to the renal pelvis. **E.** The edges of the ureter are approximated.

tomy is not warranted. Ureteral catheters are useful in some instances of severe endometriosis and adhesions.[69]

The gynecologist should note the ureter's course through the peritoneum. Endometriosis and severe pelvic adhesions can thicken the peritoneum, obscuring the location of the ureter, especially near the uterosacral ligaments. If the ureter is not identified clearly through the peritoneum, it must be located by retroperitoneal dissection. Using hydrodissection, a horizontal incision is made in the peritoneum midway between the ovary and the uterosacral ligament. The lower edge of the peritoneum is grasped and pulled medially. Blunt dissection with the suction-irrigator probe helps locate the ureter lateral to the peritoneum. If the peritoneum is involved with endometriosis and there is retroperitoneal fibrosis, the ureter can be attached to the peritoneum. The horizontal incision in the peritoneum is extended as necessary.

Until recently, most reported instances of ureteral injury during laparoscopic procedures involved electrocoagulation because that is the most reliable technique to arrest bleeding. As the use of stapling devices increases, additional injuries to the ureters are being reported.[80–82]

Nezhat and coworkers[69] reported six ureteral injuries. Four of the six injuries were intentional, occurring in the course of treating partial or complete obstruction. Unrecognized anomalies in ureteral location can predispose a patient to injury.[83]

Recognition

Early recognition intraoperatively is critical to successful treatment. Intraoperative ureteral damage is suspected if urine leakage or blood-tinged urine is noted or indigo carmine dye is seen intraperitoneally after its intravenous administration. When surgical procedures involve the ureter, postoperative ureteral patency is detected by cystoscopy, ureteral catheterization, or an intravenous retrograde pyelogram. Intraoperative recognition of these complications will minimize additional operations.[84] A new technique using transvaginal color Doppler ultrasound has been introduced for postoperative detection of ureteral jets into the bladder when ureteral integrity is in question.[85] Stenting of the ureter or repair by laparotomy is indicated, but laparoscopic repair of partial- and full-thickness injuries is an option for some laparoscopists.[72,83] Unfortunately, a diagnosis of ureteral injury usually is made postoperatively by intravenous pyelography[67] Fever, flank pain, peritonitis, and abdominal distention within 48 to 72 hours postoperatively should alert the clinician to possible ureteral injury. Leukocytosis and hematuria can be present. Some of the symptoms are present in patients who develop ileus or bowel injury so that an intravenous pyelogram (IVP) is important for diagnosis.

Management

Whether the discovery of ureteral complications is immediate or delayed, a urologist should be consulted. If the IVP indicates ureteral injury, initial therapy should involve attempts at retrograde or antegrade stenting. Therapeutic options by laparotomy include ureteroureterostomy and ureteroneocystostomy. Both require stenting and drainage with a ureteral catheter. There have been several reports of conservative and laparoscopic treatment of ureteral injuries. Winslow and associates[86] described the conservative management of a patient who sustained an electrical burn injury to the left ureter secondary to a laparoscopy that was done for an infertility evaluation. She had postoperative retrograde ureteral stenting for 18 days. After removal of the catheter, an IVP revealed grade III left hydronephrosis secondary to a ureteral stricture at the pelvic brim. The patient eventually underwent cystoscopy and left retrograde catheterization with placement of a J-stent. Her renal function improved.

Gomel and James[83] reported ureteral injury during needle electrosurgical ablation of the left uterosacral ligament. While they were examining the pelvic structures at the end of the procedure, a transverse laceration was found over the anterior aspect of the ureter, extending over more than one-half of its circumference. Notably, the ureter was medial to the uterosacral ligament, a significant variation from its normal lateral position. The edges of the laceration appeared healthy, with no blanching or irregularity. No leakage of blue-stained urine was observed after intravenous injection of methylene blue. A whistle-tip ureteral catheter was introduced through a cystoscope. The edges of the laceration were approximated with a single 4-0 plain catgut suture. Pelvic drainage was not employed, and the patient was given prophylactic antibiotics. Two weeks after the procedure, the stent was removed, and an IVP done 10 weeks postoperatively did not indicate ureteral dilation or stenosis.

A patient who had long-term ureteral obstruction caused by endometriosis needed an incidental partial resection of the ureter laparoscopically.[87]

The ureter's course was distorted by a 2-cm fibrotic nodule approximately 4 cm above the bladder, corresponding to the level of obstruction. Hydrodissection aided in entering the retroperitoneal space at the pelvic brim. The ureter was dissected with the CO_2 laser. Under cystoscopic guidance, a 7 French ureteral catheter was passed through the ureterovesical junction (Figure 20-6). The catheter was advanced through the proximal portion of the ureter to the left renal pelvis. The edges of the ureter were approximated using four interrupted 4-0 polydioxanone sutures. The postoperative course was uncomplicated, and a postoperative IVP confirmed ureteral patency.

In one woman, during the treatment of severe pelvic wall endometriosis, a 1.5-cm segment of the ureter was unintentionally completely resected midway between the pelvic brim and the uterosacral ligament.[72] After the location of the injury was identified by injecting indigo carmine intravenously, the 2 to 3 cm of the proximal and distal ureteral ends was freed from the periureteral attachments. The ends were approximated with a 4-0 polydioxanone suture (Ethicon), and a stay ureteral stent was introduced cystoscopically and passed through the proximal end of the injury into the renal pelvis.[23] The stent was secured outside and placed on continuous drainage. Repair was carried out by placing four 4-0 polydioxanone sutures at 12, 6, 9, and 3 o'clock. The lacerated edges were approximated. A Jackson-Pratt drain was inserted, and an indwelling Foley catheter was

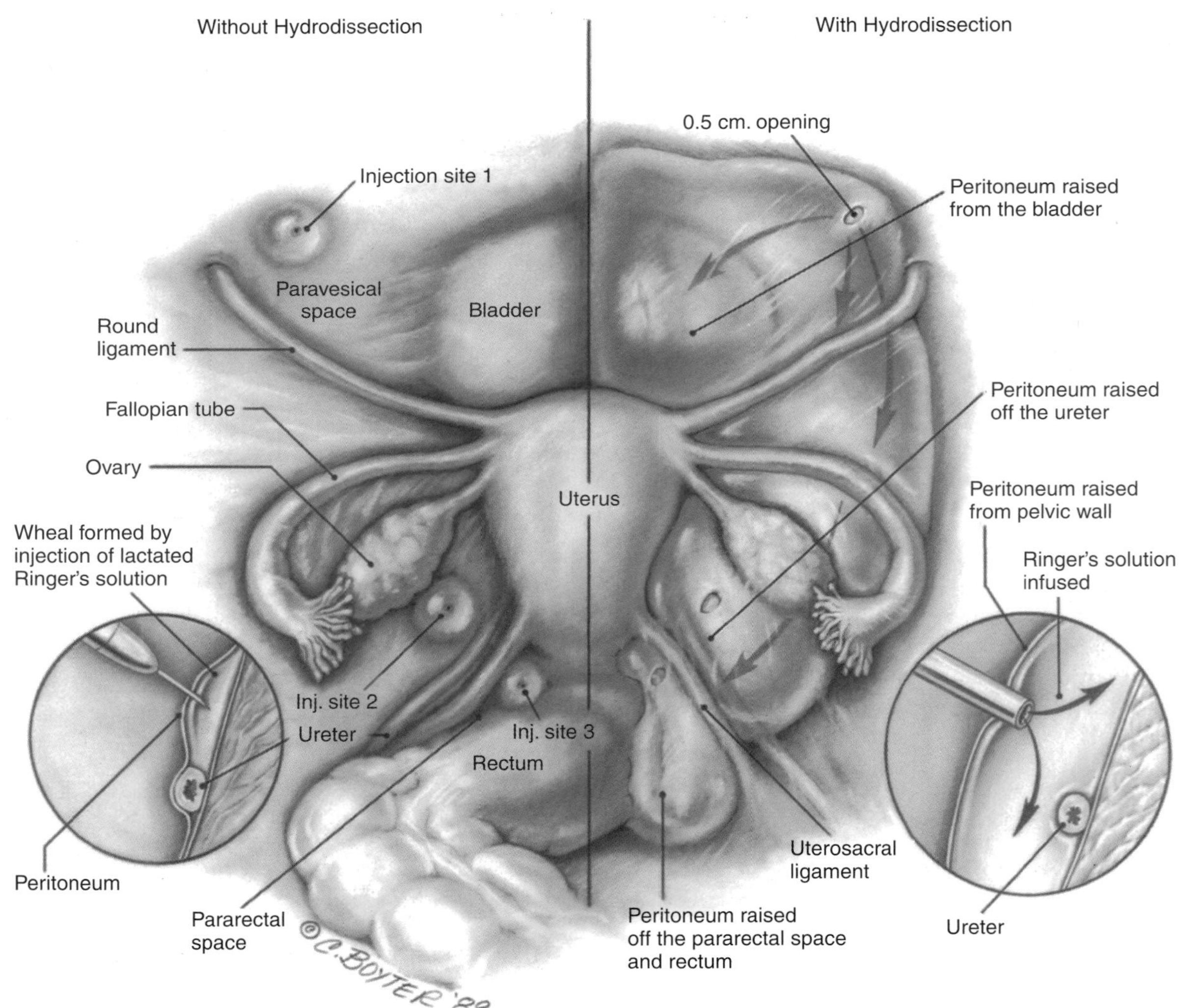

Figure 20-6. The ureter can be protected by using hydrodissection and resecting the affected peritoneum when treating endometriosis. The inset shows the forced injection of lactated Ringer's solution.

introduced into the bladder. The duration of the entire procedure was 3 hours, while the repair required 35 minutes. One gram of cefoxitin was given preoperatively and continued postoperatively until the patient was discharged from the hospital.

On the first postoperative day, there was no drainage from the Jackson-Pratt drain, and it was removed. No postoperative complications were noted. The patient remained afebrile with normal renal function tests and sterile urine. Although the ureteral stent stayed in place, the Foley catheter was removed. The patient was discharged on the second postoperative day and was prescribed prophylactic antibiotics (Septran DS; Burroughs Wellcome, Research Triangle Park, NC). Six weeks postoperatively, the ureteral catheter was removed, and no evidence of ureteral dilation or stenosis was seen. An IVP was normal.

Of the four patients who had partial resections of injured ureters, one occurred during separation of an adherent endometrioma from the pelvic side wall. The ureter was distorted, and despite retroperitoneal dissection, a 1-cm perforation was noted in the midpelvic area between the pelvic brim and the uterosacral ligament. After the ovary was removed, the ureter was freed and a stay ureteral stent was placed. The perforation was repaired with one 4-0 polydioxanone suture. No drainage was used. The patient was discharged the following day. The ureteral stent was removed 2 weeks later, after an IVP had confirmed that no leakage or stenosis was present. The other three patients had severe right pelvic side wall endometriosis with ureteral involvement, resulting in some degree of stenosis and hydroureter. The endometriosis and fibrosis were excised and removed, but ureteral resection was required. In two women, the ureter was repaired with two sutures. In one of them, the perforation was small. It was treated by inserting the stay ureteral stent for 2 weeks. No long-term complications were described by any of the six patients. Based on the authors' experience and other reports, a laparoscopist familiar with delicate laparoscopic suturing can repair ureteral injuries laparoscopically with good results.

Therapeutic options with laparotomy include ureteroureterostomy and ureteroneocystostomy.[69] A patient who had a long-term ureteral obstruction caused by endometriosis needed an incidental partial resection of the ureter laparoscopically.[87] A laparoscopist familiar with delicate laparoscopic suturing can repair ureteral injuries laparoscopically with good results.[69,88]

Small Bowel Injuries

Small bowel injuries occur if the bowel is immobilized by adhesions.[15] The bowel can be injured during insertion of the Veress needle or trocar, bowel manipulation, or enterolysis. Electrosurgery and stray laser beams can result in unrecognized thermal injuries to the bowel. Injury to the gastrointestinal tract is a serious complication. Whether discovered intraoperatively or postoperatively, small bowel injuries may necessitate a laparotomy to avoid serious morbidity and even mortality.[3]

Prevention

Direct mechanical and electrical trauma can injure the gastrointestinal tract, but a consistent difference in injury pattern has been noted. The characteristics of each pattern distinguish between the two causes.[89] Thermal burns, sharp dissection, and needle punctures create most of these injuries.[90,91]

Intestinal lacerations occur with trocars, scissors, the laser, or electricity. The risk of injury is higher if adhesions are dense and tissue planes are poorly defined. Traction on the bowel with serrated graspers can cause abrasions and lacerations. An inadvertent small bowel biopsy specimen was taken during a hysteroscopic procedure, and the diagnosis of the tissue was made by the pathologist.[92]

Intestinal inspection after sharp dissection that shows bleeding or a hematoma should alert the operator to potential intestinal injury. Manipulation of the bowel from the pelvis with a blunt metal probe is done cautiously, and blunt dissection should be avoided. Intestines trapped in incisions as trocars are withdrawn increase the risk for small bowel obstruction.[93] Some laparoscopists recommend opening the valve of the umbilical trocar as it is withdrawn to prevent the creation of a vacuum that can draw the bowel into the incision. Using a Z-track insertion may eliminate this complication.[94]

Adhesions between the small bowel and the anterior abdominal wall are associated with a risk of trocar injury, especially in patients who have had a bowel resection or exploratory laparotomy for trauma. Women who undergo a second-look laparoscopy after treatment for ovarian carcinoma by laparotomy have adhesions from previous omentectomy and debulking.[95]

Despite the use of open laparoscopy, bowel lacerations can occur when the peritoneum is entered.[96] It is difficult to decide which patients should have an open laparoscopy. In one series,[1] all 16 patients who had small bowel injuries also had had previous laparotomies and small bowel adhesions. Six were trocar injuries, eight occurred during adhesiolysis, and two occurred during open laparoscopy. When a patient is at risk for bowel adhesions, it is prudent to prepare her with a mechanical and possibly antibiotic bowel preparation preoperatively.

Recognition

Electrical injuries to the intestine are not always apparent intraoperatively, or their appearance leads the surgeon to choose conservative management.[89] Most intestinal burns less than 5 mm in diameter can be treated expectantly. If the area of blanching on the intestinal serosa exceeds 5 mm, the extent of thermal damage will exceed the apparent damage, and therapy is instituted immediately. The actual area of injury can extend up to 5 cm from the apparent injury.[97] If the small bowel is lacerated by a trocar, the laparoscopist views the mucosal surface to search for leaking intestinal contents or a hematoma on the serosa.

If the small bowel injury is not recognized intraoperatively, the patient generally presents on the third or fourth postoperative day with lower abdominal pain, fever, nausea, and anorexia. By the fifth or sixth postoperative day, increases occur in abdominal pain, nausea, vomiting, fever, and white blood cell count.[97] Radiograms reveal multiple air and fluid levels or air under the diaphragm. An unusual postoperative presentation of laparoscopic bowel injuries that were not recognized intraoperatively was reported in four patients.[98] Those patients had severe pain in a single trocar site, abdominal distention, diarrhea, and leukopenia followed by acute cardiopulmonary collapse secondary to sepsis within 96 hours. Persistent focal pain in a trocar site with abdominal distention, diarrhea, and leukopenia can present with the symptoms and signs of an unrecognized perforation.

Management

Complications from small bowel injury are related to the extent of damage and the time that elapses before the damage is discovered. Sharp trocar wounds can be limited to the serosa or involve the entire wall. Small punctures or superficial lacerations seal readily and require no further treatment, assuming that careful inspection of the affected bowel reveals no leakage or bleeding. Small (<5 mm) superficial lacerations are inspected to assure that only the serosa is involved. These patients are treated conservatively and discharged the day of the operation with instructions to report any untoward reaction.

Patients who have obvious leakage require intervention and perhaps laparotomy. The intestine should be inspected on both sides to search for through-and-through injuries, especially injuries created by a trocar. If only one entry is found and repaired, peritonitis can develop postoperatively. If the laparoscope is inserted through the laceration and a laparotomy is done, the defect is identified and closed by a purse-string suture as the laparoscope is withdrawn to decrease peritoneal contamination.[99,100]

The small intestine is repaired in one or two layers by placing an initial row of interrupted sutures to approximate the mucosa and muscularis. A reinforcing layer of 3-0 silk Lembert sutures may be used to approximate the muscularis and serosal edges.[101] All lacerations are closed transversely to lessen the occurrence of stenosis of the bowel lumen. This closure is appropriate only if the laceration is less than one-half the diameter of the bowel. When the laceration exceeds one-half the diameter of the lumen, segmental resection and anastomosis are done. If the mesenteric blood supply is interrupted by the puncture, a resection is done regardless of the size or length of the laceration to maintain blood supply to that segment of bowel.[99] Intraoperative consultation with a general surgeon is appropriate whenever significant bowel trauma occurs. Small bowel injuries caused by trocars or the CO_2 laser can be repaired in one layer by using 3-0 silk or 4-0 polydioxanone without complication or laparotomy.[102] Injuries less than 2 cm (small or large bowel) may be repaired transversely or longitudinally; however, injuries more than 2 cm should be repaired transversely. Repair of bowel perforation should be done with intraabdominal laparoscopic suturing (Figure 20-7, A and B).

After repair of a bowel laceration, the entire abdomen is irrigated. A nasogastric tube may be placed and then removed when drainage has decreased, indicating that bowel function has resumed. The patient is not given anything by mouth until she passes flatus.

When possible bowel laceration becomes apparent after the patient has been discharged, conservative management is successful in patients who have not developed peritonitis. In-hospital management consists of hydration, nothing by mouth, and close observation with white blood cell count and physical examination every 6 hours. Wheeless[97] reported that over one-half the patients

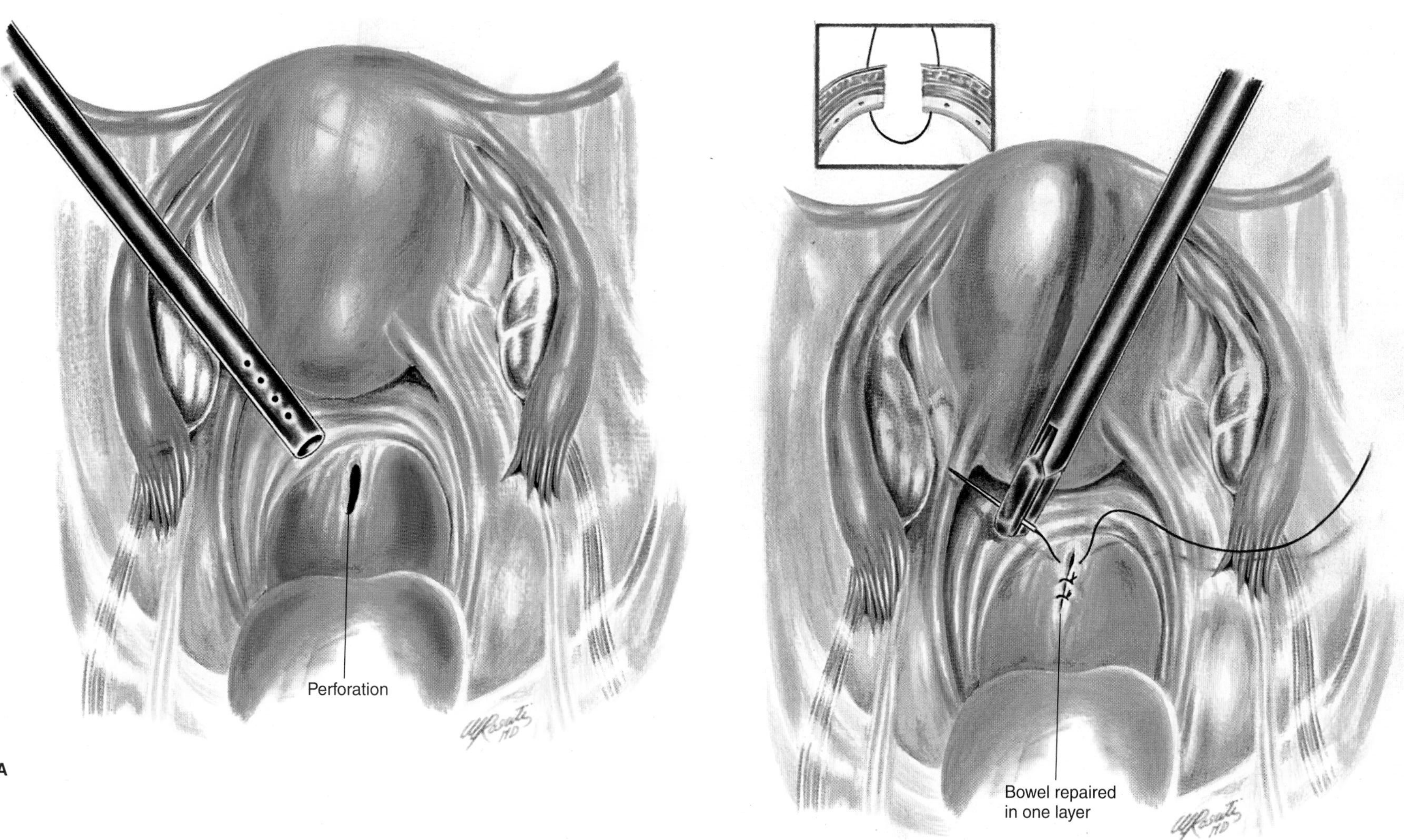

Figure 20-7 **A**. A small laceration is noted in the rectosigmoid. **B**. The bowel is repaired in one layer. The inset shows a through-and-through suture.

treated conservatively required no surgical intervention. Patients whose condition deteriorated during observation underwent laparotomy and had no complications attributable to delayed surgery.

Immediate surgical intervention and possible laparotomy are indicated in patients who present with fever, severe abdominal pain, nausea, vomiting, obstipation, or peritonitis and those whose clinical condition worsens. Surgical considerations for managing bowel injuries that are discovered postoperatively differ somewhat from those for injuries discovered and managed intraoperatively. The damaged bowel must be repaired or resected. In addition, resection of all necrotic tissue in the pelvis is mandatory even if this requires a hysterectomy and bilateral salpingo-oophorectomy. If burned or necrotic tissue that has been bathed in intestinal contents, blood, or serum is not excised, a pelvic abscess will develop.[97]

Wheeless[97] presented a seven-point plan to manage patients with peritonitis secondary to bowel perforation:

1. Preoperative stabilization with fluids, electrolytes, and nasogastric suction
2. Exploratory laparotomy with repair or resection of the injured bowel
3. Resection of all necrotic tissue
4. Copious and repeated saline lavage of the abdomen
5. Pelvic drainage through the vagina using a closed drainage system
6. Aggressive antibiotic therapy
7. Embolus prophylaxis with minidose heparin (5000 U tid).

In an AAGL membership poll, the two deaths reported from 36,928 procedures were attributed to bowel injuries. In one instance, the patient had extensive adhesions from the abdominal wall to the bowel. Although the bowel injury was recognized and repaired, the patient developed a persistent postoperative ileus and died of peritonitis. The second death was attributable to sepsis after an unrecognized small bowel perforation.[3]

Large Bowel Injuries

Colon entry is a major complication, particularly if the bowel is unprepared or the injury is not recognized. Even small perforations, such as those from the Veress needle, require attention because the high bacterial concentration of minor leaks can cause infection and abscess formation.

Prevention

Factors that contribute to an increased risk of large bowel injuries include (1) failure to establish an adequate pneumoperitoneum, (2) the use of dull trocars which require excessive force, (3) uncontrolled, sudden entry of sharp instruments, and (4) gastric distention. Poorly controlled or sudden trocar entry can result in rectosigmoid laceration. Gastric distention can displace the transverse colon toward the pelvis, where it can be punctured by the Veress needle or lacerated with the trocar. This complication can be eliminated by using a nasogastric tube intraoperatively.

The rectosigmoid can be injured if the depth of penetration by endometriosis is underestimated or the cul-de-sac is obliterated. When the rectum is adherent to the posterior aspect of the cervix or uterosacral ligaments, blunt dissection may lacerate the rectum. Sharp dissection with scissors or the CO_2 laser is recommended. The combination of high-power superpulse or ultrapulse CO_2 laser and hydrodissection is relatively safe for working around the bowel.

When the cul-de-sac is dissected, identification of the vagina and rectum is facilitated by placing a probe or an assistant's finger in both the vagina and the rectum. Dissection should begin lateral to the uterosacral ligaments, where the anatomy is less distorted, and proceed toward the obliterated cul-de-sac.[103,104] Similarly, when a posterior culdotomy is done for tissue removal or during laparoscopic hysterectomy, correct identification of the vagina and rectum is important.[80,105]

When a difficult pelvic operation is contemplated, such as cul-de-sac nodularity in a patient with endometriosis or a history suggesting significant pelvic adhesions, preoperative bowel preparation is indicated.

Recognition

Perforation of the large bowel with the Veress needle sometimes can be recognized with the saline aspiration test; recovery of brownish fluid is pathognomonic. Fecal odor may be detected. If large bowel entry is suspected on the basis of these two tests, the needle should be withdrawn promptly and another sterile Veress needle should be reinserted. Once the laparoscope is inserted, the entry site should be sought and examined.

Because of the high bacterial concentration, minor leaks of fecal material into the peritoneal cavity can be the source of serious infection. Four instances of pelvic abscess and infection were reported in a series of 187 women who underwent advanced laparoscopic treatment of infiltrative endometriosis of the bowel.[106] The "underwater" examination is recommended after the treatment of severe endometriosis and adhesions of the rectum and rectosigmoid colon.

Large bowel injuries can be serious because they may not be recognized at operation. Under these circumstances, the patient generally presents on the third or fourth postoperative day with lower abdominal pain, mild fever, slight nausea, and anorexia. By the fifth or sixth postoperative day, these symptoms progress to include fever, severe abdominal pain, nausea, vomiting, obstipation, increased white blood cell count, and peritonitis. An upright x-ray may show changes consistent with an ileus.[107] The patient appears ill with no clear explanation.

Management

For small colonic wounds associated with minimal contamination, laparotomy with primary suture closure has been the accepted therapy. In addition, copious lavage of the peritoneal cavity, broad-spectrum antibiotics, and drainage minimize the risk of infection. Under the proper circumstances, a small wound to the colon may be closed through the laparoscope. This procedure was carried out in 25 of 26 large bowel injuries without complication.[108] Copious irrigation and antibiotic coverage are essential.

Electrical injury to the right colon is managed by resecting the injured segment and doing a primary anastomosis. Diverting ileostomy facilitates healing and reduces morbidity and mortality. Injury to the descending colon, sigmoid, or rectum in unprepared bowel is not amenable to primary closure or resection with primary anastomosis. Diverting colostomy with resection of the injured portion is recommended.

Colonic lacerations in prepared bowel can be repaired laparoscopically after excising endometriosis nodules and identifying the extent of the laceration. A single-layer repair using 4-0 silk, 4-0 polydioxanone, or 0 polyglactin sutures is done.

The knowledge that the bowel can be repaired successfully by laparoscopic techniques in a properly prepared patient should increase the confidence of a surgeon operating in the deep pelvis.

Postoperative Complications

Bleeding

Hemostasis that appears adequate before closure because of the Trendelenburg position, high intraabdominal pressures, and relative hypotension may change once the patient resumes an upright position. If the patient does not respond to intravenous hydration, a repeat hematocrit may suggest hemorrhage and a physical exam may reveal abdominal distention.

Of four instances of intraabdominal bleeding,[1] one was caused by persistent ectopic pregnancy, two resulted from a blood disorder, and no source of bleeding was found for the fourth. Only two of these patients had a laparotomy. The patient with persistent ectopic pregnancy presented at another center with signs of intraabdominal bleeding and underwent a laparotomy. She had a leaking, persistent ectopic pregnancy, which was removed. A patient who had storage pool disease presented with intraabdominal bleeding 24 hours postoperatively. At laparoscopy, the source of bleeding was not located, and so a laparotomy was done. However, laparotomy failed to reveal the site. It was generalized oozing from the pelvic cavity. Postoperatively, she was treated with blood products and coagulation factors.

Nerve Injuries

Postoperative ilioinguinal neuralgia has been reported after laparoscopic ilioinguinal nerve damage caused by direct trauma from a secondary trocar placed in the right iliac fossa.[109] Neuropathy of the genitofemoral nerve may be differentiated from ilioinguinal neuralgia by diagnostic blocks and managed by laparoscopy.[110] Common postoperative neurologic syndromes include sciatic nerve injury, brachial palsy (shoulder-hand syndrome), and perineal nerve palsy. Allowing the buttocks to protrude too far off the end of the operating table may cause back injury.

Pain

Many patients still complain of moderate abdominal and shoulder pain during the first 48 to 72 hours postoperatively. Based on the theory of "dorsal horn hypersensitivity," several clinical trials have shown diminished pain with preincisional infiltration of a local anesthetic. Injection with

0.5% bupivacaine at the surgical site before incision and insertion of the trocars resulted in decreased postoperative pain.[111] Infiltrating bupivacaine at time of incision closure did not offer similar benefits in the control of pain postoperatively. Another study showed that pain is no better controlled with preincisional infiltration than with postincisional infiltration of bupivacaine.[112]

The beneficial effect of flushing 0.5% bupivacaine down the laparoscopy trocar over the peritoneal folds and into the abdominal wall after laparoscopy was small.[113] In women undergoing laparoscopic tubal sterilization with Silastic bands, topical bupivacaine decreased postoperative pain compared with placebo.[114] The addition of periportal injection of bupivacaine at the level of the parietal peritoneum under direct vision was effective in reducing pain.[112] The CO_2 commonly used for insufflation is a peritoneal irritant. Intraoperatively, this irritation can manifest as a vasovagal reaction. Postoperatively, residual gas accumulates under the diaphragm when an upright position is maintained, thus irritating the diaphragm. The pain is referred to the shoulder by the phrenic nerve.

Warming the insufflation CO_2 gas reduces postoperative pain.[55,56] Complete removal of intraabdominal CO_2 is difficult but may be facilitated by leaving the patient in the Trendelenburg position. Pressure exerted on the abdomen toward the symphysis allows the gas trapped in the lower abdomen to be expressed through the umbilical or suprapubic trocars. If pain develops, the patient can assume a supine position and use a pillow to elevate the lower abdomen, allowing gas to accumulate in the pelvis. The efficacy of intraperitoneal irrigation with a long-acting anesthetic into the subdiaphragmatic space after laparoscopic procedures reduced both the frequency and the intensity of postoperative shoulder-tip pain.[114–116] However, the effect tends to be transient and has little impact on the patient's convalescence.[117]

Infection

Urinary tract infections can be caused by instrumentation or asymptomatic bacteria. The use of advanced techniques such as laparoscopic Burch colposuspension using permanent surgical mesh can cause abscess formation.[118]

Postoperative infection is unusual after laparoscopic procedures, although the risk appears to be higher after prolonged, intricate procedures. Most infections are limited to skin or stitch abscesses and require incision and drainage. Occasionally, a pelvic infection occurs after a tubal operation, but it is not clear whether this is caused by a preexisting condition or contamination or is secondary to tissue destruction and necrosis. Urinary tract infections can be caused by instrumentation or asymptomatic bacteria.

Incisional Hernia

Herniation of the omentum or small bowel at the umbilical incision site has been reported with 5-mm or larger trocars. Patients at increased risk are those who are very thin (especially the elderly), those with chronic coughs, and those with a history of hernias. A survey of AAGL members revealed 933 hernias from an estimated 4,385,000 laparoscopic procedures, an incidence of 21 per 100,000.[119] Over two-thirds of these patients underwent subsequent surgical repair. The average time to reoperation was 8.5 days in one report.[120]

Possible preventive measures, although not proven, include Z-track insertion, avoiding trocar insertion directly through the umbilicus, and careful withdrawal of the umbilical trocar. Incisional hernia was more common in patients treated with a sharp-tip cutting single-use trocar compared with a cone-shaped noncutting reusable trocar, an incidence of 1.83% compared with 0.17%, respectively.[44]

The use of instruments for the closure of subcutaneous tissue in laparoscopic sites is gaining popularity because of the risk of incisional hernia at trocar sites.[121] However, in the AAGL survey,[119] almost one-fifth of the reported hernias occurred despite fascial closure. In such situations, incisional hernia may be attributed to infection, premature suture disruption, or failure to approximate fascial wound edges adequately.[122]

Incisional hernias occur mostly in sites where trocars 10 mm in diameter or larger were used.[119,120] Among 5300 patients who underwent laparoscopy,[123] 11 hernias occurred, an incidence of 0.2%. The 10-fold higher incidence of this complication compared with the AAGL survey was attributed to the more advanced and prolonged nature of the laparoscopic procedures in this study. Omentum herniated in seven, and bowel herniated in four others. In one patient, the sigmoid epiploica irreducibly herniated through the peritoneum, not the fascia. Six women required a laparoscopic operation to retract the entrapped omentum or bowel, and in one a laparoscopically assisted bowel resection was necessary. The hernias occurred through a 5-mm trocar incision site in half the women, and so whenever extensive manipulation is done through a 5-mm trocar port that causes extension of the incision, these ports should be closed as is done with the 10-mm ports.

A subclinical hernia with adhesions between the peritoneal incision site and the bowel may place a patient at significant risk of bowel perforation if she requires another laparoscopy. Some gynecologists advocate removing the umbilical trocar under laparoscopic observation to avoid entrapment of the bowel or removing the trocar with the valve open to avoid negative pressure that could draw omentum or small bowel into the defect.

Vaginal Cuff Dehiscence

Vaginal vault rupture with intestinal herniation is a postoperative complication of total hysterectomy. It can occur spontaneously or postcoitally. Three women, ages 40 to 43 years, presented to the emergency room with bleeding and pain 2 to 5 months after total laparoscopic hysterectomy.[124] The small bowel was visible through the introitus or protruding into the vagina. One rupture occurred after vaginal intercourse, and the other two were spontaneous. Inspection of the bowel revealed no evidence of trauma. Two vaginal cuff repairs were completed transvaginally and one laparoscopically, all with interrupted sutures of 0 polydioxanone or polyglactin.

Mortality

The AAGL 1979 membership survey, which involved primarily diagnostic laparoscopic procedures for tubal ligation, reported two deaths in 88,986 procedures, a death rate of 2 per 100,000.[2] The death rates remained essentially unchanged in subsequent AAGL surveys.[4] The 1991 AAGL membership reported one death from 56,536 laparoscopic procedures, a low death rate of 1.8 per 100,000 procedures.[5] The 1993 AAGL membership reported one death from 22,966 sterilizations and none from 36,482 diagnostic procedures.[6]

In a retrospective review of the literature and the authors' experience, data revealed 15 deaths in 501,779 laparoscopic procedures, a death rate of 3 per 100,000.[125] Surveys from France[12] and the Netherlands[11] revealed three deaths among 55,730 laparoscopic operations, a mortality rate of 5.4 per 100,000 procedures. However, in a Finish national study of laparoscopic complications, no deaths were reported in connection with 70,607 gynecologic laparoscopies.[13]

Peterson and associates[126] identified 29 deaths (3.6 per 100,000) associated with tubal sterilization: 11 resulted from anesthesia, 7 from sepsis after unrecognized bowel injury, 4 from hemorrhage after major vessel laceration, and 3 from myocardial infarction; 4 were related to other causes. Some deaths might have been prevented by the use of endotracheal intubation for general anesthesia, safer use of unipolar coagulation or alternative techniques, and careful insertion of the Veress needle and trocar.

References

1. Nezhat F, Nezhat C, Levy JS. A report of laparoscopic injuries and complications over a 10-year period. Presented at the 41st annual clinical meeting of the American College of Obstetricians and Gynecologists, Washington, D. C., 1993.
2. Phillips JM, Hulka JF, Hulka B, Corson SL. 1978 AAGL membership survey. *J Reprod Med* 1981; 26:529.
3. Peterson HB, Hulka JF, Phillips JM. American Association of Gynecologic Laparoscopists' 1988 membership survey on operative laparoscopy. *J Reprod Med* 1990; 35:587.
4. Hulka JF, Levy BS, Parker WH, Phillips JM. Laparoscopic-assisted vaginal hysterectomy: American Association of Gynecologic Laparoscopists' 1995 membership survey. *J Am Assoc Gynecol Laparosc* 1997; 4:167.
5. Hulka JF, Peterson HB, Phillips JM, Surrey MW. Operative laparoscopy: American Association of Gynecologic Laparoscopists' 1991 membership survey. *J Reprod Med* 1993; 38:569.
6. Hulka JF, Phillips JM, Peterson HB, Surrey MW. Laparoscopic sterilization: American Association of Gynecologic Laparoscopists' 1993 membership survey. *J Am Assoc Gynecol Laparosc* 1995; 2:137.
7. Lehmann-Willenbrock E, Riedel HH, Mecke H, Semm K. Pelviscopy/laparoscopy and its complications in Germany 1949–1988. *J Reprod Med* 1992; 37:671.
8. Nezhat F, Nezhat CH, Admon D, et al. Complications and results of 361 hysterectomies performed at laparoscopy. *J Am Coll Surg* 1995; 180:307.
9. Chapron CM, Dubuisson JB, Ansquer Y. Is total laparoscopic hysterectomy a safe surgical procedure? *Hum Reprod* 1996; 11:2422.

10. Querleu D, Chapron C, Chevallier L, Bruhat MA. Complications of gynecologic laparoscopic surgery—a French multicenter collaborative study (letter). *N Engl J Med* 1993; 328:1355.
11. Jansen FW, Kapiteyn K, Trimbos-Kemper T, et al. Complications of laparoscopy: A prospective multicentre observational study. *Br J Obstet Gynaecol* 1997; 104:595.
12. Chapron C, Querleu D, Bruhat MA, et al. Surgical complications of diagnostic and operative gynaecological laparoscopy: A series of 29,966 cases. *Hum Reprod* 1998; 13:867.
13. Harkki-Siren P, Kurki T. A nationwide analysis of laparoscopic complications. *Obstet Gynecol* 1997; 89:108.
14. Soderstrom RM, Butler JC. A critical evaluation of complications in laparoscopy. *J Reprod Med* 1973; 10:245.
15. Nezhat C, Nezhat F, Nezhat CH. Operative laparoscopy (minimally invasive surgery): State of the art. *J Gynecol Surg* 1992; 8:111.
16. Fried M, Peskova M, Kasalicky M. The role of laparoscopy in the treatment of morbid obesity. *Obes Surg* 1998; 8:520.
17. Pelosi MA 3rd, Pelosi MA. Alignment of the umbilical axis: An effective maneuver for laparoscopic entry in the obese patient. *Obstet Gynecol* 1998; 92:869.
18. Clough KB, Ladonne JM, Nos C, et al. Second look for ovarian cancer: Laparoscopy or laparotomy? A prospective comparative study. *Gynecol Oncol* 1999; 72:411.
19. Brill AI, Nezhat F, Nezhat CH, Nezhat C. The incidence of adhesions after prior laparotomy: A laparoscopic appraisal. *Obstet Gynecol* 1995; 85:269.
20. Amara DP, Nezhat C, Teng NN, et al. Operative laparoscopy in the management of ovarian cancer. *Surg Laparosc Endosc* 1996; 6:38.
21. Nezhat C, Seidman DS, Nezhat F, Nezhat CH. Laparoscopic surgery for gynecologic cancer, in Szabo Z, Lewis JE, Fanini GA, eds., *Surgery Technology International IV.* San Francisco: Universal Medical Press, 1995.
22. Chi DS, Curtin JP. Gynecologic cancer and laparoscopy. *Obstet Gynecol Clin North Am* 1999; 26:201.
23. Crawford DL, Phillips EH. Laparoscopic repair and groin hernia surgery. *Surg Clin North Am* 1998; 78:1047.
24. Nezhat FR, Tazuke S, Nezhat CH, et al. Laparoscopy during pregnancy: A literature review. *J Soc Laparoendosc Surg* 1997; 1:17.
25. Soriano D, Yefet Y, Oelsner G, et al. Operative laparoscopy for management of ectopic pregnancy in patients with hypovolemic shock. *J Am Assoc Gynecol Laparosc* 1997; 4:363.
26. O'Sullivan GC, Murphy D, O'Brien MG, Ireland A. Laparoscopic management of generalized peritonitis due to perforated colonic diverticula. *Am J Surg* 1996; 171:432.
27. Rizk N, Barrat C, Faranda C, et al. Laparoscopic treatment of generalized peritonitis with diverticular perforation of the sigmoid colon: Report of 10 cases. *Chirurgie* 1998; 123:358.
28. Navez B, Tassetti V, Scohy JJ, et al. Laparoscopic management of acute peritonitis. *Br J Surg* 1998; 85:32.
29. Cueto J, Diaz O, Garteiz D, et al. The efficacy of laparoscopic surgery in the diagnosis and treatment of peritonitis: Experience with 107 cases in Mexico City. *Surg Endosc* 1997; 11:366.
30. Zollinger A, Krayer S, Singer T, et al. Haemodynamic effects of pneumoperitoneum in elderly patients with an increased cardiac risk. *Eur J Anaesthesiol* 1997; 14:266.
31. Carroll BJ, Chandra M, Phillips EH, Margulies DR. Laparoscopic cholecystectomy in critically ill cardiac patients. *Am Surg* 1993; 59:783.
32. Massie MT, Massie LB, Marrangoni AG, et al. Advantages of laparoscopic cholecystectomy in the elderly and in patients with high ASA classifications. *J Laparoendosc Surg* 1993; 3:467.
33. Bateman BG, Kolp LA, Hoeger K. Complications of laparoscopy—operative and diagnostic. *Fertil Steril* 1996; 66:30.
34. Mac Cordick C, Lecuru F, Rizk E, et al. Morbidity in laparoscopic gynecological surgery: Results of a prospective single-center study. *Surg Endosc* 1999; 13:57.
35. Brill AI, Nezhat F, Nezhat CH, Nezhat C. The incidence of adhesions after prior laparotomy: A laparoscopic appraisal. *Obstet Gynecol* 1995; 85:269.
36. Servais D, Althoff H. Fatal carbon dioxide embolism as a complication of endoscopic interventions. *Chirurg* 1998; 69:773.
37. Cottin V, Delafosse B, Viale JP. Gas embolism during laparoscopy: A report of seven cases in patients with previous abdominal surgical history. *Surg Endosc* 1996; 10:166.

38. Lantz PE, Smith JD. Fatal carbon dioxide embolism complicating attempted laparoscopic cholecystectomy—case report and literature review. *J Forensic Sci* 1994; 39:1468.
39. Metzger DA. Trocar injuries to the small intestine, in Corfman RS, Diamond WP, DeCherney AH, eds., *Intraabdominal Endoscopic Complications: Prevention, Recognition, and Management.* Cambridge, UK: Blackwell, 1993.
40. Lee PI, Chi YS, Chang YK, Joo KY. Minilaparoscopy to reduce complications from cannula insertion in patients with previous pelvic or abdominal surgery. *J Am Assoc Gynecol Laparosc* 1999; 6:91.
41. Nezhat FR, Silfen SL, Evans D, Nezhat C. Comparison of direct insertion of disposable and standard reusable laparoscopic trocars and previous pneumoperitoneum with Veress needle. *Obstet Gynecol* 1991; 78:148.
42. Borgatta L, Gruss L, Barad D, Kaali SG. Direct trocar insertion versus Veress needle use for laparoscopic sterilization. *J Reprod Med* 1990; 35:891.
43. Byron JW, Markenson G, Miyazawa K. A randomized comparison of Veress needle and direct trocar insertion for laparoscopy. *Surg Gynecol Obstet* 1993; 177:259.
44. Woolcott R. The safety of laparoscopy performed by direct trocar insertion and carbon dioxide insufflation under vision. *Aust N Z J Obstet Gynaecol* 1997; 37:216.
45. Champault G, Cazacu F, Taffinder N. Serious trocar accidents in laparoscopic surgery: A French survey of 103,852 operations. *Surg Laparosc Endosc* 1996; 6:367.
46. Corson SL, Batzer FR, Gocial B, Maislin G. Measurement of the force necessary for laparoscopic trocar entry. *J Reprod Med* 1989; 34:282.
47. Leibl BJ, Schmedt CG, Schwarz J, et al. Laparoscopic surgery complications associated with trocar tip design: Review of literature and own results. *J Laparoendosc Adv Surg Tech* 1999; 9:135.
48. Hurd WW, Wang L, Schemmel MT. A comparison of the relative risk of vessel injury with conical versus pyramidal laparoscopic trocars in a rabbit model. *Am J Obstet Gynecol* 1995; 173:1731.
49. Nezhat F, Brill AI, Nezhat CH, et al. Laparoscopic appraisal of the anatomic relationship of the umbilicus to the aortic bifurcation. *J Am Assoc Gynecol Laparosc* 1998; 5:135.
50. Quint EH, Wang FL, Hurd WW. Laparoscopic transillumination for the location of anterior abdominal wall blood vessels. *J Laparoendosc Surg* 1996; 6:167.
51. Seidman DS, Nasserbakht F, Nezhat F, Nezhat C. Delayed recognition of iliac artery injury during laparoscopic surgery. *Surg Endosc* 1996; 10:1099.
52. Spitzer M, Golden P, Rehwaldt L, Benjamin F. Repair of laparoscopic injury to abdominal wall arteries complicated by cutaneous necrosis. *J Am Assoc Gynecol Laparosc* 1996; 3:449.
53. Nezhat C, Seidman DS, Vreman HJ, et al. The risk of carbon monoxide poisoning after prolonged laparoscopic surgery. *Obstet Gynecol* 1996; 88:771.
54. Healzer JM, Nezhat C, Brodsky JB, et al. Pulmonary edema after absorbing crystalloid irrigating fluid during laparoscopy. *Anesth Analg* 1994; 78:1207.
55. Moore SS, Green CR, Wang FL, et al. The role of irrigation in the development of hypothermia during laparoscopic surgery. *Am J Obstet Gynecol* 1997; 176:598.
56. Ott DE, Reich H, Love B, et al. Reduction of laparoscopic-induced hypothermia, postoperative pain and recovery room length of stay by pre-conditioning gas with the Insuflow device: A prospective randomized controlled multi-center study. *J Soc Laparoendosc Surg* 1998; 2:321.
57. Puttick MI, Scott-Coombes DM, Dye J, et al. Comparison of immunologic and physiologic effects of CO_2 pneumoperitoneum at room and body temperatures. *Surg Endosc* 1999; 13:572.
58. Mouton WG, Bessell JR, Millard SH, et al. A randomized controlled trial assessing the benefit of humidified insufflation gas during laparoscopic surgery. *Surg Endosc* 1999; 13:106.
59. Nezhat C, Childers J, Nezhat F, et al. Major retroperitoneal vascular injury during laparoscopic surgery. *Hum Reprod* 1997; 12:480.
60. Chapron CM, Pierre F, Lacroix S, et al. Major vascular injuries during gynecologic laparoscopy. *J Am Coll Surg* 1997; 185:461.
61. Geers J, Holden C. Major vascular injury as a complication of laparoscopic surgery: A report of three cases and review of the literature. *Am Surg* 1996; 62:377.
62. Nezhat F, Brill A, Nezhat C. Traumatic hypogastric artery bleeding controlled with

bipolar desiccation during operative laparoscopy. *J Am Assoc Gynecol Laparosc* 1994; 1:171.

63. Georgy FM, Fetterman HH, Chefetz MD. Complications of laparoscopy: Two cases of perforated urinary bladder. *Am J Obstet Gynecol* 1974; 120:1121.
64. Sherer DM. Inadvertent transvaginal cystotomy during laparoscopy. *Int J Gynaecol Obstet* 1990; 32:77.
65. Nezhat CH, Seidman DS, Nezhat F, et al. Laparoscopic management of intentional and unintentional cystotomy. *J Urol* 1996; 156:1400.
66. Lee CL, Lai YM, Soong YK. Management of urinary bladder injuries in laparoscopic assisted vaginal hysterectomy. *Acta Obstet Gynecol Scand* 1996; 75:174.
67. Granger DA, Soderstrom RM, Schiff SF, et al. Ureteral injuries at laparoscopy: Insights into diagnosis, management and prevention. *Obstet Gynecol* 1990; 75:839.
68. Tamussino KF, Lang PF, Breinl E. Ureteral complications with operative gynecologic laparoscopy. *Am J Obstet Gynecol* 1998; 178:967.
69. Nezhat C, Nezhat F, Nezhat CH, et al. Urinary tract endometriosis treated by laparoscopy. *Fertil Steril* 1996; 66:920.
70. Ferland RD, Rosenblatt P. Ureteral compromise after laparoscopic burch colpopexy. *J Am Assoc Gynecol Laparosc* 1999; 6:217.
71. Cheng YS. Ureteral injury resulting from laparoscopic fulguration of endometriotic implants. *Am J Obstet Gynecol* 1976; 126:1045.
72. Nezhat C, Nezhat F. Laparoscopic repair of resected ureter during operative laparoscopy to treat endometriosis: A case report. *Obstet Gynecol* 1992; 80:543.
73. Chaffkin L, Luciano LA. Ureteral injuries, in Corfman RS, Diamond WP, DeCherney AH, eds., *Complications of Laparoscopy and Hysteroscopy.* Cambridge, UK: Blackwell, 1993.
74. Nezhat C, Nezhat F. Safe laser excision or vaporization of peritoneal endometriosis. *Fertil Steril* 1989; 52:149.
75. Cook AS, Rock JA. The role of laparoscopy in the treatment of endometriosis. *Fertil Steril* 1991; 55:663.
76. Teichman JM, Lackner JE, Harrison JM. Comparison of lighted ureteral catheter luminance for laparoscopy. *Tech Urol* 1997; 3:213.
77. Quinlan DJ, Townsend DE, Johnson GH. Are ureteral catheters in gynecologic surgery beneficial or hazardous? *Am Assoc Gynecol Laparosc* 1995; 3:61.
78. Kuno K, Menzin A, Kauder HH, et al. Prophylactic ureteral catheterization in gynecologic surgery. *Urology* 1998; 52:1004.
79. Wood EC, Maher P, Pelosi MA. Routine use of ureteric catheters at laparoscopic hysterectomy may cause unnecessary complications. *J Am Assoc Gynecol Laparosc* 1996; 3:393.
80. Nezhat C, Nezhat F, Gordon S, Wilkins E. Laparoscopic versus abdominal hysterectomy. *J Reprod Med* 1992; 37:247.
81. Woodland MB. Ureter injury during laparoscopy-assisted vaginal hysterectomy with the endoscopic linear stapler. *Am J Obstet Gynecol* 1992; 176:756.
82. Nezhat C, Nezhat F, Bess O, Nezhat CH. Injuries associated with the use of a linear stapler during operative laparoscopy: Review of diagnosis, management and prevention. *J Gynecol Surg*. 1993; 9:145.
83. Gomel V, James C. Intraoperative management of ureteral injury during operative laparoscopy. *Fertil Steril* 1991; 55:416.
84. Saidi MH, Sadler RK, Vancaillie TG, et al. Diagnosis and management of serious urinary complications after major operative laparoscopy. *Obstet Gynecol* 1996; 87:272.
85. Timor-Tritsch IE, Haratz-Rubinstein N, Monteagudo A, et al. Transvaginal color Doppler sonography of the ureteral jets: A method to detect ureteral patency. *Obstet Gynecol* 1997; 89:113.
86. Winslow PH, Kreger R, Effesson B, Oster E. Conservative management of electrical burn injury of ureter secondary to laparoscopy. *Urology* 1986; 27:60.
87. Nezhat C, Nezhat F, Green B. Laparoscopic treatment of obstructed ureter due to endometriosis by resection and ureteroureterostomy: A case report. *J Urol* 1992; 148:865.
88. Nezhat CH, Nezhat FR, Freiha F, Nezhat CR. Laparoscopic vesicopsoas hitch for infiltrative ureteral endometriosis. *Fertil Steril* 1999; 71:376.
89. Levy BS, Soderstrom RM, Dail DH. Bowel injuries during laparoscopy: Gross anatomy and histology. *J Reprod Med* 1985; 30:168.
90. Chapron C, Pierre F, Harchaoui Y, et al. Gastrointestinal injuries during gynaecological laparoscopy. *Hum Reprod* 1999; 14:333.
91. Schrenk P, Woisetschlager R, Rieger R, Wayand W. Mechanism, management, and prevention of laparoscopic bowel injuries. *Gastrointest Endosc* 1996; 43:572.
92. Gentile GP, Siegler AM. Inadvertent intentional biopsy during laparoscopy and

hysteroscopy: A report of two cases. *Fertil Steril* 1981; 36:402.
93. Sauer M, Jarrett JC. Small bowel obstruction following diagnostic laparoscopy. *Fertil Steril* 1984; 42:653.
94. Corson SL, Bolognese RJ. Laparoscopy overview and results of a large series. *J Reprod Med* 1972; 9:148.
95. Loffer FD, Pent D. Indications, contraindications and complications of laparoscopy. *Obstet Gynecol Surv* 1975; 30:407.
96. Penfield AJ. How to prevent complications of open laparoscopy. *J Reprod Med* 1985; 30:660.
97. Wheeless CR. Gastrointestinal injuries associated with laparoscopy, in Phillips JM, ed., *Endoscopy in Gynecology.* Santa Fe Springs, CA: AAGL, 1978.
98. Bishoff JT, Allaf ME, Kirkels W, et al. Laparoscopic bowel injury: Incidence and clinical presentation. *J Urol* 1999; 161:887.
99. DeCherney AH. Laparoscopy with unexpected viscus penetration, in Nichols DH, ed. *Clinical Problems, Injuries and Complications of Gynecologic Surgery.* Baltimore: Williams & Wilkins, 1988.
100. Corson SL, Batzer FR, Gocial B, Maislin G. Measurement of the force necessary for laparoscopic trocar entry. *J Reprod Med* 1989; 34:282.
101. Borton M. *Laparoscopic Complication: Prevention and Management.* Philadelphia: Decker, 1986.
102. Nezhat C, Nezhat F, Ambroze W, Pennington E. Laparoscopic repair of small bowel, colon, and rectal endometriosis: A report of twenty-six cases. *Surg Endosc* 1993; 7:88.
103. Nezhat C, Nezhat F, Pennington E. Laparoscopic treatment of lower colorectal and infiltrative rectovaginal septum endometriosis by the technique of videolaseroscopy. *Br J Obstet Gynaecol* 1992; 99:664.
104. Redwine D. Laparoscopic en bloc resection for treatment of the obliterated cul-de-sac in endometriosis. *J Reprod Med* 1992; 37:696.
105. Nezhat F, Brill AI, Nezhat CH, Nezhat C. Adhesion formation after endoscopic posterior colpotomy. *J Reprod Med* 1993; 38:534.
106. Nezhat FR, Nezhat CH, Seidman DS, et al. Laparoscopic and laparoscopic assisted treatment of infiltrative endometriosis of the bowel (In Press).
107. Thompson BH, Wheeless CR. Gastrointestinal complications of laparoscopic sterilization. *Obstet Gynecol* 1973; 41:669.
108. Kirkpatrick JR, Rajpal SG. The injured colon: Therapeutic considerations. *Am J Surg* 1975; 129:187.
109. Parker J, Hayes C, Wong F, Carter J. Laparoscopic ilioinguinal nerve injury. *Gynecol Endosc* 1998; 7:327.
110. Perry CP. Laparoscopic treatment of genitofemoral neuralgia. *J Am Assoc Gynecol Laparosc* 1997; 4:231.
111. Ke RW, Portera SG, Bagous W, Lincoln SR. A randomized, double-blinded trial of preemptive analgesia in laparoscopy. *Obstet Gynecol* 1998; 92:972.
112. Alexander DJ, Ngoi SS, Lee L, et al. Randomized trial of periportal peritoneal bupivacaine for pain relief after laparoscopic cholecystectomy. *Br J Surg* 1996; 83:1223.
113. Johnson N, Onwude JL, Player J, et al. Pain after laparoscopy: An observational study and a randomized trial of local anesthetic. *J Gynecol Surg* 1994; 10:129.
114. Cunniffe MG, McAnena OJ, Dar MA, et al. A prospective randomized trial of intraoperative bupivacaine irrigation for management of shoulder-tip pain following laparoscopy. *Am J Surg* 1998; 176:258.
115. Weber A, Munoz J, Garteiz D, Cueto J. Use of subdiaphragmatic bupivacaine instillation to control postoperative pain after laparoscopic surgery. *Surg Laparosc Endosc* 1997; 7:6.
116. Tool AL, Kammerer-Doak DN, Nguyen CM, et al. Postoperative pain relief following laparoscopic tubal sterilization with silastic bands. *Obstet Gynecol* 1997; 90:731.
117. Szem JW, Hydo L, Barie PS. A double-blinded evaluation of intraperitoneal bupivacaine vs saline for the reduction of postoperative pain and nausea after laparoscopiccholecystectomy. *Surg Endosc* 1996; 10:44.
118. Balaloski SP, Richards SR, Singh E. Conservative management of delayed suprapubic abscess after laparoscopic burch colposuspension using nonabsorbable polypropylene mesh. *J Am Assoc Gynecol Laparosc* 1999; 6:225.
119. Montz FJ, Holschneider CH, Munro MG. Incisional hernia following laparoscopy: A survey of the American Association of Gynecologic Laparoscopists. *Obstet Gynecol* 1994; 84:881120.
120. Boike GM, Miller CE, Spirtos NM, et al. Incisional bowel herniations after operative laparoscopy: A series of nineteen cases and review of the literature. *Am J Obstet Gynecol* 1995; 172:1726.

121. Carter JE. A new technique of fascial closure for laparoscopic incisions. *J Laparosc Surg* 1994; 4:143.
122. Jones DB, Callery MP, Soper NJ. Strangulated incisional hernia at trocar site. *Surg Laparosc Endosc* 1996; 6:152.
123. Nezhat C, Nezhat F, Seidman DS, Nezhat C. Incisional hernias after operative laparoscopy. *J Laparoendosc Adv Surg Tech* 1997; 7:111.
124. Nezhat CH, Nezhat F, Seidman DS, Nezhat C. Vaginal vault evisceration after total laparoscopic hysterectomy. *Obstet Gynecol* 1996; 87:868.
125. Bonjer HJ, Hazebroek EJ, Kazemier G, et al. Open versus closed establishment of pneumoperitoneum in laparoscopic surgery. *Br J Surg* 1997; 84:599.
126. Peterson HB, DeStefano F, Rubin GL, et al. Deaths attributable to tubal sterilization in the United States, 1977 to 1981. *Am J Obstet Gynecol* 1983; 146:135.

21

Laparoscopy in the Pregnant Patient

The treatment of pregnant patients requires attention to the well-being of both the mother and the fetus. Abdominal and pelvic abnormalities that require operations during pregnancy represent a clinical challenge. The underlying disease or the procedure can pose risks to the mother and the fetus. Laparoscopy is safe in the absence of an inflammatory process or fever. Manipulation of the uterus and cervix should be avoided.

A retrospective case-control study compared the outcome of laparoscopic appendectomy and cholecystectomy with that of laparotomy during the first two timesters. Laparoscopic management decreased the length of hospitalization and the need for narcotics for the relief of pain. Postoperatively, no differences were noted in the length of the gestations, the 1- and 5-minute Apgar scores, or the birthweights.[1]

Nonobstetric Abdominal Operations in Pregnancy

In the United States, the most common nonobstetric abdominal operations associated with pregnancy are appendectomy, cholecystectomy, and adnexal procedures.

The specific operative risks associated with pregnancy include fetal asphyxia, fetal death in utero, premature labor, premature rupture of membranes, and thromboembolism. Perinatal mortality has been reported in 7.5% of pregnant patients who underwent abdominal operations.[2–4] After the first trimester, a patient's respiratory function is altered because of reduction in the functional residual capacity, increased oxygen consumption, physiologic hyperventilation, and a lowered oxygen reserve. Mechanical ventilation of a gravid patient during laparoscopy can be difficult because of the upwardly displaced position of the diaphragm before abdominal insufflation. The decreased respiratory reserve of pregnant patients limits the degree of the Trendelenburg position. Furthermore, physiologic hemodynamic changes in pregnant patients increase the risk of decreased cardiac output and uteroplacental blood flow after the first trimester, particularly in the supine position. These physiologic alterations put the fetus at increased risk for hypoxia. The proper maternal position should tilt the hips 15 degrees, and appropriate interpretations of hemodynamic and respiratory variables are essential.[5] Levine and Diamond[6] found that intraabdominal procedures were associated with a greater tendency for premature labor than were extraabdominal operations. Smith[7] reported that techniques requiring cervical handling increased the risk for premature labor as much as did intraabdominal manipulation.

The increase in premature labor may be caused by the underlying pathologic condition. Perforation of the appendix is associated with a risk of preterm labor four times higher than that from an appendectomy on an intact appendix.[8,9] Ahlgren[10] demonstrated that elevated temperature independently increased the motility of human myometrium in vitro. Kullander[11] noted premature labor in 50 percent of rabbits with induced fever. Pyrogens can alter the neurohypophyseal axis, causing the release of oxytocin from posterior pituitary.[12] The infectious process that requires surgical intervention or fever, rather than the operative technique, can cause uterine contractions and lead to an increased risk of preterm delivery and pregnancy loss.

The increased risk of preterm labor with surgical procedures during a pregnancy also appears to depend on the duration of the pregnancy and the acuteness of the problem. In reports of the operative management of adnexal tumors by laparotomy, preterm contractions and labor were common when the operations occurred in the third trimester. Emergency procedures had a greater risk of causing a spontaneous abortion and premature labor than did those done electively. Although there have been no controlled studies of elective procedures done at different gestational ages, Hess and associates[13] reported that operations required because of torsion and rupture of an adnexal mass after 31 weeks' gestation in two patients resulted in preterm deliveries within 72 hours. In contrast, the 39 patients who underwent elective removal of adnexal masses did not have preterm labor. Prompt, elective operations are preferable to emergency procedures.

TABLE 21-1. Laparoscopic Appendectomy

Author	Weeks of Pregnancy	Complication
Schreiber[15]	8	None
	13	Contractions before surgery, responded to tocolytics
	21	Difficulty to place Veress needle
	25	None
Cristalli[16]	14	None
Lucas[19]	18.5	None
Andreoli[20]	13	None
	15	
	19	
	21	
	24	
Amos[21]	13 to 29 weeks (3 cases)	None

Laparoscopic Procedures during Pregnancy

Gynecologists have done laparoscopy in pregnant women in the first trimester to search for an ectopic pregnancy. Although some of those procedures revealed normal intrauterine pregnancies, the laparoscopy did not have adverse effects on the pregnancy.[14]

Appendectomy

Appendicitis is the most common indication for nonobstetric abdominal surgery during pregnancy.[15–21] The diagnosis can present diagnostic and management difficulties because of displacement of the appendix by the gravid uterus.[8,22] If perforation of the appendix occurs, an increase in fetal mortality will result.[8,23,24] Case reports of laparoscopic appendectomy have been described (Table 21-1). In this group, the duration of the pregnancies ranged from 8 to 29 weeks, and none of the operations caused obstetric complications. None of them involved a perforated appendix or complicated appendicitis. Laparoscopy enables the surgeon to intervene earlier in the disease process so that the patients will experience less morbidity.[25]

Cholecystectomy

Cholecystecomy is the second most common indication for nonobstetric abdominal operations in pregnant women.[9] Dixon and coauthors[26] compared maternal morbidity, fetal outcome, and cost in 44 patients who had symptoms of cholecystitis. Twenty-six were managed conservatively, and 18 underwent cholecystectomy by laparotomy. Among those treated conservatively, 58% had recurrent symptoms and one patient developed pancreatitis. Spontaneous abortion was observed in three (12%) of the patients managed conservatively, while none occurred in the cholecystectomy group. Among the 18 who had a cholecystecomy, all the women delivered at term except one patient. She delivered prematurely because of preeclampsia during the eighth month of gestation, many weeks after the surgical procedure.[26]

Thirty-one reports involving 102 patients who had laparoscopic cholecystectomy were collected (Table 21-2).[20,21,27–57] The duration of the pregnancies ranged from 3 to 32 weeks, and obstetric complications were noted in five instances: Three spontaneous abortions occurred in the second trimester 1 week postoperatively, another occurred 2 months after the operation, and one maternal-fetal mortality occurred 15 days later from an intraabdominal hemorrhage.[21,57] While laparoscopic cholecystectomy has been successfully done in the third trimester in 12 women, the risk of uterine damage intraoperatively is increased in late pregnancies. Laparoscopic cholecystectomy during the third trimester is not advisable. In 1992, the Office of Medical Applications of Research and the National Institute of Diabetes and Digestive and Kidney Diseases of the National Institutes of Health held a consensus conference to

TABLE 21-2. **Laparoscopic Cholecystectomy**

Author	Weeks of Pregnancy	Procedure	Complication
Andreoli [20]	21–28 (5 cases)	Cholecystectomy	None
Amos et al[21]	12, 13, 15, 16	Cholecystectomy	None
Arvidsson and Gerdin[27]	22	Cholecystectomy and common bile duct stone removal	None
Milenin and Rubtsov[28]	27	Cholecystectomy and transhepatic transcutaneous drainage	None
Pucc and Seed[29]	31	Cholecystectomy	None
Weber et al[30]	13	Cholecystectomy	None
Morrell et al[31]	13, 14, 17, 18, 23	Cholecystectomy and intraoperative cholangiography	None
Soper et al[32]	23	Cholecystectomy and intraoperative cholangiography	None
Adamsen et al[33]	Second trimester	Cholecystectomy	None
Bennett and Estes[34]	19	Cholecystectomy	None
Elerding[35]	3, 14, 18, 25, 28	Cholecystectomy	None
Fabiani et al[36]	14	Cholecystectomy	None
Hart et al[37]	12, 23	Cholecystectomy	None
Jackson and Sigman[38]	17	Cholecystectomy	Not reported
Rusher et al[39]	17	Cholecystectomy	Not reported
Schorr[40]	16, 21	Cholecystectomy	Not reported
Chandra et al[41]	13	Cholecystectomy	None
Comitalo and Lynch[42]	14–19(4 cases)	Cholecystectomy	One delivered at 37 weeks RDS
Costantino et al[43]	14, 22	Cholecystectomy	None
Csaba and Orban[44]	25	Cholecystectomy	None
DePaula et al[45]	21	Common bile duct exploration, transcystic choledoscopy, intra operative cholangiography	None
Edelman[46]	15	Cholecystectomy	None
Shaked et al[47]	10	Cholecystectomy	None
Williams et al[50]	14	Cholecystectomy , laprolift	None
Davis et al[51]	18	Cholecystectomy	None
	Second trimester (2)	Cholecystectomy	None
Friedman and Friedman[52]	Third trimester (1)	Cholecystectomy	None
	Second trimester (1)	Cholecystectomy	None
Lanzaframe[53]	14, 17, 22, 27, 28	Cholecystectomy	None
Posta[54]	Second trimester (1)	Cholecystectomy	None
Eichenberg et al[55]	Second trimester (1) Third trimester (3)	Cholecystectomy	Immature deliveries in 3 women
Abuabara et al[56]	First trimester (3) Second trimester (15) Third trimester (4)	Cholecystectomy and choledocholithotomy	One premature delivery 2 months postoperatively
Barone et al[57]	9 to 32 (20 cases)	Cholecystectomy	19 none*

*One maternal-fetal death postoperatively from intraabdominal hemorrhage.
RDS—Respiratory Distress Syndrome.

evaluate the available data on laparoscopic cholecystectomy. The published guidelines include a statement addressing laparoscopic cholecystectomy during pregnancy: "Patients with acute cholecystitis, acute gallstone pancreatitis that has subsided, prior surgery in the upper abdomen, and symptomatic gallstones in the second trimester of pregnancy may be candidates for laparoscopic cholecystectomy, providing the operating surgeon is experienced in treating patients with complex

TABLE 21-3. Laparoscopic Management of Adnexal Torsion

Author	Weeks of Pregnancy	Procedure	Complications
Lucas et al[19]	8, 20	Cyst aspiration and cystectomy	None
Mage et al[84]	6	Cyst aspiration	None
Shalev et al[85]	8	Cyst aspiration	None
Ozcan et al[88]	8	Detorsion only	None
Shalev and Peleg[89]	Unknown (10 cases)	Cyst aspiration and detorsion	None
Gazarelli and Mazzuka[91]	8, 5	Cyst aspiration	None
Nagase and Konno[93]	6	Cyst drainage	None
Soriano et al[103]	First trimester (20 cases)	Cyst aspiration and detorsion	5 spontaneous abortions

laparoscopic cholecystectomy problems. The use of laparoscopic cholecystectomy in patients in the first trimester of pregnancy is controversial because of the unknown effects of carbon dioxide pneumoperitoneum on the developing fetus. Patients in the third trimester of pregnancy usually should not undergo laparoscopic cholecystectomy because of risk of damage to the uterus during the procedure."[58]

Operations on the Adnexa

Reviews of the outcome of pregnancies associated with adnexal masses found that 13 to 42% of them resulted in complications such as torsion, rupture, hemorrhage, and obstruction of labor in the second half of pregnancy, often requiring urgent surgical intervention.[59–65] Complications were more likely to occur when the mass was greater than 6 cm. These acute complications were associated with increased fetal morbidity and mortality because of premature delivery. Masses larger than 6 cm that do not regress spontaneously by 15 weeks should be removed electively. After that time, most cysts will have regressed spontaneously and fewer associated abortions will result.

In both nonpregnant and pregnant women, adnexal masses greater than 6 cm must be followed carefully. The reported prevalence of such tumors before the regular use of prenatal ultrasound ranged between 1 in 328 and 1 in 1,399 pregnancies.[16,61–69] With the routine use of early prenatal ultrasonography, the detection of incidental adnexal tumors has increased substantially.[70,71] Fewer than 8% of ovarian tumors were found to be malignant.[25,70–73] In nonpregnant women, anechoic simple cysts carry the lowest risk of being malignant. In pregnancy, these anechoic cysts, because of their size, pulsatility index, and resistive index values, are frequently in the range associated with malignancy in the nonpregnant state because of the pregnancy-related ovarian changes.[72,73] Thornton and Wells[69] collected 69 adnexal cysts larger than 5 cm detected in pregnant women by ultrasound. They noted that of the 20 cysts that did not regress, 6 of them larger than 10 cm in size contained borderline malignant features by histologic analysis. If an adnexal mass is larger than 6 cm and persists beyond 15 or 16 weeks, there is an increased risk of malignancy and removal is indicated. The accuracy of cytologic diagnosis of cyst fluid remains uncertain. There have been two reports of the development of diffuse intraabdominal dissemination of stage I ovarian cancer after cyst aspiration.[74,75]

Another indication for abdominal operations during pregnancy is a persistent adnexal mass (Table 21-3).[76–103] Torsion of the adnexa was treated mostly by detorsion and aspiration. Cystic teratomas were the most common benign tumor encountered, and functional cysts were found in 30 women (Table 21-4). Cystectomy was the procedure of choice for their management. Most operations were done in the first trimester in an emergency procedure and included laparoscopic cyst aspiration, detorsion of the adnexa, or removal of a heterotopic pregnancy. There are six instances of laparoscopic removal of heterotopic pregnancies at a gestational age between 6 and 10 weeks involving either salpingectomy or cornual resection of an interstitial pregnancy.[76,78–82] All the associated in utero pregnancies progressed normally into the third timester (Table 21-5).

Laparoscopy is feasible and safe during pregnancy in the first trimester. For laparoscopic adnexal masses, Nezhat and colleagues[83] did an elective laparoscopy at 16 weeks of gestation for the removal of a bilateral endometrioma. The authors collected eight reports of 38 laparoscopic cyst aspirations and detorsion done in the first trimester and nine other reviews of 75 laparoscopic cystectomies during the first and second

TABLE 21-4. Laparoscopic Cystectomy in Pregnancy

Author	Weeks of Pregnancy	Type of Cyst	Complication
Lucas et al[19]	16	Cystic teratoma	None
	8, 20	Torsion	None
Andreoli et al[20]	8–24 (6 cases)	Inclusion cyst, serous cyst, mucinous cyst, cystic teratoma serous cystadenoma	None
Nezhat et al[83]	16	Endometrioma	None
Howard and Tvill[90]	13	Cystic teratoma	None
	21	Paratubal cyst	None
Parker et al[96]	9–17 (12 cases)	Cystic teratoma	2 elective TOP
Nezhat et al[97]	12–22 (8 cases)	Cystic teratoma	None
		Endometrioma	
		Serous cysts	
		Corpus luteal cyst	
		Hemorrhagic cyst	
Marvelos and Mortakis[98]	12–20 (12 cases)	Functional cysts	None
Akira et al[101]	12–16 (17 cases)	Functional cysts	None
Moore and Smith[102]	12–21 (14 cases)	Serous cystadenoma, mucinous cystadenoma, mature teratoma, endometrioma, functional cyst	One fetal loss at 31 weeks postoperatively

*TOP—termination of pregnancy

trimesters. There were five first trimester pregnancy losses, two congenital anomalies resulting in second trimester termination of pregnancy, one premature delivery at 31 weeks, and one twin gestation loss at 31 weeks.[84–103] The incidence of such complications is low and most likely cannot be attributed to the laparoscopic procedure.

A questionnaire surveying the experience of laparoscopic surgeons confirmed the low complication rate. Among 189 respondents to the questionnaire, 410 laparoscopic operations involving pregnant women were reported; including 197 (48%) cholecystectomies, 66 (16.1%) appendectomies, and 115 (28%) adnexal procedures. Out of 409 of these cases, one hundred thirty-three (32.5%) occurred in the first trimester, 222 (54.1%) in the second trimester, and 54 (13.1%) in the third trimester. Among 14 complications (3.4%), there were 5 intraoperative complications, including 1 intrauterine Veress needle insertion, and 9 postoperative complications, including 5 first trimester spontaneous abortions and 1 preterm labor.[99]

TABLE 21-5. Laparoscopic Removal of a Heterotopic Pregnancy

Author	Weeks of Pregnancy	Procedure	Complication
Hanf et al[76]	7	Bilateral salpingectomy	None
Grauer and Bowditch[78]	8	Right salpingectomy	Vaginal bleeding at 29 weeks, birth at term
Bowditch[79]	9	Right salpingectomy	None
Remorgida et al[80]	10	Left salpingectomy	None
Parker et al[81]	6	Left salpingectomy	None
Sherer et al[82]	8	Cornual resection, interstitial heterotopic	None

Abdominal Pregnancy

A twenty two weeks gestational size abdominal pregnancy has been managed laparoscopically. Prior to endoscopic intervention, patient had had uterine artery embolization. Laparoscopic management included evaluation and assessment of placental site, dissection of the pregnancy sac, ligation of umblical artery and removal of demised fetus.[107]

Avoiding the Risks of Laparoscopy in Pregnant Patients

With enlarged uterine size, inadvertent uterine injuries form trocar placement may occur. The Veress needle can insufflate the intrauterine cavity, resulting in CO_2 embolism.[99,104] Numerous investigators prefer the open laparoscopic approach using a Hasson cannula to avoid such complications.[29,31,35,37,40,42,46,50,92] The authors' practice has been to modify the primary and secondary trocar insertion site to either the supraumbilical or subxiphoid midline or the left upper quadrant. Direct trocar placement rather than insufflation with a Veress needle is safer in terms of avoiding inadvertent uterine insufflation. The primary insertion site is ascertained after the uterine fundus is palpated, and the ancillary trocars can be placed safely under direct observation.

Another potential risk is the influence of pneumoperitoneum when using CO_2 on the maternal hemodynamics and possible acid-base imbalance from CO_2 absorption and hypercarbia. Both may compromise the fetus. Increased intraabdominal pressure can decrease cardiac output by several mechanisms, including direct alteration of venous resistance in the inferior vena cava, total peripheral resistance, and mean systemic pressure. Impaired venous return because of compression of the inferior vena cava is of particular concern in the second half of pregnancy, since the enlarged uterus also limits venous return. Uterine compression of the vena cava can be minimized by slight lateral positioning of the mother.[105]

In operative laparoscopy, CO_2 is the gas of choice because of its rapid rate of absorption, high solubility, rapid clearance from the body through the alveoli, and nonexplosive nature when electrosurgery is utilized. CO_2 pneumoperitoneum, however, can result in physiologically significant hypercarbia and respiratory acidosis. The risk of hypercarbia and acidosis is minimized when the intraabdominal pressure is kept below 20 mm Hg and there is a short operative time.[106] Although most pregnant patients are young and healthy, the altered physiology of pregnancy renders them susceptible to a decreased cardiopulmonary reserve.[5] CO_2 pneumoperitoneum may have significant effects. Limited studies of pneumoperitoneum in pregnant sheep demonstrated increased fetal arterial blood pressure, tachycardia, and respiratory acidosis that were corrected partially with alternation in ventilator settings based on maternal capnography results.[107–109] Two reports addressed this issue and described the use of the laparolift technique rather than insufflation with CO_2.[49,101] In one study, the fetal respiratory acidosis was not demonstrated when pneumoperitoneum was established with N_2O.[110] However, the administration of nitrous oxide as a general anesthetic to pregnant women has been controversial because of its ability to irreversibly inactivate vitamin B_{12}.[111] However, nitrous oxide for general anesthesia has been administered to women during the first two trimesters of pregnancy for many decades without any reported till effects on the fetus or neonate.

An additional potential danger is the risk of exposure to intraabdominal smoke generated by electrosurgery and lasers, with resultant production of increased levels of noxious gases, most importantly carbon monoxide.[112] The levels of serum carboxyhemoglobin in women undergoing prolonged operative laparoscopy procedures have been measured.[113] No increase in those levels was detected, and this was attributed to rapid evacuation of intraabdominal smoke generated during surgery.

Operative laparoscopy appears to be safe in pregnancy. Studies suggest that pregnant women also benefit from minimally invasive surgery. However, prospective, randomized controlled trials are needed to assess the effect of CO_2 pneumoperitoneum on maternal and fetal hemodynamics, acid-base balance, and the safety, efficacy, and advantages of operative laparoscopy over exploratory laparotomy.

References

1. Curet MJ, Allen D, Josloff RK, et al. Laparoscopy during pregnancy. *Arch Surg* 1996; 131:546.
2. Cohen EN, Bellville JW, Brown BW. Anesthesia, pregnancy and miscarriage: a study of

operating room nurses and anesthetists. Anesthesiol 1971; 35:343.

3. Duncan PG, Pope WD, Cohen M, Greer N. Fetal risk of anesthesia and surgery during pregnancy. *Anesthesiology* 1986; 64:790.
4. Mazze RI, Kallen B. Reproductive outcome after anesthesia and operation during pregnancy: A registry study of 5405 cases. *Am J Obstet Gynecol* 1989; 161:1178.
5. Barron WM. Medical evaluation of the pregnant patient requiring nonobstetric surgery. *Clin Perinatol* 1985; 12:481.
6. Levine W, Diamond B. Surgical procedures during pregnancy. *Am J Obstet Gynecol* 1961; 81:1046.
7. Smith BE. Fetal prognosis after anesthesia during gestation. *Anesth Analg* 1963; 42:521.
8. Babaknia A, Parsa H, Woodruff JD. Appendicitis during pregnancy. *Obstet Gynecol* 1977; 50:40.
9. Sharp HT. Gastrointestinal surgical conditions during pregnancy. *Clin Obstet Gynecol* 1994; 37:306.
10. Ahlgren M. The influence of temperature on the motility of the human uterus in vitro. *Acta Obstet Gynecol Scand* 1959; 38:243.
11. Kullander S. Fever and parturition: An experimental study in rabbits. *Acta Obstet Gynecol Scand* 1977; 66:77.
12. Dinarello CA. Pathogenesis of fever in man. *N Engl J Med* 1978; 298:607.
13. Hess LW, Peaceman A, O'Brien WF, et al. Adnexal mass occurring with intrauterine pregnancy: Report of fifty-four patients requiring laparotomy for definitive management. *Am J Obstet Gynecol* 1988; 158:1029.
14. Samuelsson S, Sjovall A. Laparoscopy in suspected ectopic pregnancy. *Acta Obstet Gynecol Scand* 1972; 51:31.
15. Schreiber JH. Laparoscopic appendectomy in pregnancy. *Surg Endosc* 1990; 4:100.
16. Cristalli B, Nos C, Heid M, Levardon M. Laparoscopy, appendicitis and pregnancy [letter]. *J Gynecol Obstet Biol Reprod* 1992; 21:449.
17. Dressler F, Zockler R, Raatz D, Borner P. Endoscopic appendectomy in gynecology and obstetrics. *Geburtshilfe Frauenheilkd* 1992; 52:51.
18. Korkan IP. Laparoscopy in the diagnosis of acute appendicitis in pregnant women. *Khirurgia* 1992; 2:63.
19. Lucas V, Barjot P, Allouche C, et al. Surgical laparoscopy and pregnancy: Eight cases. *J Gynecol Obstet Biol Reprod* 1994; 23:914.
20. Andreoli M, Servakov M, Meyers P, Mann WJ, Jr. Laparoscopic surgery during pregnancy. *J Am Assoc Gynecol Laparosc* 1999; 6:229.
21. Amos JD, Schorr SJ, Norman PF, et al. C. Laparoscopic surgery during pregnancy. *Am J Surg* 1996; 171:435.
22. Black WP. Acute appendicitis in pregnancy. *Br Med J* 1960; 1:1938.
23. McComb P. Luimon R. Appendicitis complicating pregnancy. *Can J Surg* 1980; 23.92.
24. Weingold AB. Appendicitis in pregnancy. *Clin Obstet Gynecol* 1983; 26:801.
25. Dufour P, Delebecq T, Vinatier D, et al. Appendicitis in pregnancy: Seven case reports. *J Gynecol Obstet Biol Reprod* 1996; 25:41.
26. Dixon NP, Faddis DM, Silberman H. Aggressive management of cholecystitis during pregnancy. *Am J Surg* 1987; 154:292.
27. Arvidsson D, Gerdin E. Laparoscopic cholecystectomy during pregnancy. *Surg Laparosc Endosc.* 1991; 1:193.
28. Milenin AV, Rubtsov MA. Therapeutic laparoscopy in cholangitis in a pregnant woman. *Khirurgia* 1991; 2:142-3.
29. Pucci RO, Seed RW. Case report of laparoscopic cholecystectomy in the third trimester of pregnancy. *Am J Obstet Gynecol* 1991; 165:401.
30. Weber AM, Bloom GP, Allan TR, Curry SL. Laparoscopic cholecystectomy during pregnancy. *Obstet Gynecol* 1991; 78:958.
31. Morrell DG, Mulins JR, Harrison PB. Laparoscopic cholecystectomy during pregnancy in symptomatic patients. *Surgery* 1992; 112:856.
32. Soper NJ, Hunter JG, Petrie RH. Laparoscopic cholecystectomy during pregnancy. *Surg Endosc* 1992; 6:115.
33. Adamsen S, Jacobsen B, Bentzon N. Laparoscopic cholecystectomy during pregnancy. *Ugeskr Laeger* 1993; 155:2215.
34. Bennett TL, Estes N. Laparoscopic cholecystectomy in the second trimester of pregnancy: A case report. *J Reprod Med* 1993; 38:833.
35. Elerding SC. Laparoscopic cholecystectomy in pregnancy. *Am J Surg* 1993; 165:625.
36. Fabiani P, Bongain A, Persch M, et al. Endoscopic surgery during pregnancy: A case report of cholecystectomy. *J Gynecol Obstet Biol Reprod* 1993; 22:317.
37. Hart RO, Tamadon A, Fitzgibbons RJ Jr, Fleming A. Open laparoscopic cholecystectomy in pregnancy. *Surg Laparosc Endosc* 1993; 3:13.
38. Jackson SJ, Sigman HH. Laparoscopic cholecystectomy in pregnancy. *J Laparoendosc Surg* 1993; 3:35.

39. Rusher AH, Fields B, Henson K. Laparoscopic cholecystectomy in pregnancy: Contraindicated or indicated? *J Arkansas Soc* 1993; 89:383.
40. Schorr RT. Laparoscopic cholecystectomy and pregnancy. *J Laparoendosc Surg* 1993; 3:291.
41. Chandra M, Shapiro SJ, Gordon LA. Laparoscopic cholecystectomy in the first trimester of pregnancy. *Surg Laparosc Endosc* 1994; 4:68.
42. Comitalo JB, Lynch D. Laparoscopic cholecystectomy in the pregnant patient. *Surg Laparosc Endosc* 1994; 4:268.
43. Constantino GN, Vincent GJ, Mukalian GG, Kliefoth WL Jr. Laparoscopic cholecystectomy in pregnancy. *J Laparoendosc Surg* 1994; 4:161.
44. Csaba J, Orban I. Laparoscopic cholecystectomy during the 25th week of pregnancy. *Orv Hetil* 1994; 135:1421.
45. DePaula AL, Hashiba K, Bafutto M. Laparoscopic management of choledocholithiasis. *Surg Endosc* 1994; 8:1399.
46. Edelman DS. Alternative laparoscopic technique for cholecystectomy during pregnancy. *Surg Endosc* 1994; 8:794.
47. Shaked G, Twena M, Charuzi I. Laparoscopic cholecystectomy for empyema of gallbladder during pregnancy. *Surg Laparosc Endosc* 1994; 4:65.
48. Wilson RB, McKenzie RJ, Fisher JW. Laparoscopic cholecystectomy in pregnancy: Two case reports. *Aust N Z J Surg* 1994; 64:647.
49. Iafrati MD, Yarnell R, Schwaitzberg SD. Gasless laparoscopic cholecystectomy in pregnancy. *J Laparoendosc Surg* 1995; 5:127.
50. Williams JK, Rosemurgy AS, Albrink MH, et al. Laparoscopic cholecystectomy in pregnancy: A case report. *J Reprod Med* 1995; 40:243.
51. Davis A, Katz VL, Cox R. Gallbladder disease in pregnancy. *J Reprod Med* 1995; 40:759.
52. Friedman RL, Friedman IH. Acute cholecystitis with calculous biliary duct obstruction in the gravid patient. *Surg Endosc* 1995; 9:910.
53. Lanzafame RJ. Laparoscopic cholecystectomy during pregnancy. *Surgery* 1995; 118:627.
54. Posta CG. Laparoscopic surgery in pregnancy: Report of two cases. *J Laparosc Surg* 1995; 5:203.
55. Eichenberg BJ, Vanderlinden J, Miguel C, et al. Laparoscopic cholecystectomy in the third tirmester of pregnancy. *Am Surg* 1996; 62:874.
56. Abuabara SR, Gross GWW, Sirinek KR. Laparoscopic cholecystectomy during pregnancy is safe for both mother and fetus. *J Gastrointest Surg* 1997; 1:48.
57. Barone JE, Bears S, Chen S, et al. Outcome study of cholecystectomy during pregnancy. *Am J Surg* 1999; 177:232.
58. NIH Consensus Development Panel on Gallstones and Laparoscopic Cholecystectomy. *JAMA* 1993; 269:1018.
59. Platek DN, Henderson CE, Golberg GL. The management of a persistent adnexal mass in pregnancy. *Am J Obstet Gynecol* 1995; 173:1236.
60. Grimes WH Jr, Bartholomew RA, Colvin ED, et al. Ovarian cyst complicating pregnancy. *Am J Obstet Gynecol* 1954; 68:594.
61. Booth RT. Ovarian tumors in pregnancy. *Obstet Gynecol* 1963; 21:189.
62. Tawa K. Ovarian tumors in pregnancy. *Am J Obstet Gynecol* 1964; 90:511.
63. Beischer NA, Battery BW, Fortune DW, Macafee AJ. Growth and malignancy of ovarian tumors in pregnancy. *Aust N Z J Obstet Gynecol* 1971; 11:208.
64. White KC. Ovarian tumors in pregnancy. *Am J Obstet Gynecol* 1973; 116:544.
65. Struyk APHB, Treffers PE. Ovarian tumors in pregnancy. *Acta Obstet Gynecol Scand* 1984; 163:421.
66. Ballard CA. Ovarian tumors associated with pregnancy termination patients. *Am J Obstet Gynecol* 1984; 149:384.
67. Koonings PP, Platt LP, Wallace R. Incidental adnexal neoplasms at Cesarean section. *Obstet Gynecol* 1988; 72:767.
68. Hopkins MP, Duchon MA. Adnexal surgery in pregnancy. *J Reprod Med* 1986; 31:1035.
69. Thornton JG, Wells M. Ovarian cysts in pregnancy: Does ultrasound make traditional management inappropriate? *Obstet Gynecol* 1987; 69:717.
70. Hogston P. Ultrasound study of ovarian cysts in pregnancy: Prevalence and significance. *Br J Obstet Gynacol* 1986; 93:625.
71. Nelson MJ, Cavalieri R, Graham D, Sanders RC. Cysts in pregnancy discovered by sonography. *J Clin Ultrasound* 1986; 14:509.
72. Salim A, Zalud I, Farmakides G, et al. Corpus luteum blood flow in normal and abnormal early pregnancy: Evaluation with transvaginal color and pulsed Doppler sonography. *J Ultrasound Med* 1994; 13:971.
73. Dillon EH, Case CQ, Ramos IM, et al. Endovaginal pulsed and color Doppler in first-trimester pregnancy. *Ultrasound Med Biol* 1993; 19:517.
74. Trimbos JB, Hacker NF. The case against aspirating ovarian cysts. *Cancer* 1993; 72: 828.

75. De Crespigny L. A comparison of ovarian cyst aspirate cytology and histology: The case against aspiration of cystic pelvic masses [letter]. *Aust N Z J Obstet Gynaecol* 1995; 35:233.
76. Hanf V, Dietl J, Gagsteiger F, Pfeiffer KH. Bilateral tubal pregnancy with intra-uterine gestation after IVF-ET: Therapy by bilateral laparoscopic salpingectomy: A case report. *Eur J Obstet Gynecol Reprod Biol* 1990; 37:87.
77. Ceci O, Caradonna F, Loizzi P, et al. Ultrasound diagnosis of heterotopic pregnancy with viable fetuses. *Eur J Obstet Gynecol Reprod Biol* 1993; 52:229.
78. Grauer S, Bowditch JDP. Laparoscopic management of heterotopic pregnancy. *Gynecol Endosc* 1993; 2:181.
79. Bowditch JDP. Heterotopic pregnancy after natural conception exhibiting the ultrasound signs of antegrade and retrograde tubal bleeding. *Aust N Z J Obstet Gynaecol* 1994; 34:614.
80. Remorgida B, Carrer C, Ferraiolo A, et al. Laparoscopic surgery in pregnancy: A case report with a brief review of the topic. *Surg Endosc* 1995; 9:195.
81. Parker J, Watkin W, Robinson H, Byrne D. Laparoscopic adnexal surgery during pregnancy: A case of heterotopic tubal pregnancy treated by laparoscopic salpingectomy. *Aust N Z J Obstet Gynaecol* 1995; 35:2:208.
82. Sherer DM, Scibetta JJ, Sanko SR. Heterotopic quadruplet gestation with laparoscopic resection of ruptured interstitial pregnancy and subsequent successful outcome of triplets. *Am J Obstet Gynecol* 1995; 172:216.
83. Nezhat F, Nezhat C, Silfen SL, Fehnel SH. Laparoscopic ovarian cystectomy during pregnancy. *J Laparoendosc Surg* 1991; 1:161.
84. Mage G, Canis M, Manhes H, et al. Laparoscopic management of adnexal torsion. *J Reprod Med* 1989; 34:520.
85. Shalev E, Rahav D, Romano S. Laparoscopic relief of adnexal torsion in early pregnancy: Case reports. *Br J Obstet Gynaecol* 1990; 97:853.
86. Cristalli B, Cayol A, Izard V, Levardon M. Value of celioscopic surgical treatment of ovarian tumors at the beginning of pregnancy. *J Gynecol Obstet Biol Reprod* 1991; 20:665.
87. Lang PF, Tamussino K, Winter R. Laparoscopic management of adnexal torsion during the second trimester [letter]. *Int J Gynaecol Obstet* 1992; 37:51.
88. Ozcan U, Vicdan K, Oguz S, et al. Torsion of the normal adnexa in early pregnancy and laparoscopic detorsion. *J Pakistan Med Assoc* 1992; 42:127.
89. Shalev E, Peleg D. Laparoscopic treatment of adnexal torsion. *Surg Gynecol Obstet* 1993; 176:448.
90. Howard FM, Vill M. Laparoscopic adnexal surgery during pregnancy. *J Am Assoc Gynecol Laparosc* 1994; 2:91.
91. Gazarelli S, Mazzuca N. One laparoscopic puncture for treatment of ovarian cysts with adnexal torsion in early pregnancy: A report of two cases. *J Reprod Med* 1994; 39:985.
92. Guerrieri JP, Thomas RL. Open laparoscopy for an adnexal mass in pregnancy: A case report. *J Reprod Med* 1994; 39:129.
93. Nagase S, Konno R. Laparoscopic treatment of adnexal torsion of hyperstimulated ovary in pregnancy. *Nippon Sanka Fujinka Gakkai Zasshi* 1994; 46:543.
94. Wittich AC, Lockrow EG, Fox JT. Laparoscopic management of adnexal torsion in early pregnancy: A case report. *Mill Med* 1994; 159:254.
95. Busine A, Murillo D. Conservative laparoscopic treatment of adnexal torsion during pregnancy. *J Gynecol Obstet Biol Reprod* 1994; 23:918.
96. Parker WH, Childers JM, Cains M, et al. Laparoscopic management of benign cystic teratomas during pregnancy. *Am J Obstet Gynecol* 1996; 1:17.
97. Nezhat FR, Tazuke S, Nezhat CH, et al. Laparoscopy during pregnancy: A literature review. *J Soc Laparoendosc Surg* 1997; 1:17.
98. Marvelos K, Mortakis A. Laparoscopic removal of ovarian cysts during pregnancy. *J Am Assoc Gynecol Laparosc* 1996; 3:S29.
99. Reedy M, Galan H, Richards W, Kuehl T. Laparoscopy during pregnancy: A survey of laparoendoscopic surgeons. *J Reprod Med* 1997; 42:33.
100. Tazuke SI, Nezhat FR, Nezhat CH, et al. Laparoscopic management of pelvic pathology during pregnancy. *J Am Assoc Gynecol Laparosc* 1997; 4:605.
101. Akira S, Yamanaka A, Ishihara T, et al. Gasless laparoscopic ovarian cystectomy during pregnancy: Comparison with laparotomy. *Am J Obstet Gynecol* 1999; 180:554.
102. Moore RD, Smith WG. Laparoscopic management of adnexal masses in pregnant women. *J Reprod Med* 1999; 44:97.
103. Soriano D, Yefet Y, Seidman DS, et al. Laparoscopy versus laparotomy in the management of adnexal masses during pregnancy. *Fertil Steril* 1999; 71:955.

104. Barnett MB, Liu DT. Complication of laparoscopy during early pregnancy [letter]. *Br Med J* 1974; 1:328.
105. Callery MP, Soper NJ. Physiology of the pneumoperitoneum. *Baillieres Clin Gastroenterol* 1993; 7:757.
106. Kashtan J, Green JF, Parsons EQ, Holocroft JW. Hemodynamic effects of increased abdominal pressure. *J Surg Res* 1981; 30:249.
107. Nezhat F, Rahman J. Laparoscopic management of a 22 weeks gestational size abdominal pregnancy. (In Press).
108. Westerband A, Van de Water JM, Amzallag M, et al. Cardiovascular changes during laparoscopic cholecystectomy. *Surg Gynecol Obstet* 1992; 175:535.
109. Barnard JM, Chaffin D, Droste S, et al. Fetal response to carbon dioxide pneumoperitoneum in the pregnant ewe. *Obstet Gynecol* 1995; 85:669.
110. Hunter JG, Swanstrom L, Thornburg K. Carbon dioxide pneumoperitoneum induces fetal acidosis in a pregnant ewe model. *Surg Endosc* 1995; 9:272.
111. Litwin DEM, Duke T, Gollagher J. Cardiopulmonary effects of abdominal insufflation in pregnancy: Fetal and maternal parameters in the sheep model [abstract]. *Surg Endosc* 1994; 8:248.
112. Baden JM, Rice SA, Serra M, et al. Thymidine and methionine syntheses in pregnant rats exposed to nitrous oxide. *Anesth Analg* 1983; 62:738.
113. Beebe DS, Swic H, Carlson N, et al. High levels of carbon monoxide are produced by electrocautery of tissue during laparoscopic cholecystectomy. *Anesth Analg* 1993; 77:338.
114. Nezhat C, Seidman DS, Vreman HJ, et al. The risk of carbon monoxide poisoning after prolonged laparoscopic surgery. *Obstet Gynecol* 1996; 88:771.

The Color Atlas

The Atlas consists of illustrations that were selected either because they are characteristic of a specific condition or they amplify material found in the text. Serous cystadenomas, polycystic ovaries, and ovarian malignancy seen at laparoscopy are illustrated. Endometriomas, implants of endometriosis involving the bowel, ureter, bladder, uterosacral ligaments, appendix, ovaries, and cul-de-sac are revealed. The laparoscopic technique for ovarian cystectomy, ovarian "drilling' myomectomy, and uterosacral ablation are shown.

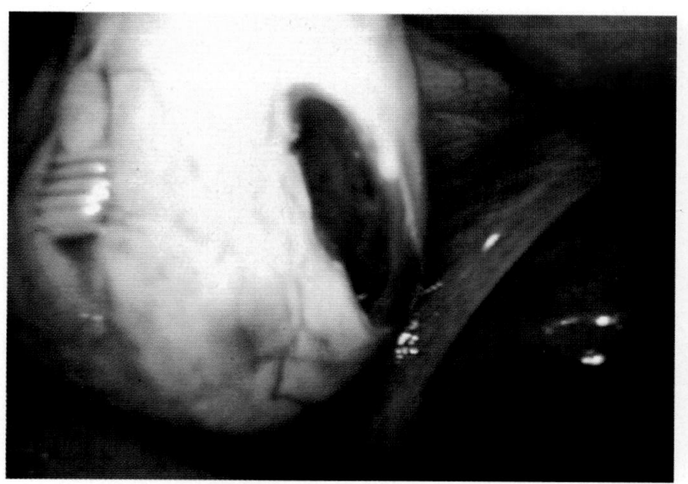

1. A hemorrhagic corpus luteum is noted.

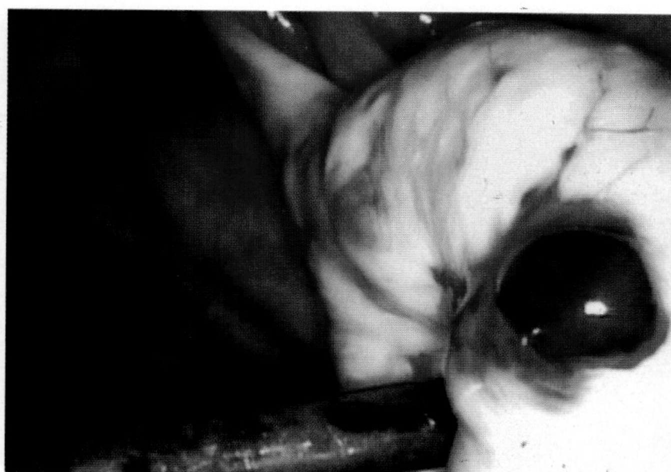

2. Endometrial implant is present on the ovary.

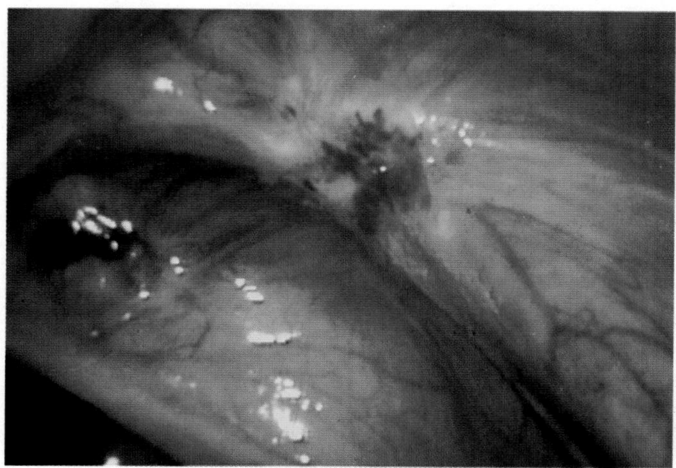

3. Endometrial implants are seen over the ureter.

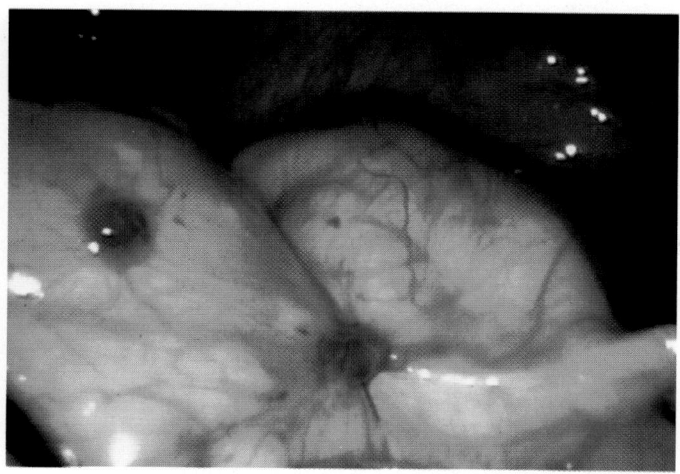

4. The rectosigmoid is involved with endometriosis.

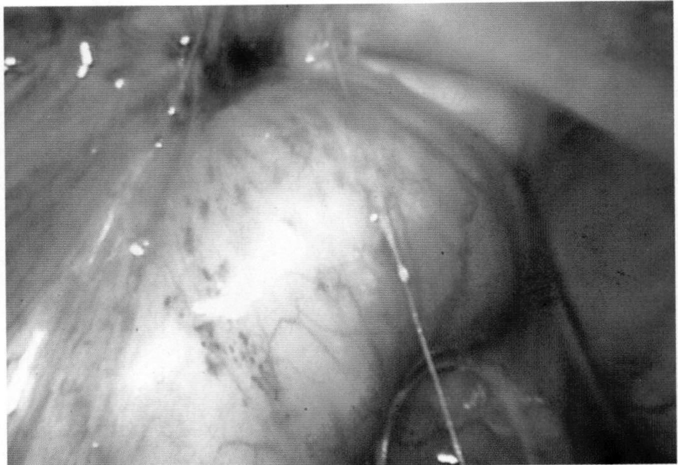

5. Rectal endometriosis is attached to the uterosacral ligaments.

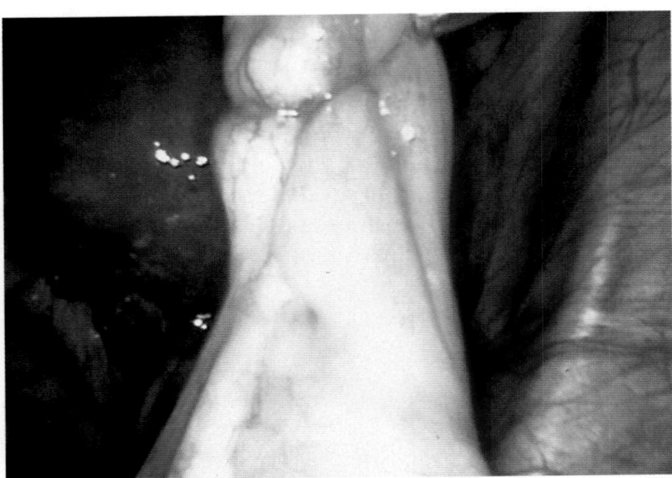

6. The appendix is involved with endometriosis.

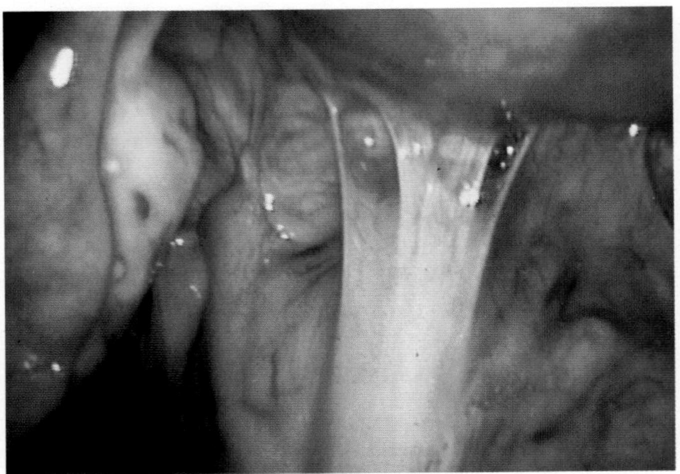

7. The cul-de-sac has been obliterated with endometrial implants and adhesions.

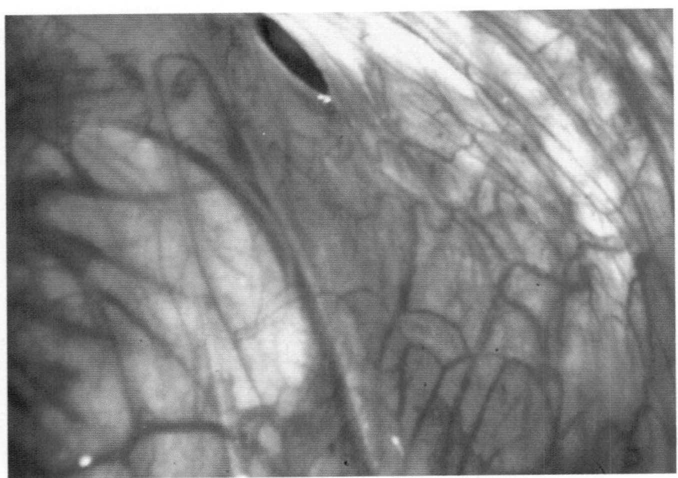

8. The peritoneal defect contained endometriosis.

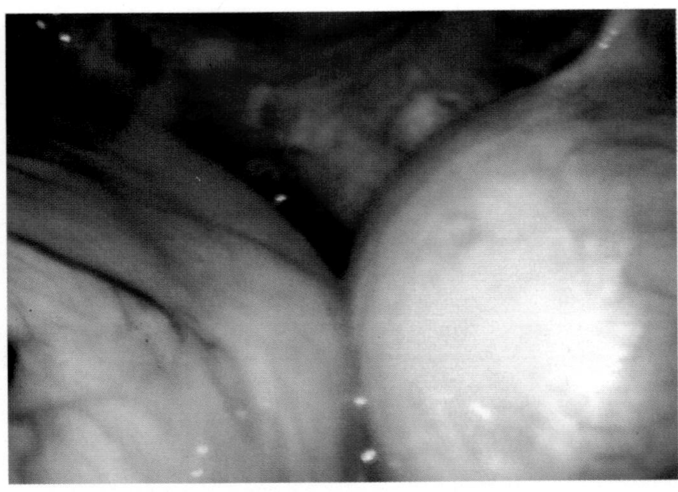

9. Endometriomas are seen in both ovaries.

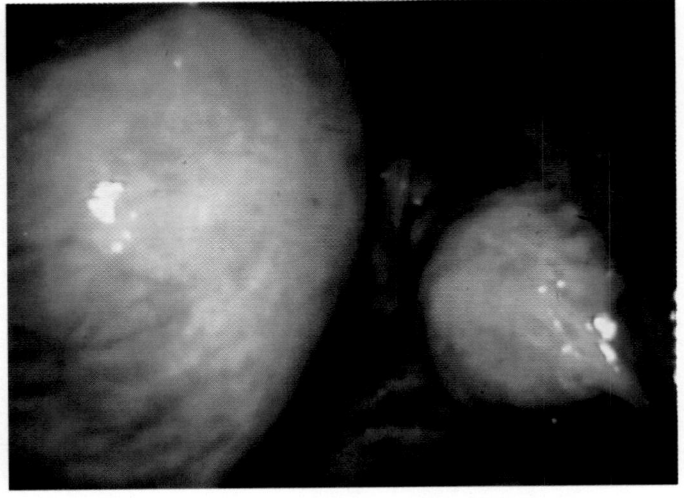

10. Cystic teratomas are present in both ovaries.

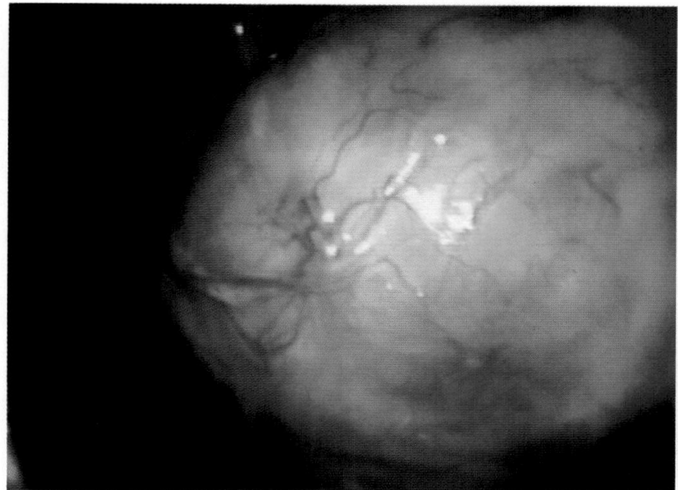

11. A benign cystadenoma was found on histologic examination.

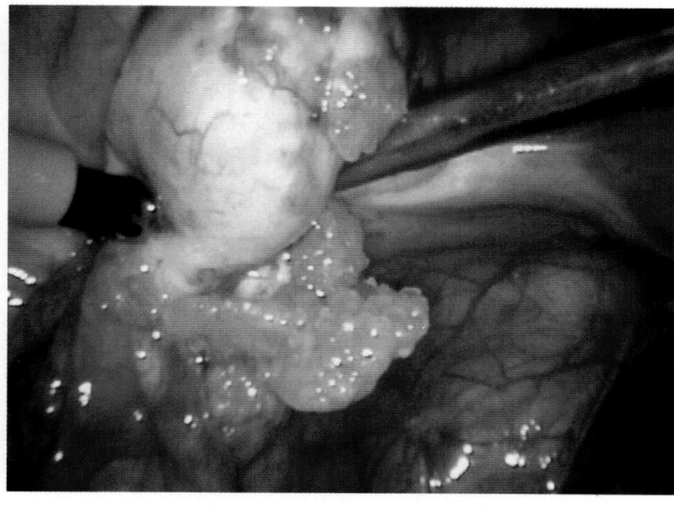

12. An ovarian malignancy is seen with excrescences.

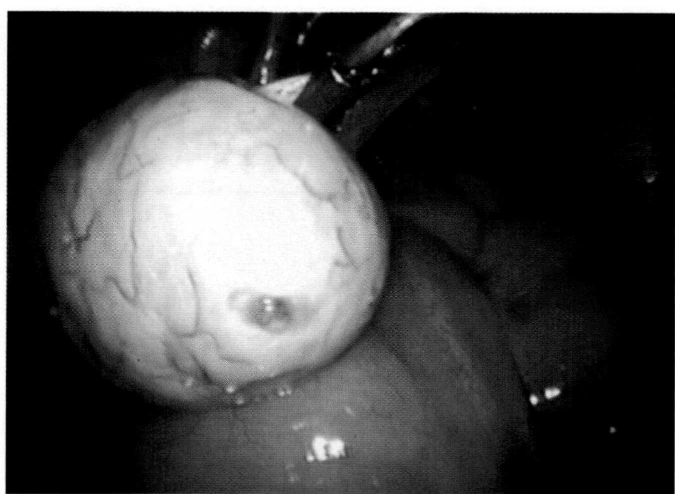

13. A polycystic ovary is noted with characteristic superficial blood vessels.

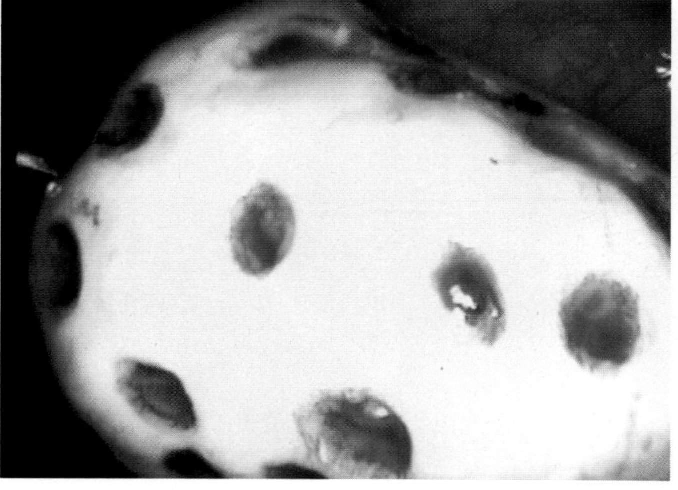

14. The appearance of the ovarian surface is seen after "drilling" with the CO_2 laser.

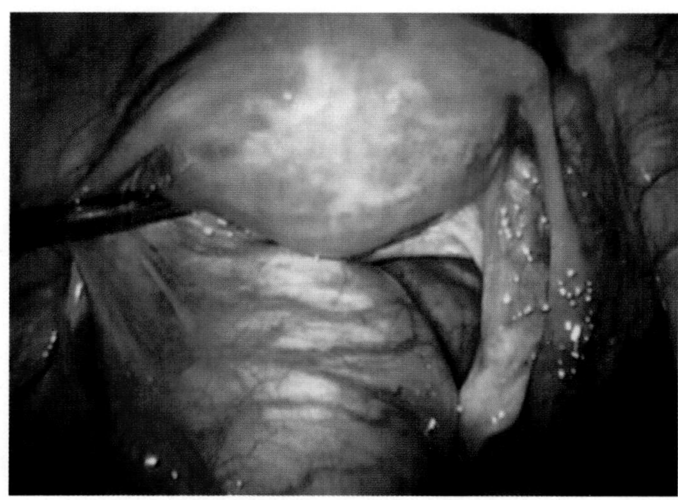

15. A large ovarian cyst was found in the left ovary.

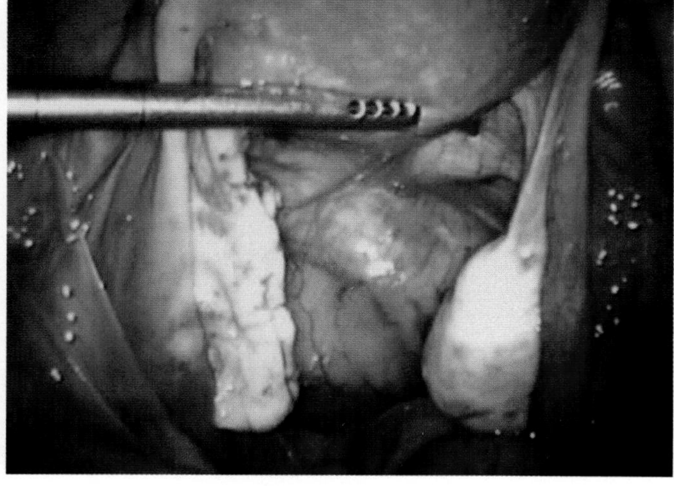

16. The cyst has been removed.

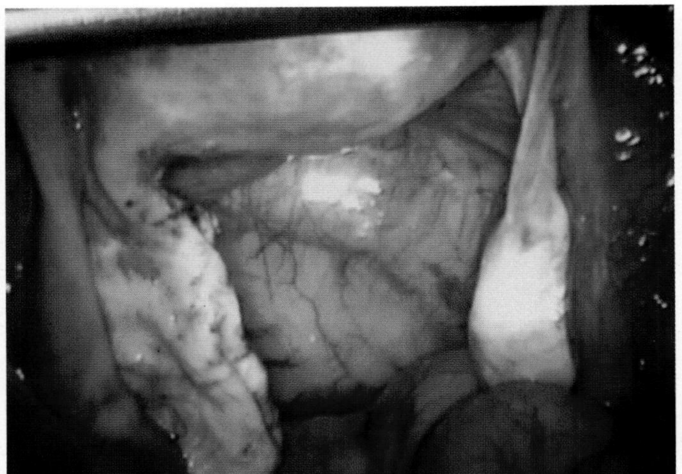

17. The ovarian edges were approximated.

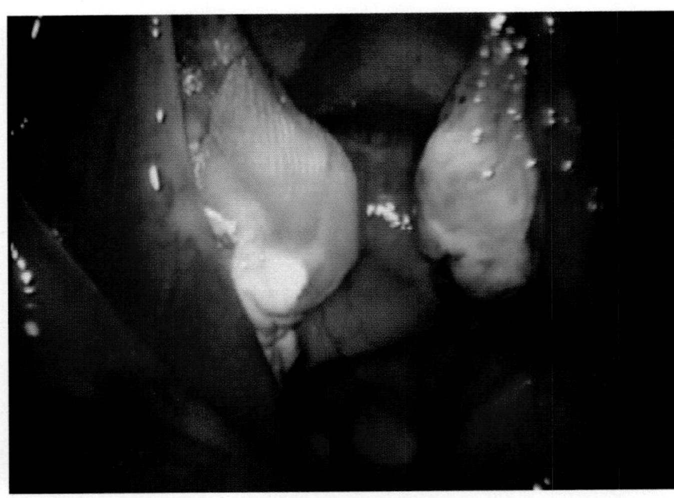

18. Interceed was placed over the ovary.

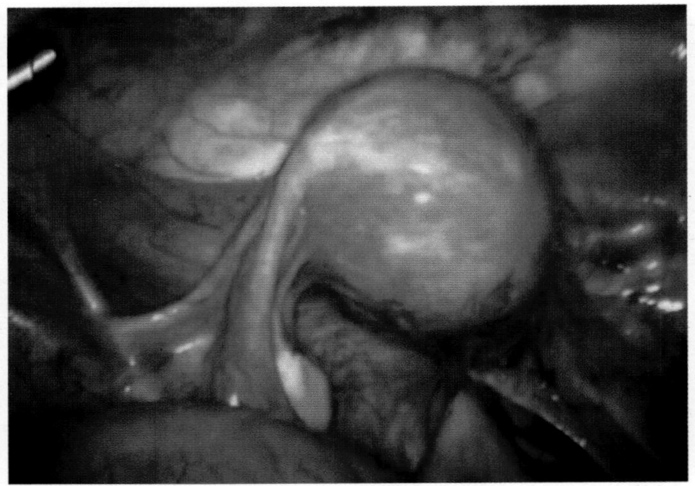

19. A unicornuate uterus is noted.

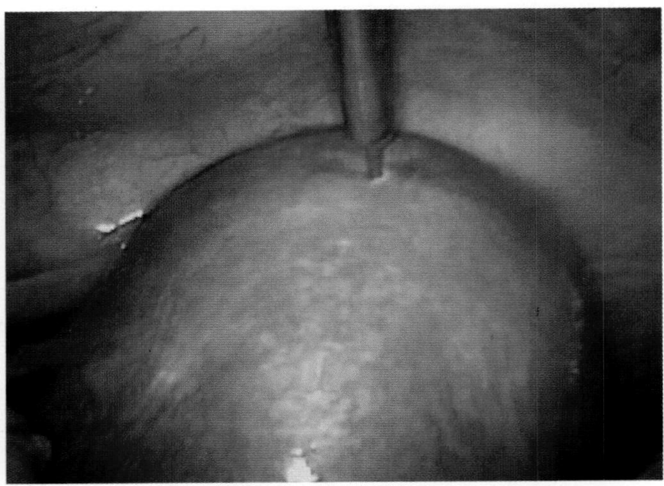

20. A "corkscrew" device is inserted into the fundal myoma.

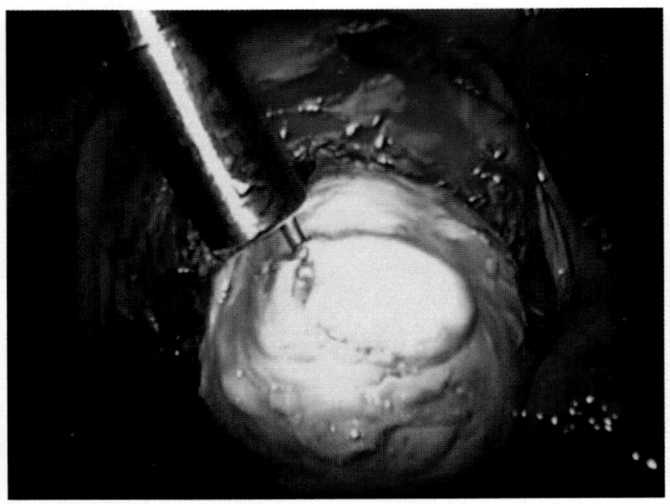

21. The myoma is being enucleated.

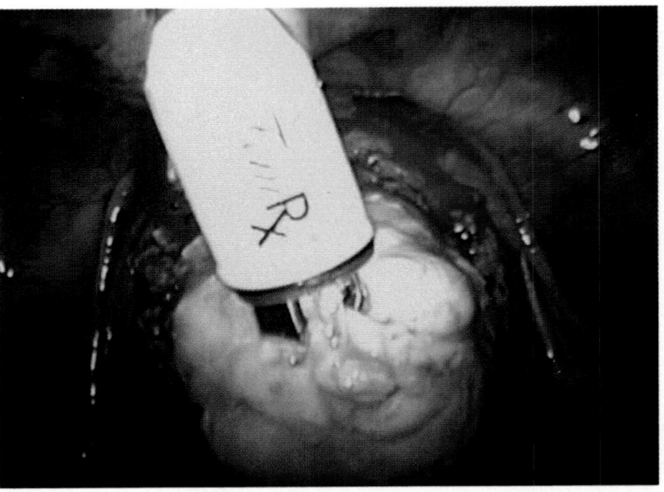

22. Myoma morcellation is beginning.

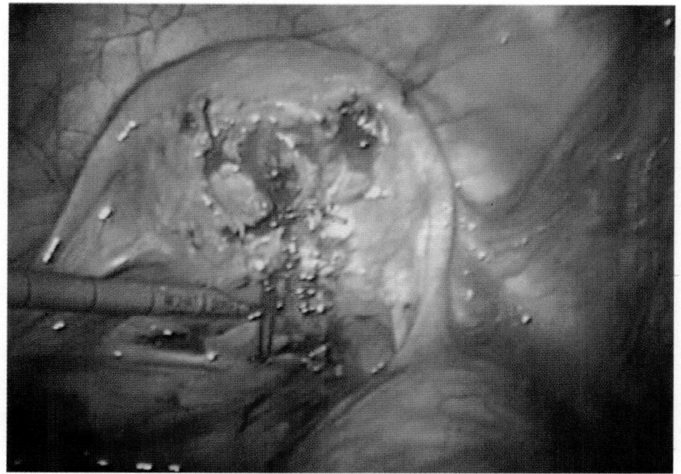

23. The uterine edges have been approximated.

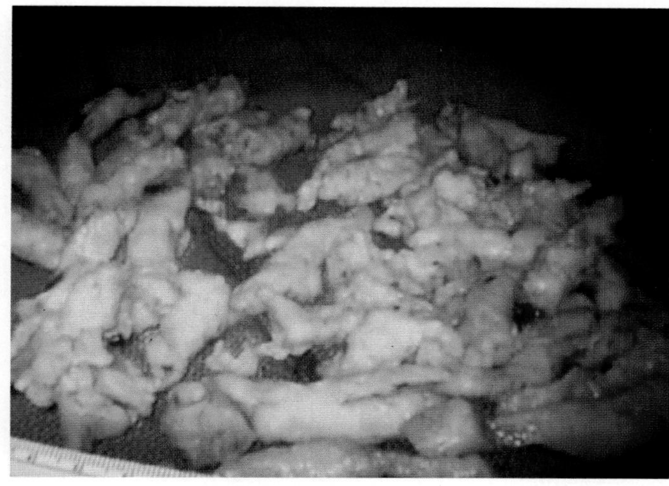

24. Myomatous fragments are seen.

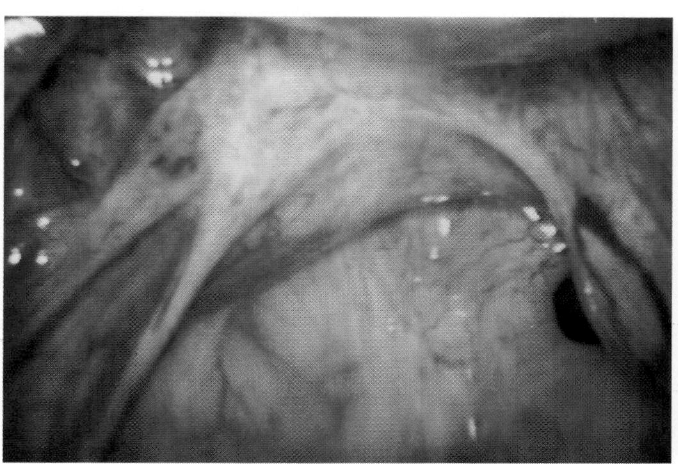

25. The uterosacral ligaments are observed.

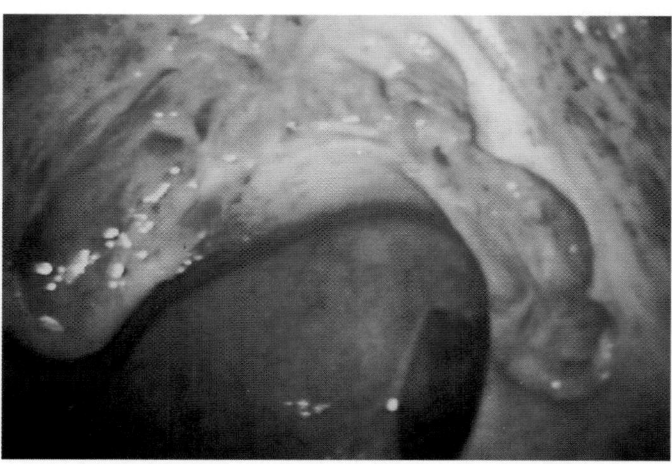

26. Note the extent of ablation of the uterosacral ligaments.

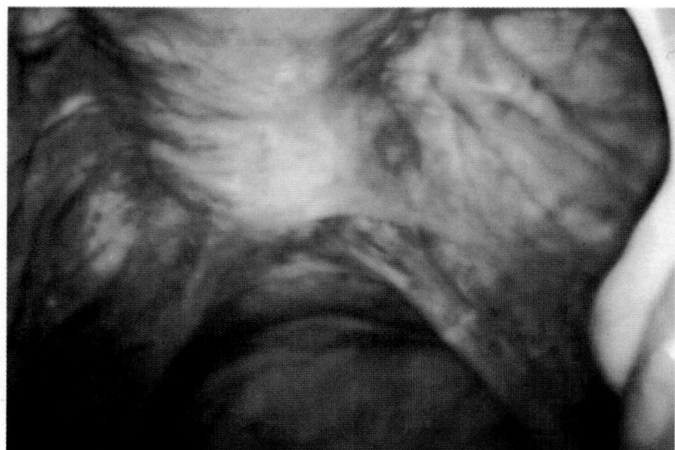

27. Two years later the area was healed without the formation of adhesions.

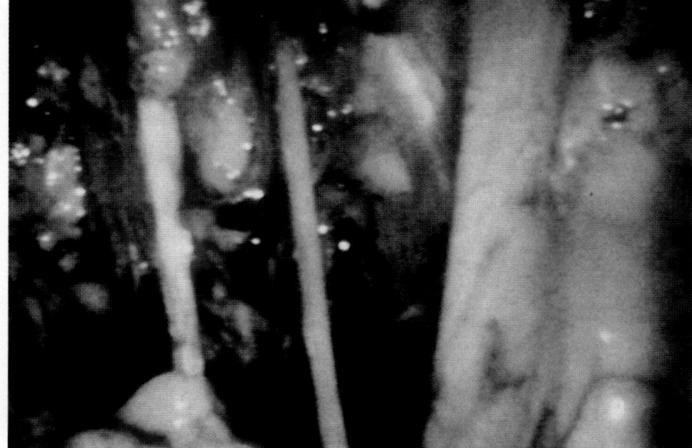

28. External iliac artery and vein are seen on the right; the obturator nerve is in the middle; the obliterated hypogastric artery is on the left.

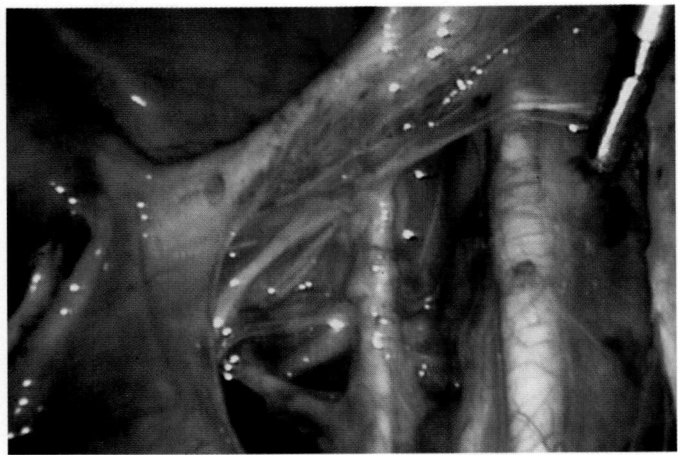

29. The uterine artery has been dissected from the hypogastric artery. The external iliac artery is on the right; the right round ligament appears in the foreground; the infundibulopelvic ligament is medial.

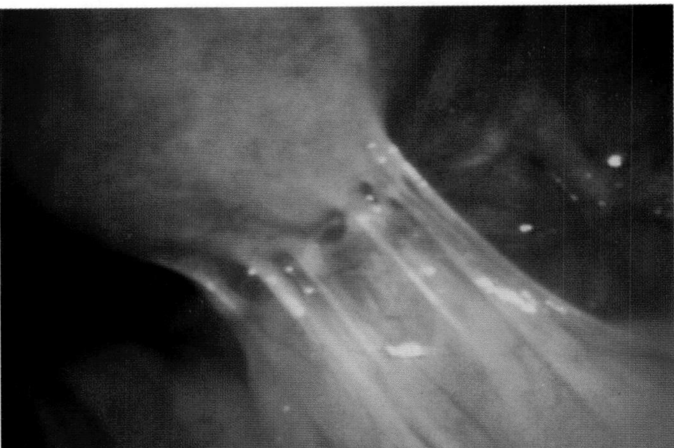

30. Avascular adhesions between the uterus and omentum are stretched before dissection with scissors.

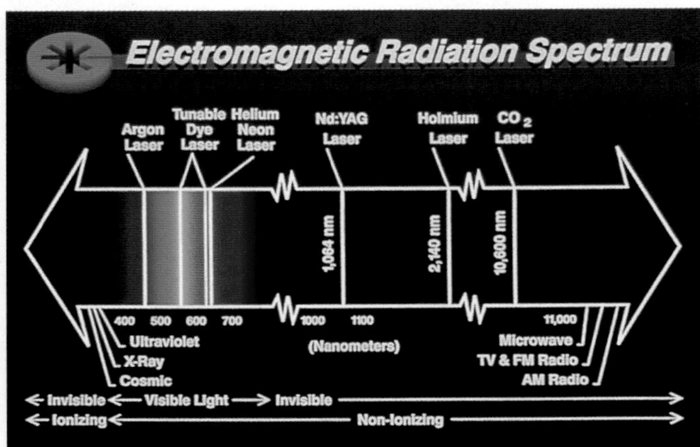

31. Laser light is unique and uniform unlike regular light which is divided into colors of the spectrum.

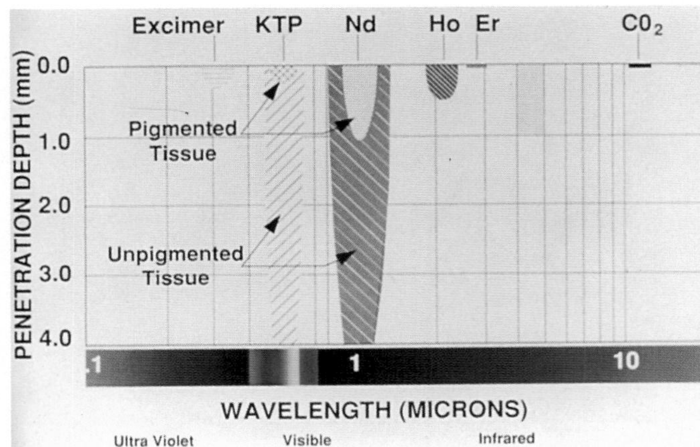

32. Argon, KTP, and Nd-YAG lasers are absorbed by pigmented tissues containing hemoglobin but pass through water and clear tissues.

INDEX

INDEX

Notes

Notes

Notes

Notes

Notes

Notes

Notes

Notes

Notes

Notes

Notes

ISBN 0-07-105431-6
90000
9 780071 054317
NEZHAT/OPERATIVE GYN
LAPAROS 2E